RN®

MAGAZINE'S

NCLEX-RN
REVIEW

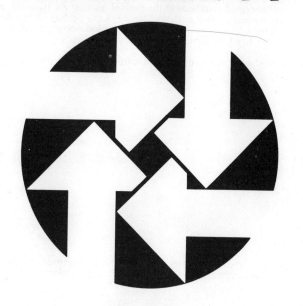

1991

EDITORS

Alice M. Stein, RN, MA
Director, Division of Continuing Nursing Education
Medical College of Pennsylvania

Nancy H. Jacobson, RN, C, MSN, CNSN
Associate Director, Division of Continuing Nursing Education
Medical College of Pennsylvania

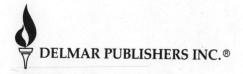

DELMAR PUBLISHERS INC.®

NOTICE TO THE READER

Cover design: John De Sieno

Delmar staff

Executive Editor: Barbara E. Norwitz
Managing Editor: Susan B. Simpfenderfer
Project Editor: Mary P. Robinson
Production Coordinator: Teresa Luterbach

For information, address Delmar Publishers Inc.,
2 Computer Drive West, Box 15-015
Albany, New York 12212

COPYRIGHT © 1991
BY DELMAR PUBLISHERS INC.

Printed in the United States of America
Published simultaneously in Canada
By Nelson Canada
A division of The Thomson Corporation

10 9 8 7 6 5 4 3 2 1

Library of Congress Cataloging-in-Publication Data
RN boards review : NCLEX-RN for 1991 / editors, Alice M. Stein, Nancy
H. Jacobson.
    p.   cm.
    "From RN magazine."
    Includes bibliographical references.
    Includes index.
    ISBN 0-8273-4646-8
    1. Nursing—Examinations, questions, etc. I. Stein, Alice M.
II. Jacobson, Nancy H. III. RN magazine.
    [DNLM: 1. Nursing—examination questions. WY 18 R6271]
RT55.R62 1990
610.73'076—dc20
DNLM/DLC
for Library of Congress
                  90-14082
                  CIP

Contents

Tables and Figures

Contributors

EDITORS

Alice M. Stein, RN, MA
Director, Division of Continuing Nursing Education, The Medical College of Pennsylvania, Philadelphia, Pennsylvania

Nancy H. Jacobson, RN, C, MSN, CNSN
Associate Director, Division of Continuing Nursing Education, The Medical College of Pennsylvania, Philadelphia, Pennsylvania

CONTRIBUTORS

Margaret Ahearn-Spera, RN, C, MSN
Associate Director, Nursing, Danbury Hospital, Danbury Connecticut; Assistant Clinical Professor, Yale School of Nursing, New Haven, Connecticut

*Margaret B. Brenner, RN, MSN
Lecturer, Division of Nursing, Holy Family College, Philadelphia, Pennsylvania

Deborah L. Dalrymple, RN, MSN, CRNI
Assistant Professor of Nursing, Montgomery County Community College, Blue Bell, Pennsylvania

Judy Donlen, RN, C, DNSc
Director of Nursing, Southern New Jersey Perinatal Cooperative, Camden, New Jersey

*Jeanne Gelman, RN, MA, MSN
Associate Professor, Widener University, Chester, Pennsylvania

Theresa M. Giglio, RD, MS
Nutrition Instructor, Albert Einstein Medical Center, Philadelphia, Pennsylvania

Holly Hillman, RN, MSN
Assistant Professor, Montgomery County Community College, Blue Bell, Pennsylvania

*Charlotte D. Kain, RN, C, EdD
Professor of Nursing, Health Care of Women, Montgomery County Community College, Blue Bell, Pennsylvania

Constance O. Kolva, RN, MSN
Faculty, Medical College of Pennsylvania, Department of Psychiatry, Division of Continuing Mental Health Education, Philadelphia, Pennsylvania; Educator and Consultant, Mental Health and Management in Nursing, Harrisburg, Pennsylvania

*Mary Lou Manning, RN, C, MSN, CPNP
Research Nurse, Division of Infectious Diseases, Children's Hospital of Philadelphia, Philadelphia, Pennsylvania

*Eileen Moran, RN, MSN
Staff Development Instructor, Fox Chase Cancer Center, American Oncologic Hospital, Philadelphia, Pennsylvania

Marie T. O'Toole, RN, MSN, CRRN
Assistant Professor, Thomas Jefferson University, College of Allied Health Sciences, Department of Nursing, Philadelphia, Pennsylvania

Janice Selekman, RN, DNSc
Associate Professor, Undergraduate Program Director, Thomas Jefferson University, College of Allied Health Sciences, Philadelphia, Pennsylvania

*Anne R. Waldman, RN, C, MSN
Clinical Nurse Specialist, Albert Einstein Medical Center, Philadelphia, Pennsylvania

*Contributors to this edition as well as to the original edition.

Preface

This book had been expressly developed to meet your needs as you study and prepare for the all important NCLEX-RN examination. Taking this exam is always a stressful event in the best of circumstance: it constitutes a major career milestone, and NCLEX success is the key to your future ability to practice as a registered nurse.

Organization, Content and Features

The content and design of this revised edition have been carefully crafted to conform to the new NCLEX-RN test plan, beginning with an introductory unit on how to prepare for NCLEX-RN. This includes:

- Explanation of the new test plan
- Information on how the test is constructed
- Data on scoring and notification of results
- Tips on how to plan your study and prepare successfully

The units that follow concentrate on adult nursing, pediatric nursing, maternity and gynecologic nursing, and psychiatric-mental health nursing. Each unit includes:

- The nursing process (utilizing all five steps) integrated with a body systems approach
  - Assessment: reviews both history and physical examination.
  - Analysis: includes appropriate NANDA nursing diagnoses.
  - Planning: discusses patient goals.
  - Implementation: provides interventions to achieve patient goals.
  - Evaluation: lists outcome criteria.
- Introductory review of anatomy and physiology, and basic theories/principles
- Review of pertinent disorders for each system including:
  - General characteristics
  - Pathophysiology/psychopathology
  - Medical management
  - Assessment data
  - Nursing intervention/patient education
- Sample test questions, structured like those on the new NCLEX-RN, so you can evaluate yourself as you study

- Pertinent journal articles on specific topics relevant to the content and level of the exam
- Updated and expanded information on selected disorders, theories, and therapies

There are two complete practice tests so that you can simulate the actual testing experience. These include:

- Practice questions similar to the NCLEX-RN
- Correct answers with rationales, and a key to categorize each question according to the new test plan including phases of the nursing process, client needs classification, and levels of cognitive ability.

The appendices provide readily accessible information on drug administration and special diets.

Contributors

The authors and editors are all experienced clinicians and educators who have extensive experience teaching nursing and helping graduates reach NCLEX success. This experience enables them to organize and present what seems to be an overwhelming amount of information very clearly and concisely. They have used an easy-to-digest outline format that emphasizes key content and frequently tested areas, as well as areas that tend to present difficulty for the graduate nurse.

We are all committed, through continuing education, to help you reach your fullest professional potential. Collectively, the authors and editors of this book have many successful years of experience helping nurses to pass their board exams. A major focus for RN magazine is the presentation of clinically relevant content, designed to help you in your nursing practice. The publisher views helping you to pass the NCLEX-RN as a major commitment. We believe that our experience, coupled with support from RN magazine, has enabled us to produce a book that will fully meet your needs.

Alice Stein
Nancy Jacobson
Editors

UNIT 1
PREPARING FOR THE
NCLEX EXAMINATION

Anne Waldman, RN, C, MSN

This first unit of the RN BOARD REVIEW FOR NCLEX-RN 1991 will provide you with the important information you need to know about the construction of the National Council Licensure Examination for Registered Nurses (NCLEX-RN, often referred to as "State Boards"), with tips on how to study, and with test-taking techniques you can use to improve your success when writing the examination.

Understanding the NCLEX Examination

THE TEST PLAN

The NCLEX-RN examination questions are based on a test plan comprised of phases of the nursing process, categories of client needs, and levels of cognitive skills.

Phases of the Nursing Process*

The phases of the nursing process to be measured in the examination for licensure are assessment, analysis, planning, implementation, and evaluation. Because all five categories are of equal importance, questions testing these nursing behaviors are distributed equally throughout the text.

Assessment

Establishing a data base.
A. Gather objective and subjective information relative to the client.
  1. Collect verbal and nonverbal information from the client, significant others, health team members, records, and other pertinent resources.
  2. Review standard data sources for information.
  3. Recognize symptoms and significant findings.
  4. Determine client's ability to assume care of daily health needs.
  5. Determine health team member's ability to provide care.
  6. Assess environment of client.
  7. Identify own or staff reactions to client, significant others, or health team members.
B. Verify data.
  1. Confirm observation or perception by obtaining additional information.
  2. Question orders and decisions by other health team members when indicated.
  3. Check condition of client personally instead of relying upon equipment.
C. Communicate information gained in assessment.

Analysis

Identifying actual or potential health care needs/problems based on assessment.

*Dvorak and Yocom, 1988, pp. 216–218. Adapted with permission.

A. Interpret data.
  1. Validate data.
  2. Organize related data.
B. Collect additional data as indicated.
C. Identify and communicate client's nursing diagnoses.
D. Determine congruency between client's needs/problems and health team member's ability to meet client's needs.

Planning

Setting goals to meet client's needs; designing strategies to achieve these goals.
A. Determine goals of care.
  1. Involve client, significant others, health team members in setting goals.
  2. Establish priorities among goals.
  3. Anticipate needs/problems according to established priorities.
B. Develop and modify plan.
  1. Involve client, significant others, health team members in designing strategies.
  2. Include all information needed to manage client's care (e.g., age, sex, culture, ethnicity, religion).
  3. Plan for client's comfort and maintenance of optimal functioning.
  4. Select nursing measures for delivery of client care.
C. Cooperate with other health team members for delivery of client care.
  1. Identify health or social resources in the community for client/significant others.
  2. Coordinate care for benefit of client.
  3. Delegate actions.
D. Formulate expected outcomes of nursing interventions.

Implementation

Initiating and completing actions necessary to accomplish the defined goals.
A. Organize and manage client's care.
B. Perform or assist in performing activities of daily living.
  1. Institute measures for client's comfort.
  2. Assist client to maintian optimal functioning.
C. Counsel and teach client, significant others, health team members.

1. Assist to recognize and manage stress.
2. Facilitate client relationships with significant others/health team members.
3. Teach correct principles, procedures, and techniques for maintenance and promotion of health.
4. Inform client about his health status.
5. Refer client, significant others, health team members to appropriate resources.

D. Provide care to achieve established goals for client.
   1. Use correct techniques in administering client care.
   2. Use precautionary and preventive measures in providing care to client.
   3. Prepare client for surgery, delivery, or other procedures.
   4. Institute action to compensate for adverse responses.
   5. Initiate necessary life-saving measures for emergency situations.

E. Provide care to optimize achievement of client's health care goals.
   1. Provide an environment conducive to attainment of client's health care goals.
   2. Adjust care in accord with client's expressed or implied needs/problems.
   3. Stimulate and motivate client to achieve self-care and independence.
   4. Encourage client to follow treatment regimen.
   5. Adapt approaches to compensate for own and health care team members' reactions to factors influencing therapeutic relationships with client.

F. Supervise, coordinate, and evaluate delivery of client's care provided by nursing staff.

G. Record and exchange information.
   1. Provide complete, accurate reports on assigned client to other team members.
   2. Record actual client responses, nursing actions, and other information relevant to implementation of care.

Evaluation

Determining the extent to which goals have been achieved.

A. Compare actual outcomes with expected outcomes of therapy.
   1. Evaluate responses (expected and unexpected) in order to determine degree of success of nursing interventions.
   2. Determine need for change in goals, environment, equipment, procedures, or therapy.

B. Evaluate compliance with prescribed/proscribed therapy.
   1. Determine impact of actions on client, significant others, or health team members.
   2. Verify that tests or measurements are done correctly.
   3. Ascertain client's, significant others', or health team members' understanding of information given.

C. Record and describe client's response to therapy/care.

D. Modify plan as indicated and reorder priorities.

Categories of Client Needs*

The health care needs of the client are grouped under four broad

*Ibid, pp. 219–220

categories, which, together with the weighting assigned to each, are: 1) safe, effective environment (25%–31%); physiologic integrity (42%–48%); psychosocial integrity (9%–15%); and health promotion/maintenance (12%–18).

Safe, Effective Care Environment

A. The nurse meets client needs for a safe and effective environment by providing and directing nursing care to promote
   1. Coordinated care
   2. Quality assurance
   3. Goal-oriented care
   4. Environmental safety
   5. Preparation for treatments and procedures
   6. Safe and effective treatments and procedures

B. In order to meet client needs for a safe, effective environment, the nurse should possess knowledge, skills, and abilities that include but are not limited to
   1. Bio/psycho/social principles
   2. Principles of teaching and learning
   3. Basic principles of management
   4. Principles of group dynamics and interpersonal communication
   5. Expected outcomes of various treatments
   6. General and specific protective measures
   7. Environmental and personal safety
   8. Client rights
   9. Confidentiality
   10. Cultural and religious influences on health
   11. Continuity of care
   12. Spread and control of infectious agents

Physiologic Integrity

A. The nurse meets the physiologic integrity needs of clients with potential life-threatening or chronically recurring physiologic conditions, or who are at risk for development of complications or untoward effects of treatments or management by providing and directing nursing care to promote
   1. Physiologic adaptation
   2. Reduction of risk potential
   3. Mobility
   4. Comfort
   5. Provision of basic care

B. In order to meet client needs for physiologic integrity, the nurse should possess knowledge, skills, and abilities that include but are not limited to
   1. Normal body structure and function
   2. Pathophysiology
   3. Drug administration and pharmacologic actions
   4. Routine nursing measures
   5. Intrusive procedures
   6. Documentation
   7. Nutritional therapies
   8. Managing emergencies, expected and unexpected response to therapies
   9. Body mechanics

10. Effects of immobility
11. Activities of daily living
12. Comfort measures
13. Uses of special equipment

Psychosocial Integrity

A. The nurse meets clients needs for psychosocial integrity in stress and crisis-related situations throughout the life cycle by providing and directing nursing care to promote
   1. Psychosocial adaptation
   2. Coping/adaptation
B. In order to meet client needs for psychosocial integrity, the nurse should possess knowledge, skills, and abilities that include but are not limited to
   1. Communication skills
   2. Mental health concepts
   3. Behavioral norms
   4. Psychodynamics of behavior
   5. Psychopathology
   6. Treatment modalities
   7. Psychopharmacology
   8. Documentation
   9. Accountability
   10. Principles of teaching and learning
   11. Appropriate community resources

Health Promotion/Maintenance

A. The nurse meets client needs for health promotion/maintenance throughout the life cycle by providing and directing nursing care to promote (for clients and their significant others)
   1. Continued growth and development
   2. Self-care
   3. Integrity of support systems
   4. Prevention and early treatment of disease
B. In order to meet client needs for health promotion/maintenance, the nurse should possess knowledge, skills, and abilities that include but are not limited to
   1. Communication skills
   2. Principles of teaching and learning
   3. Documentation
   4. Community resources
   5. Family systems
   6. Concepts of wellness
   7. Adaptation to altered health states
   8. Reproduction and human sexuality
   9. Birthing and parenting
   10. Growth and development, including dying and death
   11. Pathophysiology
   12. Body structure and function
   13. Principles of immunity

Levels of Cognitive Ability

The test also evaluates four of the cognitive abilities defined by Bloom et al. (1956): recall, comprehension, application, and analysis. While all four of these levels are evaluated, emphasis is placed on the higher functions of application and analysis. The four are defined as

A. Knowledge base: involves the ability to recall information.
B. Comprehension: involves the ability to understand what is being communicated and make use of the information without necessarily relating it to other information.
C. Application: requires the ability to remember and apply principles, procedures, and theories.
D. Analysis: requires the ability to break down a communication into the hierarchy of its parts and recognize the relationship among the ideas.

HOW THE TEST IS CONSTRUCTED

A. The National Council of State Boards of Nursing Inc. is the central organization for the independent member Boards of Nursing which includes the 50 states, the District of Columbia, Guam, and the Virgin Islands. The member boards are divided into four regional areas, which supervise the selection of test item writers (representing educators and clinicians), whose names are suggested by the individual state boards of nursing. This provides for regional representation in the testing of nursing practice.
B. The National Council contracts with a professional testing service to supervise writing and validation of test items by the item writers. This professional service works closely with the Examination Committee of the National Council in the test development process. The National Council and the state boards are responsible for the administration and security of the test.
C. The test is administered in February and July over a two-day period. It consists of four one-and-a-half-hour sections

containing approximately 90 questions each. Three hundred of the questions are actually graded and the remainder are used for experimental purposes. These experimental questions are interspersed throughout the examination so the candidate will answer all questions with equal effort.

HOW THE TEST IS SCORED

A. The NCLEX-RN is scored by machine and, effective February 1989, a pass/fail grade will be reported.
B. A criterion-referenced approach is used to set the passing score. This provides for the candidate's test performance to be compared with a consistent standard of criterion.

HOW CANDIDATES ARE NOTIFIED OF RESULTS

A. Approximately eight weeks after administration of the test, candidates are notified of their success or failure by the board of nursing of the state in which they wrote the examination.
B. Successful candidates are notified that they have passed.
C. Unsuccessful candidates are provided with a diagnostic profile that describes on a scale from low to high, their overall performance, their performance on the questions testing the phases of the nursing process, and their performance on the questions testing their abilities to meet client needs.

Preparation and Test Taking

USING THE TEST PLAN TO YOUR BEST ADVANTAGE

Performing a Self-needs Analysis

The first step to take when preparing to study for the NCLEX-RN is to perform a self-needs analysis to identify your knowledge base in relation to the information provided in the test plan.

A. Look carefully at the elements of the test plan (Phases of the Nursing Process and the Categories of Client Needs) that are reported to those failing the test.

B. Go through your notes and text references. Select what is important and star, underline, or highlight this information.

C. Categorize this information in terms of material that needs to be learned or material that needs only to be reviewed.

Planning for Study

A. Look at the period of time available to you for study between now and when you are scheduled to write the NCLEX-RN. Ideally, plan to study up to four nights before the test, allow three nights for review, and the night before the test for relaxation. If you have limited time for study, plan your time so that you have at least one night for nothing but review.

B. Identify what is your maximum concentration time for profitable study. It is better to block out short periods of time (45–60 minutes, interspersed with planned breaks) that can be quality study time, rather than setting aside three hours of time to study, which may only produce 90 minutes of quality study time.

C. When you decide what your maximum time for profitable study is, then that is the block of time you should set aside on a regular basis for study purposes. Within the confines of your allocated study time, make sure you establish a schedule that permits you to cover completely all the material identified as needing to be learned.

How to Study

A. To promote maximum concentration, ensure that your study materials are your prime area of focus.

B. Make sure you are mentally alert and in a room where you will be free from outside interruptions. If possible, choose a room with no telephone.

C. Do not smoke, do not nibble on snacks, and do not answer the telephone. This will allow you to direct your energy on the study activity.

D. Proceed with your planned study periods in an organized manner by choosing an approach that will be meaningful to you. Some content lends itself to study using concepts, while other content is best studied using systems.

E. Use methods of memory improvement that will work for you. Mnemonic devices (where a letter represents the first letter of each item in a sequence) are an effective means of retrieving material. Mental imagery can be used to form pictures in your mind to help remember details of the sequence of events, such as administration of an enema. Try practicing self-recitation to improve your study habits. Reciting to yourself the material being learned will promote retention of information being studied. Concentrate on the information you identified in your self-needs analysis as needing to be learned.

F. The final step of your study program involves a general review of all the information that you initially identified as areas for concentrated study. This consists of organizing the material so that you will be able to review all the "need to learn" and "need to review" information within the time allotted for review. Your schedule should have allowed you to complete your review so you can close your books and do something relaxing on the night before the examination.

FINAL PREPARATION FOR TEST TAKING

In addition to having studied appropriately to assure youself of a good knowledge base, there are measures you can take to be in prime physiologic and psychologic shape for writing the examination.

Physiologic Readiness

To prime yourself physiologically, you should meet your own needs for nutrition, sleep, and comfort.

A. You will function best if you are well nourished.

1. Plan to eat three well-balanced meals a day for at least three days prior to the examination as well as during the two days of the examination.
2. Be careful when choosing the food you consume at breakfast and lunch on the days of the examination.
   a. Avoid foods that will make you thirsty or cause intestinal distress.
   b. Minimize the potential for finding yourself with a full bladder midway through the examination by limiting the amount of fluids you drink and by allowing sufficient time at the test site to attend to your elimination needs before entering the room.
B. Assess your sleep needs.
   1. Determine what is the minimal amount of sleep you need in order to function effectively.
   2. Plan to allow sufficient time in your schedule the week before the examination to provide yourself with the minimum sleep you need to function effectively for at least three days prior to the examination as well as the night between the two days of the examination.
C. Plan your wardrobe ahead of time.
   1. Shoes and clothes that fit you comfortably will not distract your thought processes during the examination.
   2. Include a confortable sweater.
   3. Your clothes for the two days should be ready to wear by the night before the examination.
D. If you wear glasses or contact lenses, take along an extra pair of glasses.
E. If you are taking medications on a regular basis continue to do so during this period of time. Introduction of new medications should be avoided until after completion of the examination.

Reducing Psychologic Stress

While a certain amount of anxiety will stimulate your nervous system to focus keenly on the examination, excess anxiety will interfere with your ability to concentrate on the examination and, indeed, hinder your success. You must approach the examination with a positive attitude. You have graduated from a school of nursing that has prepared you to provide safe and effective nursing care to your clients. Trust that the curriculum in your school of nursing was designed to include all the important concepts and principles necessary for safe nursing practice. Most of the tests you wrote while in school were developed in the style used for the NCLEX-RN. Keeping these points in mind will enable you to approach the examination with a positive frame of reference for success.
A. Mininize the anxiety-producing situations related to writing the examination by carefully planning your pre-examination activities. Make a list of the important things you need to accomplish.
   1. Rehearse the route or means of transportation you plan to take to the test location, preferably at the same time of the day on which you actually will be going. Check your local resources for road conditions that might necessitate altering your planned route. In your time assessment, include parking your car, locating where you are to report for registration, and locating the bathrooms. To ensure

adequate travel time and to minimize stress related to getting to the test site on time the morning of the test, add an extra 30 minutes to the total time needed for the rehearsal run.
   2. Have your admission materials readily available.
   3. If you are staying overnight near the test site, be sure you pack everything you will need for the two days. Before retiring for the night, make your rehearsal run to the test location in preparation for the next day.
   4. Keep your anxiety under control by refraining from talking about the test with your friends until all four sections have been completed. Once you have completed your content review, you have established a positive mindset for yourself. Don't destroy that confidence. Wait until you finish writing the last examination section to rehash the questions on the test. While this is not an easy task, it is one that will, in the long run, bring positive rewards.
   5. Plan to use relaxation exercises to control your anxiety level. If you have been using a specific method of relaxation successfully, then continue using it during this period of time. If you have not, consider trying one of the following.
      a. Active progressive relaxation (Flynn, 1980): requires a quiet environment, a comfortable sitting position and progressive tension and relaxation of individual muscle groups
      b. Guided imagery: requires using your imagination to create a relaxing sensory scene on which to concentrate
      c. Breathing exercises
      d. Relaxation response (Benson, 1975): requires a quiet environment, a mental device, a passive attitude and a comfortable position.
   6. For any of the methods to achieve the desired results, you must be willing to commit the time necessary to implement their prescribed protocols.

TAKING THE TEST

While having a good knowledge base is important for success in test-taking situations, the following strategies can be used to maximize your skill in choosing the correct answers.
A. Take your seat and give yourself an opportunity to implement the method of relaxation you have been practicing.
B. Read the directions carefully, and then be sure to follow them carefully.
C. Plan to manage your time effectively. You will have 90 minutes to answer approximately 90 single multiple-choice questions. Pace yourself so that you answer about one question per minute. If you are a slow test taker, you should evaluate your progress every 15–20 minutes to prevent falling too far behind.
D. Many of the questions will be presented as part of a clinical situation. Read the conditions of the situation twice. *Do not speed read!* Use your pencil as a pointer and read each word. This will also help to control anxiety.

E. Read the stem of the question carefully. This is the part of the question that describes what is being asked. Key words which qualify what the question is asking will be typed in a manner that will make them stand out (most; best; least; contraindicated). For example

---

19. The MOST common mode of transmission of Hepatitis B is via which route?
    - o 1. Oral
    - o 2. Fecal
    - o 3. Parenteral
    - o 4. Genital

F. Read the stem a second time to be clear about what the question is asking.
G. Move to the four answer choices. One will be correct and three incorrect. Incorrect answers are called distractors.
H. Carefully evaluate the answer choices for key words. Be sure to appreciate the universality of words such as each, all, never, and none; the limitations of words such as rarely, most, and least; and the latitude offered by words such as usually, frequently, and often.
I. Read each option twice, using your pencil as a guide.
J. Answer it by saying to yourself
    1. *Yes* it answers what is being asked.
    2. *No* it does not answer what is being asked.
    3. *Maybe* it answers what is being asked.
K. Use this procedure for all four answer choices. When you first read the question, if an obvious answer comes to mind, restrain your desire to look for it in the answer choices. Read all four choices to make sure your thought was indeed the only *yes* answer. If you are fortunate enough to have only one *yes* answer, then you have eliminated the three distractors.
L. Carefully fill in the circle to the left of the answer.
M. If you identified more than one *yes* option, then evaluate those in terms of which is more *yes* than *maybe*. If you have no *yes* answer, then evaluate the *maybe* choices for which leans more toward *yes*.
N. Always choose the answer that has the highest likelihood for being *yes* (correct).
    1. Look critically at the answer choices for clues. If you see choices that are opposites, frequently one is the correct answer. For example

---

33. During insertion of a central venous catheter, the patient should be in
    - o 1. a supine position.
    - o 2. Trendelenburg's position.
    - o 3. reverse Trendelenburg's position.
    - o 4. a high-Fowler's position.

---

    2. Choices 2. and 3. are opposites, and in this case 2. is the correct answer.
O. If you have an answer that contains more than one option, all of the options must be correct for that choice to be correct. If you can eliminate one of the options in an answer, you can automatically eliminate the other answer choices with that option.

    1. For example

---

47. Metabolic complications from the administration of TPN include
    - o 1. hyperglycemia and hypokalemia.
    - o 2. hyperglycemia and hyperkalemia.
    - o 3. hypoglycemia and hypercalcemia.
    - o 4. hyperkalemia and hypercalcemia.

---

    2. Hypercalcemia and hyperkalemia are distractors. Eliminate the choices with these options and there is only one correct choice remaining.
P. Look for options that do not meet the requirements of the stem.
    1. For example

---

53. A drug that is used to lyse (break up) already formed clots is
    - o 1. warfarin sodium (Coumadin).
    - o 2. heparin sodium (Lipo-Hepin).
    - o 3. streptokinase (Kabikinase).
    - o 4. vitamin K.

---

    2. Choices 1., 2., and 3. are all used in the treatment of formed clots. Choice 4. is necessary for clot formation and therefore does not meet the requirements of the stem.
Q. If the stem asks for the exception or which choice is not the answer, you are looking for the *no* answer rather then the *yes* answer.
    1. For example

---

67. Individuals at risk of getting TB include all of the following EXCEPT
    - o 1. lower socioeconomic groups.
    - o 2. malnourished and debilitated individuals.
    - o 3. individuals on steroid therapy.
    - o 4. white females with a history of alcohol abuse.

---

    2. Choices 1., 2., and 3. are all at risk and therefore *yes* responses. Choice 4. is the *no* response and therefore the correct answer.
R. Be careful to avoid reading elements into the question that are not specifically included in the stem and answer choices.
S. Do not spend a lot of time on any one question. If you cannot clearly decide which answer is correct, skip the question. Use the note page indicated in the instructions to keep track of the question you have skipped. You will return to this after you have completed the test.
T. Unfortunately, not knowing the answer to the first question can be anxiety producing. Maintain your calm. Use your pencil to force yourself to concentrate and continue on to the next question. Should you not be able to answer this question, mark it for return on the note sheet, try to control the increasing anxiety you are feeling, and continue to the next question. When you reach the question for which you

easily obtain a single *yes* response, you will feel a physiologic relief from tension and be able to proceed more effectively with the remainder of the test.

U. Continue on through the test. Answer those questions for which you have a *yes* (correct) answer and skip those for which you are unsure of the answer. Remember to mark the note page with the numbers of the questions left unanswered.

V. After completing the test for the first time, return to answer only those questions left unanswered. While doing this second run through, be careful not to change any of your first answers. Your first answer is usually your best answer. Reread the situation and the question. If you cannot make a clear decision, then choose the answer you feel is closest to being correct. Your answers will be equally incorrect whether you choose a wrong answer or leave a blank space. *It is to your advantage to answer one choice for each question whether you are sure of the answer or not.*

W. After you have gone over the test and made sure each question has an answer, go through each page of the test and remove all stray pencil marks. While doing this, make sure all answer circles are filled in completely.

X. Then, turn in the test.

Y. A word of caution. As you are proceeding through the test booklet, you may become aware that other candidates are completing their tests and leaving the room. This can be anxiety producing to many people. Be careful not to lose valuable testing time wondering why they are finished and you are not. Reassure yourself that you are progressing satisfactorily within the framework of your individual time schedule and continue with the examination.

HOW TO USE THIS BOOK

As you go through each unit of this book, use it to perform your self-needs analysis and as a basis for study. You will make the best use of both your time and the book if you use the study skills suggested earlier in this unit.

A. For more detailed information on the particular subjects you feel need extra study, read the reprints included at the end of each section, review those subjects in current textbooks, and scan the list of recommended readings at the end of each unit for further resources.

B. The questions interspersed throughout Units 2 through 5 are typical of the board questions and they will help you to become more familiar with the style of questions found in the NCLEX-RN.

C. When setting up your study time, include at least two 90-minute blocks of time to take the two sample tests in Unit 6. You may take these tests once, before you start studying, to help you with your needs analysis. When you have completed studying, you may take them again, to evaluate for test performance. If you choose to take them both twice, you will need four 90-minute blocks of time.

D. While taking the sample tests, apply the test-taking strategies discussed earlier in this Unit.

REFERENCES

Benson, H. (1975). The relaxation response. New York: Morrow.

Bloom, B., et al. (Eds.) (1956). Taxonomy of educational objections: Handbook I, The cognitive domain. New York: Longmans, Green.

Dvorak, E., & Yocum, C. (1988). *National council licensure examination for registered nurses* (4th ed.). Chicago: Chicago Review Press.

Flynn, P. (1980) Holistic health: The art and science of care. Bowie, MD: Brady.

UNIT 2
ADULT NURSING

by

Margaret B. Brenner, RN, MSN
Eileen Moran, RN, MSN

Nursing care of the adult patient in today's changing health care environment is a challenge to the skill and knowledge of the professional nurse. Holistic care requires that nurses not only meet a patient's physical needs through technical skills and sound clinical judgment, but that they also be aware of a patient's psychosocial needs. The role of patient advocate puts the nurse in a unique position to help patients achieve the highest possible level of wellness.

This unit presents a comprehensive review of nursing care of adult patients with specific health problems. It begins with a section on introductory concepts (such as nutrition, fluid and electrolyte balance, and acid-base balance), which are basic to nursing practice, and multisystem stressors (such as infection, pain, and surgery). These concepts are common to all areas of nursing practice and may be applied to patients with various levels of health care needs.

The unit is further divided according to specific body systems. For each system there is a review of anatomy and physiology. Each step of the nursing process (assessment, analysis, planning, intervention, and evaluation) is then reviewed for the system, followed by consideration of the major health problems of that system. Congenital disorders will be discussed in Unit 3.

Introductory Concepts and Multisystem Stressors

STRESS AND ADAPTATION

Definitions

A. Stress: tension resulting from changes in the internal or external environment; either psychologic or physiologic
B. Stressors: agents or forces threatening an individual's ability to meet his or her needs
C. Adaptation: an individual's (or the body's) reaction to and attempt to deal with stress

General Characteristics

A. A certain amount of stress is necessary for life and growth, but excessive and continuous stress can be detrimental.
B. Success of adaptation depends on perception of stressor(s), the individual's coping mechanisms, and biologic adaptive resources.
C. Types of stressors: physical, chemical, microbiologic, psychologic, social.

General Adaptation Syndrome (Hans Selye)

Response to Stress

A. Caused by release of certain adaptive hormones
B. Three stages
   1. Alarm reaction
     a. Shock phase: defensive forces are mobilized; sympathetic nervous system is activated (fight or flight).
     b. Countershock phase: body returned to prealarm condition.
   2. Resistance: body adapts to stressor; uses physical, physiologic, and psychologic coping mechanisms.
   3. Exhaustion: adaptive resources are depleted, overwhelmed, or insufficient; if stress is excessive and continues, death will occur without support.

INFLAMMATORY RESPONSE

A reaction of the tissues of the body to injury in order to destroy or dilute an injurious agent, to prevent the spread of injury, and to promote repair of damaged tissue.

Causes

A. Physical irritants (e.g., trauma or a foreign body)
B. Chemical irritants (e.g., strong acids or alkalis)
C. Microorganisms (e.g., bacteria and viruses)

Components

A. Vascular response: transitory period of localized vasoconstriction, followed by vasodilatation, increased capillary permeability, and blood stasis
B. Formation of inflammatory exudate
   1. Composition: water, colloids, ions, and defensive cells
   2. Functions: dilution of toxins, transportation of nutrients to area of injury for tissue repair, transportation of protective cells that phagocytize and destroy bacteria
C. Defense cell response: migration of leukocytes to affected area for phagocytosis of foreign bodies and dead cells
D. Healing: resolution of inflammation and regeneration of tissue or replacement with scar tissue

Assessment Findings

A. Local: pain, swelling, heat, redness, and impaired function of part (five cardinal signs of inflammation)
B. Systemic (appear with moderate to severe response): fever, leukocytosis, chills, sweating, anorexia, weight loss, general malaise

IMMUNE RESPONSE

Essence of immune response is to recognize foreign substances and to neutralize, eliminate, or metabolize them with or without injury to the body's own tissues.

Functions of the Immune System

A. Defense: protection against antigens. An *antigen* is a protein or protein complex recognized as nonself.
B. Homeostasis: removal of worn out or damaged components (e.g., dead cells)
C. Surveillance: ability to perceive or destroy mutated cells or nonself cells.

Alterations in Immune Functioning

See Table 2.1.

Types of Immunity

There are two major types of immunity: natural (or innate) and acquired.

A. *Natural (innate) immunity:* immune responses that exist without prior exposure to an immunologically active substance. Genetically acquired immunity is natural immunity.

B. *Acquired immunity*
1. Immune responses that develop during the course of a person's lifetime.
2. Acquired immunity may be further classified as naturally or artificially acquired, active or passive. Active immunity results when the body produces its own antibodies in response to an antigen. Passive immunity results when an antibody is transferred artificially.
   a. *Naturally acquired active immunity:* results from having the disease and recovering successfully
   b. *Naturally acquired passive immunity:* antibodies obtained through placenta or by breast milk
   c. *Artificially acquired active immunity:* conferred by immunization with an antigen.
   d. *Artificially acquired passive immunity:* antibodies transferred from sensitized person (e.g., immune serum globulin [gamma globulin])

Components of Immune Response

A. Located throughout the body
B. Organs include thymus, bone marrow, lymph nodes, spleen, tonsils, appendix, Peyer's patches of small intestine.
C. Main cell types are WBCs (especially lymphocytes, plasma cells, and macrophages); all originate from the same stem cell in bone marrow, then differentiate into separate types.
1. Granulocytes
   a. Eosinophils: increase with allergies and parasites
   b. Basophils: contain histamine and increase with allergy and anaphylaxis
   c. Neutrophils: involved in phagocytosis
2. Monocytes (macrophages) (e.g., histiocytes, Kupffer cells): involved in phagocytosis
3. Lymphocytes (T cells and B cells): involved in cellular and humoral immunity

Classification of Immune Responses

Cellular Immunity

A. Mediated by T cells: persist in tissues for months or years
B. Functions: transplant rejection, delayed hypersensitivity, tuberculin reactions, tumor surveillance/destruction, intracellular infections

Humoral Immunity

A. Mediated by B cells
1. Production of circulating antibodies (gamma globulin)
2. Only survive for days

Table 2.1   Alterations in Immune Functioning

Immune Function	Hypofunction	Hyperfunction
Defense	Immunosuppression with increased susceptibility to infection; includes disorders such as neutropenia, AIDS, immunosuppression secondary to drugs and hypo- or agammaglobulinemia.	Inappropriate and abnormal response to external antigens; an allergy
Homeostasis	No known effect	Abnormal response where antibodies react against normal tissues and cells; an *autoimmune disease.*
Surveillance	Inability of the immune system to perceive and respond to mutated cells, suspected mechanism in cancer.	No known effect

B. Functions: bacterial phagocytosis, bacterial lysis, virus and toxin neutralization, anaphylaxis, allergic hay fever and asthma

NUTRITION*

Basic Concepts

Principles

A. Essential nutrients: carbohydrates, fats, proteins, minerals, vitamins, and water that must be supplied to the body in specified amounts.
B. Foods: the sources of nutrients, provide energy to help build, repair, and maintain tissue and regulate body processes.
C. Malnutrition: results from deficiency, excess, or imbalance of required nutrients.

Carbohydrates (Sugars and Starches)

A. Major source of food energy; 4 kcal/gm
B. Classification
1. Monosaccharides: simplest form of carbohydrate
   a. Glucose (dextrose): found chiefly in fruits and vegetables; oxidized for immediate energy
   b. Fructose: found in honey and fruits
   c. Galactose: not free in nature; part of milk sugar
2. Disaccharides: double sugars
   a. Sucrose: found in table sugar, syrups, and some fruits and vegetables

---

*The section on Nutrition was contributed by Theresa Giglio, RD, MS.

b. Lactose: found in milk
c. Maltose: intermediate product in the hydrolysis of starch
3. Polysaccharides: composed of many glucose molecules
   a. Starch: found in cereal grains, potatoes, root vegetables, and legumes
   b. Glycogen: synthesized and stored in the liver and skeletal muscles
   c. Cellulose, hemicellulose, pectins, gums, and mucilages: indigestible polysaccharides
4. Dietary fiber: includes several polysaccharides plus other substances that are not digestible by gastrointestinal (GI) enzymes.
   a. Dietary fiber (roughage) holds water so that stools are soft and bulky; increases motility of the small and large intestines and decreases transit time; reduces intraluminal pressure in the colon.
   b. Sources: wheat bran, unrefined cereals, whole wheat, raw fruits and vegetables, dried fruits
C. Functions of carbohydrates
1. Cheapest and most abundant source of energy
2. To spare protein for tissue building when sufficient carbohydrate is present
3. Necessary for the complete oxidation of fats (to prevent ketosis)
D. Dietary sources: sugars, grains, fruits, vegetables, nuts, milk

Lipids (Fats)

A. Most concentrated source of energy in foods; 9 kcal/gm
B. Include fats, oils, resins, waxes, and fatlike substances such as glycerides, phospholipids, sterols, and lipoproteins
C. Fatty acids
1. Saturated fatty acids: usually solid at room temperature; predominantly present in animal fats
2. Monounsaturated fatty acids: present in oleic acid found in olive oil, peanut oil
3. Polyunsaturated fatty acids: usually liquid at room temperature; predominantly present in plant fats and fish
4. Essential fatty acids: cannot be manufactured by the body (e.g., linoleic fatty acid)
5. Nonessential fatty acids: can be synthesized by the body
D. Functions of lipids
1. Most concentrated source of energy
2. Insulation and padding of body organs
3. Component of the cell membrane
4. Carrier of the fat-soluble vitamins A, D, E, K
5. Help maintain body temperature
E. Dietary sources: oil from seeds of grains, nuts, vegetables; milk fat, butter, cream cheese; fat in meat; lard, bacon fat; fish oil; egg yolk
F. *Cholesterol:* essential constituent of body tissues
1. A component of cell membranes
2. A precursor of steroid hormones
3. Can be manufactured in the body
4. Present in animal fats
5. Dietary sources: egg yolk, brains, liver, butter, cream, cheese, shellfish

Protein

A. Organic compounds that may be composed of hundreds of amino acids; 4 kcal/gm.
B. Classification
1. Complete protein: contains all the essential amino acids; usually from animal food sources.
2. Incomplete protein: lacks one or more essential amino acids; usually from plant food sources
C. Amino acids
1. Essential amino acids: eight amino acids that cannot be synthesized in the body and must be taken in food.
2. Nonessential amino acids: 12 amino acids that can be synthesized in the body.
D. Functions of proteins
1. Necessary for growth and continuous replacement of cells throughout life
2. Play a role in the immune processes
3. Participate in regulating body processes such as fluid balance, muscle contraction, mineral balance, iron transport, buffer actions
4. Provide energy if necessary
E. Dietary sources: meat, fish, eggs, milk, cheese, poultry, grains, vegetables, nuts
F. Deficiency diseases
1. Kwashiorkor
2. Hypoproteinemia
3. Marasmus (protein-kilocalorie malnutrition)

Energy Metabolism

A. Measurement of energy expressed in terms of heat units called kilocalories (kcal): amount of heat required to raise 1 kg water by 1°C
B. Energy expenditure
1. Basal metabolism
   a. Amount of energy expended to carry on the involuntary work of the body while at rest
   b. Factors influencing basal metabolic rate (BMR): body surface area, sex, age, body temperature, hormones, pregnancy, fasting, malnutrition
2. Physical activity: amount of energy expended depends upon the type of activity, the length of time involved, and the weight of the person
C. Factors determining total energy needs
1. Amount necessary for BMR
2. Amount required for physical activity
3. Specific dynamic action of food ingested
4. Growth
5. Climate

Weight Control

A. Underweight: 10% or more below individual's ideal weight
1. Causes: failure to ingest sufficient kcal; excess energy expenditure; irregular eating habits; GI disturbances; pathologic conditions; lack of education; economic problems; endocrine problems; emotional disturbances

Table 2.2 Minerals

Mineral	Functions	Deficiency Syndrome	Food Sources	Comments
Calcium	Development of bones and teeth Transmission of nerve impulses Muscle contraction Permeability of cell membrane Catalyze thrombin formation Maintenance of normal heart rhythm	Rickets, osteoporosis, osteomalacia, stunted growth, fragile bones, tetany	Milk, cheese, ice cream, broccoli, collard greens, kale, oysters, shrimp, salmon, clams	Needs vitamin D and parathormone for utilization. Acid, lactose and vitamin D favor absorption.
Phosphorus	Development of bones and teeth Transfer of energy in cells (ATP) Cell permeability Buffer salts Component in phospholipids	Rickets, stunted growth, poor bone mineralization	Milk, cheese, meat, fish, poultry, eggs, legumes, nuts, whole-grain cereals	Factors that affect calcium absorption also affect phosphorus.
Magnesium	Constituent of bones and teeth Cation in intracellular fluid Muscle and nerve irritability Activate enzymes in carbohydrate metabolism	Tremor observed in severe alcoholism, diabetic acidosis, severe renal disease	Milk, cheese, meat, nuts, legumes, green leafy vegetables, whole-grain cereals	Absorption similar to calcium.
Sulfur	Constituent of keratin in hair, skin, and nails Detoxification reactions Constituent of thiamin, biotin, insulin, coenzyme A, melanin, glutathione	None	Protein foods, eggs, meat, fish, poultry, milk, cheese, nuts	Diet adequate in protein provides sufficient sulfur.
Iron	Constituent of hemoglobin, myoglobin, oxidative enzymes	Anemia	Liver, organ meats, meat, poultry, egg yolk, whole-grain cereals, legumes, dark green vegetables, dried fruit	Ascorbic acid favors absorption.
Iodine	Constituent of thyroxine Regulate rate of energy metabolism	Simple goiter, cretinism, myxedema	Iodized salt, seafood	
Sodium	Principle cation of extracellular fluid Osmotic pressure Water balance Regulate nerve irritability and muscle contraction Pump for active transport of glucose	Rare	Table salt, protein foods, processed foods, baking soda	Diet usually provides excess.
Potassium	Principle cation of intracellular fluid Osmotic pressure Water balance Acid-base balance Regular heart rhythm Nerve irritability and muscle contraction	Tachycardia Deficiency may occur with diabetic acidosis Deficiency may occur with some diuretics	Oranges, bananas, dried fruits, most fruits and vegetables, whole-grain cereals	Readily absorbed.
Chlorine	Chief anion of extracellular fluid Constituent of gastric juice Acid-base balance Activate salivary amylase	Seen only after prolonged vomiting	Table salt, processed meats	Rapidly absorbed.

   2. Treatment: diet counseling, correction of underlying disease, behavior studies, social service referrals
B. Overweight: 10% above individual's ideal weight
C. Obesity: 20% or more above individual's ideal weight
   1. Causes: overeating, underactivity, genetic factors, fat cell theory, alteration in hypothalamic function, endocrine problems, emotional disturbances
   2. Treatment: diet counseling, nutritionally balanced diet, behavior modification, increased physical activity, medical treatment of any underlying disease, appropriate referrals

Minerals

Inorganic compounds that yield no energy; essential structural components involved in many body processes (see Table 2.2).

Vitamins

Organic compounds necessary in small quantities for cellular functions of the body; do not give energy; necessary in many enzyme systems (see Table 2.3).

Water

A. Distribution: present in all body tissues; accounts for 50%–60% total body weight in adults and 70%–75% in infants.
   1. Intracellular fluid: exists within the cells.
   2. Extracellular fluid: includes plasma fluid, interstitial fluid, lymph, and secretions.
B. Functions: the medium of all body fluids
   1. Necessary for many biologic reactions

Table 2.3 Vitamins

Vitamin	Function	Deficiency Syndrome	Food Sources	Comments
Vitamin A (retinol)	Maintenance of mucous membranes Visual acuity in dim light, growth and bone development	Night blindness, xerophthalmia, keratinization of epithelium, poor bone and tooth development	Fish liver oils, liver, butter, cream, whole milk, egg yolk, dark green vegetables, yellow vegetables, yellow fruits, fortified margarine	Bile necessary for absorption. Large amounts are toxic.
Vitamin B_1 (thiamin)	Involved in carbohydrate metabolism Thiamin pyrophosphate (TPP)	Beriberi, mental depression, polyneuritis, cardiac failure	Enriched cereals, whole grains, meat, organ meats, pork, fish, poultry, legumes, nuts	Very little storage.
Vitamin B_2 (riboflavin)	Coenzyme for transfer and removal of hydrogen Flavin adenine dinucleotide (FAD)	Cheilosis, photophobia, burning and itching of eyes, sore tongue and mouth	Milk, eggs, organ meats, green leafy vegetables	Limited storage.
Vitamin B_6 (pyridoxine, pyridoxal, pyridoxamine)	Coenzyme for transamination, transsulfuration, and decarboxylation	Convulsions, dermatitis, nervous irritability	Meat, poultry, fish, vegetables, potatoes	Converts glycogen to glucose.
Vitamin B_{12} (hydroxycobalamin)	Formation of mature red blood cells Synthesis of DNA and RNA	Pernicious anemia, neurologic degeneration, macrocytic anemia	Animal foods only	Intrinsic factor is necessary for absorption.
Vitamin C (ascorbic acid)	Synthesis of collagen Formation of intercellular cement Facilitation of iron absorption	Scurvy, bleeding gums, poor wound healing, cutaneous hemorrhage, capillary fragility	Citrus fruits, tomatoes, melon, raw cabbage, broccoli, strawberries	Most easily destroyed vitamin. Very little storage in body.
Vitamin D (cholecalciferol)	Increase absorption of calcium and phosphorus Bone mineralization	Rickets, osteomalacia, enlarged joints, muscle spasms, delayed dentition	Fish liver oils, fortified milk	Synthesized in skin by activity of ultraviolet light. Large amounts are toxic.
Vitamin E (tocopherol)	Reduces oxidation of vitamin A, phospholipids, and polyunsaturated fatty acids	Hemolysis of red blood cells, deficiency not likely	Vegetable oils, wheat germ, nuts, legumes, green leafy vegetables	Not toxic.
Vitamin K (phylloquinone)	Formation of prothrombin and other clotting proteins	Prolonged clotting time, hemorrhagic disease in newborn	Green leafy vegetables, cabbage, liver, alfalfa	Bile necessary for absorption. Large amounts are toxic.
Folacin (folic acid)	Maturation of red blood cells, interrelated with vitamin B_{12}	Megaloblastic anemia, tropical sprue	Organ meats, muscle meats, poultry, fish, eggs, green leafy vegetables	Ascorbic acid necessary for utilization.
Niacin (nicotinamide)	Coenzyme to accept and transfer hydrogen, coenzyme for glycolysis	Pellagra, dermatitis, neurologic degeneration, glossitis, diarrhea	Meat, poultry, fish, whole grains, enriched breads, nuts, legumes	Amino acid tryptophan is a precursor.

   2. Acts as a solvent.

   3. Transports nutrients to cells and eliminates waste.

   4. Body lubricant

   5. Regulates body temperature.

C. Sources

   1. Ingestion of water and other beverages

   2. Water content of food eaten

   3. Water resulting from food oxidation

D. Recommended daily intake

   1. Replacement of losses through the kidneys, lungs, skin, and bowel

   2. Thirst usually a good guide

   3. Approximately 48 oz/day of water from all sources is adequate; requirement is higher if physical activity is strenuous or if sweating is profuse.

Dietary Guides

A. Basic four food groups

   1. Foods are grouped in relation to composition and nutrient value: milk-cheese group, meat-fish-poultry-beans group, vegetable-fruit group, and bread-cereal group

   2. Food plan includes the minimum number of servings for the adult to obtain desired nutrients with about 1300 kcal.

B. Recommended daily allowances: established by the Food and Nutrition Board of the National Academy of Science; recommended nutrient intake is provided for infants, children, men, women, pregnant and lactating women; recommendations are stated for protein, kcal, and most vitamins and minerals.

C. Food composition tables: helpful in calculating the nutritive value of the daily diet; list nutrient content of foods.

D. Height and weight charts: ideal or desirable body weight for both men and women at specified heights with a small, medium, or large frame.

E. Exchange lists for meal planning
1. Foods are separated into six exchange lists.
2. Specific foods on each list are approximately equal in carbohydrate, protein, fat, and kcal content.
3. Individual foods on the same list may be exchanged for each other at the same meals.
4. Food lists are helpful in planning diets for weight control or diabetes (see Special Diets, Appendix 1).

Nutritional Assessment

Process that determines the state of an individual's nutritional health.

A. Anthropometric measurements: indicators of available stores in muscle and fat compartments of the body
1. Height/weight ratio
2. Midarm muscle circumference
3. Triceps skinfold (biceps, subscapular, abdominal, hip, pectoral, and calf areas may be measured in some cases)

B. Clinical findings: detected by physical exam, include assessment of the condition of skin, hair, face, eyes, teeth, nails, glands, muscle, bones

C. Laboratory biochemical studies: fluid and electrolytes, blood sugar, serum proteins (especially albumin and iron-binding capacity), total lymphocyte count, nitrogen balance studies, 24-hour urinary creatinine, feces, hair, biopsy

D. Intradermal delayed hypersensitivity testing

E. Dietary assessment: diet history includes use of food diary, 24- to 48-hour recall, calculation of nutritive value of foods eaten with evaluation and counseling.

Enteral Nutrition

Preferred method for nutritional support for the malnourished patient whose GI system is intact.

Oral Feeding

A. Always the first choice

B. Oral formula supplements may be used between meals to provide added kcal and nutrients.
1. Offer small quantities several times a day.
2. Vary flavors, avoid taste fatigue.
3. Chill and serve over ice.

Tube Feeding

A. Used for patients who have a functioning GI tract but cannot ingest food orally

1. Feeding tubes
   a. Short term: nasogastric tube
   b. Long term: esophagostomy, gastrostomy, or enterostomy tube
2. Formulas: nutritionally adequate, tolerated by patient, easily prepared, easily digested, usual concentration l kcal/cc
3. Feeding schedules
   a. Intermittent: usually 4–6 times/day, volumes up to 400 cc, by slow gravity drip over 30–60 minutes
   b. Continuous: usually administered by pump through a duodenal or proximal jejunostomy feeding tube
4. Nursing responsibilities
   a. Administer formulas at room temperature (refrigerate unused portion).
   b. Gradually increase rate and concentration until desired amount is attained if there are no signs of intolerance (e.g., gastric residual greater than 120 cc, nausea, vomiting, diarrhea, distention, diaphoresis, increased pulse, glycosuria, aspiration).
   c. Check tube placement and elevate head of bed (see also Nasogastric Tubes, page 120).
   d. Monitor intake and output (I&O), serum electrolytes, fractional urines, serum glucose, daily weights; keep a stool record as well as an ongoing assessment of tolerance.

Parenteral Nutrition

Nutrients are infused directly into a vein for patients who are unable to eat or digest food through the GI tract, who refuse to eat, or who have inadequate oral intake.

Total Parenteral Nutrition (TPN)

A. Involves the infusion of nutrients through a central vein catheter. A central vein is needed because its larger caliber and higher blood flow will quickly dilute the hypertonic hyperalimentation solution to isotonic concentrations.

B. Hyperalimentation solution: includes hypertonic glucose, amino acids, water, vitamins, and minerals (lipid emulsions are given in a separate solution).

C. Nursing responsibilities
1. For details of nursing care of the patient with a central venous line see IV Therapy, page 27.
2. Inspect solution before hanging.
   a. Check for correct solution and additives against physician's order.
   b. Check expiration date.
   c. Observe fluid for cloudiness or floating particulate matter.
3. Control flow rate of solution.
   a. Calculate correct rate.
   b. Administration via pump is preferable.
   c. Monitor flow rate.
   d. Never attempt to speed up or slow down infusion rate.
      1) speeding up infusion causes large amounts of glucose to enter body, causing hyperosmolar state.

2) slowing down infusion can cause hypoglycemic state, as it takes time for the pancreas to adjust to reduced glucose level.
4. Monitor fluid balance.
5. Obtain fractional urines every 6 hours.
6. Use Testape to detect hyperglycemia (some additives may cause false positive if Clinitest is used); cover with sliding scale insulin as ordered.
7. Provide psychologic support.
8. Encourage exercise regimen.

IV Lipid Emulsions

A. May be given through a central vein or peripherally in order to prevent essential fatty acid deficiency in long-term TPN patients, or to provide supplemental kcal IV.
B. Nursing care
1. Protect the stability of the emulsion.
   a. Administer in its own separate IV bottle and IV tubing, and piggyback the emulsion into the Y connector closest to the catheter insertion.
   b. Inspect solution for evidence of separation of oil, frothiness, inconsistency, particulate matter; discard solution if any of these signs of instability occur.
   c. Do *not* shake the bottle; this might cause aggregation of fat globules.
   d. Discard partially used bottles.
2. Control the infusion rate accurately and safely.
   a. If using gravity method, lipid emulsion must hang higher than hyperalimentation to prevent back flow.
   b. Pump is preferred, but may not be possible due to viscous nature of emulsion.
3. Prevent and assess for adverse reactions.
   a. Administer slowly according to package insert over first 30 minutes; if no adverse reactions, increase rate to complete infusion over the specified number of hours.
   b. Obtain baseline vital signs; repeat after first 30 minutes, and then every 1–2 hours until completion.
   c. Acute reactions may include: fever, chills, dyspnea, nausea, vomiting, headache, lethargy, syncope, chest or back pain, hypercoagulability, thrombocytopenia.
4. Evaluate tolerance and patient response.

Peripheral Vein Parenteral Nutrition

A. Can be used for short-term support, when the central vein is not available, and as a supplemental means of obtaining nutrients.
B. Solution contains the same components as central vein therapy, but lower concentrations.
C. Care is the same as for the patient receiving hyperalimentation centrally.
D. Phlebitis and thrombosis are common and IV sites will need frequent changing.

INFECTION

Infection is an invasion of the body by pathogenic organisms that multiply and produce injurious effects. Communicable disease is an infectious disease that may be transmitted from one person to another.

Chain of Events

A. *Causative agent:* invading organism (e.g., bacteria, virus)
B. *Reservoir:* environment in which the invading organism lives and multiplies
C. *Portal of exit:* mode of escape from reservoir (e.g., respiratory tract, GI tract)
D. *Mode of transmission:* method by which invading organism is transported to new host (e.g., direct contact, air, food)
E. *Portal of entry:* means by which organism enters new host (e.g., respiratory tract, broken skin)
F. *Susceptible host:* susceptibility determined by factors such as number of invading organisms, duration of exposure, age, state of health, nutritional status.

Nursing Responsibilities in Prevention of Spread of Infection

A. Maintain an environment that is clean, dry, and well ventilated.
B. Use proper handwashing before and after patient contact and after contact with contaminated material.
C. Disinfect and handle wastes and contaminated materials properly.
D. Prevent transmission of infectious droplets.
   1. Teach patients to cover mouth and nose when sneezing or coughing.
   2. Place contaminated tissues and articles in paper bag before disposing.
E. Institute proper isolation techniques as required by specific disease (see Isolation Procedures, page 90).
F. Use surgical aseptic technique when appropriate: caring for open wounds, irrigating or entering sterile cavities.

PAIN

Pain is an unpleasant sensation, entirely subjective, that produces discomfort, distress or suffering.

Gate Control Theory

A. Substantia gelatinosa in the dorsal horn of the spinal cord acts as a gate mechanism that can close to keep impulses from reaching the brain, or can open to allow pain impulses to ascend to the brain.
B. Most pain impulses are conducted over small-diameter fibers; if predominant nerve message is pain, the gate opens and allows pain impulses to reach the brain.
C. The gate can be closed by conflicting impulses from the skin conducted over large-diameter fibers, by impulses from the reticular formation in the brainstem, or by impulses from the entire cerebral cortex or thalamus.

Assessment of Pain

See Table 2.4.

General Nursing Interventions

A. Assess pain and evaluate response to interventions.
B. Promote rest and relaxation.
  1. Prevent fatigue.
  2. Teach relaxation techniques.
C. Institute comfort measures.
  1. Positioning: support body parts.
  2. Decrease noxious stimuli such as noise or bright lights.
D. Provide cutaneous stimulation: massage, pressure, baths, vibration, heat, cold packs; increased input of large-diameter fibers closes gate.
E. Relieve anxiety and fears.
  1. Spend time with patient.
  2. Offer reassurance, explanations.
F. Provide distraction and diversion.
G. Administer pain medication as needed.

Specific Medical and Surgical Therapies for Pain

Narcotic Analgesics

A. Examples: Brompton cocktail (a combination of a narcotic analgesic, a central nervous system [CNS] stimulant, alcohol, and an antiemetic), codeine sulfate, hydromorphone (Dilaudid), meperidine (Demerol), methadone (Dolophine), morphine sulfate, oxycodone (Percodan, Percocet), pentazocine (Talwin)
B. Mechanism of action: drug binds with opiate receptors at many sites in the CNS, altering both perception of and emotional response to pain.
C. Uses
  1. Relief of moderate to severe pain
  2. Pre-op medication to relieve anxiety and enhance effects of general anesthesia
D. Side effects
  1. CNS depression: depressed cough reflex, drowsiness, sedation, mood changes, respiratory depression
  2. Bradycardia, peripheral vasodilation, orthostatic hypotension
  3. Pupillary constriction
  4. Constipation, nausea and vomiting, dry mouth, biliary spasm
  5. Urinary retention
  6. Allergic reactions may include: pruritus, urticaria, rash.
E. Nursing interventions
  1. Assess patient's need for pain relief.
  2. Evaluate onset and duration of response to medication and record frequency of administration.
  3. Administer medication before pain becomes severe.
  4. Monitor for withdrawal symptoms and decrease dose slowly since these drugs may produce physical/psychologic dependence.
  5. Assess respiratory rate and depth before giving drug, and periodically thereafter.

Table 2.4 Pain Assessment

Influencing factors
- Past experience
- Age (tolerance generally increases with age)
- Culture and religious beliefs
- Level of anxiety
- Physical state (fatigue or chronic illness may decrease tolerance)

Characteristics of pain
- Location
- Quality
- Intensity
- Timing and duration
- Precipitating factors
- Aggravating factors
- Alleviating factors
- Interference with activities
- Patterns of response

---

  6. Encourage sighing, coughing and deep breathing.
  7. Warn ambulatory patients to avoid activities that require alertness.
  8. Advise patients to change position slowly.
  9. Observe for signs of urinary retention.
  10. Keep stool record and institute nursing measures to prevent constipation.
  11. Have narcotic antagonist (naloxone [Narcan]) available for reversal of effects if necessary.
  12. Use special caution with patients with increased intracranial pressure, chronic obstructive pulmonary disease (COPD), alcoholism, severe hepatic or renal disease, and in elderly or debilitated patients who may not metabolize the drug efficiently.

Non-narcotic Analgesics

A. Salicylates
  1. Example: acetylsalicylic acid (ASA, aspirin [Ecotrin])
  2. Mechanism of action
    a. Analgesic action: blocks prostaglandin synthesis.
    b. Antipyretic action: acts on hypothalamus promoting vasodilation, sweating, and heat loss.
    c. Anti-inflammatory action
  3. Uses
    a. Relief of mild to moderate pain
    b. Reduction of elevated body temperature
    c. Symptomatic treatment of numerous inflammatory disorders
  4. Side effects
    a. Allergic reaction: varies from rash to anaphylaxis
    b. Anemia, decreased platelet aggregation, prolonged bleeding time
    c. Nausea, vomiting, gastritis, occult GI bleeding
    d. Toxicity: tinnitus, visual changes, alterations in mental status
  5. Nursing interventions
    a. Give with food, milk, antacid or large glass of water to decrease GI irritation.

b. Check auditory and visual status periodically.

c. Instruct patient to watch for any signs of bleeding.

B. Para-aminophenol derivatives

1. Examples: acetaminophen (Datril, Tylenol)

2. Mechanism of action: elevates pain threshold.

3. Uses

a. Relief of mild to moderate pain

b. Reduction of elevated temperature

c. These drugs do *not* have any anti-inflammatory effect.

4. Side effects

a. Rash, urticaria

b. Hepatic toxicity: anorexia, nausea and vomiting, epigastric pain; progressing to encephalopathy, coma, and death

c. Allergic reaction: laryngeal edema and anaphylaxis, thrombocytopenic purpura

5. Nursing interventions

a. Advise patients that high doses or unsupervised chronic use can cause hepatic damage.

C. Nonsteroidal anti-inflammatory drugs (NSAIDs)

1. Examples: ibuprofen (Motrin, Advil, Nuprin), fenoprofen (Nalfon), naproxen (Naprosyn), sulindac (Clinoril), tolmetin (Tolectin)

2. Mechanism of action: not completely established but these drugs apparently block synthesis and possible release of prostaglandins

3. Uses

a. Relief of symptoms of rheumatoid arthritis, osteoarthritis

b. Relief of mild to moderate pain

4. Side effects

a. GI upset, nausea, vomiting, diarrhea, bloating, peptic ulceration

b. Allergic reactions: pruritus, skin rash, urticaria

c. Drowsiness, nervousness, insomnia

d. Blurred vision, diplopia, decreased hearing

e. Palpitations, tachycardia, edema

5. Nursing interventions

a. Administer with food or milk to prevent GI upset.

b. Teach patient to recognize and report signs of GI bleeding.

c. Caution patient that drowsiness and dizziness may occur and may impair ability to perform mechanical tasks.

Electrical Stimulation Techniques for Pain Control

A. *Transcutaneous electrical nerve stimulator (TENS)*

1. Noninvasive alternative to traditional methods of pain relief

2. Used in treating acute pain (e.g., post-op pain) and chronic pain (e.g., chronic low back pain)

3. Consists of impulse generator connected by wires to electrodes on skin; transmits electrical impulses to skin.

4. Mechanism based on gate-control theory: electrical impulse stimulates large diameter nerve fibers to "close the gate."

5. Nursing responsibilities

a. Do not place electrodes over incision site, broken skin, carotid sinus, eyes, laryngeal or pharyngeal muscles.

b. Do not use in patient with cardiac pacemaker.

c. Provide skin care.

1) remove electrodes once a day; wash area with soap and water and air dry.

2) wipe area with skin prep pad before reapplying electrode.

3) assess area for signs of redness; reposition electrodes if redness persists for more than 30 minutes.

B. *Dorsal column stimulator*

1. Used in selected patients for whom conventional methods of pain relief have not been effective

2. Electrode is surgically placed over the dorsal column of the spinal cord via laminectomy; connected by wires to a transmitter that may be worn externally or be implanted subcutaneously.

Neurosurgical Procedures for Pain Control

A. Performed for persistent intractable pain of high intensity

B. Involves surgical destruction of nerve pathways to block transmission of pain

C. Types

1. *Neurectomy:* interruption of cranial or peripheral nerves by incision or injection

2. *Rhizotomy:* interruption of posterior nerve root close to the spinal cord

a. Laminectomy is necessary.

b. Results in permanent loss of sensation and position sense in affected parts.

3. *Chordotomy:* interruption of pain-conducting pathways within the spinal cord

a. Laminectomy usually required.

b. May be done by percutaneous needle insertion.

c. Interrupts conduction of pain and temperature sense in affected parts.

4. *Sympathectomy:* interruption of afferent pathways in the sympathetic division of the autonomic nervous system; used to control pain from causalgia and peripheral vascular disease.

D. Nursing responsibilities

1. Provide pre- and post-op care for a laminectomy (see page 160).

2. Assess extremities for sensation (e.g., touch, pain, temperature, pressure, position sense) and movement.

3. Provide safety measures to protect patient from injury and carefully monitor skin for signs of damage or pressure.

4. Teach patient ways to compensate for loss of sensation in affected parts.

a. Visually inspect skin for signs of injury or pressure.

b. Check temperature of bath water.

c. Avoid use of hot water bottles, heating pads.

d. Avoid extremes of temperature.

Table 2.5   Physical Changes of Aging

System	Physical Change	Nursing Interventions
Special Senses *Sight*	Diminished visual acuity Reduction in visual fields Reduced accommodation to light changes Major eye problems: presbyopia (difficulty seeing clearly at close range); cataracts, glaucoma, retinal detachment, senile macular degeneration	Provide increased illumination without glare. Provide safe environment by orienting patient to surroundings and removing potential hazards.
Hearing	Decreased hearing acuity Presbycusis: hearing impairment especially in higher frequencies	Look directly at person when speaking and speak clearly. Prevent withdrawal and isolation by providing alternative forms of stimulation.
Taste/Smell	Decrease in sense of smell and number of taste buds	Provide attractive meals in comfortable social setting. Vary taste, textures, and colors of food.
Nervous	Progressive loss of number of neurons in brain and spinal cord Loss of total bulk of brain substance Slowed speed of nerve impulse and conduction Decreased blood flow to brain Behavioral changes: diminished emotional responses; lessened adaptability; decreased short-term memory; narrowed interests; confusion/disorientation	Promote independence in daily activities. Allow ample time for completion of tasks. Maintain social functioning by providing recreational and diversional activities. Prevent translocation shock, minimizing frequency of transfers. Orient to reality to prevent and treat confusion/disorientation.
Integumentary	Skin: thinning, wrinkling, loss of elasticity, dryness Decreased perspiration Increased sensitivity to cold Hair: loss of pigment (greying), thinning	Observe and assess the skin frequently. Protect the skin against trauma. Avoid overexposure to sun. Maintain adequate hydration. Keep skin clean, dry, lubricated, and pressure free. Provide adequate humidity in environment.
Musculoskeletal	Atrophy of muscles with decreased strength, endurance, and agility Bones more porous and lighter through calcium loss; falls are dangerous Enlarged, stiff joints Stooped posture	Encourage exercise program to help minimize age-related changes. Promote optimum physical activity within level of ability. Maintain optimum nutrition, especially intake of protein, calcium, and vitamins. Encourage use of appropriate adaptive or assistive devices to enhance mobility.
Cardiovascular	Decreased cardiac output Decreased endurance Arteriosclerosis, edema Increased systolic blood pressure	Assess symptoms and make appropriate modifications in care. Minimize edema and fatigue with rest periods and elevation of legs. Teach energy conservation methods in daily activities.
Respiratory	Impaired ventilation and diffusion Reduced vital capacity Reduced cough Impaired pulmonary circulation Diminished lung capacity	Manipulate environment to enhance ventilation. Position to promote optimum ventilation. Maintain tone and efficiency of respiratory muscles by encouraging exercises and prescribed pulmonary exercises.
Gastrointestinal	Reduced gastric motility and impaired absorption Diminished food appeal Reduced peristalsis and decreased excretory efficiency Constipation common problem	Assess condition of teeth and mouth, fit and comfort of dentures, and ability to chew. Encourage fluids and foods high in bulk and fiber. Encourage optimal activity. Promote independence and provide privacy in use of bathroom. Keep stool record and observe for constipation.
Urinary	Decreased kidney function. Common problems: frequency, dysuria, incontinence	Assess voiding patterns. Provide adequate fluids. Encourage independence in use of bathroom. Establish voiding schedule or bladder program as needed to control incontinence (assist to bathroom or offer bedpan every 2–3 hours). Avoid catheterization unless no other alternative.

Table 2.5   Physical Changes of Aging (continued)

System	Physical Change	Nursing Interventions
Reproductive *Female*	Atrophy and drying of vaginal canal	Promote good perineal care, treat with prescribed creams.
Male	Impaired ability to achieve full penile erection; reduced frequency of ejaculation	Provide encouragement and discuss modifications in sexual expression as necessary; rest before and after sexual activity.

Acupuncture

A. A Chinese technique of pain control by insertion of fine needles at various points on the body
B. Based on Eastern philosophy where insertion of needles is thought to block energy flow and restore the body's harmony
C. Mechanism of action: two theories
   1. Trigger points: the needles stimulate hypersensitive areas in muscle that produce local and referred pain. Extinction of the trigger point alleviates the referred pain.
   2. Endorphin system: needle insertion activates production of endorphins (body's natural opiates).
D. Acupressure: a less invasive variation; uses finger pressure and massage

Hypnosis

A. Has been used in dental procedures, labor and delivery, pain control in cancer.
B. Mechanism is thought to be that positive suggestions alter patient's perception of pain.

Behavioral Techniques

A. Types
   1. *Operant conditioning:* based on decreasing positive reinforcement for pain behaviors
   2. *Biofeedback:* teaches patients to control physiologic responses to pain (e.g., muscle tension, heart rate, blood pressure) and to replace them with a state of relaxation.
B. Work best in conjunction with other types of pain management and stress reduction techniques.

AGING

General Information

Aging is a normal process that occurs throughout the life span, causing a progressive decrease in functional capabilities. The elderly client is generally regarded as one who is 65 years of age or older.

Physical Changes of Aging

See Table 2.5.

Psychosocial Changes in the Elderly

A. Aging process is not just physical; psychologic and social factors play a crucial role.

B. Developmental tasks of the elderly
   1. Ego integrity vs despair (Erikson)
      a. Ego integrity results when the individual accepts own life as having been meaningful and appropriate.
      b. Despair results from the lack of ego integration and the feeling that time is too short to start another life and to find new means toward integrity.
   2. Other developmental tasks
      a. Successfully adjusting to retirement
      b. Making satisfactory living arrangements
      c. Adjusting to reduced income
      d. Keeping socially active
      e. Maintaining contact with friends and family members
      f. Adjusting to death of spouse
      g. Viewing own death as an appropriate outcome of life

Psychologic/Social Theories of Aging

A. Disengagement theory
   1. Aging is an inevitable mutual withdrawal or disengagement of the aging person and society from each other.
   2. The number of interrelationships with others is reduced, those remaining are altered in quality.
B. Activity theory
   1. The relationship between society and the aging individual remains fairly stable as the person passes from middle age to old age.
   2. If roles are relinquished (e.g., retirement from job) the person will substitute new roles.
C. Developmental or continuity theory
   1. As a person grows older, he or she is likely to maintain continuity in habits, preferences, commitments, etc., that are a part of personality.
   2. Because these factors are very complex and individualized, this theory implies that there are many possible adaptations to aging.

Nursing Interventions

A. Encourage effective communication and social interactions with others.
B. Promote activities that increase feelings of self-worth and self-esteem.
C. Allow for expression of feelings (e.g., loneliness, loss, grief) and provide support.

D. Provide opportunity for life review; assist individual in resolving conflicts of a lifetime in preparation for death.

FLUIDS AND ELECTROLYTES

Basic Principles

Fluids

A. Water constitutes over 50% of individual's weight; largest single component.

B. Body water divided into two compartments
   1. Intracellular: within cells
   2. Extracellular: outside cells, further divided into interstitial and intravascular fluid
C. Fluids in two compartments move among cells, tissue spaces, and plasma

Electrolytes

A. Salts or minerals in extracellular or intracellular body fluids
B. If positively charged called *cations*, if negatively charged called *anions*

Table 2.6   Fluid and Electrolyte Imbalances

Imbalance	Causes	Assessment Findings	Nursing Interventions
Hypovolemia (extracellular fluid volume deficit)	Hemorrhage, diarrhea, vomiting, kidney disease, diaphoresis, burns, fever, draining fistulas, sequestration of fluids (peritonitis, edema associated with burns)	Nausea and vomiting, weakness, weight loss, anorexia, longitudinal wrinkles of the tongue, dry skin and mucous membranes, decreased fullness of neck veins, postural hypotension, oliguria to anuria, shock	Measure I&O. Weight daily. Monitor closely and regulate isotonic IV infusion. Monitor blood pressure (determine lying down, sitting, and standing). Report urine output less than 30 cc/hr. Carefully assess skin and mucous membranes. Monitor for signs of shock.
Hypervolemia (extracellular fluid volume excess)	Excess or too rapid administration of any isotonic solution; side effect of corticosteroid administration; cardiac, liver, or renal disease; cerebral damage; stress	Weight gain, pitting edema, dyspnea, cough, diaphoresis, frothy or pink-tinged sputum, edema of the eyelids, distended neck veins, elevated blood pressure, moist rales	Weigh daily. Measure I&O. Regulate IV fluids/administration of diuretics strictly and monitor carefully. Monitor abdominal girth. Assess for pitting edema. Restrict sodium and water intake.
Water excess syndromes	Excessive intake of water, inability to excrete water due to kidney or brain damage, excessive administration of electrolyte-free solutions, poor salt intake, use of diuretics, irrigation of nasogastric tube with plain water, administration of excessive amount of ice chips to a vomiting patient or one with a nasogastric tube	Polyuria (in absence of renal disease), oliguria (with renal disease), twitching, hyperirritability, disorientation, coma, convulsions, abdominal cramps	Measure I&O. Weigh daily. Restrict oral and IV intake. Replace fluid losses with isotonic solutions. Use normal saline solution for nasogastric tube irrigation.
Water deficit syndromes	Increased water output due to watery diarrhea, diabetic acidosis, excess TPN; dysphagia; impaired thirst mechanism; coma; general debility; diaphoresis; excess protein intake without sufficient water intake	Thirst, poor skin turgor, dry skin and mucous membranes, dry furrowed tongue, sunken eyeballs, weight loss, elevated temperature, apprehension, oliguria to anuria	Measure I&O. Weigh daily. Assess skin frequently. Assure that patients with a high solute intake receive adequate water. Assess vital signs frequently, particularly temperature. Monitor TPN infusions accurately.
Hyperkalemia	Renal insufficiency, adrenocortical insufficiency, cellulose damage (burns), infection, acidotic states, rapid infusion of IV solutions with potassium, overzealous administration of potassium-conserving diuretics	Thready, slow pulse; shallow breathing; nausea and vomiting; diarrhea; intestinal colic, irritability; muscle weakness, numbness, flaccid paralysis; tingling; difficulty with phonation, respiration	Administer Kayexalate as ordered. Administer/monitor IV infusion of glucose and insulin. Control infection. Provide adequate calories and carbohydrates. Discontinue IV or oral sources of potassium.

(continued)

C. Common electrolytes
  1. Sodium (Na)
  2. Potassium (K)
  3. Calcium (Ca)
  4. Magnesium (Mg)
  5. Chloride (Cl)

Movement of Fluids and Electrolytes

A. Diffusion: movement of particles from an area of greater concentration to an area of lesser concentration as part of random activity

B. Active transport: movement across cell membranes requiring energy from an outside source

C. Osmosis: movement of water through a semipermeable membrane

Fluid and Electrolyte Imbalances

See Table 2.6.

A. *Hypovolemia:* extracellular fluid volume deficit

B. *Hypervolemia:* extracellular fluid volume excess

C. *Water excess:* hypo-osmolar imbalances; water intoxication or solute deficit

Table 2.6 Fluid and Electrolyte Imbalances (continued)

Imbalance	Causes	Assessment Findings	Nursing Interventions
Hypokalemia	Anorexia, alcoholism, gastric and intestinal suction, GI surgery, vomiting, diarrhea, laxative abuse, thiazide diuretics, steroid therapy, stress, alkalotic states	Thready, rapid, weak pulse; faint heart sounds; decreased blood pressure; skeletal muscle weakness; decreased or absent reflexes; shallow respirations; malaise; apathy; lethargy; loss of orientation; anorexia, vomiting, weight loss, gaseous intestinal distention	Be especially cautious if administering drugs that are not potassium sparing. Administer potassium supplements to replace losses. Monitor acid-base balance. Monitor pulse, blood pressure, and ECG.
Hypernatremia	Excessive/rapid IV administration of normal saline solution, inadequate water intake, kidney disease	Dry, sticky mucous membranes; flushed skin; rough, dry tongue; firm skin turgor; intense thirst; edema; oliguria to anuria	Weigh daily. Assess degree of edema frequently. Measure I&O. Assess skin frequently and institute nursing measures to prevent breakdown. Encourage sodium-restricted diet.
Hyponatremia	Decreased sodium intake, increased sodium excretion through diaphoresis or GI suctioning, adrenal insufficiency.	Nausea and vomiting; abdominal cramps; weight loss; cold, clammy skin; decreased skin turgor; fingerprinting over the sternum; shrunken tongue; apprehension; headache; convulsions; weakness; fatigue; postural hypotension; rapid, thready pulse	Provide foods high in sodium. Administer normal saline solution IV. Assess blood pressure frequently (measure lying down, sitting, and standing).
Hypercalcemia	Hyperparathyroidism, immobility, increased vitamin D intake, osteoporosis and osteomalacia (early stages)	Nausea and vomiting, anorexia, constipation, headache, confusion, lethargy, stupor, decreased muscle tone, deep bone and/or flank pain	Encourage mobilization. Limit vitamin D and calcium intake. Administer diuretics. Protect from injury.
Hypocalcemia	Acute pancreatitis, diarrhea, hypoparathyroidism, lack of vitamin D in diet, long-term steroid therapy	Painful tonic muscle spasms, facial spasms, fatigue, laryngospasm, positive Trousseau's and Chvostek's signs, convulsions, dyspnea	Administer oral calcium lactate or IV calcium chloride or gluconate. Provide safety by padding side rails. Administer dietary sources of calcium. Provide quiet environment.
Hypermagnesemia	Renal insufficiency, dehydration, excessive use of magnesium-containing antacids or laxatives	Lethargy, somnolence, confusion, nausea and vomiting, muscle weakness, depressed reflexes, decreased pulse and respirations	Withhold magnesium-containing drugs/foods. Increase fluid intake (unless contraindicated).
Hypomagnesemia	Low intake of magnesium in diet, prolonged diarrhea, massive diuresis, hypoparathyroidism	Paresthesias, confusion, hallucinations, convulsions, ataxia, tremors, hyperactive deep reflexes, muscle spasm, flushing of the face, diaphoresis	Provide good dietary sources of magnesium.

D. *Water deficit:* hyperosmolar imbalances; water depletion or solute excess

E. *Hyperkalemia:* potassium excess, serum potassium above 5.5 mEq/liter

F. *Hypokalemia:* potassium deficit, serum potassium below 3 mEq/liter

G. *Hypernatremia:* sodium excess, serum sodium level above 145 mEq/liter

H. *Hyponatremia:* sodium deficit, serum sodium level below 135 mEq/liter

I. *Hypercalcemia:* calcium excess, serum calcium level above 5.8 mEq/liter

J. *Hypocalcemia:* calcium deficit, serum calcium level below 4.5 mEq/liter

K. *Hypermagnesemia:* magnesium excess, serum magnesium level above 3 mEq/liter

L. *Hypomagnesemia:* magnesium deficit, serum magnesium level below 1.5 mEq/liter

ACID-BASE BALANCE

Basic Principles

A. Normal pH of the body is 7.35–7.45.

B. Buffer or control systems maintain normal pH. Kidneys excrete acids and reabsorb bicarbonate while the respiratory system gives off carbon dioxide in acidic states. In alkalotic states, the kidneys excrete bicarbonate and the respiratory system retains carbonic acid.

Acid-base Imbalances

See Table 2.7.

A. *Metabolic acidosis:* a primary deficit in the concentration of base bicarbonate in the extracellular fluid; decreased pH and bicarbonate, decreased pCO_2 (if lung compensation)

B. *Metabolic alkalosis:* a primary excess of base bicarbonate in the extracellular fluid; elevated pH and bicarbonate, elevated pCO_2 (if lung compensation)

C. *Respiratory acidosis:* a primary excess of carbonic acid in the extracellular fluid; decreased pH, elevated pCO_2 and bicarbonate (if renal compensation)

D. *Respiratory alkalosis:* a primary deficit of carbonic acid in the extracellular fluid; elevated pH, decreased pCO_2 and bicarbonate (if renal compensation)

INTRAVENOUS THERAPY

Purposes

A. Maintenance of fluid and electrolyte balance

Table 2.7   Acid-base Imbalances

Imbalance	Causes	Assessment Findings	Nursing Interventions
Metabolic acidosis	Diabetic ketoacidosis, uremia, starvation, diarrhea, severe infections, renal tubular acidosis	Headache, nausea and vomiting, weakness, lethargy, disorientation, tremors, convulsions, coma	Administer sodium bicarbonate as ordered and monitor for signs of excess. Monitor for signs of hyperkalemia. Provide alkaline mouthwash (baking soda and water) to neutralize acids. Lubricate lips to prevent dryness from hyperventilation. Measure I&O. Institute seizure precautions. Monitor arterial blood gases and electrolytes.
Metabolic alkalosis	Severe vomiting, nasogastric suctioning, diuretic therapy, excessive ingestion of sodium bicarbonate, biliary drainage	Nausea and vomiting, diarrhea, numbness and tingling of extremities, tetany, bradycardia, decreased respirations	Replace fluid and electrolyte losses (potassium and chloride). Institute seizure precautions. Measure I&O. Assess for signs of hypokalemia. Monitor arterial blood gases and electrolytes.
Respiratory acidosis	COPD, barbiturate or sedative overdose, acute airway obstruction, weakness of respiratory muscles, Guillain-Barré syndrome	Headache, weakness, visual disturbances, rapid respirations, confusion, drowsiness, tachycardia, coma	Position in semi-Fowler's. Maintain patent airway. Turn, cough, and deep breathe. Perform postural drainage. Administer fluids to help liquefy secretions (unless contraindicated). Administer low-concentration oxygen therapy. Monitor arterial blood gases and electrolytes. Administer prophylactic antibiotics as ordered.
Respiratory alkalosis	Hyperventilation, mechanical overventilation, encephalitis	Numbness and tingling of mouth and extremities, inability to concentrate, rapid respirations, dry mouth, coma	Offer reassurance. Encourage breathing into a paper bag or voluntary breath holding. Ensure adequate rest. Provide sedation as ordered. Monitor mechanical ventilation, arterial blood gases, and electrolytes.

B. Replacement of fluid and electrolyte loss

C. Provision of nutrients

D. Provision of a route for medications

Nursing Interventions

A. Select correct solution after checking physician's order.

B. Note clarity of solution.

C. Calculate flow rate (Intravenous Calculations, Appendix 2).

D. Assess infusion rate and site at least hourly.

E. Use infusion pump if administering medications (e.g., aminophylline, heparin, insulin).

F. Maintain I&O record.

G. Provide tubing change and IV site care or IV site change as directed: Current research recommends IV site and tubing change every 72 hours.

H. Discontinue IV if complications occur.

Complications of Intravenous Therapy

See Table 2.8.

Central Lines

Uses

A. Administration of TPN

B. Measurement of central venous pressure (CVP)

C. IV therapy when suitable peripheral veins are not available

D. Long-term antibiotic therapy

E. Chemotherapy

Types

A. Subclavian catheter

B. Multilumen catheter: has more than one lumen for simultaneous infusion of more than one solution

C. Hickman or Broviac catheters

   1. Long silicone rubber catheter tunneled under the skin to prevent infection with long-term use

   2. Inserted in cephalic vein and threaded into right atrium

D. Implanted port: totally internal device consists of subcutaneous self-sealing injection port and a silicone catheter placed in selected body site (e.g., venous, arterial, peritoneal) for long-term access

Care of the Patient with a Central Venous Line

A. Institute nursing measures to prevent infection (particularly important with TPN since high concentration of glucose encourages growth of bacteria).

   1. Change dressings

     a. Usually 3 times/week and as needed (e.g., when loose or wet) but agency policies may vary

     b. Use sterile technique and apply sterile occlusive dressing.

   2. Monitor for signs of infection: redness, drainage, odor at site, or elevated temperature.

   3. Do not piggyback anything into a TPN infusion line except intralipids.

Table 2.8	Complications of IV Therapy
Complication	**Manifestation**
Infiltration	Edema, pain, coldness at site; decreased infusion rate.
Phlebitis	Pain along course of vein, redness and swelling at site.
Pyrogenic reaction	Pain, redness, edema at site; fever, chills, general malaise.
Air embolism	Cyanosis, hypotension, tachycardia, rise in venous pressure, unconsciousness.
Circulatory overload	Shortness of breath, coughing, frothy sputum, rales, engorged neck veins, increased blood pressure.

B. Monitor for infiltration: check for swelling of neck, face, and shoulder, and pain in upper arm.

C. Prevent catheter occlusion.

   1. Keep infusion continuous.

   2. Use infusion pump.

   3. Check for kinks in tubing.

D. Prevent air embolism.

   1. Tighten and tape all tubing connections to prevent accidental disconnection of tubing.

   2. When changing or detaching tubing, instruct patient to perform Valsalva maneuver.

   3. Check tubing for cracks or perforations.

E. Maintain proper infusion rate.

   1. Monitor rate closely to prevent clotting, fluid depletion, or fluid overload.

   2. Never attempt to speed up or slow down infusion.

F. With a multilumen catheter, flush ports not being used to prevent clotting (per agency's protocol).

G. With Hickman/Broviac catheters and implanted port provide other specific care according to agency protocol.

H. If clotting occurs, try to aspirate or add a declotting agent (e.g., streptokinase) according to agency protocol. Do not irrigate.

Blood Transfusions

See page 89.

SHOCK

An abnormal physiologic state where an imbalance between the amount of circulating blood volume and the size of the vascular bed results in circulatory failure and oxygen and nutrient deprivation of tissues. See Table 2.9 for classification of shock.

Body's Response to Shock

A. Hyperventilation leading to respiratory alkalosis

B. Vasoconstriction: shunts blood to heart and brain

C. Tachycardia

D. Fluid shifts: intracellular to extracellular shift to maintain circulating blood volume

Table 2.9   Classification of Shock

Type	Characteristics	Causes
Hypovolemic	Decreased circulating blood volume	Blood loss. Plasma loss (e.g., burns). Fluid loss (e.g., excessive vomiting or diarrhea)
Cardiogenic	Failure of the heart to pump properly	Myocardial infarction Congestive heart failure Cardia arrythmias Pericardial tamponade Tension pneumothorax
Septic	Factors favoring septic shock ▪ development of antibiotic resistant organisms ▪ invasive procedures such as urinary tract instrumentation ▪ immunosuppression and old age ▪ trauma: presence of blood in peritoneal cavity greatly increases likelihood of peritonitis	Release of bacterial toxins that act directly on the blood vessels producing massive vasodilation and pooling of blood; results most frequently from gram-negative septicemia.
Neurogenic	Failure of arteriolar resistance, leading to massive vasodilation and pooling of blood.	Interruption of sympathetic impulses from ▪ exposure to unpleasant circumstances ▪ extreme pain ▪ spinal cord injury ▪ high spinal anesthesia ▪ vasomotor depression ▪ head injury
Anaphylactic	Massive vasodilation resulting from allergic reaction causing release of histamine and related substances	Allergic reaction to ▪ insect venom ▪ medications ▪ dyes used in radiologic studies

E. Impaired metabolism: tissue anoxia leads to anaerobic metabolism causing lactic acid buildup, resulting in metabolic acidosis

F. Impaired organ function
   1. Kidney: decreased perfusion can result in renal failure.
   2. Lung: shock lung (adult respiratory distress syndrome [ARDS])

Assessment Findings

A. Skin
   1. Cool, pale, moist in hypovolemic and cardiogenic shock
   2. Warm, dry, pink in septic and neurogenic shock

B. Pulse
   1. Tachycardia, due to increased sympathetic stimulation
   2. Weak and thready

C. Blood pressure
   1. Early stages: may be normal due to compensatory mechanisms
   2. Later stages: systolic and diastolic blood pressure drops.

D. Respirations: rapid and shallow, due to tissue anoxia and excessive amounts of CO_2 (from metabolic acidosis)

E. Level of consciousness: restlessness and apprehension, progressing to coma

F. Urinary output: decreases due to impaired renal perfusion

G. Temperature: decreases in severe shock (except septic shock).

Nursing Interventions

A. Maintain patent airway and adequate ventilation.
   1. Establish and maintain airway.
   2. Administer oxygen as ordered.
   3. Monitor respiratory status, blood gases.
   4. Start resuscitative procedures as necessary.

B. Promote restoration of blood volume: administer fluid and blood replacement as ordered.
   1. Electrolyte solutions (e.g., Ringer's lactate, normal saline)
   2. Blood/blood component therapy
      a. Whole blood
      b. Packed red blood cells
      c. Plasma expanders (e.g., fresh frozen plasma, albumin, dextran)

C. Administer drugs as ordered (see Table 2.10).

D. Minimize factors contributing to shock.
   1. Elevate lower extremities to 45° to promote venous return to heart, thereby improving cardiac output.
   2. Avoid Trendelenburg's position: increases respiratory impairment.
   3. Promote rest by using energy-conservation measures and maintaining as quiet an environment as possible.
   4. Relieve pain by cautious use of narcotics.
      a. Since narcotics interfere with vasoconstriction, give only if absolutely necessary, IV and in small doses.
      b. If given IM or subcutaneously, vasoconstriction may cause incomplete absorption; when circulation improves, patient may get overdose.
   5. Keep patient warm.

E. Maintain continuous assessment of the patient.
   1. Check vital signs frequently.

2. Monitor urine output: report urine output of less than 30 cc/hour.
3. Observe color and temperature of skin.
4. Monitor CVP.
5. Monitor ECG.
6. Check lab studies: CBC, electrolytes, BUN, creatinine, blood gases.
7. Monitor other parameters such as arterial blood pressures, cardiac output, pulmonary artery pressures, pulmonary artery wedge pressures.
F. Provide psychologic support: reassure patient to relieve apprehension and keep family advised.

MULTIPLE TRAUMA

Assessment and Emergency Care

Airway

A. Assess, establish, and maintain an adequate airway.
1. Do not hyperextend the neck in a patient with suspected cervical spine injury.
2. Use jaw thrust instead.
B. Administer artificial resuscitation if necessary.
C. Observe for chest trauma such as open sucking wounds or flail chest (see Chest Trauma, page 107)

Table 2.10 Drugs Used to Treat Shock

Generic (Trade) Name	Action
Dopamine (Intropin)	Stimulates myocardial contractility; increases urine output by dilating the renal vascular bed.
Dobutamine (Dobutrex)	Similar to dopamine; increases myocardial contractility without marked increase in heart rate.
Isoproterenol (Isuprel)	Increases cardiac output and reduces peripheral resistance; usefulness is limited by the tachycardia it produces.
Sodium nitroprusside (Nipride)	Decreases peripheral resistance and workload of heart, thereby increasing cardiac output; used in cardiogenic shock and hypertensive emergencies.
Norepinephrine (Levophed)	Sympathomimetic; produces vasoconstriction in all vascular beds and improves cardiac contractility.
Digitalis preparations	Improve cardiac performance.
Corticosteroids	Used especially in septic shock; help to protect cell membranes and decrease the inflammatory response to stress.
Antibiotics	Used in treating infectious processes related to septic shock.

NOTE: Vasopressors such as Levophed can cause almost complete occlusion of arterioles, causing a decrease of blood flow to larger tissue areas. Therefore, if blood pressure is adequate, a vasodilator such as Nipride could probably be given as well, to modify the vasoconstrictor effects.

D. Administer oxygen at 5 liters/minute unless patient has history of COPD.
E. Draw blood samples for ABGs.

Hemorrhage and Shock

A. Deep wounds with pulsating blood flow
1. Apply firm pressure over the wound with a sterile dressing.
2. If wound is on a limb, elevate the extremity.
3. Apply pressure with three fingers over appropriate pressure point.
4. Once bleeding is controlled, apply a pressure dressing.
5. Tourniquets should be used only when all other methods have failed.
B. Venous bleeding: apply direct pressure to bleeding site.
C. Never remove any foreign object, such as a knife, from the patient; immobilize the object with packing.
D. Assess for and treat shock (see Shock, page 27).
E. Administer tetanus booster as ordered.

Neurologic Injuries

A. Inspect the scalp, head, face, and neck for abrasions, hematomas, and lacerations.
B. Gently palpate the head for any injuries.
C. Inspect the nose and ears for leakage of cerebrospinal fluid.
D. Assess the level of consciousness.
E. Evaluate pupillary size, shape, equality, and reaction to light.
F. Assess for sensation and motor abilities.
G. Observe for signs of increased intracranial pressure (see page 48).
H. For additional details of care see Head Injury and Spinal Cord Injury, pages 56 and 57.

Abdominal Injuries

A. Keep patient NPO.
B. Assist with insertion of nasogastric tube (for assessment of stomach bleeding and aspiration of stomach contents which prevents vomiting).
C. Inspect abdomen for injuries.
D. Auscultate bowel sounds.
E. Do not palpate the abdomen (could aggravate possible internal injuries).
F. Prepare patient for peritoneal lavage if indicated.
G. Insert Foley catheter.
1. Measure urine output every 15 minutes.
2. Assess for hematuria.

Musculoskeletal Injuries

A. Observe for signs of fracture: pain, swelling, tenderness, ecchymosis, crepitation, loss of function, exposed bone fragments.
B. Cover open fracture with sterile dressing to prevent infection.
C. Immobilize any suspected fractures by splinting.
D. Perform neurovascular check of area distal to fracture: assess for color, temperature, capillary refill, sensation, movement, pulses.

Perioperative Nursing

OVERVIEW

Effects of Surgery on the Patient

Physical Effects

A. Stress response (neuroendocrine response) is activated.
B. Resistance to infection is lowered due to surgical incision.
C. Vascular system is disturbed due to severing of blood vessels and blood loss.
D. Organ function may be altered due to manipulation.

Psychologic Effects

Common fears: pain, anesthesia, loss of control, disfigurement, separation from loved ones, alterations in roles or life-style

Factors Influencing Surgical Risk

A. *Age:* very young and elderly are at increased risk.
B. *Nutrition:* malnutrition and obesity increase risk of complications.
C. *Fluid and electrolyte balance:* dehydration, hypovolemia, and electrolyte imbalances can pose problems during surgery.
D. *General health status:* infection, cardiovascular disease, pulmonary problems, liver dysfunction, renal insufficiency, or metabolic disorders create increased risk.
E. *Medications*
  1. Anticoagulants: predispose to hemorrhage; discontinue before surgery.
  2. Tranquilizers (e.g., phenothiazines) may cause hypotension and potentiate shock.
  3. Antibiotics: aminoglycosides may intensify neuromuscular blockade of anesthesia with resultant respiratory paralysis.
  4. Diuretics: may cause electrolyte imbalances.
  5. Antihypertensives: can cause hypotension and contribute to shock.
  6. Long-term steroid therapy: causes adrenocortical suppression; may need increased dosage during perioperative period.
F. *Type of surgery planned:* major surgery (e.g., thoractomy) poses greater risk than minor surgery (e.g., dental extraction).
G. *Psychologic status of patient:* excessive fear or anxiety may have adverse effect on surgery.

PREOPERATIVE PERIOD

Psychologic Support

A. Assess patient's fears, anxieties, support systems, and patterns of coping.
B. Establish trusting relationship with patient and significant others.
C. Explain routine procedures, encourage verbalization of fears, and allow patient to ask questions.
D. Demonstrate confidence in surgeon and staff.
E. Provide for spiritual care if appropriate.

Preoperative Teaching

A. Assess patient's level of understanding of surgical procedure and its implications.
B. Answer questions, clarify and reinforce explanations given by surgeon.
C. Explain routine pre- and post-op procedures and any special equipment to be used.
D. Teach coughing and deep breathing exercises, splinting of incision, turning side to side in bed, and leg exercises; explain their importance in preventing complications; provide opportunity for return demonstration.
E. Assure patient that pain medication will be available post-op.

Physical Preparation

A. Obtain history of past medical conditions, surgical procedures, allergies, dietary restrictions, and medications.
B. Perform baseline head-to-toe assessment, including vital signs, height and weight.
C. Ensure that diagnostic procedures are performed as ordered: common tests are
  1. CBC
  2. Electrolytes
  3. PT/PTT
  4. Urinalysis
  5. ECG
  6. Type and crossmatch
D. Prepare patient's skin.
  1. Shower with antibacterial soap to cleanse skin.

2. Skin prep if ordered: shave and cleanse appropriate areas to reduce bacteria on skin and minimize chance of infection.

E. Administer enema if ordered (usually for surgery on GI tract, gynecologic surgery).

F. Promote adequate rest and sleep.
   1. Provide backrub, clean linens.
   2. Administer bedtime sedation.

G. Instruct patient to remain NPO after midnight to prevent vomiting and aspiration during surgery.

Legal Responsibilities

A. Surgeon obtains operative permit (*informed consent*).
   1. Surgical procedure, alternatives, possible complications, disfigurements or removal of body parts are explained.
   2. It is part of the nurse's role as patient advocate to confirm that the patient understands information given.

B. Informed consent is necessary for any invasive procedure.

C. Adult patient (over 18 years of age) signs own permit unless unconscious or mentally incompetent.
   1. If unable to sign, relative (spouse or next of kin) or guardian will sign.
   2. In an emergency, permission via telephone or telegram is acceptable.
   3. Consents are not needed for emergency care if all four of the following criteria are met.
      a. There is an immediate threat to life.
      b. Experts agree that it is an emergency.
      c. Patient is unable to consent.
      d. A legally authorized person cannot be reached.

D. Minors (under 18) must have consent signed by an adult (i.e., parent or legal guardian). An emancipated minor (married, parent of child, college student living away from home, in military service) may sign own consent.

E. Witness to informed consent may be nurse, another physician, clerk, or other authorized person.

F. If nurse witnesses informed consent, specify whether witnessing explanation of surgery or just signature of patient.

Preparation Immediately Before Surgery

A. Obtain baseline vital signs; report any elevated temperature.

B. Provide oral hygiene and remove dentures.

C. Remove patient's clothing and dress in clean gown.

D. Remove nail polish, cosmetics, hair pins, prostheses.

E. Instruct to empty bladder.

F. Check identification band.

G. Administer pre-op medications as ordered.
   1. Narcotic analgesics (meperidine [Demerol], morphine sulfate) relax patient, relieve anxiety, and enhance effectiveness of general anesthesia.
   2. Sedatives (secobarbital sodium [Seconal]), sodium pentobarbital [Nembutal] decrease anxiety and reduce amount of general anesthesia needed.
   3. Anticholinergics (atropine sulfate, scopolamine [Hyoscine]) decrease tracheobronchial secretions to minimize danger of aspirating secretions in lungs; decrease vagal response to inhibit undesirable effects of general anesthesia (bradycardia).

H. Elevate side rails and provide quiet environment.

I. Prepare patient's chart for OR including operative permit and complete pre-op check list.

INTRAOPERATIVE PERIOD

Anesthesia

General Anesthesia

A. General information
   1. Drug-induced depression of CNS; produces decreased muscle reflex activity and loss of consciousness.
   2. Balanced anesthesia: combination of several anesthetic drugs to provide smooth induction, appropriate depth and duration of anesthesia, sufficient muscle relaxation and minimal complications.

B. Stages of general anesthesia: induction, delirium, surgical anesthesia, and danger stage (see Table 2.11)

C. Agents for general anesthesia
   1. Inhalation agents
      a. Gas anesthetics
         1) nitrous oxide: induction agent; component of balanced anesthesia; used alone for short procedures; always given in combination with oxygen

Table 2.11   Stages of Anesthesia

Stage	From	To	Patient Status
Stage I (induction)	Beginning administration of anesthetic agent	Loss of consciousness	May appear euphoric, drowsy, dizzy.
Stage II (delirium or excitement)	Loss of consciousness	Relaxation	Breathing irregular; may appear excited; very susceptible to external stimuli.
Stage III (surgical anesthesia)	Relaxation	Loss of reflexes and depression of vital functions	Regular breathing pattern; corneal reflexes absent; pupillary constriction.
Stage IV (danger stage)	Vital functions depressed	Respiratory arrest; possible cardiac arrest	No respirations; absent or minimal heartbeat; dilated pupils

2) cyclopropane: obstetric anesthesia; patients with cardiovascular complications; highly flammable and explosive
  b. Liquid anesthetics
    1) halothane (Fluothane): widely used; rapid induction, low incidence of post-op nausea and vomiting; may cause bradycardia and hypotension; contraindicated in patients with liver disease.
    2) enflurane (Ethrane): effects similar to halothane, but muscle relaxation is stronger and hepatotoxicity not a problem; use cautiously in patients with cardiac disease.
    3) ether (diethyl ether): infrequently used because of slow, unpleasant induction, excessive secretory action, increased post-op nausea and vomiting, and flammability.
    4) methoxyflurane (Penthrane): very potent agent with slow onset and recovery; circulatory depression at high concentrations; associated with liver and kidney damage; rarely used.
  2. IV anesthetics: used primarily as induction agents; produce rapid, smooth induction; may be used alone in short procedures such as dental extractions.
    a. Common IV anesthetics: methohexital (Brevital), sodium thiopental (Pentathol)
    b. Disadvantages: poor relaxation; respiratory and myocardial depression in high doses; bronchospasm, laryngospasm; hypotension
  3. Dissociative agents: produce state of profound analgesia, amnesia, and lack of awareness without loss of consciousness; used alone in short surgical and diagnostic procedures or for induction prior to administration of more potent general anesthetics.
    a. Agent: ketamine (Ketalar)
    b. Side effects: tachycardia, hypertension, respiratory depression, hallucinations, delirium
    c. Precautions: decrease verbal, tactile, and visual stimulation during recovery period
  4. Neuroleptics: produce state of neuroleptic analgesia characterized by reduced motor activity, decreased anxiety, and analgesia without loss of consciousness; used alone for short surgical and diagnostic procedures, as premedication or in combination with other anesthetics for longer anesthesia.
    a. Agent: fentanyl citrate with droperidol (Innovar)
    b. Side effects: hypotension, bradycardia, respiratory depression, skeletal muscle rigidity, twitching
    c. Precautions: reduce narcotic doses by ½ to ⅓ for at least 8 hours postanesthesia as ordered to prevent respiratory depression.
D. Adjuncts to general anesthesia: neuromuscular blocking agents: used with general anesthetics to enhance skeletal muscle relaxation.
  1. Agents: gallamine (Flaxedil), pancuronium (Pavulon), succinylcholine (Anectine), tubocurarine, atracurium besylate (Tracrium), vecuronium bromide (Norcuron)

2. Precaution: monitor patient's respirations for at least 1 hour after drug's effect has worn off.

Regional Anesthesia

A. General information (see also Table 2.12)
  1. Produces loss of painful sensation in one area of the body; does not produce loss of consciousness.
  2. Uses: biopsies, excision of moles and cysts, endoscopies, surgery on extremities
  3. Agents: lidocaine (Xylocaine), procaine (Novocain), tetracaine (Pontocaine)

POSTOPERATIVE PERIOD

Postoperative Care

Recovery Room (Immediate Postoperative Care)

A. Assess for and maintain patent airway.
  1. Position unconscious or semiconscious patient on side (unless contraindicated) or on back with head to side and chin extended forward.
  2. Check for presence/absence of gag reflex.
  3. Maintain artificial airway in place until gag and swallow reflex have returned.
B. Administer oxygen as ordered.
C. Assess rate, depth, and quality of respirations.
D. Check vital signs every 15 minutes until stable, then every 30 minutes.
E. Note level of consciousness; reorient patient to time, place, and situation.

Table 2.12	Regional Anesthesia
Types	**Method**
Topical	Cream, spray, drops, or ointment applied externally, directly to area to be anesthetized.
Local infiltration block	Injected into subcutaneous tissue of surgical area.
Field block	Area surrounding the surgical site injected with anesthetic.
Nerve block	Injection into a nerve plexus to anesthetize part of body.
Spinal	Anesthetic introduced into subarachnoid space of spinal cord producing anesthesia below level of diaphragm.
Epidural	Anesthetic injected extradurally to produce anesthesia below level of diaphragm; used in obstetrics.
Caudal	Variation of epidural block: produces anesthesia of perineum and occasionally lower abdomen; commonly used in obstetrics.
Saddle block	Similar to spinal, but anesthetized area is more limited; commonly used in obstetrics.

F. Assess color and temperature of skin, color of nailbeds and lips.

G. Monitor IV infusions: condition of site, type, and amount of fluid being infused and flow rate.

H. Check all drainage tubes and connect to suction or gravity drainage as ordered; note color, amount, and odor of drainage.

I. Assess dressings for intactness, drainage, hemorrhage.

J. Monitor and maintain patient's temperature; may need extra blankets.

K. Encourage patient to cough and deep breathe after airway is removed.

L. If spinal anesthesia used, maintain supine position and check for sensation and movement in lower extremities.

Care on Surgical Floor

A. Monitor respiratory status and promote optimal functioning.
  1. Encourage patient to cough and deep breathe every 1–2 hours.
  2. Instruct patient to splint incision while coughing.
  3. Assist patient to turn in bed every 2 hours.
  4. Encourage early ambulation.
  5. Encourage use of incentive spirometer every 2 hours: causes sustained, maximal inspiration that inflates the alveoli.
  6. Assess respiratory status and auscultate lungs every 4 hours; be alert for any signs of respiratory complications.

B. Monitor cardiovascular status and avoid post-op complications.
  1. Encourage leg exercises every 2 hours while in bed.
  2. Encourage early ambulation.
  3. Apply antiembolism stockings as ordered.
  4. Assess vital signs, color and temperature of skin every 4 hours.

C. Promote adequate fluid and electrolyte balance.
  1. Monitor IV and ensure adequate intake.
  2. Measure I&O.
  3. Irrigate NG tube properly, using normal saline solution.
  4. Observe for signs of fluid and electrolyte imbalances.

D. Promote optimum nutrition.
  1. Maintain IV infusion as ordered.
  2. Assess for return of peristalsis (presence of bowel sounds and flatus).
  3. Add progressively to diet as ordered and note tolerance.

E. Monitor and promote return of urinary function.
  1. Measure I&O.
  2. Assess patient's ability to void.
  3. Report to surgeon if patient has not voided within 8 hours after surgery.
  4. Check for bladder distention.
  5. Use measures to promote urination (e.g., assist male to sit on side of bed; pour warm water over female's perineum).

F. Promote bowel elimination.
  1. Encourage ambulation.
  2. Provide adequate food and fluid intake when tolerated.
  3. Keep stool record and note any difficulties with bowel elimination.

G. Administer post-op analgesics as ordered; provide additional comfort measures.

H. Encourage optimal activity, turning in bed every 2 hours, early ambulation if allowed (generally patient will be out of bed within 24 hours; have patient dangle legs before getting out of bed)

I. Provide wound care.
  1. Check dressings frequently to ensure they are clean, dry, and intact.
  2. Observe aseptic technique when changing dressings.
  3. Encourage diet high in protein and vitamin C.
  4. Report any signs of infection: redness, drainage, odor, fever.

J. Provide adequate psychologic support to patient/family.

K. Provide appropriate discharge teaching: dietary restrictions, medication regimen, activity limitations, wound care, and possible complications.

Postoperative Complications

Respiratory System

Common post-op complications of respiratory tract are atelectasis and pneumonia (for additional information on these disorders see pages 109 and 110).

A. Predisposing factors
  1. Type of surgery (e.g., thoracic or high abdomen surgery)
  2. Previous history of respiratory problems
  3. Age: greater risk over age 40
  4. Obesity
  5. Smoking
  6. Respiratory depression caused by narcotics
  7. Severe post-op pain
  8. Prolonged post-op immobility

B. Prevention: see Care on Surgical Floor

Cardiovascular System

Common post-op complications of the cardiovascular system are deep vein thrombosis, pulmonary embolism, and shock (for additional information on these disorders see pages 82, 83, and 27).

A. Predisposing factors to deep vein thrombosis (DVT)
  1. Lower abdominal surgery or septic diseases (e.g., peritonitis)
  2. Injury to vein by tight leg straps during surgery
  3. Previous history of venous problems
  4. Increased blood coagulability due to dehydration, fluid loss
  5. Venous stasis in the extremity due to decreased movement during surgery
  6. Prolonged post-op immobilization

B. Predisposing factors to pulmonary embolism: may occur as a complication of DVT.

C. Most common causes of shock during post-op period
  1. Hemorrhage
  2. Sepsis
  3. Myocardial infarction and cardiac arrest
  4. Drug reactions
  5. Transfusion reactions

6. Pulmonary embolism
7. Adrenal failure

D. Prevention of DVT, pulmonary embolism, and shock: see Care on Surgical Floor

Genitourinary System

Post-op complications of the genitourinary system often include urinary retention and urinary tract infection (for additional information on these disorders see pages 141 and 143).

A. Predisposing factors to urinary retention include
   1. Anxiety
   2. Pain
   3. Lack of privacy
   4. Narcotics and certain anesthetics that diminish patient's sense of a full bladder
B. Prevention and nursing interventions for urinary retention: see Care on Surgical Floor, page 33
C. Post-op urinary tract infections are most commonly caused by catheterization; prevention consists of using strict sterile technique when inserting a catheter, and appropriate catheter care (every 8 hours or according to agency protocol).

Gastrointestinal System

An important GI post-op complication is paralytic ileus (paralysis of intestinal peristalsis).

A. Predisposing factors
   1. Temporary: anesthesia, manipulation of bowel during abdominal surgery
   2. Prolonged: electrolyte imbalance, wound infection, pneumonia
B. Assessment findings
   1. Absent bowel sounds
   2. No passage of flatus
   3. Abdominal distention
C. Nursing interventions
   1. Assist with insertion of nasogastric or intestinal tube with application of suction as ordered.
   2. Keep patient NPO.
   3. Maintain IV therapy as ordered.
   4. Assess for bowel sounds every 4 hours; check for abdominal distension, passage of flatus.
   5. Encourage ambulation if appropriate.

Wound Complications

A. Wound infection
   1. Predisposing factors
      a. Obesity
      b. Diabetes mellitus
      c. Malnutrition
      d. Elderly patients
      e. Steroids and immunosuppresive agents
      f. Lowered resistance to infection, as found in cancer patients

2. Assessment findings: redness, tenderness, drainage, heat in incisional area; fever
3. Prevention: see Care on Surgical Floor, page 33
4. Nursing interventions
   a. Obtain culture and sensitivity of wound drainage *(S. aureus* most frequently cultured).
   b. Perform cleansing and irrigation of wound as ordered.
   c. Administer antibiotic therapy as ordered.

B. Wound dehiscence and evisceration
   1. Dehiscence: opening of wound edges
   2. Evisceration: protrusion of loops of bowel through incision; usually accompanied by sudden escape of profuse, pink serous drainage
   3. Predisposing factors to wound dehiscence and evisceration
      a. Wound infection
      b. Faulty wound closure
      c. Severe abdominal stretching (e.g., coughing, retching)
   4. Nursing interventions for wound dehiscence
      a. Apply Steri-Strips to incision.
      b. Notify physician.
      c. Promote wound healing.
   5. Nursing interventions for wound evisceration
      a. Place patient in supine position.
      b. Cover protruding intestinal loops with moist normal saline soaks.
      c. Notify physician.
      d. Check vital signs.
      e. Observe for signs of shock.
      f. Start IV line.
      g. Prepare patient for OR for surgical closure of wound.

Cancer Nursing

PATHOPHYSIOLOGY AND ETIOLOGY OF CANCER

Evolution of Cancer Cells

A. All cells constantly change through growth, degeneration, repair, and adaptation. Normal cells must divide and multiply to meet the needs of the organism as a whole, and this cycle of cell growth and destruction is an integral part of life processes. The activities of the normal cells in the human body are all coordinated to meet the needs of the organism as a whole, but when the regulatory control mechanisms of normal cells fail, and growth continues in excess of the body's needs, neoplasia results.

B. The term neoplasia refers to both benign and malignant growths, but malignant cells behave very differently from normal cells and have special features characteristic of the cancer process.

C. Since the growth control mechanism of normal cells is not entirely understood, it is not clear what allows the uncontrolled growth, therefore no definitive cure has been found

Characteristics of Malignant Cells

Differentiation

A. Cancer cells are mutated stem cells that have undergone structural changes so that they are unable to perform the normal functions of specialized tissue (un- or dedifferentiation).

B. They may function in a disorderly way or cease normal function completely, only functioning for their own survival and growth.

C. The most undifferentiated cells are also called *anaplastic*.

Rate of Growth

A. Cancer cells have uncontrolled growth or cell division.

B. Rate at which a tumor grows involves both increased cell division and increased survival time of cells.

C. Malignant cells do not form orderly layers, but pile on top of each other, to eventually form tumors.

Spread (Invasion and Metastasis)

A. Cancer cells are less adhesive than normal cells, more easily dissociated from their location.

B. Lack of adhesion and loss of contact inhibition make it possible for a cancer to spread to distant parts of the body (*metastasis*).

C. Malignant tumors are not encapsulated and expand into surrounding tissue (*invasion*)

Etiology (Carcinogenesis)

Actual cause of cancer is unknown but there are a number of theories; it is currently thought that there are probably multiple etiologies.

Environmental Factors

A. Majority (over 80%) of human cancers related to environmental carcinogens

B. Types
  1. Physical
    a. Radiation: x-rays, radium, nuclear explosion or waste, ultraviolet
    b. Trauma or chronic irritation
  2. Chemical
    a. Nitrites and food additives, polycyclic hydrocarbons, dyes, alkylating agents
    b. Drugs: arsenicals, stilbestrol, urethane
    c. Cigarette smoke
    d. Hormones

Genetics

A. Some cancers show familial pattern.

B. May be caused by inherited genetic defects.

Viral Theory

A. Viruses have been shown to be the cause of certain tumors in animals.

B. Oncoviruses (RNA-type viruses) thought to be culprit.

C. Two viruses (HTLV-I and Epstein-Barr) linked to human tumors.

Immunologic Factors

A. Failure of the immune system to respond to and eradicate cancer cells
B. Immunosuppressed individuals more susceptible to cancer

DIAGNOSIS OF CANCER

Classification and Staging

Tissue of Origin

A. *Carcinoma:* arises from surface, glandular, or parenchymal epithelium.
   1. *Squamous cell carcinoma:* surface epithelium
   2. *Adenocarcinoma:* glandular or parenchymal tissue
B. *Sarcoma:* arises from connective tissue.
C. *Leukemia, lymphoma,* and *multiple myeloma:* separate categories for each

Stages of Tumor Growth

A. Several staging systems, important in selection of therapy
   1. TNM system: uses letters and numbers to designate the extent of the tumor.
      a. T: stands for primary growth; 1-4 with increasing size. T1S indicates carcinoma in situ.
      b. N: stands for lymph node involvement; 0-4 indicates progressively advancing nodal disease.
      c. M: stands for metastasis; 0 indicates no distant metastases, 1 indicates presence of metastases.
   2. Stages 0-IV: all cancer divided into five stages incorporating size, nodal involvement, and spread.
B. Cytologic diagnosis of cancer (e.g., Pap smear)
   1. Involves study of shed cells
   2. Classified by degree of cellular abnormality
      a. Normal
      b. Probably normal (slight changes)
      c. Doubtful (more severe changes)
      d. Probably cancer or precancerous
      e. Definitely cancer

Patient Factors

Early detection of cancer is crucial in reducing morbidity and mortality. Patients need to be taught about
A. Seven warning signs of cancer (see Table 2.13)

Table 2.13 Seven Warning Signs of Cancer

- Change in bowel or bladder habits
- Sore that doesn't heal
- Thickening or lump in breast (or elsewhere)
- Unusual bleeding or discharge
- Indigestion or dysphagia
- Change in wart or mole
- Nagging cough or hoarseness

B. Self-breast examination (SBE)
C. Importance of rectal exam for those over age 40
D. Hazards of smoking
E. Oral self-examination as well as annual exam of mouth and teeth
F. Hazards of excess sun exposure
G. Importance of Pap smear
H. Physical exam with lab work-up: every 3 years ages 20–40; yearly age 40 and over

TREATMENT OF CANCER

Chemotherapy

Principles

A. Based on ability of drug to kill cancer cells; normal cells may also be damaged, producing side effects discussed below. Effect is greatest on rapidly dividing cells, such as bone marrow cells or the GI tract.
B. Different drugs act on tumor cells in different stages of the cell growth cycle.

Types of Chemotherapeutic Drugs

See Table 2.14.
A. Antimetabolites: foster cancer cell death by interfering with cellular metabolic process.
B. Alkylating agents: act with DNA to hinder cell growth and division.
C. Plant alkaloids: obtained from the periwinkle plant; makes the host's body a less favorable environment for the growth of cancer cells.
D. Steroids and sex hormones: alter the endocrine environment to make it less conducive to growth of cancer cells.
E. Antitumor antibiotics: affect RNA to make environment less favorable for cancer growth.

Major Side Effects and Nursing Interventions

A. GI system
   1. Nausea and vomiting
      a. Administer antiemetics routinely every 4–6 hours as well as prophylactically before chemotherapy is initiated.
      b. Withhold foods/fluids 4–6 hours before chemotherapy.
      c. Provide bland foods in small amounts after treatments.
   2. Diarrhea
      a. Administer antidiarreals.
      b. Maintain good perineal care.
      c. Give clear liquids as tolerated.
      d. Monitor potassium, sodium, and chloride levels.
   3. Stomatitis
      a. Provide and teach the patient good oral hygiene, including avoidance of commercial mouthwashes.
      b. Rinse with viscous lidocaine before meals to provide an analgesic effect.
      c. Perform a cleansing rinse with plain water or dilute hydrogen peroxide after meals.

Table 2.14 Drugs Used in Chemotherapy

Drug	Major Toxic and Side Effects	Nursing Interventions
Antimetabolites		
Methotrexate	Bone marrow depression, nausea, anorexia, diarrhea, stomatitis, alopecia	Administer oral preparations 1–2 hr before meals or 2–3 hr after meals. Provide good oral hygiene and inspect mouth daily. Assess hepatic and renal function regularly. Measure I&O. Assess for signs of thrombocytopenia (ecchymosis, petechiae, epistaxis, melena). Avoid skin exposure and inhalation of drug particles. Instruct patient to avoid self-medication with over-the-counter vitamins (folic acid and derivatives may alter methotrexate response). Treat nausea, diarrhea, and stomatitis.
5-Fluorouracil	Same as for methotrexate	Avoid skin exposure and inhalation of drug particles. Weigh every 3–4 days. Avoid extravasation at injection site. Monitor WBC, if less than 1000 μ/L institute reverse isolation. Protect from trauma, unnecessary injuries. Assess for signs and symptoms of abnormal bleeding. Instruct patient to report anorexia, vomiting, stomatitis, photophobia, or lacrimation. Assess renal and hepatic function regularly. Instruct patient to avoid exposure to sun and ultraviolet light.
ARA-C Mercaptopurine Thioguanine	Same as for methotrexate	Assess blood counts routinely. Protect patient from infection. Assess for increased bleeding tendencies. Provide adequate hydration and rest. Inspect oral cavity daily and provide good oral hygiene. Measure I&O.
Alkylating Agents		
Cyclophosphamide (Cytoxan)	Bone marrow depression, tissue destruction, nausea and vomiting, diarrhea, stomatitis	Assess for signs and symptoms of unexplained bleeding. Assess leukocyte count frequently. Monitor CBC, uric acid, electrolytes, thrombocytes, and hepatic and renal function at least twice a week. Maintain adequate hydration. Instruct patient to report hematuria or dysuria immediately.
Chlorambucil (Leukeran)	Same as for Cytoxan	Assess CBC, WBC, and serum uric acid levels routinely. Avoid IM injections when platelet count is low. Urge patient to drink 10–12 glasses of fluid/day. Provide urine alkalinization if uric acid levels are increased.
Nitrogen mustard	Same as for Cytoxan	Assess for edema, ascites, weight gain. Assess for signs and symptoms of dehydration. Monitor for abnormal bleeding. Instruct patient to report unexplained fever, chills, sore throat. Provide adequate hydration. Wear gloves if applying solid preparations.
Cisplatin (Platinol)	Mucositis, renal toxicity, ototoxicity	Monitor urine output and specific gravity. Provide a nonirritating diet. Inspect oral cavity daily and institute good oral hygiene program. Have patient void every hour or insert Foley catheter before initiating treatment. Assess for hearing deficits.

(continued)

Table 2.14 Drugs Used in Chemotherapy (continued)

Drug	Major Toxic and Side Effects	Nursing Interventions
Plant alkaloids		
Vinblastine (Velban)	Constipation, nausea and vomiting, leukopenia	Add medication to a running infusion over a period of 1 min. Assess WBC routinely. Institute measures to prevent constipation (high-fiber diet, adequate hydration)
Vincristine (Oncovin)	Alopecia, neurotoxicity	Frequent uric acid determination. Assess continually for sensory impairment/paresthesias. Assess for neuromuscular side effects, check handclasp and deep tendon reflexes daily. Monitor leukocyte counts.
Steroid Hormones		
Androgens (testosterone) and estrogens (diethylstilbestrol)	Nausea and vomiting, fluid retention; virilization of females with androgens; feminization of males with estrogens	Maintain adequate hydration. Weigh daily. Observe for peripheral edema. Measure I&O. Provide low-sodium and high-potassium diet. Advise patient of secondary sex characteristic changes (usually temporary).
Antitumor antibiotics		
Bleomycin (Blenoxane) Dactinomycin (Actinomycin-D) Daunorubicin (Cerubidine) Doxorubicin (Adriamycin) Plicamycin (Mithracin)	Bone marrow depression, nausea and vomiting, dose-related cardiac toxicity, alopecia	Monitor blood counts routinely. Measure I&O. Maintain good oral hygiene. Assess for signs of congestive heart failure. Protect patient from infection. Provide adequate hydration.

   d. Apply K-Y jelly to lubricate cracked lips.
   e. Advise patient to suck on Popsicles to provide moisture.

B. Hematologic system
   1. Thrombocytopenia
      a. Teach patient the importance of avoiding bumping or bruising the skin.
      b. Protect patient from physical injury.
      c. Avoid giving aspirin or aspirin products.
      d. Avoid giving IM injections.
      e. Monitor blood counts carefully.
      f. Assess for and teach patient signs of increased bleeding tendencies (epistaxis, petechiae, ecchymoses).
   2. Leukopenia
      a. Use careful handwashing technique.
      b. Maintain reverse isolation if white blood cell count drops below 1000 μ/liter.
      c. Assess for signs of respiratory infection.
      d. Instruct patient to avoid crowds/persons with known infection.
   3. Anemia
      a. Provide for adequate rest periods.
      b. Monitor hemoglobin and hematocrit.
      c. Protect patient from injury.
      d. Administer oxygen as necessary.
C. Integumentary System
   1. Alopecia

      a. Explain to patient that hair loss is not permanent.
      b. Offer support and encouragement.
      c. Scalp tourniquets or scalp hypothermia via ice pack may be ordered to minimize hair loss with some agents.
      d. Advise patient to obtain a wig before initiating treatments.

Radiation Therapy

Principles

A. Radiation therapy uses ionizing radiation to kill or limit the growth of cancer cells, may be internal or external.
B. It not only injures the cell membrane, but destroys or alters DNA so that the cells cannot reproduce.
C. Like chemotherapy, effect cannot be limited to cancer cells only; all exposed cells, including normal ones, will be injured, causing side effects discussed below. Localized effects are related to area of body being treated, generalized effects may be related to cellular breakdown products.
D. Types of energy emitted
   1. Alpha rays: cannot pass through skin, rarely used
   2. Beta rays: cannot pass through skin, somewhat more penetrating than alpha rays, generally emitted from radioactive isotopes, used for internal source
   3. Gamma rays (electromagnetic or x-rays): penetrate deeper areas of body, most common form of external radiotherapy.

Methods of Delivery

A. External radiation therapy: beams high-energy rays directly to the affected area.

B. Internal radiation therapy: radioactive material is injected or implanted in the patient's body for a designated period of time.

1. Sealed implants: a radioisotope enclosed in a container so it does not circulate in the body; patient's body fluids should not become contaminated with radiation.

2. Unsealed sources: a radioisotope that is not encased in a container and does circulate in the body and contaminate body fluids.

Factors Controlling Exposure

A. Half-life: time required for half of radioactive atoms to decay

1. Each radioisotope has a different half-life.

2. At the end of the half-life, the danger from exposure decreases.

B. Time: the shorter the duration, the less the exposure

C. Distance: the greater the distance from the radiation source the less the exposure

D. Shielding: all radiation can be blocked; rubber gloves stop alpha and usually beta rays; thick lead or concrete stops gamma rays

E. These factors affect health care worker's exposure as well as patient's.

1. Health care worker at greater risk from internal than from external sources

2. Film badge can measure the amount of exposure received

3. No pregnant nurses or visitors permitted near radiation source

Side Effects of Radiation Therapy and Nursing Interventions

A. Skin: itching, redness, burning, oozing, sloughing

1. Keep skin free from foreign substances.

2. Avoid use of medicated solutions, ointments, or powders that contain heavy metals such as zinc oxide.

3. Avoid pressure, trauma, infection to skin; use bed cradle.

4. Wash affected areas with plain water and pat dry; avoid soap.

5. Use cornstarch, olive oil for itching; avoid talcum powder.

6. If sloughing occurs, use a sterile dressing with micropore tape.

7. Teach patient to avoid exposing skin to heat, cold, or sunlight and to avoid constricting or irritating clothing.

B. Anorexia, nausea and vomiting

1. Arrange meal times so they do not directly precede or follow therapy.

2. Encourage bland foods.

3. Provide small, attractive meals.

4. Avoid extremes of temperature.

5. Administer antiemetics as ordered before meals.

C. Diarrhea

1. Encourage low-residue, bland, high-protein foods.

2. Administer antidiarrheal drugs as ordered.

3. Provide good perineal care.

4. Monitor electrolytes, particularly sodium, potassium, and chloride.

D. Anemia, leukopenia, and thrombocytopenia

1. Isolate from those with known infections.

2. Provide frequent rest periods.

3. Encourage high protein diet.

4. Instruct patient to avoid injury.

5. Assess for bleeding.

6. Monitor CBC, leukocytes and platelets.

SAMPLE QUESTIONS

Mr. David Latinsky is returning to the nursing unit after major abdominal surgery. He is 50 lb overweight.

1. If loops of bowel spill out through a torn incision, all of the following should be done *EXCEPT*
   - ○ 1. cover the bowel with a wet, sterile towel.
   - ○ 2. culture the protruding bowel.
   - ○ 3. insert an IV line.
   - ○ 4. administer pain medications.

Mrs. Gerald Addis, 43 years old, is undergoing treatment for uterine cancer.

2. Mrs. Addis asks the nurse how chemotherapeutic drugs work. The most accurate explanation would include which statement?
   - ○ 1. It affects all rapidly dividing cells.
   - ○ 2. Molecular structure of the DNA segment is altered.
   - ○ 3. Chemotherapy stimulates cancer cells to divide.
   - ○ 4. The cancer cells are sensitive to drug toxins.

3. Mrs. Addis experiences severe vomiting from the chemotherapy drugs. Which of the following acid-base imbalances should the nurse anticipate?
   - ○ 1. Ketoacidosis
   - ○ 2. Metabolic acidosis
   - ○ 3. Metabolic alkalosis
   - ○ 4. Respiratory alkalosis

The Nervous System

OVERVIEW OF ANATOMY AND PHYSIOLOGY

The functional unit of the nervous system is the nerve cell, or neuron. The nervous system consists of the central nervous system (CNS), which includes the brain and spinal cord, and the peripheral nervous system (PNS), which includes the cranial nerves and the spinal nerves. The autonomic nervous system (ANS) is a subdivision of the PNS that automatically controls body functions such as breathing and heart beat. It is further divided into the sympathetic and parasympathetic nervous systems. The special senses of vision and hearing are also covered in this section.

Neuron

A. Primary component of the nervous system; composed of cell body (grey matter), axon, and dendrites
B. *Axon:* elongated process or fiber extending from the cell body; transmits impulses (messages) away from the cell body to dendrites or directly to the cell bodies of other neurons; neuron usually has only one axon.
C. *Dendrites:* short, branching fibers that receive impulses and conduct them toward the nerve cell body. Neurons may have many dendrites.
D. *Synapse:* junction between neurons where an impulse is transmitted
E. *Neurotransmitters:* chemical agents (e.g., acetylcholine, norepinephrine) involved in the transmission of impulse across synapse
F. *Myelin sheath:* a wrapping of myelin (a whitish, fatty material) that protects and insulates nerve fibers and enhances the speed of impulse conduction
   1. Both axons and dendrites may or may not have a myelin sheath (myelinated/unmyelinated)
   2. Most axons leaving the CNS are heavily myelinated by *Schwann cells*

Functional Classification

A. *Afferent (sensory) neurons:* transmit impulses from peripheral receptors to the CNS

B. *Efferent (motor) neurons:* conduct impulses from CNS to muscles and glands
C. *Internuncial neurons (interneurons):* connecting links between afferent and efferent neurons

Central Nervous System: Brain and Spinal Cord

Brain

A. *Cerebrum:* outermost area (cerebral cortex) is gray matter; deeper area is composed of white matter
   1. Two hemispheres: right and left
   2. Each hemisphere divided into four lobes, many of the functional areas of the cerebrum have been located in these lobes (see Figure 2.1)
      a. *Frontal lobe*
         1) personality, behavior
         2) higher intellectual functioning
         3) precentral gyrus: motor function
         4) Broca's area: specialized motor speech area

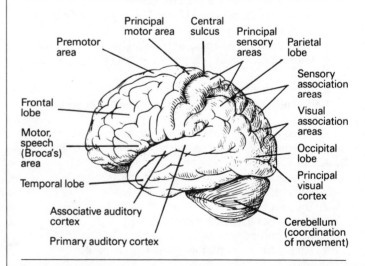

Figure 2.1 Side view of the brain, showing principal functional areas.

    b. *Parietal lobe*
       1) postcentral gyrus: registers general sensation (e.g., touch, pressure)
       2) integrates sensory information
    c. *Temporal lobe*
       1) hearing, taste, smell
       2) Wernicke's area: sensory speech area (understanding/formulation of language)
    d. *Occipital lobe:* vision
  3. *Corpus callosum:* large fiber tract that connects the two cerebral hemispheres
  4. *Basal ganglia:* islands of gray matter within white matter of cerebrum
    a. Regulate and integrate motor activity originating in the cerebral cortex
    b. Part of extrapyramidal system

B. *Diencephalon:* connecting part of the brain, between the cerebrum and the brain stem. Contains several small structures; the thalamus and hypothalamus are most important
  1. *Thalamus*
    a. Relay station for discrimination of sensory signals (e.g., pain, temperature, touch)
    b. Controls primitive emotional responses (e.g., rage, fear).
  2. *Hypothalamus*
    a. Found immediately beneath the thalamus.
    b. Plays major role in regulation of vital functions such as blood pressure, sleep, food and water intake, and body temperature.
    c. Acts as control center for pituitary gland and affects both divisions of the autonomic nervous system.

C. *Brainstem*
  1. Contains midbrain, pons, and medulla oblongata.
  2. Extends from the cerebral hemispheres to the foramen magnum at the base of the skull.
  3. Contains nucleii of the cranial nerves and the long ascending and descending tracts connecting the cerebrum and the spinal cord.
  4. Contains vital centers of respiratory, vasomotor, and cardiac functions.

D. *Cerebellum:* coordinates muscle tone and movements and maintains position in space (equilibrium).

Spinal Cord

A. Serves as a connecting link between the brain and the periphery.
B. Extends from foramen magnum to second lumbar vertebra.
C. H-shaped grey matter in the center (cell bodies) surrounded by white matter (nerve tracts and fibers).
D. *Grey matter*
  1. Anterior horns: contain cell bodies giving rise to efferent (motor) fibers
  2. Posterior horns: contain cell bodies connecting with afferent (sensory) fibers from dorsal root ganglion
  3. Lateral horns: in thoracic region, contain cells giving rise to autonomic fibers of sympathetic nervous system

E. *White matter*
  1. Ascending tracts (sensory pathways)
    a. Posterior columns: carry impulses concerned with touch, pressure, vibration, and position sense.
    b. Spinocerebellar: carry impulses concerned with muscle tension and position sense to cerebellum.
    c. Lateral spinothalamic: carry impulses resulting in pain and temperature sensations.
    d. Anterior spinothalamic: carry impulses concerned with crude touch and pressure.
  2. Descending tracts (motor pathways)
    a. Corticospinal (pyramidal, upper motor neuron): conduct motor impulses from motor cortex to anterior horn cells (cross in the medulla).
    b. Extrapyramidal: help to maintain muscle tone and to control body movement, especially gross automatic movements such as walking.

F. *Reflex arc*
  1. Reflex consists of an involuntary response to a stimulus occurring over a neural pathway called a reflex arc.
  2. Not relayed to and from brain; takes place at cord levels.
  3. Components
    a. Sensory receptor: receives/reacts to a stimulus.
    b. Afferent pathway: transmits impulses to spinal cord.
    c. Interneuron: synapses with a motor neuron (anterior horn cell).
    d. Efferent pathway: transmits impulses from motor neuron to effector.
    e. Effector: muscle or organ that responds to stimulus.

Supporting Structures

A. Skull
  1. Rigid; numerous bones fused together
  2. Protects and supports the brain.
B. Spinal column
  1. Consists of 7 cervical, 12 thoracic, and 5 lumbar vertebrae, as well as sacrum and coccyx.
  2. Supports the head and protects the spinal cord.
C. Meninges
  1. Membranes between the skull and brain and the vertebral column and spinal cord
  2. Layers
    a. *Dura mater:* outermost layer, tough, leathery
    b. *Arachnoid mater:* middle layer, weblike
    c. *Pia mater:* innermost layer, delicate, clings to surface of brain
  3. Area between arachnoid and pia mater is called *subarachnoid space.*
D. Ventricles
  1. Four fluid-filled cavities connecting with one another and the spinal canal
  2. Produce and circulate cerebrospinal fluid.
E. *Cerebrospinal fluid (CSF)*
  1. Surrounds brain and spinal cord.
  2. Offers protection by functioning as a shock absorber.
  3. Allows fluid shifts from the cranial cavity to the spinal cavity.

4. Carries nutrients to and waste products away from nerve cells.

F. Vascular supply

    1. Two *internal carotid arteries* anteriorly

    2. Two *vertebral arteries* leading to basilar artery posteriorly

    3. These arteries communicate at the base of the brain through the *circle of Willis*.

    4. Anterior, middle, and posterior cerebral arteries are the main arteries for distributing blood to each hemisphere of the brain.

    5. Brainstem and cerebellum are supplied by branches of the vertebral and basilar arteries.

    6. Venous blood drains into dural sinuses and then into internal jugular veins.

G. *Blood-brain barrier:* protective barrier preventing harmful agents from entering the capillaries of the CNS; protects brain and spinal cord.

Peripheral Nervous System

Spinal Nerves

A. 31 pairs: carry impulses to and from spinal cord.

B. Each segment of the spinal cord contains a pair of spinal nerves (one for each side of the body).

C. Each nerve is attached to the spinal cord by two roots.

    1. Dorsal (posterior) root: contains afferent (sensory) nerve whose cell body is in the dorsal root ganglion.

    2. Ventral (anterior) root: contains efferent (motor) nerve whose nerve fibers originate in the anterior horn cell of the spinal cord (lower motor neuron).

Cranial Nerves

A. 12 pairs: carry impulses to and from brain (see Table 2.15).

B. May have sensory, motor, or mixed functions.

Autonomic Nervous System

A. Part of the peripheral nervous system

B. Includes those peripheral nerves (both cranial and spinal) that regulate functions occurring automatically in the body; ANS regulates smooth muscle, cardiac muscle, and glands.

C. Components

    1. *Sympathetic nervous system:* generally accelerates some body functions in response to stress

    2. *Parasympathetic nervous system:* controls normal body functioning

D. Effects of ANS activity: see Table 2.16.

Vision

External Structures of Eye

A. Eyelids (palpebrae) and eyelashes: protect the eye from foreign particles

B. *Conjunctiva*

    1. Palpebral conjunctiva: pink; lines inner surface of eyelids.

    2. Bulbar conjunctiva: white with small blood vessels, covers anterior sclera.

Table 2.15   Cranial Nerves

Name and Number	Function
Olfactory: cranial nerve I	Sensory: carries impulses for sense of smell
Optic: cranial nerve II	Sensory: carries impulses for vision
Oculomotor: cranial nerve III	Motor: muscles for pupillary constriction, elevation of upper eyelid; 4 out of 6 extraocular movements
Trochlear: cranial nerve IV	Motor: muscles for downward, inward movement of eye
Trigeminal: cranial nerve V	Mixed: impulses from face, surface of eyes (corneal reflex); muscles controlling mastication
Abducens: cranial nerve VI	Motor: muscles for lateral deviation of eye
Facial: cranial nerve VII	Mixed: impulses for taste from anterior tongue; muscles for facial movement
Acoustic: cranial nerve VIII	Sensory: impulses for hearing (cochlear division) and balance (vestibular division)
Glossopharyngeal: cranial nerve IX	Mixed: impulses for sensation to posterior tongue and pharynx; muscles for movement of pharynx (elevation) and swallowing
Vagus: cranial nerve X	Mixed: impulses for sensation to lower pharynx and larynx; muscles for movement of soft palate, pharynx and larynx
Spinal accessory: cranial nerve XI	Motor: movement of sternomastoid muscles and upper part of trapezius muscles
Hypoglossal: cranial nerve XII	Motor: movement of tongue

C. *Lacrimal apparatus* (lacrimal gland and its ducts and passages): produces tears to lubricate the eye and moisten the cornea; tears drain into the nasolacrimal duct, which empties into nasal cavity.

D. Movement of the eye is controlled by six extraocular muscles.

Internal Structures of Eye

A. Three layers of the eyeball

    1. Outer layer

        a. *Sclera:* tough, white connective tissue ("white of the eye"); located posteriorly

        b. *Cornea:* transparent tissue through which light enters the eye; located anteriorly

    2. Middle layer

        a. *Choroid:* highly vascular layer, nourishes retina; located posteriorly

        b. *Ciliary body:* anterior to choroid, secretes aqueous humor; muscles change shape of lens

        c. *Iris:* pigmented membrane behind cornea, gives color to eye; located anteriorly. *Pupil* is a circular opening in the middle of the iris that constricts or dilates to regulate amount of light entering eye.

    3. Inner layer: *retina*

a. Light sensitive layer composed of rods and cones (visual cells)
   1) cones: specialized for fine discrimination and color vision
   2) rods: more sensitive to light than cones, aid in peripheral vision
   b. *Optic disk:* area in retina for entrance of optic nerve, has no photoreceptors
B. *Lens:* transparent body that focuses image on retina.
C. Fluids of the eye
   1. *Aqueous humor:* clear, watery fluid in anterior and posterior chambers in anterior part of eye; serves as refracting medium and provides nutrients to lens and cornea; contributes to maintenance of intraocular pressure.
   2. *Vitreous humor:* clear, gelatinous material that fills posterior cavity of eye; maintains transparency and form of eye.

Table 2.16   Effects of Autonomic Nervous System Activity

Effector	Sympathetic (Adrenergic) Effects	Parasympathetic (Cholinergic) Effects
Eye	Dilates pupil (mydriasis)	Constricts pupil (miosis)
Glands of head		
Lacrimal	No effect	Stimulates secretion
Salivary	Scanty thick, viscous secretions; dry mouth	Copious thin, watery secretions
Heart	Increases rate and force of contraction	Decreases rate
Blood vessels	Constricts smooth muscles of skin, abdominal blood vessels, and cutaneous blood vessels Dilates smooth muscle of bronchioles, blood vessels of heart, and skeletal muscles	No effect
Lungs	Bronchodilation	Bronchoconstriction
GI tract	Decreases motility Constricts sphincters Possibly inhibits secretions Inhibits activity of gallbladder and ducts Inhibits glycogenolysis in liver	Increases motility Relaxes sphincters Stimulates secretion Stimulates activity of gallbladder and ducts
Adrenal gland	Stimulates secretion of epinephrine and norepinephrine	No effects
Urinary tract	Relaxes detrusor muscle Contracts trigone sphincter (prevents voiding)	Contracts detrusor muscle Relaxes trigone sphincter (allows voiding)

Visual Pathways

A. Retina (rods and cones) translates light waves into neural impulses that travel over the optic nerves.
B. Optic nerves for each eye meet at the optic chiasm.
   1. Fibers from median halves of the retinas cross here and travel to the opposite side of the brain.
   2. Fibers from lateral halves of retinas remain uncrossed.
C. Optic nerves continue from optic chiasm as optic tracts and travel to the cerebrum (occipital lobe), where visual impulses are perceived and interpreted.

Hearing

External Ear

A. *Auricle (pinna):* outer projection of ear composed of cartilage and covered by skin; collects sound waves.
B. *External auditory canal:* lined with skin; glands secrete cerumen (wax), providing protection; transmits sound waves to tympanic membrane.
C. *Tympanic membrane (eardrum):* at end of external canal; vibrates in response to sound and transmits vibrations to middle ear.

Middle Ear

A. *Ossicles*
   1. 3 small bones: *malleus (hammer)* attached to tympanic membrane, *incus (anvil), stapes (stirrup)*
   2. Ossicles are set in motion by sound waves from tympanic membrane.
   3. Sound waves are conducted by vibration to the footplate of the stapes in the *oval window* (an opening between the middle ear and the inner ear).
B. *Eustachian tube:* connects nasopharynx and middle ear; brings air into middle ear, thus equalizing pressure on both sides of eardrum.

Inner Ear

A. *Cochlea*
   1. Contains *organ of Corti,* the receptor end-organ for hearing.
   2. Transmits sound waves from the oval window and initiates nerve impulses carried by cranial nerve VIII (acoustic branch) to the brain (temporal lobe of cerebrum).
B. *Vestibular apparatus*
   1. Organ of balance
   2. Composed of three semicircular canals and the utricle.

ASSESSMENT

Health History

Nervous System

A. Presenting problem: symptoms may include behavior changes, memory loss, mood changes, nervousness or anxiety, headache, seizures, syncope, vertigo, loss of consciousness;

problems with speech, vision, or smell; motor problems (paralysis, tremor); sensory problems (pain, paresthesias)

B. Life-style: drug and alcohol intake, exposure to toxins, recent travel, employment, stressors

C. Use of medications: prescribed and over-the-counter (OTC)

D. Past medical history
1. Perinatal exposure to toxic agents, x-rays; difficult labor and delivery
2. Childhood and adult: history of systemic diseases; seizures; loss of consciousness; head trauma

E. Family history: may uncover diseases with hereditary or congenital background.

Eye

A. Presenting problem: symptoms may include vision, glasses or contact lenses, date of last eye exam, pain, redness, excessive tearing, double vision (diplopia), drainage

B. Life-style: occupation (exposure to fumes, smoke or eye irritant); use of safety glasses

C. Use of medications: cortisone preparations may contribute to formation of glaucoma and cataracts

D. Past medical history: systemic diseases; previous childhood or adult eye disorders

E. Family history: many eye disorders may be inherited.

Ear

A. Presenting problem: symptoms may include hearing loss, tinnitus (ringing in ear), dizziness or vertigo, pain, drainage

B. Life-style: occupation (exposure to excessive noise levels), swimming habits

C. Use of medications: ototoxic drugs; aspirin (tinnitus)

D. Past medical history
1. Perinatal: rubella in first trimester of pregnancy
2. Childhood and adult: otitis media, perforated eardrum, measles, mumps, allergies, tonsillectomy and adenoidectomy

E. Family history: hearing loss in family members.

Physical Examination

Nervous System

A. Neurologic examination
1. Mental status exam (cerebral function); see also Psychiatric-Mental Health Nursing, page **489**
   a. General appearance and behavior
   b. Level of consciousness; see Neuro Check, below.
   c. Intellectual function: memory (recent and remote), attention span, cognitive skills
   d. Emotional status
   e. Thought content
   f. Language/speech
      1) *expressive aphasia:* inability to speak
      2) *receptive aphasia:* inability to understand spoken words
      3) *dysarthria:* difficult speech due to impairment of muscles involved with production of speech

2. Cranial nerves (see Table 2.15)
3. Cerebellar function: posture, gait, balance, coordination
4. Motor function: muscle size, tone, strength; abnormal or involuntary movements
5. Sensory function: light touch, superficial pain, temperature, vibration, and position sense
6. Reflexes
   a. Deep tendon: grade from 0 (no response) to 4 (hyperactive); 2 is normal
   b. Superficial
   c. Pathologic: *Babinski's reflex* (dorsiflexion of great toe with fanning of other toes) indicates damage to corticospinal tracts (see Figure 2.2)

B. Neuro check
1. *Level of consciousness (LOC)*
   a. Orientation to time, place, and person
   b. Speech: clear, garbled, rambling
   c. Ability to follow commands
   d. If patient does not respond to verbal stimuli, apply a painful stimulus (e.g., pressure on nailbeds, squeeze trapezius muscle); note response to pain
      1) appropriate: withdrawal, moaning
      2) inappropriate: nonpurposeful
   e. Abnormal posturing (may occur spontaneously or in response to stimulus)
      1) *decorticate posturing:* extension of legs, internal rotation and adduction of arms with flexion of elbows, wrists, and fingers (damage to corticospinal tracts)
      2) *decerebrate posturing:* back arched, rigid extension of all four extremities with hyperpronation of arms and plantar flexion of feet (damage to upper brainstem)
2. *Glasgow coma scale* (see Figure 2.3)
   a. Objective evaluation of LOC, motor/verbal response; a

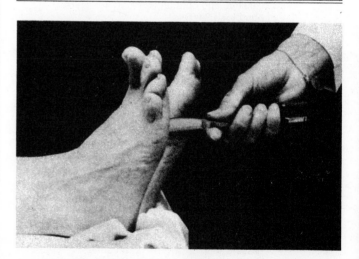

Figure 2.2 Pathologic reflex *(Babinski).*

Subscale	Response	Score
Best eye Opening (E)	Spontaneous	4
	To voice	3
	To Pain	2
	None	1
Best verbal response (V)	Oriented	5
	Confused conversation	4
	Inappropriate words	3
	Incomprehensible sounds	2
	None	1
Best motor response, Upper limb (M)	Obeys commands	6
	Localizes to pain	5
	Flexor withdrawl (decorticate posturing)	4
	Abnormal flexion (decerebrate posturing)	3
	Extension	2
	Flaccid	1

Figure 2.3 Glasgow Coma Scale.
(From "What the comatose patient can tell you," by A. Stolarik, RN, 48(4), 32.)

standardized system for assessing the degree of neurologic impairment in critically ill patients.

b. Cannot replace a complete neurologic check, but can be used as an aid in evaluation and to eliminate ambiguous terms such as stupor and lethargy.

c. A score of 15 indicates patient is awake and oriented; the lowest score, 3, is deep coma; a score of 7 or below is considered coma.

3. Pupillary reaction and eye movements
   a. Observe size, shape, and equality of pupils (note size in millimeters)
   b. Reaction to light: pupillary constriction
   c. Corneal reflex: blink reflex in response to light stroking of cornea
   d. Oculocephalic reflex (doll's eyes): present in unconscious patient with intact brainstem

4. Motor function
   a. Movement of extremities (paralysis)
   b. Muscle strength

5. Vital signs: respiratory patterns (may help localize possible lesion)
   a. *Cheyne-Stokes respiration:* regular, rhythmic alternating between hyperventilation and apnea; may be caused by structural cerebral dysfunction or by metabolic problems, such as diabetic coma.

b. *Central neurogenic hyperventilation:* sustained, rapid, regular respirations (rate of 25/minute) with normal blood oxygen levels; usually due to brainstem dysfunction.

c. *Apneustic breathing:* prolonged inspiratory phase, followed by a 2- to 3-second pause; usually indicates dysfunction of respiratory center in pons.

d. *Cluster breathing:* clusters of irregular breathing, irregularly followed by periods of apnea; usually caused by a lesion in upper medulla and lower pons.

e. *Ataxic breathing:* breathing pattern completely irregular; indicates damage to respiratory centers of the medulla.

Eye

A. Visual acuity: Snellen chart
B. Visual fields (peripheral vision)
   1. Confrontation method
   2. Perimetry: more precise method
C. External structures
   1. Position and alignment of eyes
   2. Eyebrows, eyelids, lacrimal apparatus, conjunctiva, sclera, cornea, iris, pupils (size, shape, equality and reaction to light)
D. Extraocular movements; note paralysis, nystagmus (rapid, abnormal movement of the eyeball)
E. Corneal reflex

Ear

A. Inspection and palpation of auricle, preauricular area, and mastoid area
B. Hearing acuity
   1. Whispered voice or ticking watch tests: gross estimation
   2. Audiometry: more precise method
C. Tuning fork tests distinguish between sensorineural and conductive deafness.
   1. Conductive hearing loss: secondary to problem in external or middle ear; transmission of sound waves to inner ear impaired
   2. Sensorineural (perceptive) hearing loss: disease of inner ear or cranial nerve VIII (acoustic branch)
   3. *Weber's test:* handle of vibrating tuning fork placed on midline of patient's skull, sound should be heard equally in midline or in both ears; in conductive hearing loss, sound is louder in poorer ear; in sensorineural hearing loss, sound is louder in better ear.
   4. *Rinne's test:* tuning fork placed on mastoid process (bone conduction) until sound no longer heard, then placed in front of the ear (air conduction); sound should be heard longer (almost twice as long) with air conduction than with bone conduction; bone conduction greater than air conduction indicates conductive hearing deficit.

Laboratory/Diagnostic Tests

Nervous System

A. Lumbar puncture (LP)
  1. A hollow spinal needle introduced into subarachnoid space of spinal canal between L_4/L_5 for diagnostic or therapeutic reasons
  2. Purposes
     a. Measure CSF pressure (normal opening pressure 60–150 mm H_2O)
     b. Obtain specimens for lab analysis (protein, sugar, cytology, C&S)
     c. Check color of CSF (normally clear) and check for blood
     d. Inject air, dye, or drugs into the spinal canal
  3. Nursing care: pretest
     a. Have patient empty bladder.
     b. Position patient in lateral recumbent position with head and neck flexed onto the chest and knees pulled up.
     c. Explain the need to remain still during the procedure.
  4. Nursing care: post-test
     a. Ensure labeling of CSF specimens in proper sequence.
     b. Keep patient flat for 12–24 hours as ordered.
     c. Force fluids.
     d. Check puncture site for bleeding, leakage of CSF.
     e. Assess sensation and movement in lower extremities.
     f. Monitor vital signs.
     g. Administer analgesics for headache as ordered.

B. X-rays of skull and spine
  1. Used to detect atrophy, erosion or fractures of bones; calcifications
  2. Pretest nursing care: remove hairpins, glasses, hearing aids.

C. Computerized tomography (CT scan)
  1. Skull/spinal cord are scanned in successive layers by a narrow beam of x-rays; computer uses information obtained to construct a picture of the internal structure of the brain; contrast medium may or may not be used.
  2. Used to detect intracranial and spinal cord lesions and monitor effects of surgery or other therapy.
  3. Nursing care
     a. Explain appearance of scanner.
     b. Instruct patient to lie still during procedure.
     c. Check for allergy to iodine if contrast material is used.
     d. Remove hairpins, etc.

D. Magnetic resonance imaging (MRI)
  1. Also known as nuclear magnetic resonance (NMR)
  2. Computer-drawn, detailed pictures of structures of the body through use of large magnet, radio waves
  3. Used to detect intracranial and spinal abnormalities associated with disorders such as cerebrovascular disease, tumors, abscesses, cerebral edema, hydrocephalus, multiple sclerosis
  4. Nursing care
     a. Instruct patient to remove jewelry, hairpins, glasses, wigs (with metal clips), and other metallic objects.
     b. Be aware that this test cannot be performed on anyone with pacemaker, internal surgical clips, or other fixed metallic objects in the body.
     c. Inform patient of need to remain still while completely enclosed in scanner throughout the procedure, which lasts 45–60 minutes.
     d. Teach relaxation techniques to assist patient to remain still and to help prevent claustrophobia.
     e. Warn patient of normal audible humming and thumping noises from the scanner during test.
     f. Have patient void before test.
     g. Sedate patient if ordered.

E. Brain scan
  1. Injection of radioactive isotope, followed by scanning of head; isotopes will accumulate in abnormal lesions and be recorded by the scanner.
  2. Used to detect intracranial masses, vascular lesions, infarcts, hemorrhage
  3. Nursing care: check for allergy to iodine.

F. Myelography (see page 152)

G. Cerebral angiography
  1. Injection of radiopaque substance into the cerebral circulation via carotid, vertebral, femoral or brachial artery followed by x-rays
  2. Used to visualize cerebral vessels and detection of tumors, aneurysms, occlusions, hematomas, or abscesses
  3. Nursing care: pretest
     a. Explain that patient may have warm flushed feeling and salty taste in mouth during procedure.
     b. Check for allergy to iodine.
     c. Keep NPO after midnight or offer clear liquid breakfast only.
     d. Take baseline vital signs and neuro check.
     e. Administer sedation if ordered.
  4. Nursing care: post-test
     a. Maintain pressure dressing over site if femoral or brachial artery used; apply ice as ordered.
     b. Maintain bedrest until next morning as ordered.
     c. Monitor vital signs and neuro checks frequently; report any changes immediately.
     d. Check site frequently for bleeding or hematoma; if carotid artery used, assess for swelling of neck, difficulty swallowing or breathing.
     e. Check pulse, color, and temperature of extremity distal to site used.
     f. Keep extremity extended and avoid flexion.

H. Ventriculography
  1. Injection of air directly into ventricles via burr hole or craniotomy flap, followed by x-rays
  2. Used to visualize ventricles, detect tumors; preferred over pneumoencephalography in presence of increased intracranial pressure; virtually replaced now by CT scanning
  3. Nursing care: post-test
     a. Elevate head of bed 15°–20°.
     b. Keep on bedrest for 24 hours.

c. Monitor vital signs frequently.

d. Check needle entry site frequently.

e. Use aseptic technique to prevent infection.

f. Administer analgesics and icebags for headache as needed.

g. Offer food/fluids as tolerated.

I. Pneumoencephalography

  1. Introduction of air into subarachnoid spaces and ventricles through a lumbar puncture, followed by x-rays

  2. Used to detect brain tumors, hydrocephalus and brain atrophy; rarely used now because safer and less painful tests available

  3. Nursing care: pretest

   a. Explain that patient will be strapped in chair and turned upside down.

   b. Keep NPO after midnight.

  4. Nursing care: post-test

   a. Keep patient flat and turn frequently.

   b. Force fluids.

   c. Monitor vital signs and neuro checks.

   d. Administer analgesics and antiemetics as ordered.

J. Echoencephalography: use of ultrasound to detect midline shift of intracranial contents due to brain tumors, hematomas.

K. Electroencephalography (EEG)

  1. Graphic recording of electrical activity of the brain by several small electrodes placed on the scalp

  2. Used to detect focus or foci of seizure activity, and to quantitatively evaluate level of brain function (determine brain death)

  3. Pretest nursing care: withhold sedatives, tranquillizers, stimulants for 2–3 days.

  4. Post-test nursing care: remove electrode paste with acetone and shampoo hair.

Eye

A. Ophthalmoscopic exam

B. Refraction: detects refractive errors and provides information for prescription of eye glasses and contact lenses

C. Perimetry: assesses peripheral vision, visual fields

D. Tonometry: measures intraocular pressure (normal: 12–20 mm Hg)

Ear

A. Otoscopic exam

B. Audiometry: screening test for hearing loss and diagnostic test to determine degree and type of hearing loss

C. Vestibular function

  1. Caloric test

  2. Electronystagmography (ENG)

ANALYSIS

Nursing diagnoses for patients with disorders of the nervous system, eye, or ear may include

A. Alteration in bowel elimination: constipation, incontinence

B. Potential for injury related to sensory, motor, or visual deficits

C. Impaired physical mobility

D. Potential alteration in nutrition: less than body requirements

E. Alteration in respiratory function: ineffective airway clearance related to immobility, muscular weakness, or unconsciousness; ineffective breathing patterns related to neurologic dysfunction

F. Self-care deficit

G. Sensory-perceptual alteration: visual, auditory, kinesthetic, gustatory, tactile, olfactory

H. Sexual dysfunction

I. Impairment of skin integrity related to immobility, sensory deficits

J. Alteration in thought processes

K. Alteration in tissue perfusion: cerebral

L. Alteration in patterns of urinary elimination

M. Impaired verbal communication

PLANNING AND IMPLEMENTATION

Goals

A. Adequate respiratory function will be maintained.

B. Constipation will be prevented.

C. Adequate urinary elimination will be maintained.

D. Ability to communicate will be improved.

E. Patient will remain free from any injury resulting from neurologic deficits.

F. Mobility will be restored to optimum level.

G. Nutritional state will be optimal.

H. Performance of self-care activities will be improved.

I. Sensory perception will be improved.

J. Sexual health will return to optimum level.

K. Skin integrity will be maintained.

L. Optimal level of orientation will be achieved.

M. Cerebral perfusion will be improved.

Interventions

Care of the Unconscious Patient

A. Maintain a clear, patent airway.

  1. Place patient in a side-lying or three-quarters prone position to prevent tongue from obstructing airway.

  2. If tongue is obstructing, insert oral airway.

  3. Prepare for insertion of a cuffed endotracheal or tracheostomy tube as the patient's condition requires.

  4. Suction as needed.

  5. Check respiratory rate, depth, and quality every 1–2 hours and as needed.

  6. Auscultate breath sounds for rales, rhonchi, or absent breath sounds every 4 hours and before and after suctioning.

B. Take vital signs and perform neuro checks at specified intervals as ordered; report any significant changes immediately.

C. Maintain fluid and electrolyte balance and ensure adequate nutrition.
   1. Administer IV fluids, nasogastric tube feedings as ordered.
   2. Maintain accurate I&O.
   3. Assess patient's hydration status: skin turgor, check for dry mucous membranes.
   4. Provide mouth care to keep mucous membranes clean, moist, and intact.

D. Provide for patient's safety.
   1. Keep side rails up at all times.
   2. Avoid restraints if at all possible.
   3. Observe patient carefully for seizures and intervene to avoid precipitating factors: fever, hypoxia, electrolyte imbalance.
   4. Protect patient if seizure occurs.
   5. Speak softly and use patient's name during nursing care.
   6. Touch patient as gently as possible.
   7. Protect patient's eyes from corneal irritation.
      a. Check for corneal reflex.
      b. Instill artificial tears as ordered; patch eye.

E. Prevent complications of immobility.
   1. Keep skin clean, dry, and pressure free.
   2. Turn and reposition patient every 2 hours.
   3. Perform passive range-of-motion (ROM) exercises every 4 hours.
   4. Use nursing measures to prevent deformities: footboard/high-topped sneakers to prevent foot drop, splint to prevent wrist drop

F. Maintain adequate bladder and bowel elimination.
   1. Urinary: indwelling catheter (may use external device in male)
   2. Bowel: stool softeners and suppositories as ordered.

Care of the Patient with Increased Intracranial Pressure (ICP)

A. General information
   1. An increase in intracranial bulk due to an increase in any of the major intracranial components: brain tissue, CSF, or blood
   2. Increased ICP may be caused by tumors, abscesses, hemorrhage, edema, hydrocephalus, inflammation.
   3. Untreated increased ICP can lead to displacement of brain tissue (*herniation*).
   4. Presents life-threatening situation because of pressure on vital structures in the brainstem, nerve tracts, and cranial nerves.

B. Assessment findings
   1. Most sensitive sign: decrease in LOC; progresses from restlessness to confusion and disorientation to lethargy and coma
   2. Changes in vital signs
      a. Systolic blood pressure rises while diastolic pressure remains the same (widening pulse presence)
      b. Pulse slows
      c. Abnormal respiratory patterns (e.g., Cheyne-Stokes respirations)
      d. Elevated temperature
   3. Pupillary changes
      a. Ipsilateral dilation of pupil with sluggish reaction to light from compression of cranial nerve III
      b. Pupil eventually becomes fixed and dilated.
   4. Motor abnormalities
      a. Contralateral hemiparesis from compression of corticospinal tracts
      b. Decorticate or decerebrate rigidity
   5. Headache, projectile vomiting, papilledema (edema of the optic disc)

C. Nursing care
   1. Maintain patent airway and adequate ventilation.
      a. Prevention of hypoxia and hypercarbia (increased CO_2) important: hypoxia may cause brain swelling and hypercarbia causes cerebral vasodilation, which increases ICP.
      b. Assist with mechanical hyperventilation as indicated: produces hypocarbia (decreased CO_2) causing cerebral vasoconstriction and decreased ICP.
   2. Monitor vital sign and neuro checks frequently to detect rises in ICP.
   3. Maintain fluid balance: fluid restriction to 1200–1500 ml/day may be ordered.
   4. Position patient with head of bed elevated to 30°–45° and neck in neutral position unless contraindicated (improves venous drainage from brain).
   5. Prevent further increases in ICP.
      a. Maintain quiet, comfortable environment.
      b. Avoid use of restraints.
      c. Prevent straining at stool; administer stool softeners and mild laxatives as ordered.
      d. Prevent vomiting; administer antiemetics as ordered.
      e. Prevent excessive coughing.
      f. Avoid clustering nursing care activities together.
   6. Prevent complications of immobility.
   7. Administer medications as ordered.
      a. Hyperosmotic agents (mannitol [Osmitrol]) to reduce cerebral edema; monitor urine output every hour (should increase).
      b. Corticosteroids (dexamethasone [Decadron]): anti-inflammatory effect reduces cerebral edema.
      c. Diuretics (furosemide [Lasix]) to reduce cerebral edema.
      d. Anticonvulsants (phenytoin [Dilantin]) to prevent seizures.
      e. Analgesics for headache as needed
         1) small doses of codeine
         2) stronger opiates are contraindicated since they potentiate respiratory depression, alter LOC, and cause pupillary changes.
   8. Assist with ICP monitoring when indicated.
      a. *Ventriculostomy:* insertion of catheter into lateral ventricle for monitoring ICP/removing CSF

b. Monitoring devices in subarachnoid, epidural, or subdural spaces

c. Normal pressure: 5–10 mm Hg

Care of the Patient with Hyperthermia

A. General information

1. Abnormal elevation of body temperature to 41°C (106°F) or above
2. Caused by dysfunction of hypothalamus (temperature regulating center) from edema, head injury, hemorrhage, CVA, brain tumor, or intracranial surgery
3. Hyperthermia increases cerebral metabolism; predisposes to seizures; may cause neurologic damage if prolonged.

B. Nursing care

1. Remove blankets and excess clothing if temperature rises above 38.4°C (101°F)
2. Maintain room temperature at 21.1°C (70°F)
3. Administer antipyretic drugs (aspirin, acetaminophen [Tylenol]) orally or rectally every 4 hours as ordered
4. Increase fluid intake to 3000 cc/day unless contraindicated (in increased ICP).
5. Monitor vital signs, especially temperature, every 2–4 hours (more often if hypothermia is used).
6. Monitor urine output and assess for signs of dehydration.
7. Observe for seizure activity and protect patient if seizures occur.
8. Change linen frequently if patient is diaphoretic (sweating profusely).
9. Apply methods for inducing hypothermia as ordered: cool or tepid sponge baths, fans, ice bags, hypothermia blanket.
10. Provide special care for the patient with a hypothermia blanket.
    a. Reduce temperature gradually to prevent shivering and serious arrhythmias; chlorpromazine (Thorazine) may be given for shivering.
    b. Provide frequent skin care to prevent breakdown.
       1) check every hour for signs of tissue damage or frostbite.
       2) apply lotion to skin to prevent drying.
       3) turn every 2 hours.
    c. Monitor temperature with rectal probe.

Removal of Foreign Body from Eye

A. Instruct patient to look upward.
B. Evert lower lid to expose the conjunctival sac.
C. Gently remove the particle with a cotton applicator dipped in sterile normal saline using a twisting motion
D. If particle is not found, examine the upper lid.
E. Place cotton applicator stick or tongue blade horizontally on outer surface of upper lid; grasp upper eyelashes with fingers of other hand and pull the upper lid outward and upward over the cotton stick.
F. Gently remove the particle as above.

Irrigation of the Ear

A. Introduction of fluid into external auditory canal for cleansing purposes; may be used to apply antiseptic solutions.
B. Nursing care

1. Explain procedure to the patient.
2. Prepare supplies needed: irrigating solution (about 500 cc normal saline at body temperature), irrigating syringe, basin, towel, cotton-tipped applicators, cotton balls.
3. Assist patient to a sitting or lying position with head tilted toward the affected ear.
4. Straighten ear canal by pulling auricle upward and backward (down and forward on a child).
5. Insert tip of syringe into auditory meatus and direct the solution gently upward toward the top of the canal.
6. Collect returning fluid in basin.
7. Dry the outer ear with cotton balls.
8. Instruct patient to lie on affected side to encourage drainage of solution.
9. Record the procedure and results.

EVALUATION

A. Patient's breath sounds are clear and respiratory function adequate.
B. Patient is well nourished; has regular bowel movements.
C. Patient has adequate patterns of urinary elimination.
D. Patient communicates effectively, responds appropriately to others.
E. No contractures or limitations on motor function have occurred or loss of motor function has been kept to a minimum.
F. Sensory dysfunction is corrected or compensated for.
G. Patient experiences satisfying sexual activity/expression.
H. Patient is oriented to time, place, and person; able to evaluate reality.
I. Cerebral perfusion is improved.

DISORDERS OF THE NERVOUS SYSTEM

Headache

A. General information

1. Diffuse pain in different parts of the head
2. Types
   a. Functional
      1) tension (muscle contraction): associated with tension or anxiety
      2) migraine: recurrent throbbing headache
         a) often starts in adolescence
         b) affects women more than men
         c) vascular origin: vasoconstriction or spasm of cerebral blood vessels (producing an aura) then vasodilation

3) cluster: similar to migraine (vascular origin); recur several times a day over a period of weeks followed by remission lasting for weeks or months

b. Organic: secondary to intracranial or systemic disease (e.g., brain tumor, sinus disease)

B. Assessment findings

1. Tension headache: pain usually bilateral, often occurring in the back of the neck and extending diffusely over top of head

2. Migraine headache: severe, throbbing pain, often in temporal or supraorbital area, lasting several hours to days; may be an aura (e.g., visual disturbance) preceding the pain; nausea and vomiting; pallor; sweating; irritability

3. Cluster headache: intense, throbbing pain, usually affecting only one side of face and head; abrupt onset, lasts 30–90 minutes; eye and nose water on side of pain; skin reddens

4. Diagnostic tests may be used to rule out organic causes.

C. Nursing interventions

1. Carefully assess details regarding the headache.

2. Provide quiet, dark environment.

3. Administer medications as ordered.

   a. Symptomatic during acute attack

      1) nonnarcotic analgesics (aspirin, acetaminophen [Tylenol])

      2) Fiorinal (analgesic-sedative/tranquilizer combination)

      3) for migraines, ergotamine tartate (Gynergen) or ergotamine with caffeine (Cafergot); vasoconstrictors given during aura may prevent the headache

      4) Midrin (vasoconstrictor and sedative)

   b. Prophylactic to prevent migraine attacks

      1) methysergide maleate (Sansert): after 6 months' use, drug should be discontinued for a 2-month period before resuming

      2) propranolol (Inderal) and amytriptyline (Elavil): have also been used in migraine prevention

4. Provide additional nursing interventions for pain (see page 19).

5. Provide patient teaching and discharge planning concerning

   a. Identification of factors that appear to precipitate attacks

   b. Examination of life-style, identification of stressors, and development of more positive coping behaviors

   c. Importance of daily exercise and relaxation periods

   d. Relaxation techniques

   e. Use and side effects of prescribed medications

   f. Alternative ways of handling the pain of headache: meditation, relaxation, self-hypnosis, yoga.

Meningitis

A. General information

1. Inflammation of the meninges of the brain and spinal cord

2. Caused by bacteria, viruses, or other microorganisms

3. May reach CNS

   a. Via the blood, CSF, lymph

   b. By direct extension from adjacent cranial structures (nasal sinuses, mastoid bone, ear, skull fracture)

   c. By oral or nasopharyngeal route

4. Most common organisms: meningococcus, pneumococcus, *H. influenzae,* streptococcus

B. Assessment findings

1. Headache, photophobia, malaise, irritability

2. Chills and fever

3. Signs of meningeal irritation

   a. Nuchal rigidity: stiff neck

   b. *Kernig's sign:* contraction or pain in the hamstring muscle when attempting to extend the leg when the hip is flexed

4. *Brudzinski's sign:* flexion at the hip and knee in response to forward flexion of the neck

5. Vomiting

6. Possible seizures and decreasing LOC

7. Diagnostic test: lumbar puncture (measurement and analysis of CSF shows increased pressure, elevated WBC and protein, decreased glucose and culture positive for specific microorganism)

C. Nursing interventions

1. Administer large doses of antibiotics IV as ordered.

2. Enforce strict isolation for 24–48 hours after initiation of antibiotic therapy.

3. Provide nursing care for increased ICP, seizures, and hyperthermia if they occur.

4. Provide nursing care for delirious or unconscious patient as needed.

5. Provide bedrest; keep room quiet and dark if patient has headache or photophobia.

6. Administer analgesics for headache as ordered.

7. Maintain fluid and electrolyte balance.

8. Prevent complications of immobility.

9. Monitor vital signs and neuro checks frequently.

10. Provide patient teaching and discharge planning concerning

   a. Importance of good diet: high protein, high calorie with small, frequent feedings

   b. Rehabilitation program for residual deficits.

Encephalitis

A. General information

1. Inflammation of the brain usually caused by a virus

2. May occur as a sequela of other diseases such as measles, mumps, chickenpox.

B. Assessment findings

1. Headache

2. Fever, chills, vomiting

3. Signs of meningeal irritation

4. Possibly seizures

5. Alterations in LOC

C. Nursing interventions

1. Monitor vital signs and neuro checks frequently.

2. Administer antibiotics as ordered.

3. Provide nursing measures for increased ICP, seizures, hyperthermia if they occur.

4. Provide nursing care for confused or unconscious patient as needed.

5. Provide patient teaching and discharge planning: same as for Meningitis.

Brain Abscess

A. General information
  1. Collection of free or encapsulated pus within the brain tissue
  2. Usually follows an infectious process elsewhere in the body (ear, sinuses, mastoid bone).

B. Assessment findings
  1. Headache, malaise, anorexia
  2. Vomiting
  3. Signs of increased ICP
  4. Focal neurologic deficits (hemiparesis, seizures)

C. Nursing interventions
  1. Administer large doses of antibiotics as ordered.
  2. Monitor vital signs and neuro checks.
  3. Provide symptomatic and supportive care.
  4. Prepare patient for surgery if indicated (see Craniotomy, page 58).

Brain Tumors

A. General information
  1. Tumor within the cranial cavity; may be benign or malignant
  2. Types
    a. Primary: originates in brain tissue (e.g., glioma, meningioma)
    b. Secondary: metastasizes from tumor elsewhere in the body (e.g., lung, breast)

B. Medical management
  1. Craniotomy: to remove the tumor when possible
  2. Radiation therapy and chemotherapy: may follow surgery; also for inaccessible tumors and metastatic tumors
  3. Drug therapy: hyperosmotic agents, corticosteroids, diuretics to manage increased ICP

C. Assessment findings
  1. Headache: worse in the morning and with straining and stooping
  2. Vomiting
  3. Papilledema
  4. Seizures (focal or generalized)
  5. Changes in mental status
  6. Focal neurologic deficits (e.g., aphasia, hemiparesis, sensory problems)
  7. Diagnostic tests
    a. Skull x-ray, CT scan, brain scan: reveal presence of tumor
    b. Abnormal EEG

D. Nursing interventions
  1. Monitor vital signs and neuro checks; observe for signs and symptoms of increased ICP.
  2. Administer medications as ordered.
    a. Drugs to decrease ICP

b. Anticonvulsants
    c. Analgesics for headache
  3. Provide supportive care for any neurologic deficit (see Cerebrovascular Accident).
  4. Prepare patient for surgery (see Craniotomy, page 58).
  5. Provide care for effects of radiation therapy or chemotherapy (see Cancer Nursing, page 36).
  6. Provide psychologic support to patient/family.
  7. Provide patient teaching and discharge planning concerning
    a. Use and side effects of prescribed medications
    b. Rehabilitation program for residual deficits.

Cerebrovascular Accident (CVA)

A. General information
  1. Destruction (infarction) of brain cells caused by a reduction in cerebral blood flow and oxygen
  2. Affects men more than women; incidence increases with age
  3. Caused by thrombosis, embolism, hemorrhage
  4. Risk factors
    a. Hypertension, diabetes mellitus, arteriosclerosis/atherosclerosis, cardiac disease (valvular disease/replacement, chronic atrial fibrillation, myocardial infarction)
    b. Life-style: obesity, smoking, inactivity, stress, use of oral contraceptives
  5. Pathophysiology
    a. Interruption of cerebral blood flow for 5 minutes or more causes death of neurons in affected area with irreversible loss of function
    b. Modifying factors
      1) cerebral edema: develops around affected area causing further impairment
      2) vasospasm: constriction of cerebral blood vessel may occur causing further decrease in blood flow
      3) collateral circulation: may help to maintain cerebral blood flow when there is compromise of main blood supply
  6. Stages of development
    a. *Transient ischemic attack (TIA)*
      1) warning sign of impending CVA
      2) brief period of neurologic deficit: visual loss, hemiparesis, slurred speech, aphasia, vertigo
      3) may last less than 30 seconds, but no more than 24 hours with complete resolution of symptoms
    b. *Stroke in evolution:* progressive development of stroke symptoms over a period of hours to days
    c. *Completed stroke:* neurologic deficit remains unchanged for a 2- to 3-day period.

B. Assessment findings
  1. Headache
  2. Generalized signs: vomiting, seizures, confusion, disorientation, decreased LOC, nuchal rigidity, fever, hypertension, slow bounding pulse, Cheyne-Stokes respirations

3. Focal signs (related to site of infarction): hemiplegia, sensory loss, aphasia, homonymous hemianopsia

4. Diagnostic tests

    a. CT and brain scan: reveal lesion

    b. EEG: abnormal changes

    c. Cerebral arteriography: may show occlusion or malformation of blood vessels

C. Nursing interventions: acute stage

    1. Maintain patent airway and adequate ventilation.

    2. Monitor vital signs and neuro checks and observe for signs of increased ICP, shock, hyperthermia, and seizures.

    3. Provide complete bedrest as ordered.

    4. Maintain fluid and electrolyte balance and ensure adequate nutrition.

        a. IV therapy for the first few days

        b. Nasogastric tube feedings if patient unable to swallow

        c. Fluid restriction as ordered to decrease cerebral edema

    5. Maintain proper positioning and body alignment.

        a. Head of bed may be elevated 30°–45° to decrease ICP

        b. Turn and reposition every 2 hours (only 20 minutes on the affected side)

        c. Passive ROM exercises every 4 hours.

    6. Promote optimum skin integrity: turn patient and apply lotion every 2 hours

    7. Maintain adequate elimination.

        a. Offer bedpan or urinal every 2 hours, catheterize only if absolutely necessary.

        b. Administer stool softeners and suppositories as ordered to prevent constipation and fecal impaction.

    8. Provide a quiet, restful environment.

    9. Establish a means of communicating with the patient.

    10. Administer medications as ordered.

        a. Hyperosmotic agents, corticosteroids to decrease cerebral edema

        b. Anticonvulsants to prevent or treat seizures

        c. Anticoagulants for stroke in evolution or embolic stroke (hemorrhage must be ruled out)

            1) heparin

            2) warfarin (Coumadin) for long-term therapy

            3) aspirin and dipyridamole (Persantine) to inhibit platelet aggregation in treating TIAs

        d. Antihypertensives if indicated for elevated blood pressure.

D. Nursing interventions: rehabilitation

    1. *Hemiplegia:* results from injury to cells in the cerebral motor cortex or to corticospinal tracts (causes contralateral hemiplegia since tracts cross in medulla)

        a. Turn every 2 hours (20 minutes only on affected side).

        b. Use proper positioning and repositioning to prevent deformities (foot drop, external rotation of hip, flexion of fingers, wrist drop, abduction of shoulder and arm).

        c. Support paralyzed arm on pillow or use sling while out of bed to prevent subluxation of shoulder.

        d. Elevate extremities to prevent dependent edema.

        e. Provide active and passive ROM exercises every 4 hours.

    2. Susceptibility to hazards

        a. Keep side rails up at all times.

        b. Institute safety measures.

        c. Inspect body parts frequently for signs of injury.

    3. *Dysphagia* (difficulty swallowing)

        a. Check gag reflex before feeding patient.

        b. Maintain a calm, unhurried approach.

        c. Place patient in upright position.

        d. Place food in unaffected side of mouth.

        e. Offer soft foods.

        f. Give mouth care before and after meals.

    4. *Homonymous hemianopsia:* loss of half of each visual field

        a. Approach patient on unaffected side.

        b. Place personal belongings, food, etc., on unaffected side.

        c. Gradually teach patient to compensate by scanning, i.e., turning the head to see things on affected side.

    5. Emotional lability: mood swings, frustration

        a. Create a quiet, restful environment with a reduction in excessive sensory stimuli.

        b. Maintain a calm, nonthreatening manner.

        c. Explain to family that the patient's behavior is not purposeful.

    6. *Aphasia:* most common in right hemiplegics; may be receptive/expressive

        a. Receptive aphasia

            1) give simple, slow directions.

            2) give one command at a time; gradually shift topics.

            3) use nonverbal techniques of communication (e.g., pantomime, demonstration).

        b. Expressive aphasia

            1) listen and watch very carefully when the patient attempts to speak.

            2) anticipate patient's needs to decrease frustration and feelings of helplessness.

            3) allow sufficient time for patient to answer.

    7. *Sensory/perceptual deficits:* more common in left hemiplegics; characterized by impulsiveness, unawareness of disabilities, visual neglect (neglect of affected side and visual space on affected side)

        a. Assist with self-care.

        b. Provide safety measures.

        c. Initially arrange objects in environment on unaffected side.

        d. Gradually teach patient to take care of the affected side and to turn frequently and look at affected side.

    8. *Apraxia:* loss of ability to perform purposeful, skilled acts

        a. Guide patient through intended movement (e.g., take object such as washcloth and guide patient through movement of washing).

        b. Keep repeating the movement.

Cerebral Aneurysm

A. General information

    1. Dilation of the walls of a cerebral artery, resulting in a saclike, outpouching of vessel

2. Caused by congenital weakness in the vessel, trauma, arteriosclerosis, hypertension
3. Pathophysiology
  a. Aneurysm compresses nearby cranial nerves or brain substance producing dysfunction
  b. Aneurysm may rupture, causing subarachnoid hemorrhage or intracerebral hemorrhage
  c. Initially a clot forms at the site of rupture, but fibrinolysis (dissolution of the clot) tends to occur within 7–10 days and may cause rebleeding.
B. Assessment findings
  1. Severe headache and pain in the eyes
  2. Diplopia, tinnitus, dizziness
  3. Nuchal rigidity, ptosis, decreasing LOC, hemiparesis, seizures
C. Nursing interventions
  1. Maintain a patent airway and adequate ventilation.
    a. Instruct patient to take deep breaths, but to avoid coughing.
    b. Suction only with a specific order.
  2. Monitor vital signs and neuro checks and observe for signs of vasospasm, increased ICP, hypertension, seizures, and hyperthermia.
  3. Enforce strict bedrest and provide complete care.
  4. Keep head of bed flat or elevated to 20°–30° as ordered.
  5. Maintain a quiet, darkened environment.
  6. Avoid taking temperature rectally and instruct patient to avoid sneezing, coughing, and straining at stool.
  7. Enforce fluid restriction as ordered; maintain accurate I&O.
  8. Administer medications as ordered.
    a. Antihypertensive agents to maintain normotensive levels
    b. Corticosteroids to prevent increased ICP
    c. Anticonvulsants to prevent seizures
    d. Stool softeners to prevent straining
    e. Aminocaproic acid (Amicar) to decrease fibrinolysis of the clot (administered IV).
  9. Prevent complications of immobility.
  10. Institute seizure precautions.
  11. Provide nursing care for the unconscious patient if needed.
  12. Prepare the patient for surgery if indicated (see Craniotomy, page 58).

Parkinson's Disease

A. General information
  1. A progressive disorder with degeneration of the nerve cells in the basal ganglia resulting in generalized decline in muscular function; disorder of the extrapyramidal system
  2. Usually occurs in the older population
  3. Cause unknown; predominantly idiopathic, but sometimes disorder is postencephalitic, toxic, arteriosclerotic, traumatic, or drug-induced (reserpine, methyldopa [Aldomet], haloperidol [Haldol], phenothiazines)
  4. Pathophysiology
    a. Disorder causes degeneration of the dopamine-producing neurons in the substantia nigra in the midbrain
    b. Dopamine influences purposeful movement
    c. Depletion of dopamine results in degeneration of the basal ganglia.
B. Assessment findings
  1. Tremor: mainly of the upper limbs, "pill-rolling," resting tremor; most common initial symptom
  2. Rigidity: cogwheel type
  3. Bradykinesia: slowness of movement
  4. Fatigue
  5. Stooped posture; shuffling, propulsive gait
  6. Difficulty rising from sitting position
  7. Masklike face with decreased blinking of eyes
  8. Quiet, monotone speech
  9. Emotional lability, depression
  10. Increased salivation, drooling
  11. Cramped, small handwriting
  12. Autonomic symptoms: excessive sweating, seborrhea, lacrimation, constipation; decreased sexual capacity
C. Nursing interventions
  1. Administer medications as ordered
    a. Levodopa (L-dopa)
      1) increases level of dopamine in the brain; relieves tremor, rigidity, and bradykinesia
      2) side effects: anorexia; nausea and vomiting; postural hypotension; mental changes such as confusion, agitation, and hallucinations; cardiac arrhythmias; dyskinesias.
      3) contraindications: narrow-angle glaucoma; patients taking MAO inhibitors, reserpine, guanethidine, methyldopa, antipsychotics; acute psychoses.
      4) avoid multiple vitamin preparations containing vitamin B_6 (pyridoxine) and foods high in vitamin B_6.
      5) be aware of any worsening of symptoms with prolonged high-dose therapy: "on-off" syndrome.
      6) administer with food or snack to decrease GI irritation.
      7) inform patient that urine and sweat may be darkened.
    b. Carbidopa-levodopa (Sinemet): prevents breakdown of dopamine in the periphery and causes fewer side effects.
    c. Amantadine (Symmetrel): used in mild cases or in combination with L-dopa.
    d. Anticholinergic drugs: benztropine mesylate (Cogentin), procyclidine (Kemadrin), trihexyphenidyl (Artane)
      1) inhibit action of acetylcholine
      2) used in mild cases or in combination with L-dopa
      3) relieve tremor and rigidity
      4) side effects: dry mouth, blurred vision, constipation, urinary retention, confusion, hallucinations, tachycardia
    e. Antihistamines: diphenhydramine (Benadryl)
      1) decrease tremor and anxiety
      2) side effect: drowsiness

f. Bromocriptine (Parlodel)
  1) stimulates release of dopamine in the substantia nigra.
  2) often employed when L-dopa loses effectiveness.
2. Provide a safe environment.
  a. Side rails on bed; rails and handlebars in toilet, bathtub, and hallways; no scatter rugs
  b. Hard-back or spring-loaded chair to make getting up easier
3. Provide measures to increase mobility.
  a. Physical therapy: active and passive ROM exercises; stretching exercises; warm baths
  b. Assistive devices
  c. If patient "freezes," suggest thinking of something to walk over.
4. Encourage independence in self-care activities: alter clothing for ease in dressing; use assistive devices; do not rush patient.
5. Improve communication abilities: instruct patient to practice reading aloud, to listen to own voice, and enunciate each syllable clearly.
6. Refer for speech therapy when indicated.
7. Maintain adequate nutrition.
  a. Cut food into bite-sized pieces.
  b. Provide small, frequent feedings.
  c. Allow sufficient time for meals, use warming tray.
8. Avoid constipation and maintain adequate bowel elimination.
9. Provide psychologic support to patient/family; depression is common due to changes in body-image and self-concept.
10. Provide patient teaching and discharge planning concerning
  a. Nature of the disease
  b. Use of prescribed medications and side effects
  c. Importance of daily exercise: walking, swimming, gardening as tolerated; balanced activity and rest
  d. Activities/methods to limit postural deformities: firm mattress with a small pillow; keep head and neck as erect as possible; use broad-based gait; raise feet while walking
  e. Promotion of active participation in self-care activities.

Multiple Sclerosis (MS)

A. General information
  1. Chronic, intermittently progressive disease of the CNS, characterized by scattered patches of demyelination within the brain and spinal cord
  2. Incidence
    a. Affects women more than men
    b. Usually occurs from 20–40 years of age
    c. More frequent in cool or temperate climates
  3. Cause unknown; may be a slow-growing virus or possibly of autoimmune origin
  4. Signs and symptoms are varied and multiple, reflecting the location of demyelination within the CNS
  5. Characterized by remissions and exacerbations
B. Assessment findings

1. Visual disturbances: blurred vision, scotomas (blind spots), diplopia
2. Impaired sensation: touch, pain, temperature, or position sense; paresthesias such as numbness, tingling
3. Euphoria or mood swings
4. Impaired motor function: weakness, paralysis, spasticity
5. Impaired cerebellar function: scanning speech, ataxic gait, nystagmus, dysarthria, intention tremor
6. Bladder: retention or incontinence
7. Constipation
8. Sexual impotence in the male
9. Diagnostic tests: supportive only; MS is clinically diagnosed by two separate episodes with history of exacerbation and remission
  a. CSF studies: increased protein and IgG (immunoglobulin)
  b. Visual evoked response (VER) determined by EEG: may be delayed
  c. CT scan: increased density of white matter
  d. MRI: shows areas of demyelination
C. Nursing interventions
  1. Assess the patient for specific deficits related to location of demyelinization.
  2. Promote optimum mobility.
    a. Muscle-stretching and strengthening exercises
    b. Walking exercises to improve gait: use wide-based gait
    c. Assistive devices: canes, walker, rails, wheelchair as necessary
  3. Administer medications as ordered.
    a. For acute exacerbations: corticosteroids (ACTH [IV], prednisone) to reduce edema at sites of demyelinization
    b. For spasticity: baclofen (Lioresal), dantrolene (Dantrium), diazepam (Valium)
  4. Encourage independence in self-care activities.
  5. Prevent complications of immobility.
  6. Maintain bowel elimination.
  7. Maintain urinary elimination.
    a. Urinary retention
      1) administer bethanecol choride (Urecholine) as ordered.
      2) perform intermittent catheterization as ordered.
      3) use Credé maneuver or reflex stimulation.
    b. Urinary incontinence
      1) establish voiding schedule.
      2) administer propantheline bromide (Pro-Banthine) if ordered.
    c. Force fluids to 3000 cc/day.
    d. Promote use of acid-ash foods like cranberry or grape juice.
  8. Prevent injury related to sensory problems.
    a. Test bath water with thermometer.
    b. Avoid heating pads, hot-water bottles.
    c. Inspect body parts frequently for injury.
    d. Make frequent position changes.
  9. Prepare patient for plasmapheresis (plasma exchange to remove antibodies) if indicated.

10. Provide psychologic support to patient/family.
    a. Encourage positive attitude and assist patient in setting realistic goals.
    b. Provide compassion in helping patient adapt to changes in body image and self-concept.
    c. Do not encourage false hopes during remission.
    d. Refer to MS societies and community agencies.
11. Provide patient teaching and discharge planning concerning
    a. General measures to ensure optimum health
       1) balance between activity and rest
       2) regular exercise such as walking, swimming, biking in mild cases
       3) use of energy conservation techniques
       4) well-balanced diet
       5) fresh air and sunshine
       6) avoiding fatigue, overheating or chilling, stress, infection
    b. Use of medications and side effects
    c. Alternative methods for sexual gratification; refer for sexual counseling if indicated.

Myasthenia Gravis

A. General information
   1. A neuromuscular disorder in which there is a disturbance in the transmission of nerve impulses at the myoneural junction causing extreme muscle weakness
   2. Incidence
      a. Highest between ages 20–30 for women, 60–70 for men
      b. Affects women more than men
   3. Cause unknown; may be autoimmune disorder whereby antibodies destroy acetylcholine receptor sites in the postsynaptic cleft
   4. Voluntary muscles are affected, especially those muscles innervated by the cranial nerves.
B. Medical management
   1. Drug therapy
      a. Anticholinesterase drugs: ambenonium (Mytelase), neostigmine (Prostigmin), pyridostigmine (Mestinon)
         1) block action of cholinesterase and increase levels of acetycholine at the myoneural junction
         2) side effects: excessive salivation and sweating, abdominal cramps, nausea and vomiting, diarrhea, fasciculations (muscle twitching)
      b. Corticosteroids: prednisone
         1) used if other drugs are not effective
         2) suppress autoimmune response
   2. Surgery *(thymectomy)*
      a. Surgical removal of the thymus gland
      b. Used in selected patients who do not respond to anticholinesterase drugs
   3. Plasmapheresis
      a. Removal of plasma to lower levels of circulating antibodies
      b. Used in patients who do not respond to other types of therapy

C. Assessment findings
   1. Diplopia, dysphagia
   2. Extreme muscle weakness, increased with activity and reduced with rest
   3. Ptosis, masklike facial expression
   4. Weak voice, hoarseness
   5. Diagnostic tests
      a. Tensilon test: IV injection of Tensilon provides spontaneous relief of symptoms (lasts 5–10 minutes)
      b. Electromyography (EMG): amplitude of evoked potentials decreases rapidly
D. Nursing interventions
   1. Administer anticholinesterase drugs as ordered.
      a. Give medication exactly on time.
      b. Give with milk and crackers to decrease GI upset.
      c. Monitor effectiveness of drugs: assess muscle strength and vital capacity before and after medication.
      d. Avoid use of the following drugs: morphine, quinine, curare, procainamide, neomycin, streptomycin, kanamycin and other aminoglycosides, strong sedatives.
      e. Observe for side effects.
   2. Promote optimal nutrition.
      a. Mealtimes should coincide with the peak effects of the drugs: give medications 30 minutes before meals.
      b. Check gag reflex and swallowing ability before feeding.
      c. Provide a mechanical soft diet.
      d. If the patient has difficulty chewing and swallowing, do not leave alone at mealtimes; keep emergency airway and suction equipment nearby.
   3. Monitor respiratory status frequently: rate, depth; vital capacity; ability to deep breathe and cough
   4. Assess muscle strength frequently; plan activity to take advantage of energy peaks and provide frequent rest periods.
   5. Observe for signs of myasthenic or cholinergic crisis.
      a. *Myasthenic crisis*
         1) abrupt onset of severe, generalized muscle weakness with inability to swallow, speak, or maintain respirations
         2) caused by undermedication, physical or emotional stress, infection
         3) symptoms will improve temporarily with Tensilon test.
      b. *Cholinergic crisis*
         1) symptoms similar to myasthenic crisis and in addition, the side effects of anticholinesterase drugs (e.g., excessive salivation and sweating, abdominal cramps, nausea and vomiting, diarrhea, fasciculations)
         2) caused by overmedication with the cholinergic (anticholinesterase) drugs
         3) symptoms worsen with Tensilon test; keep atropine sulfate and emergency equipment on hand.

c. Nursing care in crisis
   1) maintain tracheostomy or endotracheal tube with mechanical ventilation as indicated (see Mechanical Ventilation, page 103).
   2) monitor arterial blood gases and vital capacities.
   3) administer medications as ordered.
      a) *myasthenic crisis:* increase doses of anticholinesterase drugs as ordered.
      b) *cholinergic crisis:* discontinue anticholinesterase drugs as ordered until the patient recovers.
   4) establish a method of communication.
   5) provide support and reassurance.
6. Provide nursing care for the patient with a thymectomy.
7. Provide patient teaching and discharge planning concerning
   a. Nature of the disease
   b. Use of prescribed medications, their side effects and signs of toxicity
   c. Importance of checking with physician before taking any OTC drugs
   d. Importance of planning activities to take advantage of energy peaks and of scheduling frequent rest periods
   e. Need to avoid fatigue, stress, people with upper-respiratory infections
   f. Use of eye patch for diplopia (alternate eyes)
   g. Need to wear Medic-Alert bracelet
   h. Myasthenia Gravis Foundation and other community agencies.

Epilepsy

See Seizure Disorders, page **304**.

Head Injury

A. General information
1. Usually caused by car accidents, falls, assaults
2. Types
   a. *Concussion:* severe blow to the head jostles brain causing it to strike the skull; results in temporary neural dysfunction
   b. *Contusion:* results from more severe blow that bruises the brain and disrupts neural function
   c. Hemorrhage
      1) *epidural hematoma:* accumulation of blood between the dura mater and skull; commonly results from laceration of middle meningeal artery during skull fracture; blood accumulates rapidly
      2) *subdural hematoma:* accumulation of blood between the dura and arachnoid; venous bleeding that forms slowly; may be acute, subacute, or chronic
      3) *subarachnoid hematoma:* bleeding in subarachnoid space
      4) *intracerebral hematoma:* accumulation of blood within the cerebrum ·
   d. Fractures: linear, depressed, comminuted, compound

B. Assessment findings (depend on type of injury)
1. Concussion: headache, transient loss of consciousness, retrograde or post-traumatic amnesia, nausea, dizziness, irritability
2. Contusion: neurologic deficits depend on the site and extent of damage; include decreased LOC, aphasia, hemiplegia, sensory deficits
3. Hemorrhages
   a. Epidural hematoma: brief loss of consciousness followed by lucid interval; progresses to severe headache, vomiting, rapidly deteriorating LOC, possible seizures, ipsilateral pupillary dilation
   b. Subdural hematoma: alterations in LOC, headache, focal neurologic deficits, personality changes, ipsilateral pupillary dilation
   c. Intracerebral hematoma: headache, decreased LOC, hemiplegia, ipsilateral pupillary dilation
4. Fractures
   a. Headache, pain over fracture site
   b. Compound fractures: rhinorrhea (leakage of CSF from nose); otorrhea (leakage of CSF from ear)
5. Diagnostic tests
   a. Skull x-ray: reveals skull fracture or intracranial shift
   b. CT scan: reveals hemorrhage

C. Nursing interventions (see also Care of the Unconscious Patient [page 47] and Care of the Patient with Increased ICP [page 48])
1. Maintain a patent airway and adequate ventilation.
2. Monitor vital signs and neuro checks; observe for changes in neurologic status, signs of increased ICP, shock, seizures and hyperthermia.
3. Observe for CSF leakage.
   a. Check discharge for positive Testape reaction for glucose; bloody spot encircled by watery, pale ring.
   b. Never attempt to clean the ears or nose of a head-injured patient or use nasal suction unless cleared by physician.
4. If a CSF leak is present
   a. Instruct the patient not to blow nose.
   b. Elevate the head of bed 30° as ordered.
   c. Observe for signs of meningitis and administer antibiotics to prevent meningitis as ordered.
   d. Place a cotton ball in the ear to absorb otorrhea; replace frequently.
   e. Gently place a sterile gauze pad at the bottom of the nose for rhinorrhea; replace frequently.
5. Prevent complications of immobility.
6. Prepare the patient for surgery if indicated.
   a. Depressed skull fracture: surgical removal or elevation of splintered bone; debridement and cleansing of area; repair of dural tear if present; cranioplasty (if necessitated for large cranial defect)
   b. Epidural or subdural hematoma: evacuation of the hematoma
7. Provide psychologic support to patient/family.
8. Observe for hemiplegia, aphasia, sensory problems, and plan care accordingly (see Cerebrovascular Accident, page 51)

9. Provide patient teaching and discharge planning concerning rehabilitation for neurologic deficits; note availability of community agencies.

Spinal Cord Injuries

A. General information
1. Occurs most commonly in young adult males between ages 15 and 29
2. Common traumatic causes: motor vehicle accidents, diving in shallow water, falls, industrial accidents, sports injuries, gunshot or stab wounds
3. Nontraumatic causes: tumors, hematomas, aneurysms, congenital defects (spina bifida)
4. Classified by extent, level, and mechanism of injury
   a. Extent of injury
      1) may affect the vertebral column: fracture, fracture/dislocation
      2) may affect anterior or posterior ligaments, causing compression of spinal cord
      3) may be to the spinal cord and its roots: concussion, contusion, compression or laceration by fracture/dislocation or penetrating missiles
   b. Level of injury: cervical, thoracic, lumbar
   c. Mechanism of injury
      1) hyperflexion
      2) hyperextension
      3) axial loading (force exerted straight up or down spinal column as in a diving accident)
      4) penetrating wounds
5. Pathophysiology: hemorrhage and edema cause ischemia, leading to necrosis and destruction of the cord
B. Medical management: immobilization and maintenance of normal spinal alignment to promote fracture healing
1. Horizontal turning frames (Stryker frame)
2. Skeletal traction: to immobilize the fracture and maintain alignment of the cervical spine
   a. *Cervical tongs (Crutchfield, Gardner-Wells, Vinke)*: inserted through burr holes; traction is provided by a rope extended from the center of tongs over a pully with weights attached at the end
   b. *Halo traction*
      1) stainless steel halo ring fits around the head and is attached to the skull with four pins; halo is attached to plastic body cast or plastic vest
      2) permits early mobilization, decreased period of hospitalization and reduces complications of immobility
3. Surgery: decompression laminectomy, spinal fusion
   a. Depends on type of injury and the preference of the surgeon
   b. Indications: unstable fracture, cord compression, progression of neurologic deficits
C. Assessment findings
1. Spinal shock
   a. Occurs immediately after the injury as a result of the insult to the CNS

b. Temporary condition lasting from several days to three months
c. Characterized by absence of reflexes below the level of the lesion, flaccid paralysis, lack of temperature control in affected parts, hypotension with bradycardia, retention of urine and feces
2. Symptoms depend on the level and the extent of the injury.
   a. Level of injury
      1) *quadriplegia:* cervical injuries (C_1–C_8) cause paralysis of all four extremities; respiratory paralysis occurs in lesions above C_4 due to lack of innervation to the diaphragm.
      2) *paraplegia:* thoraco/lumbar injuries (T_1–L_4) cause paralysis of the lower half of the body involving both legs.
   b. Extent of injury
      1) complete cord transection
         a) loss of all voluntary movement and sensation below the level of the injury; reflex activity below the level of the lesion may return after spinal shock resolves.
         b) lesions in the conus medullaris or cauda equina result in permanent flaccid paralysis and areflexia.
      2) incomplete lesions: varying degrees of motor or sensory loss below the level of the lesion depending on which neurologic tracts are damaged and which are spared.
3. Diagnostic test: spinal x-rays may reveal fracture.
D. Nursing interventions: emergency care
1. Assess airway, breathing, circulation
   a. Do not move the patient during assessment.
   b. If airway obstruction or inadequate ventilation exists: do not hyperextend neck to open airway, use jaw thrust instead.
2. Perform a quick head-to-toe assessment: check for LOC, signs of trauma to the head or neck, leakage of clear fluid from ears or nose, signs of motor or sensory impairment.
3. Immobilize the patient in the position found until help arrives.
4. Once emergency help arrives, assist in immobilizing the head and neck with a cervical collar and place the patient on a spinal board; avoid any movement during transfer, especially flexion of the spinal column.
5. Have suction available to clear the airway and prevent aspiration if the patient vomits; patient may be turned slightly to the side if secured to a board.
6. Evaluate respiration and observe for weak or labored respirations.
E. Nursing interventions: acute care
1. Maintain optimum respiratory function.
   a. Observe for weak or labored respirations; monitor arterial blood gases.
   b. Prevent pneumonia and atelectasis: turn every 2 hours; cough and deep breathe every hour; use incentive spirometry every 2 hours.

   c. Tracheostomy and mechanical ventilation may be necessary if respiratory insufficiency occurs.

2. Maintain optimal cardiovascular function.
   a. Monitor vital signs; observe for bradycardia, arrhythmias, hypotension.
   b. Apply thigh-high elastic stockings or Ace bandages.
   c. Change position slowly and gradually elevate the head of the bed to prevent postural hypotension.
   d. Observe for signs of thrombophlebitis.

3. Maintain fluid and electrolyte balance and nutrition.
   a. Nasogastric tube may be inserted until bowel sounds return.
   b. Maintain IV therapy as ordered; avoid overhydration (can aggravate cord edema).
   c. Check bowel sounds before feeding patient (paralytic ileus is common).
   d. Progress slowly from clear liquid to regular diet.
   e. Provide diet high in protein, carbohydrates, calories.

4. Maintain immobilization and spinal alignment always.
   a. Turn every hour on turning frame.
   b. Maintain cervical traction at all times if indicated.

5. Prevent complications of immobility; use footboard/high-topped sneakers to prevent foot drop; provide splint for quadriplegic patient to prevent wrist drop.

6. Maintain urinary elimination.
   a. Provide intermittent catheterization or maintain indwelling catheter as ordered.
   b. Increase fluids to 3000 cc/day.
   c. Provide acid-ash foods/fluids to acidify urine and prevent infection.

7. Maintain bowel elimination: administer stool softeners and suppositories to prevent impaction as ordered.

8. Monitor temperature control.
   a. Check temperature every 4 hours.
   b. Regulate environment closely.
   c. Avoid excessive covering or exposure.

9. Observe for and prevent infection.
   a. Observe tongs or pin site for redness, drainage.
   b. Provide tong- or pin-site care.
   c. Observe for signs of respiratory or urinary infection.

10. Observe for and prevent stress ulcers.
   a. Assess for epigastic or shoulder pain.
   b. If corticosteroids are ordered, give with food or antacids; administer cimetidine (Tagamet) as ordered.
   c. check nasogastric tube contents and stools for blood.

F. Nursing interventions: chronic care
1. *Neurogenic bladder*
   a. Reflex or upper motor neuron bladder: reflex activity of the bladder may occur after spinal shock resolves; the bladder is unable to store urine very long and empties involuntarily
   b. Nonreflexic or lower motor neuron bladder: reflex arc is disrupted and no reflex activity of the bladder occurs, resulting in urine retention with overflow
   c. Management of reflex bladder
     1) intermittent catheterization every 4 hours and gradually progress to every 6 hours.

     2) regulate fluid intake to 1800–2000 cc/day.
     3) bladder taps or stimulating trigger points to cause reflex emptying of the bladder.
   d. Management of nonreflexic bladder
     1) intermittent catheterization every 6 hours.
     2) Credé maneuver or rectal stretch.
     3) regulate intake to 1800–2000 cc/day to prevent overdistension of bladder.
   e. Management depends on life-style, age, sex, home care, and availability of care giver.

2. *Spasticity*
   a. Return of reflex activity may occur after spinal shock resolves; severe spasticity may be detrimental
   b. Drug therapy: baclofen (Lioresal), dantrolene (Dantrium), diazepam (Valium)
   c. Physical therapy: stretching exercises, warm tub baths, whirlpool
   d. Surgery: chordotomy

3. *Autonomic dysreflexia*
   a. Rise in blood pressure, sometimes to fatal levels
   b. Reflex response to stimulation of the sympathetic nervous system
   c. Stimulus may be overdistended bladder or bowel, decubitus ulcer, chilling, pressure from bedclothes
   d. Symptoms: severe headache, hypertension, bradycardia, sweating, goose bumps, nasal congestion, blurred vision, convulsions
   e. Interventions
     1) raise patient to sitting position.
     2) check for source of stimulus (bladder, bowel, skin).
     3) remove offending stimulus (e.g., catheterize patient, digitally remove impacted feces, reposition patient).
     4) monitor blood pressure.
     5) administer antihypertensives (hydralazine HCl [Apresoline], diazoxide [Hyperstat]) as ordered.

G. Nursing interventions: general rehabilitative care
1. Provide psychologic support to patient/family.
   a. Support during grieving process.
   b. Assist patient to adjust to effects of injury.
   c. Encourage independence.
   d. Involve the patient in decision making.

2. Provide sexual counseling.
   a. Work with the patient and partner.
   b. Explore alternative methods of sexual gratification.

3. Initiate rehabilitation program.
   a. Physical therapy
   b. Vocational rehabilitation
   c. Psychologic counseling
   d. Use of braces, electronic wheelchair, and other assistance devices to maximize independence.

Intracranial Surgery

A. Types
1. *Craniotomy:* surgical opening of skull to gain access to intracranial structures; used to remove a tumor, evacuate

blood clot, control hemorrhage, relieve increased ICP
2. *Craniectomy:* excision of a portion of the skull; sometimes used for decompression
3. *Cranioplasty:* repair of a cranial defect with a metal or plastic plate
B. Nursing interventions: preoperative
1. Routine pre-op care (see Perioperative Nursing, page 30).
2. Provide emotional support; explain post-op procedures and that patient's head will be shaved, there will be a large bandage on head, possibly temporary swelling and discoloration around the eye on the affected side, and possible headache.
3. Shampoo the scalp and check for signs of infection.
4. Save hair.
5. Evaluate and record baseline vital signs and neuro checks.
6. Avoid enemas unless directed (straining increases ICP).
7. Give pre-op steroids as ordered to decrease brain swelling.
8. Insert Foley catheter as ordered.
C. Nursing interventions: postoperative
1. Provide nursing care for the unconscious patient (page 47).
2. Maintain a patent airway and adequate ventilation.
   a. Supratentorial incision: elevate head of bed 15°–45° as ordered; position on back (if intubated or conscious) or on unaffected side; turn every 2 hours to facilitate breathing and venous return.
   b. Infratentorial incision: keep head of bed flat or elevate 20°–30° as ordered; do not flex head on chest; turn side to side every 2 hours using a turning sheet; check respirations closely and report any signs of respiratory distress.
   c. Instruct the conscious patient to breathe deeply but not to cough; avoid vigorous suctioning.
3. Check vital signs and neuro checks frequently; observe for decreasing LOC, increased ICP, seizures, hyperthermia.
4. Monitor fluid and electrolyte status.
   a. Maintain accurate I&O.
   b. Restrict fluids to 1500 cc/day or as ordered to decrease cerebral edema.
   c. Avoid overly rapid infusions.
   d. Watch for signs of diabetes insipidus (severe thirst, polyuria, dehydration) and inappropriate ADH secretion (decreased urine output, hunger, thirst, irritability, decreased LOC, muscle weakness).
   e. For infratentorial surgery: may be NPO for 24 hours due to possible impaired swallowing and gag reflexes.
5. Assess dressings frequently and report any abnormalities.
   a. Reinforce as needed with sterile dressings.
   b. Check dressings for excessive drainage, CSF, infection, displacement and report to physician.
   c. If surgical drain is in place, note color, amount, and odor of drainage.
6. Administer medications as ordered.
   a. Corticosteroids: to decrease cerebral edema
   b. Anticonvulsants: to prevent seizures
   c. Stool softeners: to prevent straining
   d. Mild analgesics
7. Apply ice to swollen eyelids; lubricate lids and areas around eyes with petrolatum jelly.
8. Refer patient for rehabilitation for residual deficits.

Specific Disorders of the Peripheral Nervous System

Trigeminal Neuralgia (Tic Douloureux)
A. General information
1. Disorder of cranial nerve V causing disabling and recurring attacks of severe pain along the sensory distribution of one or more branches of the trigeminal nerve
2. Incidence increased in elderly women
3. Cause unknown
B. Medical management
1. Anticonvulsant drugs: carbamazepine (Tegretol), phenytoin (Dilantin)
2. Nerve block: injection of alcohol or phenol into one or more branches of the trigeminal nerve; temporary effect, lasts 6–18 months
3. Surgery
   a. Peripheral: avulsion of peripheral branches of trigeminal nerve
   b. Intracranial
      1) craniotomy: division of the sensory root of the trigeminal nerve intracranially; results in permanent anesthesia, numbness, heaviness, and stiffness in affected part; loss of corneal reflex
      2) microsurgery: uses more precise cutting and may preserve sensation and corneal reflex
      3) percutaneous radiofrequency rhizotomy: placement of needle in trigeminal rootlets and destruction of the area by means of radio frequency; produces permanent numbness; may preserve sensation and corneal reflex.
C. Assessment findings
1. Sudden paroxysms of extremely severe shooting pain in one side of the face
2. Attacks may be triggered by a cold breeze, foods/fluids of extreme temperature, toothbrushing, chewing, talking, or touching the face
3. During attack: twitching, grimacing, and frequent blinking/tearing of the eye
4. Poor eating and hygiene habits
5. Withdrawal from interactions with others
6. Diagnostic tests: x-rays of the skull, teeth, and sinuses may identify dental or sinus infection as an aggravating factor.
D. Nursing interventions
1. Assess characteristics of the pain including triggering factors, trigger points, and pain management techniques.

2. Administer medications as ordered; monitor response.
3. Maintain room at an even, moderate temperature, free from drafts.
4. Provide small, frequent feedings of lukewarm, semiliquid, or soft foods that are easily chewed.
5. Provide the patient with a soft washcloth and lukewarm water and perform hygiene during periods when pain is decreased.
6. Prepare the patient for surgery if indicated.
7. Provide patient teaching and discharge planning concerning
   a. Need to avoid outdoor activities during cold, windy or rainy weather
   b. Importance of good nutrition and hygiene
   c. Use of medications, side effects, and signs of toxicity
   d. Specific instructions following surgery for residual effects of anesthesia and loss of corneal reflex
      1) protective eye care
      2) chew on unaffected side only
      3) avoid hot fluids/foods
      4) mouth care after meals to remove particles
      5) good oral hygiene; visit dentist every 6 months
      6) protect the face during extremes of temperature.

Bell's Palsy

A. General information
   1. Disorder of cranial nerve VII resulting in the loss of ability to move the muscles on one side of the face
   2. Cause unknown; may be secondary to brain tumor, trauma, meningitis
   3. Complete recovery in 3–4 months in majority of patients
B. Assessment findings
   1. Loss of taste over anterior two-thirds of tongue on affected side
   2. Complete paralysis of one side of face
   3. Loss of expression, displacement of mouth toward unaffected side, and inability to close eyelid (all on affected side)
C. Nursing interventions
   1. Assess facial nerve function regularly (see Table 2.15).
   2. Administer medications as ordered.
      a. Corticosteroids: to decrease edema and pain
      b. Mild analgesics as necessary
   3. Provide facial sling to prevent stretching of weakened muscles and loss of tone, and to improve lip alignment and facilitate eating.
   4. Provide soft diet with supplementary feedings as indicated.
   5. Instruct to chew on unaffected side, avoid hot fluids/foods, and perform mouth care after each meal.
   6. Provide special eye care to protect the cornea.
      a. Dark glasses (cosmetic and protective reasons) or eyeshield
      b. Artificial tears to prevent drying of the cornea
      c. Ointment and eye patch at night
   7. Provide support and reassurance.

Guillain-Barré Syndrome

A. General information
   1. Symmetrical, bilateral, peripheral polyneuritis characterized by ascending paralysis
   2. Can occur at any age; affects women and men equally
   3. Cause unknown; may be an autoimmune process
   4. Precipitating factors: antecedent viral infection, malignancy, immunization
   5. Progression of disease is highly individual; 90% of patients stop progression in 4 weeks; recovery is usually from 3–6 months; may have residual deficits.
B. Assessment findings
   1. Mild sensory changes; in some patients severe misinterpretation of sensory stimuli resulting in extreme discomfort
   2. Clumsiness: usually first symptom
   3. Progressive motor weakness in more than one limb (classically is ascending and symmetrical)
   4. Cranial nerve involvement (dysphagia)
   5. Ventilatory insufficiency if paralysis ascends to respiratory muscles
   6. Absence of deep tendon reflexes
   7. Autonomic dysfunction (sympathetic overload)
   8. Diagnostic tests
      a. CSF studies: increased protein
      b. EMG: slowed nerve conduction
C. Nursing interventions
   1. Maintain adequate ventilation.
      a. Monitor rate and depth of respirations; serial vital capacities.
      b. Observe for ventilatory insufficiency.
      c. Maintain mechanical ventilation as needed; keep airway free of secretions and prevent pneumonia.
   2. Check individual muscle groups every 2 hours in acute phase to check for progression of muscle weakness.
   3. Assess cranial nerve function: check gag reflex and swallowing ability; ability to handle secretions; check voice.
   4. Monitor vital signs and observe for signs of autonomic dysfunction such as acute periods of hypertension fluctuating with hypotension, tachycardia, arrhythmias.
   5. Administer corticosteroids to suppress immune reaction as ordered.
   6. Prevent complications of immobility.
   7. Promote comfort (especially in patients with sensory changes): foot cradle, sheepskin, guided imagery, relaxation techniques.
   8. Promote optimum nutrition.
      a. Check gag reflex before feeding.
      b. Start with pureed foods.
      c. Assess need for nasogastric tube feedings if unable to swallow.
   9. Provide psychologic support and encouragement to patient/family.
   10. Refer for rehabilitation to regain strength and to treat any residual deficits.

Amyotrophic Lateral Sclerosis (Lou Gehrig's Disease)

A. General information
  1. Progressive motor neuron disease, which usually leads to death in 2–6 years
  2. Onset usually between ages 40–70; affects men more than women
  3. Cause unknown
  4. There is no cure or specific treatment; death usually occurs as a result of respiratory infection secondary to respiratory insufficiency.
B. Assessment findings
  1. Progressive weakness and atrophy of the muscles of the arms, trunk, or legs
  2. Dysarthria, dysphagia
  3. Fasciculations
  4. Respiratory insufficiency
  5. Diagnostic tests: EMG and muscle biopsy can rule out other diseases.
C. Nursing interventions
  1. Provide nursing measures for muscle weakness and dysphagia.
  2. Promote adequate ventilatory function.
  3. Prevent complications of immobility.
  4. Encourage diversional activities; spend time with the patient.
  5. Provide compassion and intensive support to patient/family.
  6. Provide or refer for physical therapy as indicated.
  7. Promote independence for as long as possible.

DISORDERS OF THE EYE

Cataracts

A. General information
  1. Opacity of the ocular lens
  2. Incidence increases with age
  3. May be caused by changes associated with aging ("senile" cataract); may be congenital; or may develop secondary to trauma, radiation, infection, certain drugs (corticosteroids)
B. Assessment findings
  1. Blurred vision
  2. Progressive decrease in vision
  3. Glare in bright lights
  4. Pupil may develop milky white appearance
  5. Diagnostic test: ophthalmoscopic exam confirms presence of cataract
C. Nursing interventions: prepare patient for cataract surgery.

Cataract Surgery

A. General information
  1. Performed when patient can no longer remain independent because of reduced vision
  2. Surgery performed on one eye at a time
  3. Local anesthesia usually used

  4. Types
     a. *Intracapsular extraction:* lens is totally removed within its capsule, may be delivered from eye by *cryoextraction* (lens is frozen with a metal probe and removed).
     b. *Extracapsular extraction:* lens capsule is excised and the lens is expressed; posterior capsule is left in place (may be used to support new artificial lens implant).
     c. *Phacoemulsification:* a type of extracapsular extraction; a hollow needle capable of ultrasonic vibration is inserted into lens, vibrations emulsify the lens, which is then aspirated.
  5. *Peripheral iridectomy* often performed at the time of surgery; small hole cut in iris to prevent development of secondary glaucoma
  6. *Intraocular lens implant* may also be performed at the time of surgery.
B. Nursing interventions: preoperative (see also Perioperative Nursing, page 30)
  1. Assess vision in the unaffected eye since the affected eye will be patched post-op.
  2. Provide pre-op teaching regarding measures to prevent increased intraocular pressure post-op.
  3. Administer medications as ordered.
     a. Topical mydriatics and cycloplegics to dilate the pupil
     b. Topical antibiotics to prevent infection
     c. Acetazolamide (Diamox) and osmotic agents (oral glycerin or mannitol [IV]) to decrease intraocular pressure to provide a soft eyeball for surgery
C. Nursing interventions: postoperative
  1. Reorient the patient to surroundings.
  2. Provide safety measures: elevate side rails, provide call bell, assist with ambulation (usually out of bed the day of surgery).
  3. Prevent increased intraocular pressure and stress on the suture line.
     a. Elevate head of bed 30°–40°.
     b. Have patient lie on back or unaffected side.
     c. Avoid having patient cough, sneeze, bend over, or move head too rapidly.
     d. Treat nausea with antiemetics as ordered to prevent vomiting.
     e. Give stool softeners as ordered to prevent straining.
     f. Observe for and report signs of increased intraocular pressure: severe eye pain, restlessness, increased pulse.
  4. Protect eye from injury.
     a. Dressings are usually removed the day after surgery.
     b. Eyeglasses or eye shield used during the day.
     c. Always use eye shield during the night.
  5. Administer medications as ordered.
     a. Topical mydriatics and cycloplegics to decrease spasm of ciliary body and relieve pain
     b. Topical antibiotics and corticosteroids
     c. Mild analgesics as needed
  6. Provide patient teaching and discharge planning concerning

a. Technique of eyedrop administration
b. Use of eye shield at night
c. No bending, stooping or lifting
d. Cataract glasses/contact lenses
   1) if a lens implant has not been performed, the patient will need glasses or contact lenses.
   2) temporary glasses are worn for 1–4 weeks, then permanent glasses fitted.
   3) cataract glasses magnify objects by $\frac{1}{3}$ and distort peripheral vision; have patient practice manual coordination with assistance until new spatial relationships become familiar; have patient practice walking, using stairs, reaching for articles.
   4) contact lenses cause less distortion of vision; prescribed at one month.

Glaucoma

A. General information
1. Characterized by increased intraocular pressure resulting in progressive loss of vision; may cause blindness if not recognized and treated
2. Risk factors: age over 40, diabetes, hypertension, heredity; history of previous eye surgery, trauma, or inflammation
3. Types
   a. *Chronic (open-angle) glaucoma*: most common form, due to obstruction of the outflow of aqueous humor, in trabecular meshwork or canal of Schlemm
   b. *Acute (closed-angle) glaucoma:* due to forward displacement of the iris against the cornea obstructing the outflow of the aqueous humor; occurs suddenly and is an emergency situation; if untreated, blindness will result
   c. *Chronic (closed-angle) glaucoma:* similar to acute (closed-angle) glaucoma, with the potential for an acute attack
4. Early detection is very important; regular eye exams including tonometry for persons over age 40 is recommended.
B. Medical management
1. Chronic (open-angle) glaucoma
   a. Drug therapy: one or a combination of the following
      1) miotic eye drops (pilocarpine) to increase outflow of aqueous humor
      2) epinephrine eye drops to decrease aqueous humor production
      3) acetazolamide (Diamox): carbonic anhydrase inhibitor to decrease aqueous humor production
      4) timolol maleate (Timoptic): topical beta-adrenergic blocker to decrease intraocular pressure
   b. Surgery (if no improvement with drugs)
      1) filtering procedure (trabeculectomy, trephining) to create artificial openings for the outflow of aqueous humor
      2) cyclotherapy: heat, cold, or laser to damage ciliary body and decrease aqueous humor production

2. Acute (closed-angle) glaucoma
   a. Drug therapy (before surgery)
      1) miotic eye drops (e.g., pilocarpine) to cause pupil to contract and draw iris away from cornea
      2) osmotic agents (e.g., glycerin [oral], mannitol [IV]) to decrease intraocular pressure
      3) narcotic analgesics for pain
   b. Surgery
      1) peripheral iridectomy: portion of the iris is excised to facilitate outflow of aqueous humor
      2) iridectomy usually performed on second eye later since a large number of patients have an acute attack in the other eye
3. Chronic (closed-angle) glaucoma
   a. Drug therapy: miotics (pilocarpine)
   b. Surgery: bilateral peripheral iridectomy to prevent acute attacks
C. Assessment findings
1. Chronic (open-angle) glaucoma: symptoms develop slowly; impaired peripheral vision (tunnel vision); loss of central vision if unarrested; mild discomfort in the eyes; halos around lights
2. Acute (closed-angle) glaucoma: severe eye pain; blurred, cloudy vision; halos around lights; nausea and vomiting; steamy cornea; moderate pupillary dilation
3. Chronic (closed-angle) glaucoma: transient blurred vision; slight eye pain; halos around lights
4. Diagnostic tests
   a. Visual acuity: reduced
   b. Tonometry: reading of 24–32 mm Hg suggests glaucoma; may be 50 mm Hg or more in acute (closed-angle) glaucoma
   c. Ophthalmoscopic exam: reveals narrowing of small vessels of optic disk, cupping of optic disk
   d. Perimetry: reveals defects in visual fields
   e. Gonioscopy: examine angle of anterior chamber
D. Nursing interventions
1. Administer medications as ordered.
2. Provide quiet, dark environment.
3. Maintain accurate I&O with the use of osmotic agents.
4. Prepare the patient for surgery if indicated.
5. Provide post-op care (see Cataract Surgery above).
6. Provide patient teaching and discharge planning concerning.
   a. Self-administration of eye drops
   b. Need to avoid stooping, heavy lifting or pushing, emotional upsets, excessive fluid intake, constrictive clothing around the neck
   c. Need to avoid the use of antihistamines or sympathomimetic drugs (found in cold preparations) in closed-angle glaucoma since they may cause mydriasis
   d. Importance of follow-up care
   e. Need to wear Medic-Alert tag.

Detached Retina

A. General information

1. Detachment of the sensory retina from the pigment epithelium of the retina
2. Caused by trauma, aging process, severe myopia, postcataract extraction, severe diabetic retinopathy
3. Pathophysiology: tear in the retina allows vitreous humor to seep behind the sensory retina and separate it from the pigment epithelium

B. Medical management
   1. Bedrest with eyes patched and detached areas dependent to prevent further detachment
   2. Surgery: necessary to repair detachment
      a. *Photocoagulation:* light beam (argon laser) through dilated pupil creates an inflammatory reaction and scarring to heal the area
      b. *Cryosurgery* or *diathermy:* application of extreme cold or heat to the external globe; inflammatory reaction causes scarring and healing of area
      c. *Scleral buckling:* shortening of sclera to force pigment epithelium close to retina

C. Assessment findings
   1. Flashes of light, floaters
   2. Visual field loss, veil-like curtain coming across field of vision
   3. Diagnostic test: ophthalmoscopic examination confirms diagnosis.

D. Nursing interventions: preoperative
   1. Maintain bedrest as ordered with head of bed flat and detached area in a dependent position.
   2. Use bilateral eye patches as ordered; elevate side rails to prevent injury.
   3. Identify yourself when entering the room.
   4. Orient the patient frequently to time, date and surroundings; explain procedures.
   5. Provide diversional activities to provide sensory stimulation.

E. Nursing interventions: postoperative (see also Cataract Surgery, page 61)
   1. Check orders for positioning and activity level.
      a. May be on bedrest for 1–2 days.
      b. May need to position patient so that detached area is in dependent position.
   2. Administer medications as ordered: topical mydriatics, analgesics as needed.
   3. Provide patient teaching and discharge planning concerning
      a. Technique of eye drop administration
      b. Use of eye shield at night
      c. No bending from waist; no heavy work or lifting for 6 weeks
      d. Restriction of reading for 3 weeks or more
      e. May watch television
      f. Need to check with physician regarding combing and shampooing hair and shaving
      g. Need to report complications such as recurrence of detachment.

DISORDERS OF THE EAR

Otosclerosis

A. General information
   1. Formation of new spongy bone in the labyrinth of the ear causing fixation of the stapes in the oval window; this prevents transmission of auditory vibration to the inner ear
   2. Found more often in females
   3. Cause unknown, but there is a familial tendency.

B. Medical management: stapedectomy is the procedure of choice.

C. Assessment findings
   1. Progressive loss of hearing
   2. Tinnitus
   3. Diagnostic tests
      a. Audiometry: reveals conductive hearing loss
      b. Weber's and Rinne's tests: show bone conduction is greater than air conduction

D. Nursing interventions: see Stapedectomy.

Stapedectomy

A. General information
   1. Removal of diseased portion of stapes and replacement with a prosthesis to conduct vibrations from the middle ear to inner ear; usually performed under local anesthesia
   2. Used to treat otosclerosis

B. Nursing interventions: preoperative
   1. Provide general pre-op nursing care, including an explanation of post-op expectations.
   2. Explain to the patient that hearing may improve during surgery and then decrease due to edema and packing.

C. Nursing interventions: postoperative
   1. Position the patient according to the surgeon's orders (possibly with operative ear uppermost to prevent displacement of the graft).
   2. Have patient deep breathe every 2 hours while in bed, but no coughing.
   3. Elevate side rails; assist the patient with ambulation and move slowly (may have some vertigo).
   4. Administer medications as ordered: analgesics, antibiotics, antiemetics, anti-motion sickness drugs.
   5. Check dressings frequently for excessive drainage or bleeding.
   6. Question patient about pain, headache, vertigo, and unusual sensations in the ear; report existence to physician.
   7. Provide patient teaching and discharge planning concerning
      a. Warnings against smoking, blowing nose, or coughing; sneeze with the mouth open
      b. Need to keep ear dry in the shower; no shampooing until allowed
      c. No flying for 6 months, especially if an upper respiratory tract infection is present
      d. Placement of cotton ball in auditory meatus after packing is removed, change twice a day.

Ménière's Disease

A. General information
1. Disease of the inner ear resulting from dilation of the endolymphatic system and increased volume of endolymph; characterized by recurrent and usually progressive triad of symptoms: vertigo, tinnitus, and hearing loss
2. Incidence highest between ages 30 and 60
3. Cause unknown; theories include allergy, toxicity, localized ischemia, hemorrhage, viral infection, or edema.

B. Medical management
1. Acute: atropine (decreases autonomic nervous system activity), diazepam (Valium), fentanyl and droperidol (Innovar)
2. Chronic
   a. Drug therapy: vasodilators (nicotinic acid), diuretics, mild sedatives or tranquilizers (diazepam [Valium]), antihistamines (diphenhydramine [Benedryl])
   b. Low-sodium diet and restricted fluid intake
3. Surgery
   a. Surgical destruction of labyrinth causing loss of vestibular and cochlear function (if disease is unilateral)
   b. Intracranial division of vestibular portion of cranial nerve VIII

C. Assessment findings
1. Sudden attacks of vertigo lasting hours or days; attacks occur several times a year
2. Nausea, tinnitus, progressive hearing loss
3. Vomiting, nystagmus
4. Diagnostic tests
   a. Audiometry: reveals sensorineural hearing loss
   b. Vestibular tests: reveal decreased function

D. Nursing interventions
1. Maintain bedrest in a quiet, darkened room in position of choice; elevate side rails as needed.
2. Only move the patient for essential care (bath may not be essential).
3. Provide an emesis basin for vomiting.
4. Monitor IV therapy; maintain accurate I&O.
5. Assist with ambulation when the attack is over.
6. Administer medications as ordered.
7. Prepare the patient for surgery as indicated (post-op care includes using above measures).
8. Provide patient teaching and discharge planning concerning
   a. Use of medication and side effects
   b. Low-sodium diet and decreased fluid intake
   c. Importance of eliminating smoking.

SAMPLE QUESTIONS

Mr. Henry Wilson has a medical diagnosis of increased intracranial pressure and is being cared for on the neurology unit. The nursing care plan includes elevating the head of the bed and positioning Mr. Wilson's head in proper alignment.

4. The nurse recognizes that these actions are effective because they act by
   o 1. making it easier for the patient to breathe.
   o 2. preventing a Valsalva maneuver.
   o 3. promoting venous drainage.
   o 4. reducing pain.

5. Mr. Wilson begins to have Cheyne-Stokes respirations. This type of breathing pattern is best explained as
   o 1. completely irregular breathing pattern with random deep and shallow respirations.
   o 2. prolonged inspirations with inspiratory and/or expiratory pauses.
   o 3. Rhythmic waxing and waning of both rate and depth of respiration with brief periods of interspersed apnea.
   o 4. Sustained, regular, rapid respirations of increased depth.

The Cardiovascular System

OVERVIEW OF ANATOMY AND PHYSIOLOGY

The cardiovascular system consists of the heart, arteries, veins, and capillaries. The major functions are circulation of blood, delivery of oxygen and other nutrients to the tissues of the body, and removal of carbon dioxide and other products of cellular metabolism.

Heart

The heart is a muscular pump that propels blood into the arterial system and receives blood from the venous system.

Heart Wall

A. *Pericardium:* composed of fibrous (outermost layer) and serous pericardium (parietal and visceral); a sac that functions to protect the heart from friction.
B. *Epicardium:* covers surface of heart, becomes continuous with visceral layer of serous pericardium.
C. *Myocardium:* middle, muscular layer
D. *Endocardium:* thin, inner membranous layer lining the chambers of the heart
E. *Papillary muscles:* arise from the endocardial and myocardial surface of the ventricles and attach to the chordae tendinae.
F. *Chordae tendinae:* attach to the tricuspid and mitral valves and prevent eversion during systole.

Chambers

A. *Atria:* two chambers, function as receiving chambers, lie above the the ventricles
   1. Right atrium: receives systemic venous blood through the superior vena cava, inferior vena cava, and coronary sinus.
   2. Left atrium: receives oxygenated blood returning to the heart from the lungs through the pulmonary veins.
B. *Ventricles:* two thick-walled chambers; major responsibility for forcing blood out of the heart; lie below the atria
   1. Right ventricle: contracts and propels deoxygenated blood into the pulmonary circulation via the pulmonary artery.
   2. Left ventricle: propels blood into the systemic circulation via the aorta during ventricular systole.

Valves

See Figure 2.4.
A. Atrioventricular (AV) valves
   1. *Mitral valve:* located between the left atrium and left ventricle; contains two leaflets attached to the chordae tendinae.
   2. *Tricuspid valve:* located between the right atrium and right ventricle; contains three leaflets attached to the chordae tendinae.
   3. Functions
      a. Permit unidirectional flow of blood from specific atrium to specific ventricle during ventricular diastole
      b. Prevent reflux flow during ventricular systole
      c. Valve leaflets open during ventricular diastole and close during ventricular systole; valve closure produces *first heart sound (S_1)*.

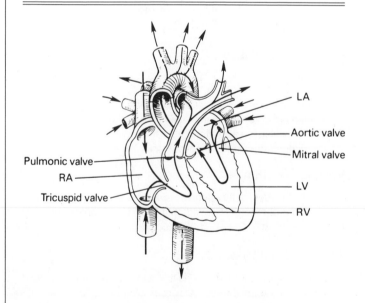

Figure 2.4 The valves of the heart. *Arrows indicate direction of blood flow.*

B. Semilunar valves
   1. *Pulmonary valve:* located between right ventricle and pulmonary artery
   2. *Aortic valve:* located between left ventricle and aorta
   3. Functions
      a. Permit unidirectional flow of blood from specific ventricle to arterial vessel during ventricular systole
      b. Prevent reflux blood flow during ventricular diastole
      c. Valves open when ventricles contract and close during ventricular diastole; valve closure produces *second heart sound (S$_2$).*

Conduction System

A. *Sinoatrial (SA) node:* the pacemaker of the heart; initiates the cardiac impulse, which spreads across the atria and into AV node.
B. *Atrioventricular (AV) node:* delays the impulse from the atria while the ventricles fill.
C. *Bundle of His:* arises from the AV node and conducts impulse to the bundle branch system.
   1. Right bundle branch: divided into anterior, lateral, and posterior; transmits impulses down the right side of the interventricular septum toward the right ventricular myocardium
   2. Left bundle branch: divided into anterior and posterior
      a. Anterior portion transmits impulses to the anterior endocardial surface of the left ventricle.
      b. Posterior portion transmits impulses over the posterior and inferior endocardial surfaces of the left ventricle.
D. *Purkinje fibers:* transmit impulses to the ventricles and provide for depolarization after ventricular contraction.
E. Electrical activity of heart can be visualized by attaching electrodes to the skin and recording activity by electrocardiograph (see page 67).

Coronary Circulation

See Figure 2.5.
A. Coronary arteries: branch off at the base of the aorta and supply blood to the myocardium and the conduction system; three main coronary arteries are *right, left,* and *circumflex.*
B. Coronary veins: return blood from the myocardium back to the right atrium via the coronary sinus.

Vascular System

The major function of the blood vessels is to supply the tissues with blood and to remove wastes and carry unoxygenated blood back to the heart.

Types of Blood Vessels

A. *Arteries:* elastic walled vessels that can stretch during systole and recoil during diastole; they carry blood away from the heart and distribute oxygenated blood throughout the body.
B. *Arterioles:* small arteries that distribute blood to the capillaries and function in controlling systemic vascular resistance and, therefore, arterial pressure.

C. *Capillaries:* the following exchanges occur in the capillaries
   1. Oxygen and carbon dioxide
   2. Solutes between the blood and tissues
   3. Fluid volume transfer between the plasma and interstitial spaces.
D. *Venules:* small veins that receive blood from the capillaries and function as collecting channels between the capillaries and veins
E. *Veins:* low-pressure vessels with thin walls and less muscle than arteries, most contain valves that prevent retrograde blood flow; they carry deoxygenated blood back to the heart. When skeletal muscles surrounding veins contract, the veins are compressed promoting movement of blood back to the heart.

ASSESSMENT

Health History

A. Presenting problem
   1. Nonspecific symptoms may include fatigue, shortness of breath, cough, dizziness, syncope, headache, palpitations, weight loss/gain, anorexia, difficulty sleeping.
   2. Specific signs and symptoms
      a. Chest pain: note character, quality, location, radiation, frequency, and whether it is associated with precipitating factors (exertion, eating, excitement).
      b. Dyspnea (shortness of breath): note kind and extent of precipitating activities.
      c. Orthopnea (form of dyspnea that develops when patient lies down): determine how many pillows are used when sleeping; note any paroxysmal nocturnal dyspnea (PND) (patient awakens suddenly in the night, breathing with difficulty).
      d. Palpitations (awareness of heartbeat, fluttering feeling): assess precipitating factors (anxiety, caffeine, nicotine, stress); ask patient to tap out the rhythm.
      e. Edema (abnormal accumulation of fluid in tissues):

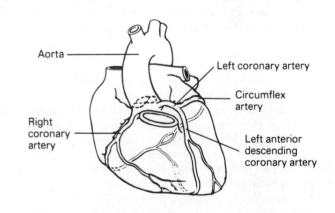

Figure 2.5 The coronary circulation.

note whether unilateral/bilateral, location, time of day when most apparent.

   f. Cyanosis (dusky, bluish coloration to the skin): note whether peripheral or central.

B. Life-style: occupation, hobbies, financial status, stressors, unusual life patterns, relaxation time, exercise, living conditions, smoking, sleep habits

C. Use of medications: over-the-counter (OTC) drugs, contraceptives, cardiac drugs

D. Personality profile: Type A, manic-depressive, anxieties

E. Nutrition: dietary habits; calorie, cholesterol, salt intake; alcohol consumption

F. Past medical history

   1. Heart murmurs, rheumatic fever, sexually transmitted diseases, angina, myocardial infarction (MI), hypertension, CVA, alcoholism, obesity, hyperlipidemia, varicose veins, claudication

   2. Pregnancies, contraceptive use

G. Family history: heart disease (congenital, acute, chronic); risk factors (diabetes, hypertension, obesity)

Physical Examination

A. Skin and mucous membranes: note color/texture, temperature, hair distribution on extremities, atrophy or edema, venous pattern, petechiae, lesions, ulcerations or gangrene; examine nails.

B. Peripheral pulses: palpate and rate all arterial pulses (temporal, carotid, brachial, radial, femoral, popliteal, dorsalis pedis, and posterior tibial) on scale of: 0 = absent, 1 = palpable, 2 = normal, 3 = full, 4 = full and bounding.

C. Assess for arterial insufficiency and venous impairment.

D. Measure and record blood pressure.

E. Inspect and palpate the neck vessels.

   1. Jugular veins: note location, characteristics; measure jugular venous pressure.

   2. Carotid arteries: note location, characteristics

F. Precordium

   1. Inspect and palpate sternoclavicular, aortic, pulmonic, Erb's point, tricuspid, apical, epigastric sites.

   2. Note point of maximum impulse (PMI), pulsations, thrills.

G. Auscultate aortic, pulmonic, Erb's point, tricuspid, mitral or apical, xiphoid areas; note heart rate and rhythm (see Figure 2.6).

   1. Normal heart sounds (S_1 and S_2): note location, intensity, splitting.

   2. Abnormal heart sounds (S_3, S_4: note location, occurrence in cardiac cycle

   3. Murmurs: note location, occurrence in cardiac cycle

   4. Friction rubs

Laboratory/Diagnostic Tests

A. Blood chemistry and electrolyte analysis

   1. Cardiac enzymes: creatine phosphokinase (CPK) and CPK-MB fraction; lactic acid dehydrogenase (LDH) and electrophoresis of LDH_1 and LDH_2; serum glutamic oxaloacetic transaminase (SGOT)

   2. Electrolytes: sodium, potassium, magnesium, calcium, phosphorus

   3. Serum lipids: cholesterol, triglycerides

   4. Uric acid levels

B. Hematologic studies

   1. CBC

   2. Coagulation time

   3. Clotting profile

   4. Erythrocyte sedimentation rate (ESR)

   5. Partial thromboplastin time (PTT)

   6. Activated partial thromboplastin time (APTT)

   7. Prothrombin time (PT)

   8. WBC

C. Urine studies: routine urinalysis

D. *Electrocardiogram (ECG or EKG):* a noninvasive test that produces a graphic record of the electrical activity of the heart. In addition to determining cardiac rhythm, pattern variations may reveal pathologic processes (MI and ischemia, electrolyte and acid-base imbalance, chamber enlargement, block of the right or left bundle branch); see also Cardiac Monitoring, page 68.

E. *Exercise ECG (stress test):* the ECG is recorded during prescribed exercise such as climbing a set of stairs, walking a treadmill, or riding a stationary bicycle; stress tests may show heart disease when resting ECG does not.

F. *Phonocardiogram:* noninvasive device to amplify and record heart sounds and murmurs.

G. *Echocardiogram:* noninvasive recording of the cardiac structures using ultrasound

H. *Cardiac catheterization:* invasive, but often definitive test for diagnosis of cardiac disease

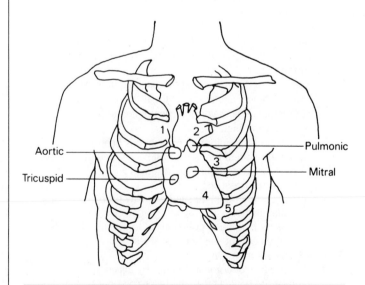

Figure 2.6 The heart valves and areas of auscultation: **(1)** aortic area. **(2)** pulmonic area. **(3)** Erb's point. **(4)** tricuspid area. **(5)** mitral area.

1. A catheter is inserted into the right or left side of the heart to obtain information.
   a. Right-sided catheterization: the catheter is inserted into an antecubital vein and advanced into the vena cava, right atrium, and right ventricle with further insertion into the pulmonary artery.
   b. Left-sided catheterization: performed by inserting the catheter into a brachial or femoral artery; the catheter is passed retrograde up the aorta and into the left ventricle.
2. Purpose: to measure intracardiac pressures and oxygen levels in various parts of the heart; with injection of a dye, it allows visualization of the heart chambers, blood vessels and course of blood flow *(angiography)*.
3. Nursing care: pretest
   a. Confirm that informed consent has been signed.
   b. Ask about allergies, particularly to iodine, if dye being used.
   c. Keep patient NPO for 8–12 hours prior to test.
   d. Record height and weight, take baseline vital signs, and monitor peripheral pulses.
   e. Inform patient that a feeling of warmth and fluttering sensation as catheter is passed is common.
4. Nursing care: post-test
   a. Assess circulation to extremity used for catheter insertion.
   b. Keep affected extremity straight for approximately 8 hours.
   c. Check peripheral pulses, color, and sensation of affected extremity every 15 minutes for 4 hours.
   d. Observe catheter insertion site for swelling and bleeding; a sandbag or pressure dressing may be over insertion site.
   e. Assess vital signs and report significant changes from baseline.

I. *Aortography*
   1. Injection of radiopaque contrast medium into the aorta to visualize the aorta, valve leaflets, and major vessels on a movie film.
   2. Purpose: to determine and diagnose aortic valve incompetence, aneurysms of the ascending aorta, abnormalities of major branches of the aorta.
   3. Nursing care: pretest
      a. Confirm that informed consent has been signed.
      b. Inform patient that a dye will be injected and to report any dyspnea, numbness, or tingling.
   4. Nursing care: post-test
      a. Assess the puncture site frequently for bleeding or inflammation.
      b. Assess peripheral pulses distal to the injection site every hour for 4–8 hours post-test.

J. *Coronary arteriography*
   1. Visualization of coronary arteries by injection of radiopaque contrast dye and recording on a movie film.
   2. Purpose: evaluation of heart disease and angina, location of areas of infarction and extent of lesions, ruling out coronary artery disease in patients with myocardial disease
   3. Nursing care: same as for Aortography (above).

ANALYSIS

Nursing diagnoses for the patient with a cardiovascular dysfunction may include
A. Alteration in comfort: pain
B. Potential for injury
C. Anxiety
D. Fear
E. Alteration in cardiac output: decreased
F. Alteration in fluid volume: excess
G. Impairment of skin integrity
H. Alteration in thought processes
I. Alteration in tissue perfusion
J. Ineffective individual coping

PLANNING AND IMPLEMENTATION

Goals

A. Pain in the chest or in the affected extremity will be diminished.
B. Regular cardiac rhythm will be regained (no myocardial ischemia/damage or thromboembolus formation).
C. Patient's level of fear and anxiety will be decreased.
D. Cardiac output will be improved.
E. Fluid imbalance will be resolved, edema minimized.
F. Adequate skin integrity will be maintained.
G. Usual thought processes will be regained.
H. Adequate tissue perfusion will be maintained.
I. Patient will be able to use effective coping skills.

Interventions

Cardiac Monitoring

A. The cardiac monitor provides continuous information regarding the cardiac rhythm and rate (ECG). Constant surveillance and understanding of the basic electrocardiographic system is imperative to avoid/treat arrhythmias (see Figure 2.7).
   1. ECG strip: each small square represents 0.04 seconds, each large square 0.2 seconds.
   2. P wave: produced by atrial depolarization; indicates SA node function.
   3. P-R interval
      a. Indicates atrioventricular conduction time or the time it takes an impulse to travel from the atria down and through the AV node
      b. Measured from beginning of P wave to beginning of QRS complex
      c. Normal: 0.12–0.20 seconds
   4. QRS complex
      a. Indicates ventricular depolarization
      b. Measured from onset of Q wave to end of S wave
      c. Normal: 0.06–0.10 seconds
   5. ST segment
      a. Indicates time interval between complete depolarization of ventricles and repolarization of the ventricles
      b. Measured after QRS complex to beginning of T wave

6. T wave
   a. Represents ventricular repolarization
   b. Follows ST segment

Swan-Ganz Catheter (Hemodynamic Monitoring)

A. A multilumen catheter with a balloon tip that is advanced through the superior vena cava into the right atrium, right ventricle, and pulmonary artery. When it is wedged it is in the distal arterial branch of the pulmonary artery.

B. Purposes
   1. Proximal port: measures right atrial pressure
   2. Distal port
      a. Measures pulmonary artery (PA) pressure (reflects left and right heart pressures) and pulmonary capillary wedge pressure (PCWP) (reflects left atrial and left ventricular end diastolic pressure).
      b. Normal values: PA systolic and diastolic less than 20 mm Hg; PCWP 4–12 mm Hg
   3. Balloon port: inflated with 1–2 cc air to obtain PWCP
   4. Thermistor lumen: used to measure cardiac output if ordered

C. Nursing care
   1. A sterile dry dressing should be applied to site and changed every 24 hours; inspect site daily and report signs of infection.
   2. If catheter is inserted via an extremity, immobilize extremity to prevent catheter dislodgment or trauma.
   3. Observe catheter site for leakage.
   4. Ensure that balloon is deflated with a syringe attached, except when PCWP is read.
   5. Continuously monitor PA systolic and diastolic pressures and report significant variations.
   6. Irrigate line before each reading of PCWP.
   7. Maintain patient in same position for each reading.
   8. Maintain pressure bag at 300 mm Hg.
   9. Record PA systolic and diastolic readings at least every hour and PCWP as ordered, noting position of patient.

Central Venous Pressure (CVP)

A. Obtained by inserting a catheter into the external jugular, antecubital, or femoral vein and threading it into the vena

cava. The catheter is attached to an IV infusion and H_2O manometer by a three-way stopcock.

B. Purposes
   1. Reveals right atrial pressure, reflecting alterations in the right ventricular pressure
   2. Provides information concerning blood volume and adequacy of central venous return
   3. Provides an IV route for drawing blood samples, administering fluids or medication, and possibly inserting a pacing catheter.

C. Normal range is 4–10 cm H_2O; elevation indicates hypervolemia, decreased level indicates hypovolemia.

D. Nursing care
   1. Ensure patient is relaxed.
   2. Maintain zero point of manometer always at level of right atrium (midaxillary line).
   3. Determine patency of catheter by opening IV infusion line.
   4. Turn stopcock to allow IV solution to run into manometer to a level 10–20 cm above expected pressure reading.
   5. Turn stopcock to allow IV solution to flow from manometer into catheter; fluid level in manometer fluctuates with respiration.
   6. Stop ventilatory assistance during measurement of CVP.
   7. After CVP reading, return stopcock to IV infusion position.
   8. Record CVP reading and position of patient.

EVALUATION

A. Patient expresses relief from pain, has relaxed facial expression, depth and rate of respiration are normal for patient; demonstrates an increase in activity tolerance.

B. Patient's apical pulse is regular; ECG demonstrates a normal sinus rhythm; blood pressure is stable and within normal range; peripheral pulses are palpable; skin warm, dry, and usual color; usual skin temperature and color in the extremities; patient does not experience syncope or lightheadedness.

C. Patient states that he is less anxious; can express understanding of hospital routines, procedures, and treatments.

D. Capillary refill is less than 3 seconds, balanced I&O with urine output at least 30 cc/hour, hemodynamic measurements within normal range, usual mental status.

E. Resolution of peripheral edema and neck vein distension.

F. Patient's skin shows absence of redness and irritation.

G. Patient shows improved memory and level of orientation.

H. Patient is willing to participate in treatment plan and self-care activities, recognizes and uses available support systems.

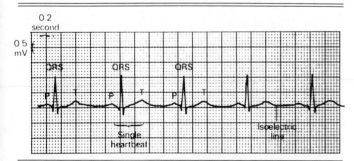

Figure 2.7 A typical ECG. *All beats appear as a similar pattern, equally spaced, and have three major units: P wave, QRS complex, and T wave.*

DISORDERS OF THE CARDIOVASCULAR SYSTEM

The Heart

Coronary Artery Disease (CAD)

A. General information

1. CAD refers to a variety of pathologic conditions that cause narrowing or obstruction of the coronary arteries resulting in decreased blood supply to the myocardium.
2. *Atherosclerosis* (deposits of cholesterol and lipids within the walls of the artery) is the major causative factor.
3. Occurs most often between ages 30 and 50; men affected more often than women; nonwhites have higher mortality rates.
4. May manifest as angina pectoris or MI.
5. Risk factors: family history of CAD, elevated serum lipoproteins, cigarette smoking, diabetes mellitus, hypertension, obesity, sedentary and/or stressful/competitive life-style, elevated serum uric acid levels

B. Medical management, assessment findings, and nursing interventions: see Angina Pectoris (below) and Myocardial Infarction (page 72).

Angina Pectoris

A. General information
1. Transient, paroxysmal chest pain produced by insufficient blood flow to the myocardium resulting in myocardial ischemia.
2. Risk factors: CAD, atherosclerosis, hypertension, diabetes mellitus, thromboangiitis obliterans, severe anemia, aortic insufficiency
3. Precipitating factors: physical exertion, consumption of a heavy meal, extremely cold weather, strong emotions, cigarette smoking, sexual activity

B. Medical management
1. Drug therapy: nitrates, beta-adrenergic blocking agents, and/or calcium-blocking agents
2. Modification of diet and other risk factors
3. Surgery: coronary artery bypass surgery (page 72)

C. Assessment findings
1. Pain: substernal with possible radiation to the neck, jaw, back, and arms; relieved by rest
2. Palpitations, tachycardia
3. Dyspnea
4. Diaphoresis
5. Increased serum lipid levels
6. Diagnostic tests
   a. ECG may reveal S-T segment depression and T-wave inversion during chest pain.
   b. Stress test may reveal an abnormal ECG during exercise.

D. Nursing interventions
1. Administer oxygen.
2. Give prompt pain relief with nitrates or narcotic analgesics as ordered.
3. Monitor vital signs, status of cardiopulmonary function.
4. Monitor ECG.
5. Place patient in semi- to high-Fowler's position.
6. Provide emotional support.
7. Provide patient teaching and discharge planning concerning

   a. Proper use of nitrates
      1) nitroglycerin tablets (sublingual)
         a) allow tablet to dissolve.
         b) relax for 15 minutes after taking tablet to prevent dizziness.
         c) if no relief with 1 tablet, take additional tablets at 5-minute intervals, but no more than 3 tablets within a 15-minute period.
         d) know that transient headache is a frequent side effect.
         e) keep bottle tightly capped and prevent exposure to air, light, heat.
         f) ensure tablets are within reach at all times.
         g) check shelf life, expiration date of tablets.
      2) nitroglycerin ointment (topical)
         a) rotate sites to prevent dermal inflammation.
         b) remove previously applied ointment.
         c) avoid massaging/rubbing as this increases absorption and interferes with the drug's sustained action.
   b. Ways to minimize precipitating events
      1) reduce stress and anxiety (relaxation techniques, guided imagery)
      2) avoid overexertion and smoking
      3) maintain low-cholesterol, low-saturated fat diet and eat small, frequent meals
      4) avoid extremes of temperature
      5) dress warmly in cold weather
   c. Gradual increase in activities and exercise
      1) participate in regular exercise program
      2) space exercise periods and allow for rest periods.
8. Instruct patient to notify physician immediately if pain occurs and persists, despite rest and medication administration.

Arrhythmias

An arrhythmia is a disruption in the normal events of the cardiac cycle. It may take a variety of forms. Treatment varies depending on the type of arrhythmia; commonly used drugs are summarized in Table 2.17.

Sinus Tachycardia

A. General information
1. A heart rate of over 100 beats/minute, originating in the SA node
2. May be caused by fever, apprehension, physical activity, anemia, hyperthyroidism, drugs (epinephrine, theophylline), myocardial ischemia, caffeine

B. Assessment findings
1. Rate: 100–160 beats/minute
2. Rhythm: regular
3. P wave: precedes each QRS complex with normal contour
4. P-R interval: normal (0.08 second)
5. QRS complex: normal (0.06 second)

C. Treatment: correction of underlying cause, elimination of stimulants; sedatives, propranolol (Inderal).

Table 2.17 Antiarrhythmic Drugs

Drug	Action	Side Effects	Nursing Responsibilities
Quinidine	Depresses myocardial excitability; slows conduction time in atria and ventricles, prolongs P-R interval and QRS complex; prolongs refractory period; depresses myocardial contractility, reduces vagal tone. Used in atrial fibrillation and ventricular dysrhythmias.	*Hypersensitivity:* fever, rash, hypotension CNS: tinnitus, diplopia, confusion, headache, delirium GI: anorexia, nausea, vomiting, diarrhea CV: heart block, nodal rhythm, ventricular arrhythmias; emboli when heart is converting to normal rhythm	Administer drug with food to minimize GI symptoms (nausea and vomiting). Carefully monitor electrolyte levels, blood counts, and kidney and liver function. Count apical pulse for 1 min. before administering drug. Instruct patient to report tinnitus, breathlessness, palpitations, or faintness. Instruct patient to avoid fatigue, excessive caffeine, alcohol, smoking, heavy meals, stressful situations, OTC medications.
Procainamide (Pronestyl)	Depresses ectopic pacemakers; action on the heart similar to quinidine. Used to treat PVCs, ventricular tachycardia, and some atrial dysrhythmias.	Same as quinidine, plus severe hypotension with parenteral use, possible development of a erythematosus-like syndrome in some patients	Administer PO preparations on an empty stomach 1 hr before or 2 hr after means. Constantly monitor an IV infusion of drug. Check apical/radial pulse before each dose during adjustment period. Teach patient to take own pulse. Instruct patient to report immediately changes in ratio of intake to output, signs of local edema, weakness or irregularity of pulse. Instruct patient to store drug in dark, airtight container.
Lidocaine (Xylocaine)	Rapid-acting local or topical anesthetic; depresses myocardium; decreases excitability, conduction, and force of contraction. Used for acute ventricular dysrhythmias.	CNS: dizziness, blurred vision, sweating, progressing to coma and convulsions CV: hypotension; large doses occasionally cause decreased myocardial contractility	Constantly monitor ECG and blood pressure during IV administration. Observe for neurotoxic effects (drowsiness, confusion, paresthesias, visual disturbances, excitement, behavioral changes).
Verapamil (Isoptin)	Inhibits calcium influx into conductile and contractile myocardial cells and vascular smooth muscle cells; slows AV conduction	CV: hypotension, edema, flushing, congestive heart failure, AV block CNS: vertigo, syncope, headache GI: nausea, constipation	Establish baseline date for blood pressure, pulse, hepatic and renal function before treatment is started. Instruct patient to remain recumbent for at least 1 hr after dose is given to decrease change of hypotension. Teach patient to take own pulse. Explain that dizziness during early treatment is common.
Nifedipine (Procardia)	Calcium ion antagonist; selectively blocks calcium ion influx across cell membrane of cardiac muscle and smooth muscle	CV: hypotension, edema, flushing, tachycardia, palpitations CNS: vertigo, syncope, headache, weakness, nervousness GI: nausea, heartburn, diarrhea, constipation ENT: nasal congestion	Warn patient not to omit or change dosage. Protect drug from exposure to light. Instruct patient to keep a record of use and report if changes occur.
Digitalis	Decreases heart rate and increases force of contraction.	*Digitalis toxicity:* CNS: headache, fatigue, malaise, drowsiness, muscle weakness, insomnia, agitation, seizures, paresthesias of hands and feet, personality changes, impaired memory, hallucinations CV: arrhythmias (PVCs, supraventricular tachycardia, congestive heart failure ENT: yellow-green halos GI: anorexia, nausea and vomiting, abdominal distension and pain	Count apical pulse for 1 min.; note rate, rhythm, and quality before administration. Instruct patient to be alert for signs and symptoms of digitalis toxicity. Monitor digitalis/electrolyte levels frequently.

Sinus Bradycardia

A. General information
 1. A slowed heart rate initiated by SA node
 2. Caused by excessive vagal or decreased sympathetic tone, MI, intracranial tumors, meningitis, myxedema, cardiac fibrosis; a normal variation of the heart rate in well-trained athletes
B. Assessment findings
 1. Rate: less than 60 beats/minute
 2. Rhythm: regular
 3. P wave: precedes each QRS with a normal contour
 4. P-R interval: normal
 5. QRS complex: normal
C. Treatment: usually not needed; if cardiac output is inadequate, atropine and isoproterenol (Isuprel) are usually prescribed; if drugs are not effective, a pacemaker may need to be inserted (see page 75).

Atrial Fibrillation

A. General information
 1. An arrhythmia in which ectopic foci cause rapid, irregular contractions of the heart
 2. Commonly seen in patients with rheumatic mitral stenosis, thyrotoxicosis, cardiomyopathy, hypertensive heart disease, pericarditis, and coronary heart disease
B. Assessment findings
 1. Rate
  a. Atrial: 350–600 beats/minute
  b. Ventricular: varies between 100–160 beats/minute
 2. Rhythm: atrial and ventricular irregularly irregular
 3. P wave: no definite P wave; rapid undulations called fibrillatory (F) waves
 4. P-R interval: not measurable
 5. QRS complex: generally normal
C. Treatment: digitalis preparations, propranolol, verapamil in conjunction with digitalis; direct current cardioversion

Premature Ventricular Contractions (PVCs)

A. General information
 1. Irritable impulses originate in the ventricles
 2. Caused by electrolyte imbalance (hypokalemia); digitalis drug therapy; myocardial disease; stimulants (caffeine, epinephrine, isoproterenol); hypoxia; congestive heart failure
B. Assessment findings
 1. Rate: varies according to number of PVCs
 2. Rhythm: irregular because of PVCs
 3. P wave: normal; however, often lost in QRS complex
 4. P-R interval: often not measurable
 5. QRS complex: wide and distorted in shape, greater than 0.12 seconds
C. Treatment
 1. IV push of lidocaine (50–100 mg) followed by IV drip of lidocaine at rate of 1–4 mg/minute
 2. Procainamide (Pronestyl), quinidine
 3. Treatment of underlying cause

Ventricular Tachycardia

A. General information
 1. A run of three or more consecutive PVCs; occurs from repetitive firing of an ectopic focus in the ventricles.
 2. Caused by acute MI, CAD, digitalis intoxication, hypokalemia
B. Assessment findings
 1. Rate
  a. Atrial: 60–100 beats/minute
  b. Ventricular: 110–250 beats/minute
 2. Rhythm: atrial (regular), ventricular (occasionally irregular)
 3. P wave: often lost in QRS complex
 4. P-R interval: usually not measurable
 5. QRS complex: greater than 0.12 seconds, wide
C. Treatment
 1. IV push of lidocaine (50–100 mg), then IV drip of lidocaine 1–4 mg/minute
 2. Procainamide via IV infusion of 2–6 mg/minute
 3. Direct current cardioversion
 4. Bretylium, propranolol (Inderal)

Myocardial Infarction (MI)

A. General information
 1. The death of myocardial cells from inadequate oxygenation, often caused by a sudden complete blockage of a coronary artery; characterized by localized formation of necrosis (tissue destruction) with subsequent healing by scar formation and fibrosis.
 2. Risk factors: atherosclerotic CAD, thrombus formation, hypertension, diabetes mellitus
B. Assessment findings (see also Angina Pectoris, page 70)
 1. Pain usually substernal with radiation to the neck, arm, jaw or back; severe, crushing, viselike with sudden onset; *unrelieved by rest or nitrates*
 2. Nausea and vomiting
 3. Dyspnea
 4. Skin: cool, clammy, ashen
 5. Elevated temperature
 6. Initial increase in blood pressure and pulse, with gradual drop in blood pressure
 7. Restlessness
 8. Occasional findings: rales; presence of S_1; pericardial friction rub; split S_1, S_2
 9. Diagnostic tests
  a. Elevated WBC
  b. Elevated CPK and CPK-MB
  c. Elevated SGOT
  d. Elevated LDH, LDH_1, and LDH_2
  e. ECG changes (specific changes dependent on location of myocardial damage and phase of the MI)
  f. Increased ESR, elevated serum cholesterol
C. Nursing interventions
 1. Establish a patent IV line.
 2. Provide pain relief: morphine sulfate IV (given IV

because after an infarction there is poor peripheral perfusion and because serum enzymes would be affected by IM injections) as ordered.

3. Administer oxygen as ordered to relieve dyspnea and prevent arrhythmias.
4. Provide bedrest with semi-Fowler's position.
5. Monitor ECG and hemodynamic procedures.
6. Administer antiarrhythmics as ordered.
7. Perform complete lung/cardiovascular assessment.
8. Monitor urinary output and report output of less than 30 cc/hour.
9. Maintain full liquid diet with gradual increase to soft; low sodium.
10. Maintain quiet environment.
11. Administer stool softeners as ordered to facilitate bowel evacuation and prevent straining.
12. Relieve anxiety associated with coronary care unit (CCU) environment.
13. Administer anticoagulants as ordered.
14. Provide patient teaching and discharge planning concerning
    a. Effects of MI, healing process, and treatment regimen
    b. Medication regimen including name, purpose, schedule, dosage, side effects
    c. Risk factors, with necessary life-style modifications
    d. Dietary restrictions: low sodium, low cholesterol, avoidance of caffeine
    e. Importance of participation in a progressive activity program
    f. Resumption of sexual activity according to physician's orders (usually 4–6 weeks)
    g. Need to report the following symptoms: increased persistent chest pain, dyspnea, weakness, fatigue, persistent palpitations, lightheadedness
    h. Enrollment of patient in a cardiac rehabilitation program.

Coronary Artery Bypass Surgery

A. General information
  1. A coronary artery bypass graft is the surgery of choice for patients with severe CAD.
  2. New supply of blood brought to diseased/occluded coronary artery by bypassing the obstruction with a graft that is attached to the aorta proximally and to the coronary artery distally.
  3. Several bypasses can be performed depending on the location and extent of the blockage.
  4. Procedure requires use of extracorporeal circulation (heart-lung machine, cardiopulmonary bypass)
B. Nursing interventions: preoperative
  1. Explain anatomy of the heart, function of coronary arteries, effects of CAD.
  2. Explain events of the day of surgery: length of time in surgery, length of time until able to see family.
  3. Orient to the critical and coronary care units and introduce to staff.
  4. Explain equipment to be used (monitors, hemodynamic procedures, ventilator, endotracheal tube, drainage tubes).

5. Demonstrate activity and exercises (turning from side to side, dangling, sitting in a chair, ROM exercises for arms and legs, effective deep breathing and coughing).
6. Reassure patient that pain medication is available.

C. Nursing interventions: postoperative
  1. Maintain patent airway.
  2. Promote lung reexpansion.
     a. Monitor drainage from chest/mediastinal tubes, and check patency of chest drainage system.
     b. Assist patient with turning, coughing, and deep breathing.
  3. Monitor cardiac status.
     a. Monitor vital signs and cardiac rhythm and report significant changes, particularly temperature elevation.
     b. Perform peripheral pulse checks.
     c. Carry out hemodynamic monitoring.
     d. Administer anticoagulants as ordered and monitor hematologic test results carefully.
  4. Maintain fluid and electrolyte balance.
     a. Maintain accurate I&O with hourly outputs; report if less than 30 cc/hour urine.
     b. Assess color, character, and specific gravity of urine.
     c. Daily weights.
     d. Assess lab values, particularly BUN, creatinine, sodium, and potassium levels.
  5. Maintain adequate cerebral circulation: frequent assessment of pupillary size and reaction, LOC and orientation, motor functioning.
  6. Provide pain relief.
     a. Administer narcotics cautiously and monitor effects.
     b. Assist with positioning for maximum comfort.
     c. Teach relaxation techniques.
  7. Prevent abdominal distension.
     a. Monitor nasogastric drainage and maintain patency of system.
     b. Assess for bowel sounds every 2–4 hours.
     c. Measure abdominal girths if necessary.
  8. Monitor for and prevent the following complications.
     a. Thrombophlebitis/pulmonary embolism
     b. Cardiac tamponade (see page 77)
     c. Arrhythmias
        1) maintain continuous ECG monitoring and report changes.
        2) assess electrolyte levels daily and report significant changes, particularly potassium.
        3) administer antiarrhythmics as ordered.
     d. Congestive heart failure (see below)
  9. Provide patient teaching and discharge planning concerning
     a. Limitation with progressive increase in activities
        1) encourage daily walking with gradual increase in distance weekly
        2) avoid heavy lifting and activities that require continuous arm movements (vacuuming, playing golf, bowling)
        3) avoid driving a car until physician permits

b. Sexual intercourse: can usually be resumed by third or fourth week post-op; avoid sexual positions in which the patient would be supporting weight

c. Medication regimen: ensure patient/family are aware of drugs, dosages, proper time of administration, and side effects

d. Meal planning with prescribed modifications (decreased sodium, cholesterol, and possibly carbohydrates)

e. Wound cleansing daily with mild soap and H_2O and to report signs of infection

f. Symptoms to be reported: fever, dyspnea, chest pain with minimal exertion.

Congestive Heart Failure (CHF)

A. General information: inability of the heart to pump an adequate supply of blood to meet the metabolic needs of the body.

B. Types

1. *Left-sided heart failure*
   a. Left ventricular damage causes blood to back up through the left atrium and into the pulmonary veins. Increased pressure causes transudation into the interstitial tissues of the lungs with resultant pulmonary congestion.
   b. Caused by left ventricular damage (usually due to an MI), hypertension, ischemic heart disease, aortic valve disease, mitral stenosis
   c. Assessment findings
      1) dyspnea, orthopnea, PND, tiredness, muscle weakness, cough
      2) tachycardia, PMI displaced laterally, possible S_3, bronchial wheezing, rales, cyanosis, pallor
      3) decreased pO_2, increased pCO_2
      4) diagnostic tests
         a) chest x-ray: shows cardiac hypertrophy
         b) PAP and PCWP usually increased; however, this is dependent on the degree of heart failure
      5) Echocardiography: shows increased size of cardiac chambers

2. *Right-sided heart failure*
   a. Weakened right ventricle is unable to pump blood into the pulmonary system; systemic venous congestion occurs as pressure builds up.
   b. Caused by left-sided heart failure, right ventricular infarction, atherosclerotic heart disease, COPD, pulmonic stenosis, pulmonary embolism.
   c. Assessment findings
      1) anorexia, nausea, weight gain
      2) dependent pitting edema, jugular venous distension, bounding pulses, hepatomegaly, cool extremities, oliguria
      3) elevated CVP, decreased pO_2, increased SGPT
      4) diagnostic tests
         a) chest x-ray: reveals cardiac hypertrophy
         b) Echocardiography: indicates increased size of cardiac chambers.

3. *High-output failure*

a. Cardiac output is adequate, but exceeded by the metabolic needs of the tissues; the exorbitant demands made on the heart eventually cause ventricular failure.
   b. Caused by hyperthyroidism, anemia, AV fistula, pregnancy

C. Medical management (all types)
   1. Determination and elimination/control of underlying cause
   2. Drug therapy: digitalis preparations, diuretics, vasodilators
   3. Sodium-restricted diet
   4. If medical therapies unsuccessful, mechanical assist devices (intra-aortic balloon pump), cardiac transplantation, or mechanical hearts may be employed.

D. Nursing interventions
   1. Monitor respiratory status and provide adequate ventilation (when CHF progresses to pulmonary edema).
      a. Administer oxygen therapy.
      b. Maintain patient in semi- or high-Fowler's position.
      c. Monitor ABGs.
      d. Assess for breath sounds, noting any changes.
   2. Provide physical and emotional rest.
      a. Constantly assess level of anxiety.
      b. Maintain bedrest with limited activity.
      c. Maintain quiet, relaxed environment.
      d. Organize nursing care around rest periods.
   3. Increase cardiac output.
      a. Administer digitalis as ordered and monitor effects.
      b. Monitor ECG and hemodynamic monitoring.
      c. Administer vasodilators as ordered.
      d. Monitor vital signs.
   4. Reduce/eliminate edema.
      a. Administer diuretics (usually thiazide derivatives) as ordered.
      b. Daily weights.
      c. Maintain accurate I&O.
      d. Assess for peripheral edema.
      e. Measure abdominal girths daily.
      f. Monitor electrolyte levels.
      g. Monitor CVP and Swan-Ganz readings.
      h. Provide sodium-restricted diet as ordered.
      i. Provide meticulous skin care.
   5. Provide patient teaching and discharge planning concerning
      a. Need to monitor self daily for signs and symptoms of CHF (pedal edema, weight gain of 1–2 kg in a 2-day period, dyspnea, loss of appetite, cough)
      b. Medication regimen including name, purpose, dosage, frequency, and side effects (digitalis, diuretics)
      c. Prescribed dietary plan (low sodium; small, frequent meals)
      d. Need to avoid fatigue and plan for rest periods.

Pulmonary Edema

A. General information
   1. A medical emergency that usually results from left-sided

heart failure. The capillary pressure within the lungs becomes so great that fluid pours from the blood into the alveoli, bronchi, and bronchioles. Death occurs by suffocation if this condition is untreated.

2. Caused by left-sided heart failure, rapid administration of IV fluids

B. Medical management

1. Oxygen therapy
2. Endotracheal/nasotracheal intubation (possible)
3. Drug therapy
   a. Morphine sulfate to induce vasodilation and decrease anxiety; 5 mg IV, administer slowly
   b. Digitalis to improve cardiac output
   c. Diuretics (furosemide [Lasix] is drug of choice) to relieve fluid retention
   d. Aminophylline to relieve bronchospasm and increase cardiac output; 250–500 mg IV, administer slowly
   e. Vasodilators (nitroglycerin, isosorbide dinitrate) to dilate the vessels, thereby reducing amount of blood returned to the heart
4. Rotating tourniquets or phlebotomy

C. Assessment findings

1. Dyspnea
2. Cough with large amounts of blood-tinged sputum
3. Tachycardia, pallor, wheezing, rales, diaphoresis
4. Restlessness, fear/anxiety
5. Jugular vein distension
6. Decreased pO_2, increased pCO_2, elevated CVP

D. Nursing interventions

1. Assist with intubation (if necessary) and monitor mechanical ventilation.
2. Administer oxygen by mask in high concentrations (40%–60%) if not intubated.
3. Place patient in semi-Fowler's position or over bedside table to ease dyspnea.
4. Administer medications as ordered.
5. Apply and monitor *rotating tourniquets.*
   a. Occlude vessels of each limb for no more than 45 minutes at a time.
   b. Rotate in a clockwise fashion every 15 minutes.
   c. Assess continuously for presence of arterial pulses.
   d. Observe skin for signs of irritation.
   e. When discontinuing, remove 1 tourniquet every 15 minutes to avoid rapid influx of fluid to the heart.
6. Assist with phlebotomy (removal of 300–500 cc of blood from a peripheral vein) if performed.
7. CVP/hemodynamic monitoring.
8. Provide patient teaching and discharge planning concerning
   a. Prescribed medications, including name, purpose, schedule, dosage, and side effects
   b. Dietary restrictions: low sodium, low cholesterol
   c. Importance of adhering to planned rest periods with gradual progressive increase in activities
   d. Daily weights
   e. Need to report the following symptoms to physician immediately: dyspnea, persistent productive cough, pedal edema, restlessness.

Pacemakers

A. General information

1. A pacemaker is an electronic device that delivers an electrical stimulation to the heart through electrodes sewn directly in the epicardium or placed in contact with the endocardium.
2. Today most pacemakers are demand type (programmed to stimulate a contraction when needed).
3. May be temporary or permanent.

B. Indications for use

1. Temporary pacemakers: bradycardia, anterior MI with heart block, conversion of arrhythmias, control of drug-resistant tachyarrhythmias, electrophysiologic studies, prophylactically after open-heart surgery
2. Permanent pacemakers: heart block with low cardiac output, heart failure, tachyarrhythmias, symptomatic sinus bradycardia (sick-sinus syndrome), syncope (Adams-Stokes attacks)

C. Nursing interventions: temporary pacemaker

1. Assess pacemaker function: monitor heart rate and rhythm, noting any deviations from preset level.
2. Maintain the integrity of the system.
   a. Ensure that catheter terminals are attached securely to the pulse generator.
   b. Attach pulse generator to the patient securely to prevent accidental dislodgment.
3. Provide safety and comfort.
   a. Provide safe environment by properly grounding all equipment in the room.
   b. Prevent infection by maintaining sterile technique and assessing site daily.
   c. Encourage ROM in extremity to which pulse generator is attached when permitted.
   d. Observe daily for electrolyte changes that may change myocardial conduction.

D. Nursing interventions: permanent pacemaker

1. Monitor cardiac rhythm and rate, noting any deviations from preset levels.
2. Prevent catheter displacement (activity restricted for the first few days after insertion).
3. Prevent infection.
   a. Assess vital signs, particularly temperature changes.
   b. Maintain sterile dressings over operative site.
   c. Administer antibiotics as prescribed.
   d. Inspect site daily, noting signs of infection.

E. Provide patient teaching and discharge planning concerning

1. Fundamental concepts of cardiac physiology
2. How to monitor pulse daily and to report deviations to physician
3. Ability to carry out usual physical activity with avoidance of contact sports (direct blows to pacemaker)
4. Need to avoid high-output electrical generators and possibly microwave ovens (many pacemakers today are not affected, patient should check with physician)
5. Need to carry identification at all times that includes
   a. Type of pacemaker and model number
   b. Heart rate

c. Manufacturer's name

d. Physician's name and phone number

6. Need for regular medical follow-up

7. Signs of infection and need to report immediately.

Cardiac Arrest

A. General information: sudden, unexpected cessation of breathing and adequate circulation of blood by the heart

B. Medical management

1. Cardiopulmonary resuscitation (CPR); see page 76

2. Drug therapy

a. Lidocaine, procainamide, verapamil

b. Dopamine (Intropin), isoproterenol (Isuprel), norepinephrine (Levophed): see also Drugs Used to Treat Shock, Table 2.10)

c. Epinephrine to enhance myocardial automaticity, excitability, conductivity, and contractility

d. Atropine sulfate to reduce vagus nerve's control over the heart, thus increasing the heart rate

e. Sodium bicarbonate: administered during first few moments of a cardiac arrest to correct respiratory and metabolic acidosis

f. Calcium chloride: calcium ions help the heart beat more effectively by enhancing the myocardium's contractile force

3. Defibrillation (electrical countershock)

C. Assessment findings: unresponsiveness, cessation of respiration, pallor, cyanosis, absence of heart sounds/blood pressure/palpable pulses, dilation of pupils, ventricular fibrillation (if patient on a monitor)

D. Nursing interventions: monitored arrest caused by ventricular fibrillation

1. Begin precordial thump and, if successful, administer lidocaine.

2. If unsuccessful, defibrillation.

3. If defibrillation unsuccessful, initiate CPR immediately.

4. Assist with administration of and monitor effects of additional emergency drugs.

Cardiopulmonary Resuscitation (CPR)

A. General information: process of externally supporting the circulation and respiration of a person who has had a cardiac arrest

B. Nursing interventions: unwitnessed cardiac arrest

1. Assess LOC.

a. Shake victim's shoulder and shout.

b. If no response, summon help.

2. Position victim supine on a firm surface.

3. Open airway.

a. Use chin lift maneuver.

b. Place ear over nose and mouth.

1) look to see if chest is moving.

2) listen for escape of air.

3) feel for movement of air against face.

c. If no respiration, proceed to #4.

4. Ventilate twice, allowing for deflation between breaths.

5. Assess circulation: palpate for carotid pulse; if not present, proceed to #6.

6. Initiate external cardiac compressions.

a. One rescuer: 15 compressions (at rate of 80–100/minute) with 2 ventilations

b. Two rescuers: 5 compressions (at rate of 80–100/minute) with 1 ventilation

7. Simultaneous switch occurs with two-rescuer CPR when compressor is fatigued.

Endocarditis

A. General information

1. Inflammation of the endocardium; platelets and fibrin deposit on the mitral and/or aortic valves causing deformity, insufficiency, or stenosis.

2. Caused by bacterial infection: commonly *S. aureus, S. viridans,* B-hemolytic streptococcus, gonococcus

3. Precipitating factors: rheumatic heart disease, open-heart surgery procedures, GU/Ob-Gyn instrumentation/surgery, dental extractions, invasive monitoring, septic thrombophlebitis

B. Medical management

1. Drug therapy

a. Antibiotics specific to sensitivity of organism cultured

b. Penicillin G and streptomycin if organism not known

c. Antipyretics

2. Cardiac surgery to replace affected valve

C. Assessment findings

1. Fever, malaise, fatigue, dyspnea and cough (if extensive valvular damage), acute upper quadrant pain (if splenic involvement), joint pain

2. Petechiae, murmurs, edema (if extensive valvular damage), splenomegaly, hemiplegia and confusion (if cerebral infarction), hematuria (if renal infarction)

3. Elevated WBC and ESR, decreased Hgb and Hct

4. Diagnostic tests: positive blood culture for causative organism

D. Nursing interventions

1. Administer antibiotics as ordered to control the infectious process.

2. Control temperature elevation by administration of antipyretics.

3. Assess for vascular complications (see Thrombophlebitis, page 82, and Pulmonary Embolism, page 83).

4. Provide patient teaching and discharge planning concerning

a. Types of procedures/treatments (e.g., tooth extractions, GU instrumentation) that increase the chances of recurrences

b. Antibiotic therapy, including name, purpose, dose, frequency, side effects

c. Signs and symptoms of recurrent endocarditis (persistent fever, fatigue, chills, anorexia, joint pain)

d. Avoidance of individuals with known infections.

Pericarditis

A. General information
1. An inflammation of the visceral and parietal pericardium
2. Caused by a bacterial, viral, or fungal infection; collagen diseases; trauma; acute MI; neoplasms; uremia; radiation therapy; drugs (procainamide, hydralazine, doxorubicin HCl [Adriamycin])

B. Medical management
1. Determination and elimination/control of underlying cause
2. Drug therapy
   a. Medication for pain relief
   b. Corticosteroids, salicylates (aspirin) and indomethacin (Indocin) to reduce inflammation
   c. Specific antibiotic therapy against the causative organism may be indicated.

C. Assessment findings
1. Chest pain with deep inspiration (increasing pain when supine), cough, hemoptysis, malaise
2. Tachycardia, fever, pleural friction rub, cyanosis or pallor, accentuated component of S_2, pulsus paradoxus, jugular vein distension
3. Elevated WBC and ESR, normal or elevated SGOT
4. Diagnostic tests
   a. Chest x-ray may show increased heart size if effusion occurs
   b. ECG changes: ST elevation (precordial leads and 2- or 3-limb heads), T wave inversion

D. Nursing interventions
1. Ensure comfort: bedrest with semi- or high-Fowler's position.
2. Monitor hemodynamic parameters carefully.
3. Administer medications as ordered and monitor effects.
4. Provide patient teaching and discharge planning concerning
   a. Signs and symptoms of pericarditis indicative of a recurrence (chest pain that is intensified by inspiration and position changes, fever, cough)
   b. Medication regimen including name, purpose, dosage, frequency, side effects.

Cardiac Tamponade

A. General information
1. An accumulation of fluid/blood in the pericardium that prevents adequate ventricular filling; without emergency treatment patient will die in shock.
2. Caused by blunt or penetrating chest trauma, malignant pericardial effusion; can be a complication of cardiac surgery

B. Medical management: emergency treatment of choice is *pericardiocentesis* (insertion of a needle into the pericardial sac to aspirate fluid/blood and relieve the pressure on the heart)

C. Assessment findings
1. Chest pain
2. Hypotension, distended neck veins, tachycardia, muffled or distant heart sounds, paradoxical pulse, pericardial friction rub
3. Elevated CVP, decreased Hgb and Hct if massive hemorrhage
4. Diagnostic test: chest x-ray reveals enlarged heart and widened mediastinum.

D. Nursing interventions
1. Administer oxygen therapy.
2. Monitor CVP/IVs closely.
3. Assist with pericardiocentesis.
   a. Monitor ECG, blood pressure, and pulse.
   b. Assess aspirated fluid for color, consistency.
   c. Send specimen to lab immediately.

Cardiogenic Shock

See page 28.

The Blood Vessels

Hypertension

A. General information
1. According to the World Health Organization, hypertension is a persistent elevation of the systolic blood pressure above 140 mm Hg and of the diastolic above 90 mm Hg.
2. Types
   a. Essential (primary, idiopathic): marked by loss of elastic tissue and arteriosclerotic changes in the aorta and larger vessels coupled with decreased caliber of the arterioles
   b. Benign: a moderate rise in blood pressure marked by a gradual onset and prolonged course
   c. Malignant: characterized by a rapid onset and short dramatic course with a diastolic blood pressure of more than 150 mm Hg
   d. Secondary: elevation of the blood pressure as a result of another disease such as renal parenchymal disease, Cushing's disease, pheochromocytoma, primary aldosteronism, coarctation of the aorta
3. Essential hypertension usually occurs between ages 35 and 50; more common in men over 35, women over 45; black men affected twice as often as white men/women
4. Risk factors for essential hypertension include positive family history, obesity, stress, cigarette smoking, hypercholesteremia, increased sodium intake

B. Medical management
1. Diet and weight reduction (restricted sodium, kcal, cholesterol)
2. Life-style changes: alcohol moderation, exercise regime, cessation of smoking
3. Antihypertensive drug therapy (see Table 2.18)

C. Assessment findings
1. Pain similar to anginal pain; pain in calves of legs after ambulation or exercise *(intermittent claudication);* severe occipital headaches, particularly in the morning;

Table 2.18   Antihypertensive Drugs

Drug	Action	Side Effects	Nursing Interventions
Diuretics			
Thiazide diuretics Chlorothiazide (Diuril), Hydrochlorothiazide (Esidrix, HydroDIURIL, Oretic)	Block sodium reabsorption in ascending tubule of kidney; water excreted with sodium, producing decreased blood volume	Common: increased BUN, uric acid, blood glucose, and calcium; decreased potassium Less common: sensitivity reactions, GI irritation, rashes, anemia, thrombocytopenia, purpura, pancreatitis *Note:* Thiazides are ineffective if patient has renal failure.	Monitor I&O. Establish a baseline weight prior to initiation of therapy, then weigh daily. Monitor serum electrolytes, BUN, creatinine, uric acid, blood sugar; be particularly alert for hypokalemia. Schedule doses to avoid nocturia and interrupted sleep. Advise patients to change position slowly and to avoid standing still for prolonged periods of time to avoid orthostatic hypotension. Take frequent blood pressure readings, be consistent in method used. Instruct patients about foods high in potassium.
Loop diuretics Furosemide (Lasix) Ethacrynic acid (Edecrin)	Inhibit reabsorption of sodium and chloride at the proximal portion of ascending loop of Henle	Same as for thiazides, but more likely to result in hypovolemia and dehydration.	Observe closely patients on concomitant digitalis therapy for signs of hypokalemia.
Chlorthalidone (Hygroton)		Same as for thiazides, but more likely to result in hypovolemia and dehydration	
Potassium-sparing diuretic Spironolactone (Aldactone)	Antagonizes the effect of aldosterone on the tubular cells of the kidney; sodium excreted in exchange for potassium	Hyperkalemia, gynecomastia, hirsutism, irregular menses, rash, drowsiness or confusion	Monitor serum electrolytes and I&O. Establish baseline weight prior to initiation of drug therapy and then weigh daily. Be particularly alert for signs and symptoms of hyperkalemia/hyponatremia. Observe for and immediately report onset of mental changes.

(continued)

polyuria; nocturia; fatigue; dizziness; epistaxis; dyspnea on exertion

2. Blood pressure consistently above 140/90, retinal hemorrhages and exudates, edema of extremities (indicative of right-sided heart failure)
3. Rise in systolic blood pressure from supine to standing position (indicative of essential hypertension)
4. Diagnostic tests: elevated serum uric acid, sodium, cholesterol levels

D. Nursing interventions
   1. Record baseline blood pressure in three positions (lying, sitting, standing) and in both arms.
   2. Continuously assess blood pressure and report any variables that relate to changes in blood pressure (positioning, restlessness).
   3. Administer antihypertensive agents as ordered; monitor closely and assess for side effects.
   4. Monitor intake and hourly outputs.
   5. Provide patient teaching and discharge planning concerning
      a. Risk factor identification and development/implementation of methods to modify them

   b. Restricted sodium, kcal, cholesterol diet; include family in teaching (see Appendix 1)
   c. Antihypertensive drug regimen (include family)
      1) names, actions, dosages, and side effects of prescribed medications
      2) take drugs at regular times and avoid omission of any doses
      3) never abruptly discontinue the drug therapy
      4) supplement diet with potassium-rich foods if taking potassium-wasting diuretics
      5) avoid hot baths, alcohol, or strenuous exercise within 3 hours of taking medications that cause vasodilation
   d. Development of a graduated exercise program
   e. Importance of routine follow-up care.

Arteriosclerosis Obliterans

A. General information
   1. A chronic occlusive arterial disease that may affect the abdominal aorta or the lower extremities. The obstruction to blood flow with resultant ischemia usually affects the femoral, popliteal, aortal, and iliac arteries.

Table 2.18 Antihypertensive Drugs (continued)

Drug	Action	Side Effects	Nursing Interventions
Drugs acting on CNS			
Guanethidine (Ismelin)	Blocks norepinephrine release from adrenergic nerve endings	Orthostatic hypotension (very common), diarrhea, impotence or loss of ejaculation *Note:* Poor, inconsistent absorption from GI tract	Instruct patients to avoid rapid position changes, prolonged standing, alcohol ingestion, and excess physical exercise. Advise patients to lie or sit down at onset of dizziness, weakness or fatigue. Instruct to report diarrhea.
Methyldopa (Aldomet)	Metabolized into a false neurotransmitter displacing norepinephrine from its receptor sites; sympathetic activity reduced	Orthostatic hypotension, drowsiness, fever, liver damage, anemia, impotence *Note:* methyldopa is the drug of choice in patients with renal disease	Instruct patients to report fever, diarrhea. Advise patients to make position changes slowly, and to lie or sit down at onset of dizziness or lightheadedness. Monitor blood pressure frequently, in both lying and standing positions.
Propranolol (Inderal)	Beta-adrenergic blocker at peripheral outonomic site	GI disturbances, thrombocytopenia, rash, congestive heart failure, aggravation of asthma, fever, severe bradycardia	Instruct patients to take medication before meals. Teach how to take own pulse and to monitor before each dose. Advise to make position changes slowly and to avoid prolonged standing. Counsel to avoid alcohol, coffee, and smoking. Instruct to report dizziness and lightheadedness.
Nadolol (Corgard)	Beta-adrenergic blocking agent; acts by blocking catecholamine-induced increases in heart rate, blood pressure, force of contraction	Bradycardia, postural hypotension; peripheral vascular insufficiency; nasal stuffiness; nausea, vomiting, anorexia	Instruct patient to check pulse before taking each dose. Monitor weight; report weight gain of 3–4 lb/day. Protect drug from light.
Clonidine (Catapres)	Stimulates alpha-adrenergic receptor in brain, causing inhibition of sympathetic vasoconstriction	Orthostatic hypotension, dry mouth, sedation, headache, constipation, fatigue	Monitor I&O during period of dosage adjustment. Closely supervise patients with history of mental depression. Advise patients to change position slowly and to dangle feet a few minutes before standing. Advise patients of possible sedative affect.
Vasodilators			
Hydralazine (Apresoline), Prazosin (Minipress)	Direct relaxation of arteriolar smooth muscle causing vasodilation	Headache, tachycardia, nausea, weakness, angina, rash, dizziness, fever	Note mental status, particularly anxiety, depression, or obtundation. Check blood pressure and pulse, particularly during IV administration. Advise patients to make position changes slowly and to avoid standing still for prolonged periods. Advise patients to avoid alcohol.

   2. Occurs most often in men ages 50–60
   3. Caused by atherosclerosis
   4. Risk factors: cigarette smoking, hyperlipidemia, hypertension, diabetes mellitus
B. Medical management
   1. Drug therapy
      a. Vasodilators: papaverine, isoxsuprine HCl (Vasodilan), nylidrin HCl (Arlidin), nicotinyl alcohol (Roniacol), cyclandelate (Cyclospasmol), tolazoline HCl (Priscoline) to improve arterial circulation; effectiveness questionable
      b. Analgesics to relieve ischemic pain
      c. Anticoagulants to prevent thrombus formation
      d. Lipid-reducing drugs: cholestyramine (Questran),

   colestipol HCl (Cholestid), dextrothyroxine sodium (Choloxin), clofibrate (Atromid-S), gemfibrozil (Lopid), niacin
   2. Surgery: bypass grafting, endarterectomy, balloon catheter dilation; lumbar sympathectomy (to increase blood flow), amputation may be necessary
C. Assessment findings
   1. Pain, both intermittent claudication and rest pain, numbness or tingling of the toes
   2. Pallor after 1–2 minutes of elevating feet, and dependent hyperemia/rubor; diminished or absent dorsalis pedis, posterior tibial and femoral pulses; trophic changes; shiny, taut skin with hair loss on lower legs
   3. Diagnostic tests

a. Oscillometry may reveal decrease in pulse volume
b. Doppler ultrasound reveals decreased blood flow through affected vessels
c. Angiography reveals location and extent of obstructive process
4. Elevated serum tryglicerides; sodium

D. Nursing interventions
1. Encourage slow, progressive physical activity (out of bed at least 3–4 times/day, walking 2 times/day).
2. Administer medications as ordered.
3. Assess for sensory function and trophic changes.
4. Protect patient from injury
5. Provide patient teaching and discharge planning concerning
   a. Restricted kcal, low-saturated fat diet; include family (see Appendix 1)
   b. Importance of continuing with established exercise program
   c. Measures to reduce stress (relaxation techniques, biofeedback)
   d. Importance of avoiding smoking, constrictive clothing, standing in any position for a long time, injury
   e. Importance of foot care, immediately taking care of cuts, wounds, injuries
6. Prepare patient for surgery if necessary.

Thromboangiitis Obliterans (Buerger's Disease)

A. General information
1. Acute, inflammatory disorder affecting medium/smaller size arteries and veins of the lower extremities. Occurs as focal, obstructive process; results in occlusion of a vessel with subsequent development of collateral circulation.
2. Most often affects men ages 25–40
3. Disease is idiopathic; high incidence among smokers.

B. Medical management: see Arteriosclerosis Obliterans, page 79; only really effective treatment is cessation of smoking.

C. Assessment findings
1. Intermittent claudication, sensitivity to cold (skin of extremity may at first be white, changing to blue, then red)
2. Decreased or absent peripheral pulses (posterior tibial and dorsalis pedis), trophic changes, ulceration and gangrene (advanced)
3. Diagnostic tests: same as in Arteriosclerosis Obliterans except no elevation in serum triglycerides

D. Nursing interventions
1. Prepare patient for surgery.
2. Provide patient teaching and discharge planning concerning
   a. Drug regimen (vasodilators, anticoagulants, analgesics) to include names, dosages, frequency, and side effects
   b. Need to avoid trauma to the affected extremity
   c. Need to maintain warmth, especially in cold weather
   d. Importance of stopping smoking.

Raynaud's Phenomenon

A. General information
1. Intermittent episode of arterial spasms, most frequently involving the fingers
2. Most often affects women between the teenage years and age 40
3. Cause unknown
4. Predisposing factors: collagen diseases (systemic lupus erythematosus, rheumatoid arthritis), trauma (e.g., from typing, piano playing, operating a chain saw)

B. Medical management: vasodilators, catecholamine-depleting antihypertensive drugs (reserpine, guanethidine monosulfate (Ismelin)

C. Assessment findings
1. Coldness, numbness, tingling in one or more digits; pain (usually precipitated by exposure to cold, emotional upsets, tobacco use)
2. Intermittent color changes (pallor, cyanosis, rubor); small ulcerations and gangrene at tips of digits (advanced)

D. Nursing interventions
1. Provide patient teaching concerning
   a. Importance of stopping smoking
   b. Need to maintain warmth, especially in the cold weather
   c. Need to use gloves when handling cold objects/opening freezer or refrigerator door
   d. Drug regimen.

Aneurysms

An aneurysm is a sac formed by dilation of an artery secondary to weakness and stretching of the arterial wall. The dilation may involve one or all layers of the arterial wall.

Classification

A. *Fusiform:* uniform spindle shape involving the entire circumference of the artery
B. *Saccular:* outpouching on one side only, affecting only part of the arterial circumference
C. *Dissecting:* separation of the arterial wall layers to form a cavity that fills with blood
D. *False:* the vessel wall is disrupted, blood escapes into surrounding area but is held in place by surrounding tissue.

Thoracic Aortic Aneurysm

A. General information
1. An aneurysm, usually fusiform or dissecting, in the descending, ascending, or transverse section of the thoracic aorta.
2. Usually occurs in men ages 50–70
3. Caused by arteriosclerosis, infection, syphilis, hypertension

B. Medical management
1. Control of underlying hypertension
2. Surgery: resection of the aneurysm and replacement with a Teflon/Dacron graft; patients will need extracorporeal circulation (heart-lung machine).
C. Assessment findings
1. Often asymptomatic
2. Deep, diffuse chest pain; hoarseness; dysphagia; dyspnea
3. Pallor, diaphoresis, distended neck veins, edema of head and arms
4. Diagnostic tests
   a. Aortography shows exact location of the aneurysm
   b. X-rays: chest film reveals abnormal widening of aorta; abdominal film may show calcification within walls of aneurysm
D. Nursing interventions: see Cardiac Surgery, page 73.

Abdominal Aortic Aneurysm

A. General information
1. Most aneurysms of this type are saccular or dissecting and develop just below the renal arteries but above the iliac bifurcation
2. Occur most often in men over age 60
3. Caused by arteriosclerosis, atherosclerosis, hypertension, trauma, syphilis, other types of infectious processes
B. Medical management: surgical resection of the lesion and replacement with a graft (extracorporeal circulation not needed)
C. Assessment findings
1. Severe mid- to low-abdominal pain, low-back pain
2. Mass in the periumbilical area or slightly to the left of the midline with bruits heard over the mass
3. Pulsating abdominal mass
4. Diminished femoral pulses
5. Diagnostic tests: same as for Thoracic Aneurysms.
D. Nursing interventions: preoperative
1. Prepare patient for surgery: routine pre-op care.
2. Assess rate, rhythm, character of the peripheral pulses and mark all distal pulses.
E. Nursing interventions: postoperative
1. Provide routine post-op care.
2. Monitor the following parameters
   a. Hourly circulation checks noting rate, rhythm, character of all pulses distal to the graft
   b. CVP/PAP/PCWP
   c. Hourly outputs through Foley catheter (report less than 30 cc/hour)
   d. Daily BUN/creatinine/electrolyte levels
   e. Presence of back pain (may indicate retroperitoneal hemorrhage)
   f. IV fluids
   g. Neuro status including LOC, pupil size and response to light, hand grasp, movement of extremities
   h. Heart rate and rhythm via monitor.

3. Maintain patient flat in bed without sharp flexion of hip/knee (avoid pressure on femoral/popliteal arteries).
4. Auscultate lungs and encourage turning, coughing, and deep breathing.
5. Assess for signs and symptoms of paralytic ileus (see page 34).
6. Prevent thrombophlebitis.
   a. Encourage patient to dorsiflex foot while in bed.
   b. Use elastic stockings.
   c. Assess for signs and symptoms (see Thrombophlebitis, page 82).
7. Provide patient teaching and discharge planning concerning
   a. Importance of changes in color/temperature of extremities
   b. Avoidance of prolonged sitting, standing, and smoking
   c. Need for a gradual progressive activity regimen
   d. Adherence to low-cholesterol, low-saturated fat diet.

Femoral-Popliteal Bypass Surgery

A. General information
1. Most common type of surgery to correct arterial obstructions of the lower extremities
2. Procedure involves bypassing the occluded vessel with a graft, such as Teflon, Dacron, or an autogenous artery or vein (saphenous).
B. Nursing interventions: preoperative
1. Provide routine pre-op care.
2. Monitor and correct potassium imbalances to prevent cardiac arrhythmias.
3. Assess for focus of infection (infected tooth) or infectious processes (urinary tract infections).
4. Mark distal peripheral pulses.
C. Nursing interventions: postoperative
1. Provide routine post-op care.
2. Assess the following
   a. Circulation, noting rate, rhythm and quality of peripheral pulses distal to the graft, color, temperature and sensation
   b. Signs and symptoms of thrombophlebitis (see page 82)
   c. Neuro checks including LOC and pupillary reaction to light
   d. Hourly outputs
   e. CVP
   f. Wound drainage, noting amount, color, and characteristics.
3. Elevate legs above the level of the heart.
4. Encourage turning, coughing, and deep breathing while splinting incision.

Venous Stasis Ulcers

A. General information
1. Usually a complication of thrombophlebitis and varicose veins.

2. Ulcers result from incompetent valves in the veins, causing high pressure with rupture of small skin veins and venules.
B. Medical management
 1. Antibiotic therapy (specific to organism cultured); topical bacteriocidal solutions
 2. Skin grafting
C. Assessment findings
 1. Pain in the limb in dependent position or during ambulation
 2. Skin of leathery texture, brownish pigment around ankles; positive pulses but edema makes palpation difficult
D. Nursing interventions
 1. Provide bedrest, elevating extremity.
 2. Provide a balanced diet with added protein and vitamin supplements.
 3. Administer antibiotics as ordered to control infection.
 4. Promote healing by cleansing ulcer with prescribed agents.
 5. Provide patient teaching and discharge planning concerning
  a. Importance of avoiding trauma to affected limb
  b. Skin care regimen
  c. Use of elastic support stockings (after ulcer is healed)
  d. Need for planned rest periods with elevation of the extremities
 6. Adherence to balanced diet with vitamin supplements.

Thrombophlebitis

A. General information
 1. Inflammation of the vessel wall with formation of a clot (thrombus); may affect superficial or deep veins.
 2. Most frequent veins affected are the saphenous, femoral, and popliteal.
 3. Can result in damage to the surrounding tissues, ischemia and necrosis.
 4. Risk factors: obesity, CHF, prolonged immobility, MI, pregnancy, oral contraceptives, trauma, sepsis, cigarette smoking, dehydration, severe anemias, venous cannulation, complication of surgery
B. Medical management
 1. Anticoagulant therapy
  a. Heparin
   1) blocks conversion of prothrombin to thrombin and reduces formation or extension of thrombus
   2) side effects: spontaneous bleeding, injection site reactions, ecchymoses, tissue irritation and sloughing, reversible transient alopecia, cyanosis, pain in arms or legs, thrombocytopenia
  b. Warfarin (Coumadin)
   1) blocks prothrombin synthesis by interfering with vitamin K synthesis
   2) side effects

   a) GI: anorexia, nausea and vomiting, diarrhea, stomatitis
   b) hypersensitivity: dermatitis, urticaria, pruritus, fever
   c) other: transient hair loss, burning sensation of feet, bleeding complications
 2. Surgery
  a. Vein ligation and stripping (see page 83)
  b. *Venous thrombectomy:* removal of a clot in the iliofemoral region
  c. *Plication of the inferior vena cava:* insertion of an umbrella-like prosthesis into the lumen of the vena cava to filter incoming clots
C. Assessment findings
 1. Pain in the affected extremity
 2. Superficial vein: tenderness, redness, induration along course of the vein
 3. Deep vein: swelling, venous distension of limb, tenderness over involved vein, positive Homan's sign, cyanosis
 4. Elevated WBC and ESR
 5. Diagnostic tests
  a. Venography (phlebography): increased uptake of radioactive material
  b. Doppler ultrasonography: impairment of blood flow ahead of thrombus
  c. Venous pressure measurements: high in affected limb until collateral circulation is developed.
D. Nursing interventions
 1. Provide bedrest, elevating involved extremity to increase venous return and decrease edema.
 2. Apply continuous warm, moist soaks to decrease lymphatic congestion.
 3. Administer anticoagulants as ordered
  a. Heparin
   1) monitor PTT; dosage should be adjusted to keep PTT between 1.5–2.5 times normal control level.
   2) use infusion pump to administer IV heparin.
   3) ensure proper injection technique.
    a) use 26- or 27-gauge tuberculin syringe with $\frac{1}{2}$–$\frac{5}{8}$ in needle, inject into fatty layer of abdomen above iliac crest.
    b) avoid injecting within 2 inches of umbilicus.
    c) insert needle at 90° to skin.
    d) do not withdraw plunger to assess blood return.
    e) apply gentle pressure after removal of needle, avoid massage.
   4) assess for increased bleeding tendencies (hematuria; hematemesis; bleeding gums; petechiae of soft palate, conjunctiva, retina; ecchymoses, epistaxis, bloody sputum, melena) and instruct patient to observe for and report these.
   5) have antidote (protamine sulfate) available.
   6) instruct patient to avoid aspirin, antihistamines, cough preparations containing glyceryl

guaiacolate, and to obtain physician's permission before using other OTC drugs.
  b. Warfarin (Coumadin)
  1) assess PT daily; dosage should be adjusted to maintain PT at 1.5–2.5 times normal control level.
  2) obtain careful medication history, there are many drug-drug interactions.
  3) advise patient to withhold dose and notify physician immediately if bleeding or signs of bleeding occur (see Heparin, above).
  4) instruct patient to use a soft toothbrush and to floss gently.
  5) have antidote (vitamin K) available.
  6) alert patient to factors that may affect the anticoagulant response (high-fat diet or sudden increases in vitamin K-rich foods.
  7) instruct patient to wear Medic-Alert bracelet .
4. Assess vital signs every 4 hours.
5. Monitor for chest pain or shortness of breath (possible pulmonary embolism).
6. Measure thighs, calves, ankles, and instep every morning.
7. Provide patient teaching and discharge planning concerning
  a. Need to avoid standing, sitting for long periods; constrictive clothing; crossing legs at the knees; smoking and oral contraceptives
  b. Importance of adequate hydration to prevent hypercoagability
  c. Use of elastic stockings when ambulatory
  d. Importance of planned rest periods with elevation of the feet
  e. Drug regimen
  f. Plan for exercise/activity
  1) begin with dorsiflexion of the feet while sitting or lying down
  2) swim several times weekly
  3) gradually increase walking distance
  g. Importance of weight reduction if obese.

Pulmonary Embolism

A. General information
  1. Most pulmonary emboli arise as detached portions of venous thrombi formed in the deep veins of the legs, right side of the heart, or pelvic area.
  2. Distribution of emboli is related to blood flow; emboli involve the lower lobes of the lung because of higher blood flow.
  3. Embolic obstruction to blood flow increases venous pressure in the pulmonary artery and pulmonary hypertension.
  4. Risk factors: venous thrombosis, immobility, pre- and post-op states, trauma, pregnancy, CHF, use of oral contraceptives, obesity
B. Medical management

1. Drug therapy
  a. Anticoagulants (see Thrombophlebitis, page 82)
  b. Fibrinolytics: streptokinase or urokinase
  c. Dextran 70 to decrease blood viscosity and aggregation of blood cells
  d. Narcotics for pain relief
  e. Vasopressors (in the presence of shock)
2. Surgery: *embolectomy* (surgical removal of an embolus from the pulmonary arteries)
C. Assessment findings
  1. Chest pain (pleuritic), severe dyspnea, feeling of impending doom
  2. Tachypnea, tachycardia, anxiety, hemoptysis, shock symptoms (if massive)
  3. Decreased pCO_2; increased pH (due to hyperventilation)
  4. Increased temperature
  5. Intensified pulmonic S_2; crackles
  6. Diagnostic tests
    a. Pulmonary angiography: reveals location/extent of embolism
    b. Lung scan reveals adequacy/inadequacy of pulmonary circulation.
D. Nursing interventions
  1. Administer medications as ordered; monitor effects and side effects.
  2. Administer oxygen therapy to correct hypoxemia.
  3. Assist with turning, coughing, deep breathing, and passive ROM exercises.
  4. Provide adequate hydration to prevent hypercoagulability.
  5. Offer support/reassurance to patient/family.
  6. Elevate head of bed to relieve dyspnea.
  7. Provide patient teaching and discharge planning: same as for Thrombophlebitis.

Varicose Veins

A. General information
  1. Dilated veins that occur most often in the lower extremities and trunk. As the vessel dilates, the valves become stretched and incompetent with resultant venous pooling/edema
  2. Most common between ages 30 and 50
  3. Predisposing factors: congenital weakness of the veins, thrombophlebitis, pregnancy, obesity, heart disease
B. Medical management: vein ligation (involves ligating the saphenous vein where it joins the femoral vein and stripping the saphenous vein system from groin to ankle).
C. Assessment findings
  1. Pain after prolonged standing (relieved by elevation)
  2. Swollen, dilated, tortuous skin veins
  3. Diagnostic tests
    a. Trendelenburg test: varicose veins distend very quickly (less than 35 seconds)
    b. Doppler ultrasound: decreased or no blood flow heard after calf or thigh compression
D. Nursing interventions

1. Elevate legs above heart level.
2. Measure circumference of ankle and calf daily.
3. Apply knee-length elastic stockings.
4. Provide adequate rest.
5. Prepare patient for vein ligation, if necessary.
   a. Provide routine pre-op care.
   b. In addition to routine post-op care
      1) keep affected extremity elevated above the level of the heart to prevent edema.
      2) apply elastic bandages and stockings, which should be removed every 8 hours for short periods and reapplied.
      3) assist out of bed within 24 hours, ensuring that elastic stockings are applied.
      4) assess for increased bleeding, particularly in the groin area.
6. Provide patient teaching and discharge planning: same as for Thrombophlebitis, page 82.

Amputation

A. General informatiuon
   1. Surgical procedure done for peripheral vascular disease if medical management is ineffective and the symptoms become worse.
   2. The level of amputation is determined by the extent of the disease process.
      a. Above knee (AK): performed between the lower third to the middle of the thigh
      b. Below knee (BK): usually done in middle third of leg, leaving a stump of 12.5–17.5 cm
B. Nursing interventions: preoperative
   1. Provide routine pre-op care.
   2. Offer support/encouragement and accept patient's response of anger/grief.
   3. Discuss
      a. Rehabilitation program and use of prosthesis
      b. Upper extremity exercises such as push-ups in bed
      c. Crutch walking
      d. Amputation dressings/cast
      e. Phantom limb sensation as a normal occurrence.
C. Nursing interventions: postoperative
   1. Provide routine post-op care.
   2. Prevent hip/knee contractures
   3. Avoid letting patient sit in chair with hips flexed for long periods of time.
   4. Have patient assume prone position several times a day and position hip in extension (unless otherwise ordered).
   5. Avoid elevation of the stump after 12-24 hours.
   6. Observe stump dressing for signs of hemorrhage and mark outside of dressing so rate of bleeding can be assessed.
   7. Administer pain medication as ordered.
   8. Ensure that stump bandages fit tightly and are applied properly to enhance prosthesis fitting.
   9. Initiate active ROM exercises of all joints (when

medically advised), crutch walking and arm/shoulder exercises.
10. Provide stump care.
   a. Inspect daily for signs of skin irritation.
   b. Wash thoroughly daily with warm water and bacteriostatic soap; rinse and dry thoroughly.
   c. Avoid use of irritating substances such as lotions, alcohol, powders.

SAMPLE QUESTIONS

Mrs. Jane Heath is admitted to the critical care unit to rule out a myocardial infarction. She tells the nurse she is sure it is just angina and cannot understand what the difference is between angina and infarct pain.

6. Which of the following responses made by the nurse demonstrates the best understanding of Mrs. Heath's confusion?
   o a. Anginal pain usually lasts only 3-5 minutes.
   o b. Anginal pain produces clenching of the fists over the chest while acute MI pain does not.
   o c. Anginal pain requires morphine for relief.
   o d. Anginal pain radiates to the left arm while acute MI pain does not.

7. The morning after admission, Mrs. Heath and her husband tell the nurse that Mrs. Heath must be home tonight to care for the children when Mr. Heath goes to work. The problem identified at this point would be
   o a. anxiety related to physical limitations.
   o b. alteration in cardiac output.
   o c. inability of patient/family to understand disease process.
   o d. safety needs related to inability to cope.

The Hematologic System

This section contributed by Margaret Ahearn Spera, RNC, MSN.

OVERVIEW OF ANATOMY AND PHYSIOLOGY

The structures of the hematologic or hematopoietic system include the blood, blood vessels, and blood-forming organs (bone marrow, spleen, liver, lymph nodes, and thymus gland). The major function of blood is to carry necessary materials (oxygen, nutrients) to cells and to remove carbon dioxide and metabolic waste products. The hematologic system also plays an important role in hormone transport, the inflammatory and immune responses, temperature regulation, and fluid and electrolyte and acid-base balances.

Bone Marrow

A. Contained inside all bones, occupies interior of spongy bones and center of long bones; collectively one of the largest organs of the body (4%–5% of total body weight)
B. Primary function is hematopoiesis (the formation of blood cells)
C. Two kinds of bone marrow, red and yellow
  1. Red (functioning) marrow
    a. Carries out hematopoiesis; production site of erythroid, myeloid, and thrombocytic components of blood; one source of lymphocytes and macrophages
    b. Found in ribs, vertebral column, other flat bones
  2. Yellow marrow: red marrow that has changed to fat; found in long bones; does not contribute to hematopoiesis
D. All blood cells start as stem cells in the bone marrow; these mature into the different, specific types of cells, collectively referred to as formed elements of blood or blood components: erythrocytes, leukocytes, and thrombocytes.

Blood

A. Composed of plasma (55%) and cellular components (45%)
B. *Hematocrit*
  1. Reflects portion of blood composed of red blood cells
  2. Centrifugation of blood results in separation into top layer of plasma, middle layer of leukocytes and platelets, and bottom layer of erythrocytes.
  3. Majority of formed elements is erythrocytes; volume of leukocytes and platelets is negligible.
C. Distribution
  1. 1300 cc in pulmonary circulation
    a. 400 cc arterial
    b. 60 cc capillary
    c. 840 cc venous
  2. 3000 cc in systemic circulation
    a. 550 cc arterial
    b. 300 cc capillary
    c. 2150 cc venous

Plasma

A. Liquid part of blood; yellow in color because of pigments
B. Consists of serum (liquid portion of plasma) and fibrinogen
C. Contains plasma proteins such as albumin, serum globulins, fibrinogen, prothrombin, plasminogen
  1. Albumin: largest of plasma proteins, involved in regulation of intravascular plasma volume and maintenance of osmotic pressure
  2. Serum globulins: alpha, beta, gamma
    a. Alpha: role in transport of steroids, lipids, bilirubin
    b. Beta: role in transport of iron and copper
    c. Gamma: role in immune response, function of antibodies
  3. Fibrinogen, prothrombin, plasminogen (see Coagulation, page 86).

Cellular Components

Cellular components or formed elements of blood are erythrocytes (red blood cells [RBCs]), which are responsible for oxygen transport; leukocytes (white blood cells [WBCs]), which play a major role in defense against microorganisms; and thrombocytes (platelets), which function in hemostasis.
A. *Erythrocytes*
  1. Bioconcave disc shape, no nucleus, chiefly sacs of hemoglobin
  2. Cell membrane is highly diffusible to O_2 and CO_2
  3. RBCs are responsible for oxygen transport via *hemoglobin (Hgb)*

a. Two portions: iron carried on heme portion; second portion is protein

b. Normal blood contains 12–18 gm Hgb/100 cc blood; higher (14–18 gm) in men than in women (12–14 gm)

4. Production

a. Start in bone marrow as stem cells, released as reticulocytes (immature cells), mature into erythrocytes

b. Erythropoietin stimulates differentiation; produced by kidneys and stimulated by hypoxia

c. Iron, vitamin B_{12}, folic acid, pyridoxine (vitamin B_6) and other factors required for erythropoiesis.

5. Hemolysis (destruction)

a. Average life span 120 days

b. Immature RBCs destroyed in either bone marrow or other reticuloendothelial organs (blood, connective tissue, spleen, liver, lungs, and lymph nodes)

c. Mature cells removed chiefly by liver and spleen

d. *Bilirubin:* byproduct of Hgb released when RBCs destroyed, excreted in bile

e. Iron: freed from Hgb during bilirubin formation; transported to bone marrow via transferrin and reclaimed for new Hgb production

f. Premature destruction: may be caused by RBC membrane abnormalities, Hgb abnormalities, extrinsic physical factors (such as the enzyme defects found in G_6PD)

g. Normal age RBCs may be destroyed by gross damage as in trauma or extravascular hemolysis (in spleen, liver, bone marrow).

B. *Leukocytes:* granulocytes and mononuclear cells; involved in protection from bacteria and other foreign substances

1. Granulocytes: eosinophils, basophils, and neutrophils

a. *Eosinophils:* involved in phagocytosis and allergic reactions

b. *Basophils:* involved in prevention of clotting in microcirculation and allergic reactions

c. Eosinophils and basophils are reservoirs of histamine, serotonin, and heparin

d. *Neutrophils:* involved in short-term phagocytosis

1) mature neutrophils: polymorphonuclear leukocytes

2) immature neutrophils: band cells (bacterial infection usually produces increased numbers of band cells [shift to the left])

2. Mononuclear cells: monocytes and lymphocytes; large nucleated cells

a. *Monocytes:* involved in long-term phagocytosis; play a role in immune response

1) largest leukocyte

2) produced by bone marrow: give rise to histiocytes (Kupffer cells of liver), macrophages, and other components of reticuloendothelial system

b. *Lymphocytes:* immune cells; produce substances against foreign cells; produced primarily in lymph tissue (B cells) and thymus (T cells) (see also Immune Response, page 13)

C. *Thrombocytes (platelets)*

1. Fragments of megakaryocytes formed in bone marrow

2. Production regulated by thrombopoietin

3. Essential factor in coagulation via adhesion, aggregation, and plug formation

4. Release substances involved in coagulation.

Blood Groups

A. Erythrocytes carry antigens, which determine the different blood groups.

B. Blood-typing systems are based on the many possible antigens, but the most important are the antigens of the ABO and Rh blood groups because they are most likely to be involved in transfusion reactions.

1. ABO typing

a. Antigens of system are labelled A and B.

b. Absense of both antigens results in type O blood.

c. Presense of both antigens is type AB.

d. Presence of either A or B results in type A and type B respectively.

e. Nearly half the population is type O, the *univeral donor.*

f. Antibodies are automatically formed against the ABO antigens not on person's own RBCs; transfusion with mismatched or incompatible blood results in a transfusion reaction (Table 2.19).

2. Rh typing

a. Identifies presence or absence of Rh antigen (Rh positive or Rh negative).

b. Anti-Rh antibodies not automatically formed in Rh-negative person, but if Rh-positive blood is given antibody formation starts and a second exposure to Rh antigen will trigger a transfusion reaction.

c. Important for Rh-negative woman carrying Rh-positive baby; first pregnancy not affected, but in a subsequent pregnancy with an Rh-positive baby mother's antibodies attack baby's RBCs (see Hemolytic Disease of the Newborn, page **422**).

Blood Coagulation

Conversion of fluid blood to a solid clot to reduce blood loss when blood vessels are ruptured.

A. Systems that initiate clotting

1. *Intrinsic system:* initiated by contact activation following endothelial injury ("intrinsic" to vessel itself)

a. Factor XII initiates as contact made between damaged vessel and plasma protein

b. Factors VIII, IX, and XI activated

2. *Extrinsic system*

a. Initiated by tissue thromboplastins, released from injured vessels ("extrinsic" to vessel)

b. Factor VII activated

B. Common pathway: activated by either intrinsic or extrinsic pathways

1. Platelet factor 3 (PF3) and calcium react with factors X and V.

2. Prothrombin converted to thrombin via thromboplastin.

3. Thrombin acts on fibrinogen forming soluble fibrin.

4. Soluble fibrin polymerized by factor XIII to produce a stable, insoluble fibrin clot.

C. Clot resolution: takes place via fibrinolytic system by plasmin and proteolytic enzymes; clot dissolves as tissue repairs.

Spleen

A. Largest lymphatic organ; functions as blood filtration system and reservoir

B. Vascular, bean shaped; lies beneath the diaphragm, behind and to the left of the stomach; composed of a fibrous tissue capsule surrounding a network of fiber

C. Contains two types of pulp
   1. Red pulp: located between the fibrous strands, composed of RBCs, WBCs, and macrophages
   2. White pulp: scattered throughout the red pulp, produces lymphocytes and sequesters lymphocytes, macrophages, and antigens

D. 1%–2% of red cell mass or 200 cc blood/minute stored in spleen; blood comes via the splenic artery to the pulp for cleansing, then passes into splenic venules that are lined with phagocytic cells, and finally to the splenic vein to the liver.

E. Important hematopoietic site in fetus; postnatally produces lymphocytes and monocytes

F. Important in phagocytosis; removes misshapen erythrocytes, unwanted parts of erythrocytes

G. Also involved in antibody production by plasma cells and iron metabolism (iron released from Hgb portion of destroyed erythrocytes returned to bone marrow)

H. In the adult, functions of the spleen can be taken over by the reticuloendothelial system.

Liver

See also Gastrointestinal Tract, page 116.

A. Involved in bile production (via erythrocyte destruction and bilirubin production) and erythropoiesis (during fetal life and when bone marrow production is insufficient).

B. Kupffer cells of liver have reticuloendothelial function as histiocytes; phagocytic activity and iron storage

C. Liver also involved in synthesis of clotting factors, synthesis of antithrombins.

ASSESSMENT

Health History

A. Presenting problem
   1. Nonspecific symptoms may include: chills, fatigue, fever, weakness, weight loss, night sweats, delayed wound healing, malaise, lethargy, depression, cold/heat intolerance
   2. Note specific signs and symptoms
      a. Skin: prolonged bleeding, petechiae, jaundice, ecchymosis, pruritus, pallor
      b. Eyes: visual disturbance, yellowed sclera
      c. Ears: vertigo, tinnitus
      d. Mouth and nose: epistaxis; gingival bleeding, ulceration, pain; dysphagia, hoarseness
      e. Neck: nuchal rigidity, lymphadenopathy
      f. Respiratory: dyspnea, orthopnea, palpitations, chest discomfort or pain, cough (productive or dry), hemoptysis
      g. GI: melena, abdominal pain, change in bowel habits
      h. GU: hematuria, recurrent infection, amenorrhea, menorrhagia
      i. CNS: confusion, headache, paresthesias, syncope
      j. Musculoskeletal: joint, back, or bone pain

B. Life-style: exposure to chemicals, occupational exposure to radiation

C. Use of medications
   1. Iron, vitamins (B_6, B_{12}, folic acid)
   2. Corticosteroids
   3. Anticoagulants
   4. Antibiotics
   5. Aspirin or aspirin-containing compounds
   6. Cold or allergy preparations
   7. Antiarrhythmics
   8. Blood transfusions (cryoprecipitates)
   9. Cancer chemotherapy drugs
   10. Immunosuppressant drugs

D. Medical history
   1. Surgery: splenectomy, tumor resection, cardiac valve replacement, GI tract resection
   2. Allergies: multiple transfusions with whole blood or blood products, other known allergies
   3. Mononucleosis; radiation therapy; recurrent infections; malabsorption syndrome; anemia; delayed wound healing; thrombophlebitis, pulmonary embolism, deep vein thrombosis (DVT); liver disease, ETOH abuse, vitamin K deficiency; angina pectoris, atrial fibrillation

E. Family history: jaundice, anemia, bleeding disorders (hemophilia, polycythemia), malignancies, congenital blood dyscrasias

Physical Examination

A. Auscultate for heart murmurs; bruits (cerebral, cardiac, carotid); pericardial or pleural friction rubs; bowel sounds.

B. Inspect for
   1. Flush or pallor of mucous membranes, nail beds, palms, soles of feet
   2. Injection or pallor of sclera, conjunctiva
   3. Cyanosis
   4. Jaundice of skin, mucous membranes, conjunctiva
   5. Signs of bleeding, petechiae, ecchymoses, oral mucosal bleeding (especially gums), epistaxis, hemorrhage from any orifice
   6. Ulcerations or lesions
   7. Swelling or erythema
   8. Neurologic changes: pain and touch, position and vibratory sense, superficial and deep tendon reflexes.

C. Palpate lymph nodes; note location, size, texture, sensation, fixation; palpate the ribs for sternal, bone tenderness.

D. Evaluate joint range of motion and tenderness.
E. Percuss for lung excursion, splenomegaly, hepatomegaly.

Laboratory/Diagnostic Tests

A. Blood
   1. Complete blood count (CBC) with differential and peripheral smear
      a. White blood cell count (WBC) with differential
      b. Hgb and Hct
      c. Platelet and reticulocyte count
      d. Red blood cell count (RBC) with peripheral smear
   2. Coagulation studies
      a. Prothrombin time (PT)
      b. Partial thromboplastin time (PTT)
      c. Fibrin split products (FSP)
      d. Lee-White clotting time (whole blood clotting time)
   3. Blood chemistry
      a. Blood urea nitrogen (BUN)
      b. Creatinine
      c. Bilirubin: direct and indirect
      d. Uric acid
   4. Miscellaneous
      a. Erythrocyte sedimentation rate (ESR)
      b. Serum protein electrophoresis
      c. Serum iron and total iron-binding capacity
      d. Plasma protein assays
      e. Direct and indirect Coombs' tests
B. Urine and stool
   1. Urinalysis
   2. Hematest
   3. Bence Jones protein assay (urine)
C. Radiologic
   1. Chest or other x-ray as indicated by history and physical exam
   2. Radionuclide scans (e.g., bone scan)
   3. Lymphangiography
D. *Bone marrow aspiration and biopsy*
   1. Puncture, usually of sternum, vertebral body, iliac crest, or tibia (in infants) to collect tissue from bone marrow
   2. Purpose: study cells involved in blood production
   3. Nursing care
      a. Confirm that consent form has been signed.
      b. Allay patient anxiety; prepare patient for a sharp, brief pain when bone marrow is aspirated into syringe.
      c. Position patient and assist physician to maintain sterile field.
      d. Send specimen to laboratory.

ANALYSIS

Nursing diagnoses for the patient with a disorder of the blood or blood-forming organs may include
A. Alteration in tissue perfusion
B. Impaired gas exchange
C. Potential activity intolerance
D. Potential self-care deficit
E. Potential impairment of skin integrity
F. Potential alteration in fluid volume (excess or deficit)
G. Potential alteration in oral mucous membranes
H. Alteration in nutrition: less than body requirements

PLANNING AND IMPLEMENTATION

Goals

A. Patient will have increased strength and endurance.
B. Patient will be free from infection.
C. Patient will be free from bleeding.
D. Pain will be relieved/controlled.
E. Patient will be able to cope with the diagnosis and prognosis.
F. Circulatory overload will be prevented.
G. Patient will be free from febrile reaction.
H. Patient will be free from allergic reaction.
I. Hemolytic reaction will be prevented.
J. Delayed hemolytic reaction will not occur.
K. Disease will not be transmitted through blood transfusion.
L. Adequate nutrition will be maintained.

Interventions

Blood Transfusion and Component Therapy

A. Purpose: improve oxygen transport (RBCs); volume expansion (whole blood, plasma, albumin); provision of proteins (fresh frozen plasma, albumin, plasma protein fraction); provision of coagulation factors (cryoprecipitate, fresh frozen plasma, fresh whole blood); provision of platelets (platelet concentrate, fresh whole blood)
B. Blood and blood products
   1. Whole blood: provides all components
      a. Large volume can cause difficulty: 12–24 hours for Hgb and Hct to rise
      b. Complications: volume overload, transmission of hepatitis or AIDS, transfusion reaction, infusion of excess potassium and sodium, infusion of anticoagulant (citrate) used to keep stored blood from clotting, calcium binding and depletion (citrate) in massive transfusion therapy
   2. Red blood cells
      a. Provide twice the amount of Hgb as an equivalent amount of whole blood
      b. Indicated in cases of blood loss, pre- and post-op patients, and those with incipient congestive failure
      c. Complications: transfusion reaction (less common than with whole blood due to removal of plasma proteins)
   3. Fresh frozen plasma
      a. Contains all coagulation factors including V and VIII
      b. Can be stored frozen for 12 months; takes 20 minutes to thaw
      c. Hang immediately upon arrival to unit (loses its coagulation factors rapidly).
   4. Platelets

a. Will raise recipient's platelet count by 10,000 μ/liter

b. Pooled from 4–8 units of whole blood

c. Single-donor platelet transfusions may be necessary for patients who have developed antibodies; compatibility testing may be necessary.

5. Factor VIII fractions (cryoprecipitate): contains Factors VIII, fibrinogen, and XIII

6. Granulocytes

a. Do not increase WBC; increases marginal pool (at tissue level) rather than circulating pool

b. Premedication with steroids, antihistamines, and acetaminophen

c. Respiratory distress with shortness of breath, cyanosis, and chest pain may occur; requires cessation of transfusion and immediate attention

d. Shaking chills or rigors common, require brief cessation of therapy, administration of meperidine IV until rigors are diminished, and resumption of transfusion when symptoms relieved.

7. Volume expanders: albumin; percentage concentration varies (50–100 cc/unit); hyperosmolar solutions should not be used in dehydrated patients.

C. Nursing care

1. Assess patient for history of previous blood transfusions and any adverse reactions.

2. Ensure that the adult patient has an 18- or 19-gauge IV catheter in place.

3. Use 0.9% sodium chloride.

4. At least two nurses should verify the ABO group, Rh type, patient and blood numbers, and expiration date.

5. Take baseline vital signs before initiating transfusion.

6. Start transfusion slowly (2 cc/minute).

7. Stay with the patient during the first 15 minutes of the transfusion and take vital signs frequently.

8. Maintain the prescribed transfusion rate.

a. Whole blood: approximately 3–4 hours

b. RBCs: approximately 2–4 hours

c. Fresh frozen plasma: as quickly as possible

d. Platelets: as quickly as possible

e. Cryoprecipitate: rapid infusion

f. Granulocytes: usually over 2 hours

g. Volume expanders: volume dependent rate

9. Monitor for adverse reactions (see Table 2.19).

10. Document the following

a. Blood component unit number (apply sticker if available)

b. Date infusion starts and ends

c. Type of component and amount transfused

d. Patient reaction and vital signs

e. Signature of transfusionist.

Isolation Techniques

A. General information

1. Used to prevent the spread of communicable disease within the hospital environment

2. Three elements in spread of infection

a. Source of infection: patient, visitor, employee, inanimate object

b. Means of transmission: contact (direct, indirect, droplet spread), vehicle (airborne, vectorborne)

c. Host factors: susceptibility vs resistance

3. Differences in infectivity and in mode of transmission of various agents form the basis for the categories of isolation and precautions.

4. Infectious agent and host factors are difficult to control; efforts to interrupt the chain of infection directed at transmission.

5. Requirements vary depending on type of isolation; strict isolation requires

a. A private room with the door closed

b. Gowns, masks, and gloves worn by all who enter the room

c. Hand washing upon entering and leaving the room

d. Articles, including linen, to be double bagged for disinfection, sterilization, or disposal.

6. Disadvantages: procedures are time-consuming and expensive, make visits by health care personnel inconvenient, and make delivery of care more difficult; private rooms occupy space that could otherwise accommodate more than one patient, deprive patient of normal social contacts.

B. Categories of Isolation

1. *Strict isolation*: recommended for highly communicable diseases spread by direct contact and airborne routes

2. *Enteric isolation*: designed to prevent transmission of disease through direct or indirect contact with infected feces or heavily contaminated articles

3. *Respiratory isolation* and *special respiratory isolation for pulmonary tuberculosis* : to prevent transmission of organisms by droplets or droplet nuclei (coughed, sneezed, or breathed into environment)

4. *Neutropenic precautions (reverse isolation)*: indicated for protection of patients with absolute granulocyte counts below 1000 μ/liter or for those in whom granulocytopenia is anticipated (patients receiving chemotherapeutic drugs)

5. *Skin and wound isolation*: necessary to prevent cross-contamination where infective material is present in wounds, on body surfaces, or on heavily contaminated articles

6. *Blood and needle precautions*: necessary for conditions spread through contact with blood or blood-contaminated excreta or articles

7. *Secretion-excretion precautions*: necessary for conditions spread through contact with bodily secretions or excretions except as noted with enteric precautions

8. *Caution to pregnant women:* for diseases such as rubella and varicella (chickenpox), pregnant women should not enter the patient's room

9. *Antibiotic resistance precautions:* necessary for patients with organisms known to be resistant to antibiotic therapy

10. *AIDS precautions:* for patient with proven or suspected AIDS or HIV-associated illness.

Table 2.19 Complications of Blood Transfusion

Type	Causes	Mechanism	Occurrence	Signs and Symptoms	Intervention
Hemolytic	ABO incompatibility; Rh incompatibility; use of dextrose solutions; wide temperature fluctuations	Antibodies in recipient plasma react with antigen in donor cells. Agglutinated cells block capillary blood flow to organs. Hemolysis (Hgb into plasma and urine).	*Acute:* first 5 min after completion of transfusion *Delayed:* days to 2 weeks after	Headache, lumbar or sternal pain, nausea, vomiting, diarrhea, fever, chills, flushing, heat along vein, restlessness, anemia, jaundice, dyspnea, signs of shock, renal shutdown, DIC	Stop transfusion. Continued saline IV. Send blood unit and patient blood sample to lab. Watch for hemoglobin-urea. Treat or prevent shock, DIC, and renal shutdown.
Allergic	Transfer of an antigen or antibody from donor to recipient; allergic donors	Immune sensitivity to foreign serum protein	Within 30 min of start of transfusion	Urticaria, laryngeal edema, wheezing, dyspnea, bronchospasm, headache, anaphylaxis	Stop transfusion. Administer antihistamine and/or epinephrine. Treat life-threatening reactions.
Pyrogenic	Recipient possesses antibodies directed against WBCs; bacterial contamination; multitransfused patients; multiparous patients	Leukocyte agglutination. Bacterial organisms.	Within 15–90 min after initiation of transfusion	Fever, chills, flushing, palpitations, tachycardia, occasional lumbar pain	Stop transfusion. Treat temperature. Transfuse with leukocyte-poor blood or washed RBCs. Administer antibiotics PRN.
Circulatory overload	Too rapid infusion in susceptible patients	Fluid volume overload	During and after transfusion	Dyspnea, tachycardia, orthopnea, increased blood pressure, cyanosis, anxiety	Slow infusion rate. Use packed cells instead of whole blood. Monitor CVP through a separate line.
Air embolism	Blood given under air pressure following severe blood loss	Bolus of air blocks pulmonary artery outflow	Any time	Dyspnea, increased pulse, wheeze, chest pain, decreased blood pressure, apprehension	Clamp tubing. Turn patient on left side.
Thrombocytopenia	Use of large amounts of banked blood	Platelets deteriorate rapidly in stored blood	When large amounts of blood given over 24 hr	Abnormal bleeding	Assess for signs of bleeding. Initiate bleeding precautions. Use fresh blood.
Citrate intoxication	Large amounts of citrated blood in patients with decreased liver function	Citrate binds ionic calcium	After large amounts of banked blood	Neuromuscular irritability Bleeding due to decreased calcium	Monitor/treat hypocalcemia. Avoid large amounts of citrated blood. Monitor liver function.
Hyperkalemia	Potassium levels increase in stored blood	Release of potassium into plasma with red cell lysis	In patients with renal insufficiency	Nausea, colic, diarrhea, muscle spasms, ECG changes (tall peaked T-wave, short Q–T segment)	Administer blood less than 5–7 days old in patients with impaired potassium excretion.

EVALUATION

A. Patient experiences increased strength and endurance.
  1. Describes causes for weakness and fatigue.
  2. Staggers activity throughout the day.
  3. Plans rest periods at specified intervals.
  4. Alters life-style to accommodate reduced activity tolerance.
  5. Improves endurance progressively.
B. Patient remains free from infection.
  1. Maintains adequate nutritional intake.
  2. Practices regular and routine oral hygiene.
  3. States signs and symptoms of infection and preventive measures.
  4. Avoids sources of infection.
  5. Reports signs and symptoms of infection immediately.
C. Patient is free from bleeding.
  1. Manages established therapeutic regimen.
  2. Avoids trauma.
  3. Utilizes atraumatic oral hygiene.
  4. Monitors self for evidence of excessive bleeding (e.g., menses, urine, stool).
  5. Reports signs and symptoms of infection immediately.
D. Patient reports relief/control of pain.
  1. Uses analgesics as instructed.
  2. Uses positioning techniques to decrease pain.
  3. Uses comfort measures to relieve pain (e.g., heat or cold compress).
E. Patient is able to cope with diagnosis and prognosis.
  1. Verbalizes to family/significant others concerns about diagnosis.
  2. Sets realistic goals.
  3. Explains basis for anemia or other disorder.
  4. Plans to obtain Medic-Alert identification if needed.
F. Patient remains free from circulatory overload.
  1. Maintains normal vital signs.
  2. Lungs clear to auscultation.
  3. Respiratory rate normal and unlabored.
  4. Blood pressure within normal limits.
  5. Pulse within normal limits.
G. Patient is free from febrile reaction.
  1. Maintains normal pulse rate and temperature.
  2. Is without chills, headache, or flushing.
H. Patient remains free from allergic reaction.
  1. Is without rash, pruritus, or skin eruptions.
  2. Respiratory rate normal and unlabored.
I. Patient is free from hemolytic reaction.
  1. Maintains normal vital signs: temperature, pulse, blood pressure within normal limits.
  2. Urine amber color.
J. Patient remains free from delayed hemolytic reaction (5–10 days after transfusion).
  1. Maintains normal vital signs: temperature within normal limits.
  2. Hgb and Hct within normal limits.
  3. Absence of jaundice.
K. Patient is free from disease transmitted by blood transfusions: absence of hepatitis, AIDS.
L. Patient maintains adequate nutrition.
  1. Describes appropriate dietary modifications.
  2. Describes components of a well-balanced diet.
  3. Plans menus based on inclusion of deficient nutrients (e.g., iron, B-complex vitamins, folic acid).
  4. Maintains adequate hydration.

DISORDERS OF THE HEMATOLOGIC SYSTEM

Anemias

Iron-deficiency Anemia

A. General information
  1. Chronic microcytic, hypochromic anemia caused by either inadequate absorption or excessive loss of iron
  2. Acute or chronic bleeding principal cause in adults (chiefly from trauma, excessive menses, and GI bleeding)
  3. May also be caused by inadequate intake of iron-rich foods or by inadequate absorption of iron (from chronic diarrhea, malabsorption syndromes, high cereal-product intake with low animal protein ingestion, partial or complete gastrectomy, pica)
  4. Incidence related to geographic location, economic class, age group, and sex
    a. More common in developing countries and tropical zones (blood-sucking parasites)
    b. Women between ages 15–45 and children affected more frequently, as are the poor
  5. In iron-deficiency states, iron stores are depleted first, followed by a reduction in Hgb formation.
B. Assessment findings
  1. Mild cases usually asymptomatic
  2. Palpitations, dizziness, and cold sensitivity
  3. Brittleness of hair and nails; pallor
  4. Dysphagia, stomatitis, and atrophic glossitis
  5. Dyspnea, weakness
  6. Laboratory findings
    a. RBCs small (microcytic) and pale (hypochromic)
    b. Hgb markedly decreased
    c. Hct moderately decreased
    d. Serum iron markedly decreased
    e. Hemosiderin absent from bone marrow
    f. Serum ferritin decreased
    g. Reticulocyte count decreased
C. Nursing interventions
  1. Monitor for signs and symptoms of bleeding through hematest of all elimination including stool, urine, and gastric contents.
  2. Provide for adequate rest: plan activities so as not to overtire.
  3. Provide a thorough explanation of all diagnostic tests used to determine sources of possible bleeding (helps allay anxiety and ensure cooperation).
  4. Administer iron preparations as ordered.
    a. Oral iron preparations: route of choice

1) give following meals or a snack.

2) dilute liquid preparations well and administer using a straw to prevent staining teeth.

3) when possible administer with orange juice as vitamin C (ascorbic acid) enhances iron absorption.

4) warn patients that iron preparations will change stool color and consistency (dark and tarry) and may cause constipation.

b. Parenteral: used in patients intolerant to oral preparations, who are noncompliant with therapy, or who have continuing blood losses.

1) use one needle to withdraw and another to administer iron preparations as tissue staining and irritation are a problem.

2) use the "Z" track injection technique to prevent leakage into tissues.

3) do not massage injection site but encourage ambulation as this will enhance absorption; advise against vigorous exercise and constricting garments.

4) observe for local signs of complications: pain at the injection site, development of sterile abscesses, lymphadenitis as well as fever, headache, urticaria, hypotension, or anaphylactic shock.

5. Provide dietary teaching regarding foods high in iron.

6. Encourage ingestion of roughage and increase fluid intake to prevent constipation if oral iron preparations being taken.

Pernicious Anemia

A. General information

1. Chronic progressive, macrocytic anemia caused by a deficiency of intrinsic factor; the result is abnormally large erythrocytes and hypochlorhydria (a deficiency of hydrochloric acid in gastric secretions)

2. Characterized by neurologic and GI symptoms; death usually results if untreated

3. Lack of intrinsic factor is caused by gastric mucosal atrophy (possibly due to heredity, prolonged iron deficiency, or an autoimmune disorder); can also result in patients who have had a total gastrectomy if vitamin B_{12} not administered.

4. Usually occurs in men and women over age 50, with an increase in blue-eyed persons of Scandinavian descent

5. Pathophysiology

a. Intrinsic factor is necessary for the absorption of vitamin B_{12} by the small intestine.

b. B_{12} deficiency diminishes DNA synthesis, which results in defective maturation of cells (particularly rapidly dividing cells such as blood cells and GI tract cells).

c. B_{12} deficiency can alter structure and function of peripheral nerves, spinal cord, and the brain.

B. Medical management

1. Drug therapy

a. Vitamin B_{12} injections: monthly maintenance

b. Iron preparations (if Hgb level inadequate to meet increased numbers of erythroctyes)

c. Folic acid

1) controversial

2) reverses anemia and GI symptoms but may intensify neurologic symptoms

3) may be safe if given in small amounts in addition to vitamin B_{12}

2. Transfusion therapy

C. Assessment findings

1. Anemia, weakness, pallor, dyspnea, palpitations, fatigue

2. GI symptoms: sore mouth; smooth, beefy, red tongue; weight loss; dyspepsia; constipation or diarrhea; jaundice

3. CNS symptoms: tingling, paresthesias of hands and feet, paralysis, depression, psychosis

4. Laboratory tests

a. Erythrocyte count decreased

b. Blood smear: oval, macrocytic erythrocytes with a proportionate amount of Hgb

c. Bone marrow

1) increased megaloblasts (abnormal erythrocytes)

2) few normoblasts or maturing erythrocytes

3) defective leukoctye maturation

d. Bilirubin (indirect): elevated unconjugated fraction

e. Serum LDH elevated

f. Positive *Schilling test*

1) measures absorption of radioactive vitamin B_{12} both before and after parenteral administration of intrinsic factor

2) definitive test for pernicious anemia

3) used to detect lack of intrinsic factor

g. Gastric analysis: decreased free hydrochloric acid

h. Large numbers of reticulocytes in the blood following parenteral vitamin B_{12} administration

D. Nursing interventions

1. Provide a nutritious diet high in iron, protein, and vitamins (fish, meat, milk/milk products, and eggs).

2. Avoid highly seasoned, coarse, or very hot foods if patient has mouth sores.

3. Provide mouth care before and after meals using a soft tooth brush and nonirritating rinses.

4. Bedrest may be necessary if anemia is severe.

5. Provide safety when ambulating (especially if carrying hot items, etc.).

6. Provide patient teaching and discharge planning concerning

a. Dietary instruction

b. Importance of lifelong vitamin B_{12} therapy

c. Rehabilitation and physical therapy for neurologic deficits, as well as instruction regarding safety.

Aplastic Anemia

A. General information

1. Pancytopenia or depression of granulocyte, platelet, and erythrocyte production due to fatty replacement of the bone marrow

2. Bone marrow destruction may be idiopathic or secondary

3. Secondary aplastic anemia may be caused by

a. Chemical toxins (e.g., benzene)
b. Drugs (e.g., chloramphenicol, cytotoxic drugs)
c. Radiation
d. Immunologic injury

B. Medical management
1. Blood transfusions (see page 88): key to therapy until patient's own marrow begins to produce blood cells
2. Aggressive treatment of infections
3. Bone marrow transplantation
4. Drug therapy
   a. Corticosteroids and/or androgens to stimulate bone marrow function and to increase capillary resistance (effective in children, but not usually in adults)
   b. Estrogen and/or progesterone to prevent amenorrhea in female patients
5. Identification and withdrawal of offending agent or drug

C. Assessment findings
1. Fatigue and dyspnea
2. Increased susceptibility to infection
3. Bleeding tendencies and hemorrhage
4. Laboratory findings: normocytic anemia, granulocytopenia, thrombocytopenia
5. Bone marrow biopsy: marrow is fatty and contains very few developing cells.

D. Nursing interventions
1. Administer blood transfusions as ordered.
2. Provide nursing care for patient with bone marrow transplantation.
3. Administer medications as ordered.
4. Monitor for signs of infection and provide care to minimize risk.
   a. Maintain neutropenic isolation.
   b. Encourage high-protein, high-vitamin diet to help reduce incidence of infection.
   c. Provide mouth care before and after meals.
5. Monitor for signs of bleeding and provide measures to minimize risk.
   a. Use a soft toothbrush and electric razor.
   b. Avoid intramuscular injections.
   c. Hematest urine and stool.
   d. Observe for oozing from gums, petechiae, or ecchymoses.
6. Provide patient teaching and discharge planning concerning
   a. Self-care regimen
   b. Identification of offending agent and importance of avoiding it (if possible) in future.

Hemolytic Anemia

A. General information
1. A category of diseases in which there is an increased rate of RBCs destruction.
2. May be congenital or acquired.
   a. Congenital: includes hereditary spherocytosis, G_6PD deficiency, sickle cell anemia, thalassemia
   b. Acquired: includes transfusion incompatibilities,

thrombotic thrombocytopenic purpura, disseminated intravascular clotting, spur cell anemia
3. Cause often unknown, but erythrocyte life span is shortened and hemolysis occurs at a rate that the bone marrow cannot compensate for.
4. The degree of anemia is determined by the lag between erythrocyte hemolysis and the rate of bone marrow erythropoiesis.
5. Diagnosis is based on laboratory evidence of an increased rate of erythrocyte destruction and a corresponding compensatory effort by bone marrow to increase production.

B. Medical management
1. Identify and eliminate (if possible) causative factors.
2. Drug therapy
   a. Corticosteroids in autoimmune types of anemia
   b. Folic acid supplements
3. Blood transfusion therapy
4. Splenectomy (below)

C. Assessment findings
1. Clinical manifestations vary depending on severity of anemia and the rate of onset (acute vs chronic)
2. Pallor, scleral icterus, and slight jaundice (chronic)
3. Chills, fever, irritability, precordial spasm, and pain (acute)
4. Abdominal pain and nausea, vomiting, diarrhea, melena
5. Hematuria, marked jaundice, and dyspnea
6. Splenomegaly and symptoms of cholelithiasis, hepatomegaly
7. Laboratory tests
   a. Hgb and Hct decreased
   b. Reticulocyte count decreased
   c. Coombs' test (direct): positive if autoimmune features present
   d. Bilirubin (indirect): elevated unconjugated fraction

D. Nursing interventions
1. Monitor for signs and symptoms of hypoxia including confusion, cyanosis, shortness of breath, tachycardia, and palpitations.
2. Note that the presence of jaundice may make assessment of skin color in hypoxia unreliable.
3. If jaundice and associated pruritus are present, avoid soap during bathing and use cool or tepid water.
4. Frequent turning and meticulous skin care are important as skin friability is increased.
5. Teach patients about the nature of the disease and identification of factors that predispose to episodes of hemolytic crisis.

Splenectomy

A. General information
1. Indications
   a. Rupture of the spleen caused by trauma, accidental tearing during surgery, diseases causing softening or damage (e.g., infectious mononucleosis)
   b. Hypersplenism: excessive splenic damage of cellular blood components

c. As the spleen is a major source of antibody formation in children, splenectomy is not recommended during the early years of life; if absolutely necessary, patient should receive prophylactic antibiotics post-op.

2. Primary hypersplenism can be alleviated with splenectomy; procedure is palliative only in secondary hypersplenism.

B. Nursing interventions

1. Be aware that it is crucial to monitor carefully for hemorrhage and shock as patients with pre-op bleeding tendencies will remain at risk post-op.
2. Monitor post-op temperature elevation: fever may not be the best indicator of post-op complications such as pneumonia or urinary tract infection, as fever without concomitant infection is common following splenectomy.
3. Observe for abdominal distension and discomfort secondary to expansion of the intestines and stomach; an abdominal binder may reduce distension.
4. Know that post-op infection in a child is considered life threatening; administer prophylactic antibiotics as ordered.
5. Ambulate early and provide chest physical therapy as location of the incision makes post-op atelectasis or pneumonia a risk.

Sickle Cell Anemia

See page 319.

Disorders of Platelets and Clotting Mechanism

Disseminated Intravascular Coagulation (DIC)

A. General information

1. Diffuse fibrin deposition within arterioles and capillaries with widespread coagulation all over the body, and subsequent depletion of clotting factors.
2. Hemorrhage from kidneys, brain, adrenals, heart, and other organs.
3. Cause unknown
4. Patients are usually critically ill with an obstetric, surgical, hemolytic, or neoplastic disease.
5. May be linked with entry of thromboplastic substances into the blood.
6. Pathophysiology
   a. Underlying disease (e.g., toxemia of pregnancy, cancer) causes release of thromboplastic substances that promote the deposition of fibrin throughout the microcirculation.
   b. Microthrombi form in many organs causing microinfarcts and tissue necrosis.
   c. RBCs are trapped in fibrin strands and are hemolysed.
   d. Platelets, prothrombin, and other clotting factors are destroyed, leading to bleeding.
   e. Excessive clotting activates the fibrinolytic system, which inhibits platelet function causing further bleeding.
7. Mortality rate is high, usually because underlying disease cannot be corrected.

B. Medical management

1. Identification and control of underlying disease is key
2. Blood transfusions: include whole blood, packed RBCs, platelets, plasma, cryoprecipitates, and volume expanders.
3. Heparin administration
   a. Somewhat controversial
   b. Inhibits thrombin thus preventing further clot formation, allowing coagulation factors to accumulate

C. Assessment findings

1. Petechiae and ecchymoses on the skin, mucous membranes, heart, lungs, and other organs
2. Prolonged bleeding from breaks in the skin (e.g., IV or venipuncture sites)
3. Severe and uncontrollable hemorrhage during childbirth or surgical procedures
4. Oliguria and acute renal failure
5. Convulsions, coma, death
6. Laboratory findings
   a. PT prolonged
   b. PTT usually prolonged
   c. Thrombin time usually prolonged
   d. Fibrinogen level usually depressed
   e. Platelet count usually depressed
   f. Fibrin split products elevated
   g. Protamine sulfate test strongly positive
   h. Factor assays (II, V, VII) depressed

D. Nursing interventions

1. Monitor blood loss and attempt to quantify.
2. Observe for signs of additional bleeding or thrombus formation.
3. Monitor appropriate laboratory data.
4. Prevent further injury.
   a. Avoid IM injections.
   b. Apply pressure to bleeding sites.
   c. Turn and position patient frequently and gently.
   d. Provide frequent nontraumatic mouth care (e.g., soft tooth brush or gauze sponge).
5. Provide emotional support.
6. Administer blood transfusions and medications as ordered.
7. Teach patients the importance of avoiding aspirin or aspirin-containing compounds.

Hemophilia

See page 320.

Idiopathic Thrombocytopenic Purpura

See page 320.

Immunologic Disorders

Acquired Immune Deficiency Syndrome (AIDS)

A. General information

1. Characterized by severe deficits in cellular immune function; manifested clinically by opportunistic infection or unusual neoplasms

2. Etiologic factors
  a. Results from infection with human immunodeficiency virus (HIV), an RNA virus that preferentially infects helper T-lymphocytes
  b. Transmissible through sexual contact, contaminated blood or blood products, and from infected woman to child in utero or through breast-feeding
  c. HIV is present in an infected person's blood, semen, and other body fluids
3. Epidemiology is similar to that of hepatitis B; increased incident in populations in which sexual promiscuity is common and in IV drug abusers
4. Most individuals with AIDS fall into one or more of the following categories
  a. Homosexual or bisexual men
  b. IV drug abusers
  c. Hemophiliacs or other recipients of blood transfusions
  d. Heterosexual partners of infected individuals
  e. Newborn children of infected women
5. At this time disease is 100% fatal within 2–3 years of diagnosis.

B. Assessment findings
  1. AIDS-related complex: nonspecific symptoms such as fatigue, weakness, anorexia, weight loss, diarrhea, pallor, fever, night sweats
  2. Dyspnea and progressive hypoxemia secondary to infection (pneumonia)
  3. Progressive weight loss secondary to diarrhea and a general wasting syndrome
  4. Temperature elevation (intermittent or persistent)
  5. Neurologic dysfunction secondary to acute meningitis, progressive dementia, encephalopathy, encephalitis
  6. Presence of opportunistic infection
    a. Pneumocystis carinii pneumonia
    b. Herpes simplex, cytomegalovirus, and Epstein-Barr viruses
    c. Candidiasis: oral or esophageal
  7. Neoplasms
    a. Kaposi's sarcoma
    b. CNS lymphoma
    c. Burkitt's lymphoma
    d. Diffuse undifferentiated non-Hodgkin's lymphoma
  8. Laboratory findings: diagnosis based on clinical criteria and positive HIV antibody test (confirmed by Western blot assay). Other lab findings may include
    a. Leukopenia with profound lymphopenia
    b. Anemia
    c. Thrombocytopenia
    d. Decreased circulatory T_4 lymphocyte cells
    e. Low T_4:T_8 lymphocyte ratio

C. Nursing interventions
  1. Administer medications as ordered for concomitant disease; monitor for signs of medication toxicity, including neutropenia and nephrotoxicity.
  2. If leukopenia develops, institute precautions appropriate for an immunosuppressed patient.
    a. Single room.
    b. Avoid IM injections.
    c. Limit staff and visitors with upper respiratory or other active infections.
    d. No rectal temperatures.
  4. Institute AIDS precautions.
    a. Single room required.
    b. Gowns required during contact with body fluids, blood, secretions, and excretions; masks not necessary unless unless patient infected with an organism requiring them, goggles/mask needed if aerolization of blood or secretions likely (e.g., suctioning a patient, dialysis); gloves required during contact with body fluids, blood, secretions, and excretions as well as when handling any articles or surfaces exposed to them.
    c. Handwashing required upon entering and leaving and after contact with patient's blood, body fluid, or blood-contaminated articles.
    d. Articles contaminated with blood, secretions, excretions, or body fluids are double bagged.
    e. All laboratory specimens must be bagged and labeled.
    f. Articles contaminated with blood, secretions, excretions, or body fluids are washed thoroughly with 1:10 solution of household bleach and water.
  5. Provide emotional support for patient/significant others.
  6. Provide patient teaching and discharge planning concerning
    a. Communicability and routes of transmission (e.g., shared syringes, sexual intercourse either vaginal or anal)
    b. Use of condoms for sexual intercourse
    c. Community resources including support groups, local church groups, gay rights groups, drug rehabilitation programs.

Malignancies

Multiple Myeloma

A. General information
  1. A neoplastic condition characterized by the abnormal proliferation of plasma cells in the bone marrow, causing the development of single or multiple tumors composed of abnormal plasma cells. Disease disseminates into lymph nodes, liver, spleen, and kidneys and causes bone destruction throughout the body.
  2. Cause unknown, but environmental factors thought to be involved
  3. Disease occurs after age 40; affects men twice as often as women
  4. Pathophysiology
    a. Bone demineralization and destruction with osteoporosis and a negative calcium balance
    b. Disruption of erythrocyte, leukocyte, and thrombocyte production

B. Medical management
  1. Drug therapy

    a. Analgesics for bone pain
    b. Chemotherapy (melphalan [Alkeran] and cyclophosphamide [Cytoxan]) to reduce tumor mass; may intensify the pancytopenia to which these patients are prone; requires careful monitoring of laboratory studies
    c. Antibiotics to treat infections
    d. Gammaglobulin for infection prophylaxis
    e. Corticosteroids and mithramycin for severe hypercalcemia
  2. Radiation therapy to reduce tumor mass
  3. Transfusion therapy
C. Assessment findings
  1. Headache and bone pain increasing with activity
  2. Pathologic fractures
  3. Skeletal deformities of sternum and ribs
  4. Loss of height (spinal column shortening)
  5. Osteoporosis
  6. Renal calculi
  7. Anemia, hemorrhagic tendencies, and increased susceptibility to infection
  8. Hypercalcemia
  9. Renal dysfunction secondary to obstruction of convoluted tubules by coagulated protein particles
  10. Neurologic dysfunction: spinal cord compression and paraplegia
  11. Laboratory tests
    a. Radiologic: diffuse bone lesions, widespread dimineralization, osteoporosis, osteolytic lesions of skull
    b. Bone marrow: many immature plasma cells; depletion of other cell types
    c. CBC: reduced Hgb, WBC, and platelet counts
    d. Serum globulins elevated
    e. Bence Jones protein: positive (abnormal globulin that appears in the urine of patients with multiple myeloma and other bone tumors)
D. Nursing interventions
  1. Provide comfort measures to help alleviate bone pain.
  2. Encourage ambulation to slow dimineralization process.
  3. Promote safety as patients are prone to pathologic and other fractures.
  4. Encourage fluids: 3000–4000 cc/day to counteract calcium overload and to prevent protein from precipitating in the renal tubules.
  5. Provide nursing care for patients with bleeding tendencies and susceptibility to infection.
  6. Provide a supportive atmosphere to enhance communication and reduce anxiety.
  7. Provide patient teaching and discharge planning concerning
    a. Crucial importance of long-term hydration to prevent urolithiasis and renal obstruction
    b. Safety measures vital to decrease the risk of injury
    c. Avoidance of crowds or sources of infection if leukopenic.

Polycythemia Vera

A. General information
  1. An increase in both the number of circulating erythrocytes and the concentration of Hgb within the blood
  2. Three forms: polycythemia vera, secondary polycythemia, and relative polycythemia
  3. Classified as a myeloproliferative disorder (bone marrow overgrowth)
  4. Cause unknown, but thought to be a form of malignancy similar to leukemia
  5. Usually develops in middle age, common in Jewish men
  6. Pathophysiology
    a. A pronounced increase in the production of erythrocytes accompanied by an increase in the production of myeloctyes (leukocytes within bone marrow) and thrombocytes.
    b. The consequences of this overproduction are an increase in blood viscosity, an increase in total blood volume (2–3 times greater than normal), and severe congestion of all tissues and organs with blood.
B. Assessment findings
  1. Ruddy complexion and duskiness of mucosa secondary to capillary congestion in the skin and mucous membranes
  2. Hypertension associated with vertigo, headache, and "fullness" in the head secondary to increased blood volume
  3. Symptoms of CHF secondary to overwork of the heart
  4. Thrombus formation: CVA, MI, gangrene of the extremities, DVT, and pulmonary embolism can occur
  5. Bleeding and hemorrhage secondary to congestion and overdistension of capillaries and venules
  6. Hepatomegaly and splenomegaly
  7. Peptic ulcer secondary to increased gastric secretions
  8. Gout secondary to increased uric acid released by nucleoprotein breakdown
  9. Laboratory tests
    a. CBC: increase in all mature cell forms (erythrocytes, leukocytes, and platelets)
    b. Hct: increased
    c. Bone marrow: increase in immature cell forms
    d. Bilirubin (indirect): increase in unconjugated fraction
    e. Liver enzymes may be increased
    f. Uric acid increased
    g. Hematuria and melena possible
C. Nursing interventions
  1. Monitor for signs and symptoms of bleeding complications.
  2. Force fluids and record I&O.
  3. Prevent development of DVT.
  4. Monitor for signs and symptoms of CHF.
  5. Provide care for the patient having a phlebotomy.
  6. Prevent/provide care for bleeding or infection complications.
  7. Administer medications as ordered.
    a. Radioactive phosphorus (^{32}P): reduction of

erythrocyte production, produces a remission of 6 months to 2 years

b. Nitrogen mustard, busulfan (Myleran), chlorambucil, cyclophosphamide to effect myelosuppression

c. Anti-gout and peptic ulcer drugs as needed.

8. Provide patient teaching and discharge planning concerning

a. Decrease in activity tolerance, need to space activity with periods of rest

b. Phlebotomy regimens: outpatient frequency is determined by Hct; importance of long-term therapy

c. High fluid intake

d. Avoidance of iron-rich foods to avoid counteracting the therapeutic effects of phlebotomy

e. Recognition and reporting of bleeding

f. Need to avoid persons with infections, especially in leukopenic patients.

Leukemia

See page 321.

Hodgkin's and Non-Hodgkin's Lymphoma

See pages 322.

The Respiratory System

OVERVIEW OF ANATOMY AND PHYSIOLOGY

Upper Respiratory Tract

Structures of the respiratory system, primarily an air conduction system, include the nose, pharynx, and larynx. Air is filtered, warmed, and humidified in the upper airway before passing to lower airway (see Figure 2.8).

Nose

A. External nose is a framework of bone and cartilage, internally divided into two passages or *nares (nasal cavities)* by the septum; air enters the system through the nares.
B. The *septum* is covered with a mucous membrane, where the olfactory receptors are located. Turbinates, located internally, assist in warming and moistening the air.
C. The major functions of the nose are warming, moistening, and filtering the air.

Pharynx

A. Muscular passageway commonly called the throat.
B. Air passes through the nose to the pharynx, composed of three sections
    1. *Nasopharynx:* located above the soft palate of the mouth, contains the adenoids and openings to the eustachian tubes.
    2. *Oropharynx:* located directly behind the mouth and tongue, contains the palatine tonsils; air and food enter body through oropharynx.
    3. *Laryngopharynx:* extends from the epiglottis to the sixth cervical level.

Larynx

A. Sometimes called "voice box," connects upper and lower airways; framework is formed by the hyoid bone, epiglottis, and thyroid, cricoid, and arytenoid cartilages. The opening of the larynx is called the glottis.
B. Larynx opens to allow respiration and closes to prevent aspiration when food passes through the pharynx.

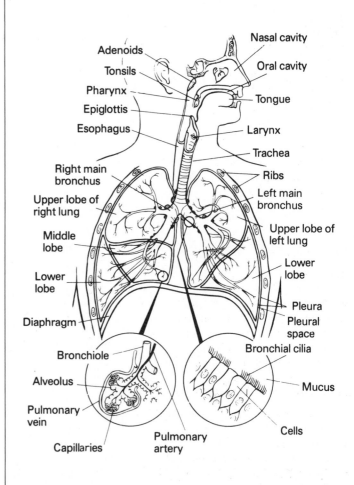

Figure 2.8 The respiratory system.
(Reproduced with permission from Basics of RD, New York, The American Lung Association, 1980.)

C. Vocal cords of larynx permit speech and are involved in the cough reflex.

Lower Respiratory Tract

Consists of the trachea, bronchi and branches, and the lungs and associated structures (see Figure 2.8).

Trachea

A. Air moves from the pharynx to larynx to trachea (length ll–l3 cm, diameter 1.5–2.5 cm in adult).
B. Extends from the larynx to the second costal cartilage, where it bifurcates and is supported by 16–20 C-shaped cartilage rings.
C. The area where the trachea divides into two branches is called the *carina.*

Bronchi

A. Formed by the division of the trachea into two branches (bronchi)
  1. *Right mainstem bronchus:* larger and straighter than the left; further divides into three lobar branches (upper, middle, and lower lobar bronchi) to supply the three lobes of right lung. If passed too far, endotracheal tube might enter right mainstem bronchus; only right lung is then intubated.
  2. *Left mainstem bronchus:* divides into the upper and lower lobar bronchi, to supply two lobes of left lung.
B. At the point a bronchus reaches about 1 mm in diameter it no longer has a connective tissue sheath and is called a *bronchiole.*

Bronchioles

A. In the bronchioles, airway patency is primarily dependent upon elastic recoil formed by network of smooth muscles.
B. The tracheobronchial tree ends at the terminal bronchioles. Distal to the terminal bronchioles the major function is no longer air conduction, but gas exchange between blood and alveolar air. The *respiratory bronchioles* serve as the transition to the alveolar epithelium.

Lungs (Right and Left)

A. Main organs of respiration, lie within the thoracic cavity on either side of the heart.
B. Broad area of lung resting on diaphragm is called the base; the narrow, superior portion is the apex.
C. Each lung is divided into lobes: three in the right lung, two in the left.
D. *Pleura:* serous membrane covering the lungs; continuous with the parietal pleura that lines the chest wall.
E. Lungs and associated structures are protected by the chest wall.

Chest Wall

A. Includes the rib cage, intercostal muscles, and diaphragm

B. Parietal pleura lines the chest wall and secretes small amounts of lubricating fluid into the intrapleural space (space between the visceral and parietal pleura). This fluid holds the lung and chest wall together as a single unit while allowing them to move separately.
C. The chest is shaped and supported by 12 pairs of ribs and costal cartilages; the ribs have several attached muscles.
  1. Contraction of the external intercostal muscles raises the rib cage during inspiration and helps increase the size of the thoracic cavity.
  2. The internal intercostal muscles tend to pull ribs down and in and play a role in forced expiration.
D. The *diaphragm* is the major muscle of ventilation (the exchange of air between the atmosphere and the alveoli). Contraction of muscle fibers causes the dome of the diaphragm to descend thereby increasing the volume of the thoracic cavity. As exertion increases, additional chest muscles or even abdominal muscles may be employed in moving the thoracic cage.

Pulmonary Circulation

A. Provides for reoxygenation of blood and release of CO_2; gas transfer occurs in the pulmonary capillary bed.
B. Pulmonary arteries arise from the right ventricle of the heart and continue to the bronchi and alveoli, gradually decreasing in size to capillaries.
C. The capillaries, after contact with the gas-exchange surface of the alveoli, reform to form the pulmonary veins.
D. The two pulmonary veins, superior and inferior, empty into the left atrium.

Gas Exchange

Alveolar Ducts and Alveoli

A. Alveolar ducts arise from the respiratory bronchioles and lead to the alveoli.
B. *Alveoli* are the functional cellular units of the lungs; about half arise directly from the alveolar ducts and are responsible for about 35% of alveolar gas exchange.
C. Alveoli produce *surfactant,* a phospholipid substance found in the fluid lining the alveolar epithelium. Surfactant reduces surface tension and increases the stability of the alveoli and prevents their collapse.
D. *Alveolar sacs* form the last part of the airway; functionally the same as the alveolar ducts, they are surrounded by alveoli and are responsible for 65% of the alveolar gas exchange.

ASSESSMENT

Health History

A. Presenting problem
  1. Nose/nasal sinuses: symptoms may include colds, discharge, epistaxis, sinus problems (swelling, pain)
  2. Throat: symptoms may include sore throats, hoarseness, difficulty swallowing, strep throat

3. Lungs: symptoms may include
   a. Cough: note duration; frequency; type (dry, hacking, bubbly, barky, hoarse, congested); sputum (productive vs nonproductive); circumstances related to cough (time of day, positions, talking, anxiety); treatment.
   b. Dyspnea: note onset, severity, duration, efforts to treat, whether associated with radiation, if accompanied by cough or diaphoresis, time of day when it most likely occurs, interference with ADL, whether precipitated by any specific activities, whether accompanied by cyanosis.
   c. Wheezing
   d. Chest pain
   e. Hemoptysis
B. Life-style: smoking (note type of tobacco, duration, number per day, number of years of smoking, inhalation, related cough, desire to quit); occupation (work conditions that could irritate respiratory system [asbestos, chemical irritants, dry cleaning fumes] and monitoring or protection of exposure conditions), geographic location (environmental conditions that could irritate respiratory system [chemical plants/industrial pollutants]); type and frequency of exercise/recreation.
C. Nutrition/diet: fluid intake per 24-hour period; intake of vitamins
D. Past medical history: immunizations (yearly immunizations for colds/flu; frequency and results of tuberculin skin testing); allergies (foods, drugs, contact or inhalant allergens, precipitating factors, specific treatment, desensitization)

Physical Examination

A. Inspect for configuration of the chest (kyphosis, scoliosis, barrel chest) and cyanosis.
B. Determine rate and pattern of breathing (normal rate 12–18/minute); note tachypnea, hyperventilation, or labored breathing pattern.
C. Palpate skin, subcutaneous structures, and muscles for texture, temperature, and degree of development.
D. Palpate for tracheal position, respiratory excursion (symmetric or asymmetric movement of the chest), and for fremitus.
   1. Fremitus is normally increased in intensity at second intercostal spaces at sternal border and interscapular spaces only.
   2. Increased intensity elsewhere may indicate pneumonia, pulmonary fibrosis, or tumor.
   3. Decreased intensity may indicate pneumothorax, pleural effusion, COPD.
E. Percuss lung fields (should find resonance over normal lung tissue, note hyperresonance or dullness) and for diaphragmatic excursion (normal distance between levels of dullness on full expiration and full inspiration is 6–12 cm).
F. Auscultate for normal (vesicular, bronchial, bronchovesicular) and adventitious (rales, rhonchi, pleural friction rub) breath sounds (see Figure 2.9).

Laboratory/Diagnostic Tests

A. *Arterial blood gases (ABGs)*
   1. Measure base excess/deficit, blood pH, CO_2, total CO_2, O_2 content, O_2 saturation (SO_2), pCO_2 (partial pressure carbon dioxide), pO_2 (partial pressure of oxygen)
   2. Nursing care
      a. If drawn by arterial stick, place a 4x4 bandage over puncture site after withdrawal of needle and maintain pressure with two fingers for at least 2 minutes.
      b. Gently rotate sample in test tube to mix heparin with the blood.
      c. Place sample in ice-water container until it can be analyzed.
B. *Pulmonary function studies*
   1. Evaluation of lung volume and capacities by spirometry: tidal volume (TV), vital capacity (VC), inspiratory and expiratory reserve volume (IRV and ERV), residual volume (RV), inspiratory capacity (IC), functional residual capacity (FRC)
   2. Involves use of a spirometer to diagram movement of air as patient performs various respiratory maneuvers; shows restriction or obstruction to air flow, or both.
   3. Nursing care
      a. Carefully explaining procedure will help allay anxiety and assure cooperation.

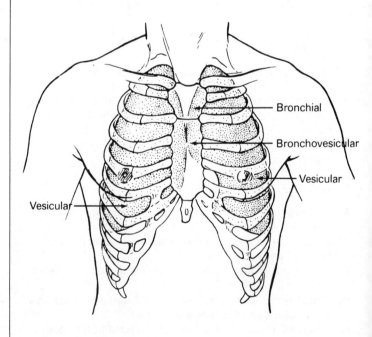

Figure 2.9 Locations for hearing normal breath sounds.

b. Perform tests before meals.

c. Withhold medication that may alter respiratory function unless otherwise ordered.

d. After procedure assess pulse and provide for rest period.

C. Hematologic studies (ESR, Hgb and Hct, WBC)

D. *Sputum culture and sensitivity*

1. Culture: isolation and identification of specific microorganism from a specimen

2. Sensitivity: determination of antibiotic agent effective against organism (sensitive or resistant)

3. Nursing care

a. Explain necessity of effective coughing.

b. If patient unable to cough, heated aerosoi will assist with obtaining a specimen.

c. Collect specimen in a sterile container that can be capped afterwards.

d. Volume need not exceed l–3 cc.

e. Deliver specimen to lab rapidly.

E. *Tuberculin skin test*

1. Intradermal test done to detect tuberculosis infection; does not differentiate active from dormant infections

2. Purified protein derivative (PPD) tuberculin administered to determine any previous sensitization to tubercle bacillus

3. Several methods of administration

a. *Mantoux test:* 0.l cc solution containing 0.5 tuberculin units of PPD-tuberculin is injected into the forearm.

b. *Tine test:* a stainless steel disc with 4 tines impregnated with PPD-tuberculin is pressed into the skin.

4. Results: read within 48–72 hours; inspect skin and circle zone of induration with a pencil; measure diameter in mm.

a. Negative: zone diameter less than 5 mm

b. Doubtful or probable: zone diameter 5–l0 mm

c. Positive: zone diameter l0 mm or more

F. *Thoracentesis*

1. Insertion of a needle through the chest wall into the pleural space to obtain a specimen for diagnostic evaluation, removal of pleural fluid accumulation, or to instill medication into the pleural space

2. Nursing care: pretest

a. Confirm that a signed permit has been obtained.

b. Explain procedure; instruct patient not to cough or talk during procedure.

c. Position patient at side of bed, with upper torso supported on overbed table, feet and legs well supported.

d. Assess vital signs.

3. Nursing care: post-test

a. Observe for signs and symptoms of pneumothorax, shock, leakage at puncture site.

b. Auscultate chest to ascertain breath sounds.

G. *Bronchoscopy*

1. Insertion of a fiberscope into the bronchi for diagnosis, biopsy, specimen collection, examination of structures/tissues, removal of foreign bodies

2. Nursing care: pretest

a. Confirm that a signed permit has been obtained.

b. Explain procedure, remove dentures, and provide good oral hygiene.

c. Keep patient NPO 6–12 hours pretest.

3. Nursing care post-test

a. Position patient on side or in semi-Fowler's.

b. Keep NPO until return of gag reflex.

c. Assess for and report frank bleeding.

d. Apply ice bags to throat for comfort; discourage talking, coughing, smoking for a few hours to decrease irritation.

ANALYSIS

Nursing diagnoses for the patient with a respiratory dysfunction may include

A. Anxiety

B. Alteration in respiratory functions: ineffective airway clearance, ineffective breathing pattern, impaired gas exchange, mechanical ventilation

C. Impaired verbal communication

D. Alteration in nutrition: less than body requirements

E. Impairment of skin integrity

F. Activity intolerance

G. Potential for injury

H. Alteration in comfort: pain

PLANNING AND IMPLEMENTATION

Goals

A. Patient's fear and anxiety will be reduced.

B. Adequate respiratory function will be maintained.

C. Patient will be able to communicate needs/desires effectively.

D. Adequate nutritional status will be maintained.

E. Patient's skin integrity will be adequate.

F. Patient will have increased tolerance for activity.

G. Patient will experience no falls or injury.

H. Patient's chest pain will be decreased.

Interventions

Chest Tubes/Water-seal Drainage

A. Insertion of a catheter into the intrapleural space to maintain constant negative pressure when air/fluid have accumulated

B. Chest tube is attached to underwater drainage to allow for the escape of air/fluid and to prevent reflux of air into the chest.

C. For evacuation of air, chest tube is placed in the second or third intercostal space, anterior or midaxillary line (air rises to the upper chest).

D. For drainage of fluid, chest tube is placed in the eighth or ninth intercostal space, midaxillary line.

E. Chest tube is connected to tubing for the collection system; the distal end of the collection tubing must be placed below the water level in order to prevent atmospheric air from entering the pleural space.

F. Drainage systems: a water-seal drainage system can be set up using one, two, or three bottles; or a commercial, disposable device (e.g., Pleur-evac) may be used.

1. *One-bottle system* (Figure 2.10a)
  a. Operates by gravity, not suction; the bottle serves as both collection chamber and water seal.
  b. Two hollow tubes (glass rods) are inserted into the stopper of the bottle; the drainage tube is connected to the glass rod that is submerged approximately 2 cm below the water level; the second glass tube allows for the escape of air.
  c. If considerable drainage accumulates it is difficult for the patient to expel air and fluid from the pleural space. If this occurs, the glass rod may be pulled up or a new drainage bottle may be set up (according to physician's orders).

2. *Two-bottle system* (Figure 2.10bc)
  a. One bottle serves as a drainage collection chamber, the other as the water seal.
  b. The first bottle is the drainage collection chamber and has two short tubes in the rubber stopper. One of these tubes is attached to the drainage tubing coming from the patient; the other is attached to the underwater tube

of the second bottle (the water-seal bottle). The air vent of the water-seal bottle must be left open to atmospheric air. If suction is used, the first bottle serves as drainage collection and water-seal chamber, and the second bottle serves as the suction chamber.

3. *Three-bottle system* (Figure 2.10d)
  a. This system has a drainage collection, a water-seal, and a suction-control bottle.
  b. The third bottle controls the amount of pressure in the system. The suction-control bottle has three tubes inserted in the stopper, two short and one long. One short tube is joined with the tubing to the former air vent of the water-seal bottle; the second short tube is connected to suction. The third (long) tube (or suction-control tube) is located between the short tubes, and has one end open to the atmosphere and the other below the water level.
  c. The depth to which the suction-control tube is immersed controls the amount of pressure within the system. The pressure is determined by the physician.

4. *Commercial water-seal units:* most popular is *Pleur-evac* (Figure 2.10e); lightweight, disposable; functions like a three-bottle system, may be used with or without suction.

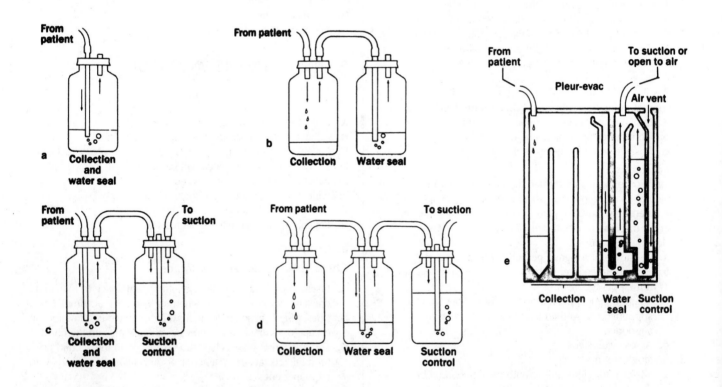

Figure 2.10 Water-seal drainage systems.
    a. One-bottle system.   **b.** Two-bottle system without suction.   **c.** Two-bottle system with suction.
    d. Three-bottle system.   **e.** Pleur-evac.
    (Adapted from "You can manage chest tubes confidently," by B. Mims, RN, 48(1), 39–44.)

G. Nursing care: without suction
1. Prepare the unit for use and connect the chest catheter to the drainage tubing.
2. Examine the entire system to ensure airtightness and absence of obstruction from kinks or dependent loops of tubing.
3. Note oscillation of the fluid level within the water-seal tube. It will rise on inspiration and fall on expiration due to changes in the intrapleural pressure. If oscillation stops and system is intact, notify physician.
4. Milk the chest tubes and drainage tubing every 1–2 hours as ordered to dislodge mucus and blood clots. Hold the proximal part of tubing with one hand and squeeze the distal portion in a downward direction.
5. Check the amount, color, and characteristics of the drainage. If drainage ceases and system is not blocked, assess for signs of respiratory distress from fluid/air accumulation.
6. Always keep drainage system lower than the level of the patient's chest.
7. Keep Vaseline gauze at bedside at all times in case chest tube falls out.
8. Encourage coughing and deep breathing to facilitate removal of air and drainage from pleural cavity.
9. Provide ROM exercises.

H. Nursing care: with suction
1. Attach suction tubing to suction apparatus, and chest catheter to drainage tubing.
2. Open suction slowly until a stream of bubbles is seen in the suction chamber. There should be continuous bubbling in this chamber and intermittent bubbling in the water seal. Check for an air leak in the system if bubbling in water seal is constant; notify physician if no air leak.
3. Milk chest tubes, check drainage, keep drainage system below level of patient's chest, keep Vaseline gauze at bedside, encourage coughing and deep breathing, and provide ROM exercises as noted above.

I. Never clamp chest tubes unless a specific order is written by the physician. Clamping the chest tubes of a patient with air in the pleural space will cause increased pressure buildup and possible tension pneumothorax.

J. Removal of the chest tube: instruct the patient to perform Valsalva maneuver; apply a Vaseline pressure dressing to the site.

K. If the water-seal bottle should break, immediately obtain some type of fluid-filled container to create an emergency water seal until a new unit can be obtained.

Chest Physiotherapy

A. General information
1. Used for individuals with increased production of secretions or thick, sticky secretions, and for patients with impaired removal of secretions or with ineffective cough. May also be used as a preventive measure for patients with weakness of the muscles of respiration or a predisposition to increased production or thickness of secretions.

2. Includes the techniques of postural drainage, percussion, and vibration.
   a. *Postural drainage:* uses gravity and various positions to stimulate the movement of secretions.
      1) postural drainage positions are determined by the areas of involved lung, assessed by chest x-ray and physical assessment findings.
      2) careful positioning is required to help secretions flow from smaller airways into the segmental bronchus and larger airways where secretions can be coughed up.
   b. *Percussion:* involves clapping with cupped hands on the chest wall over the segment to be drained.
      1) the hand is cupped by holding the fingers together so that the shape of the hand conforms with chest wall.
      2) clapping should be vigorous but not painful.
   c. *Vibration:* in this technique the hand is pressed firmly over the appropriate segment of chest wall, and muscles of upper arm and shoulder are tensed (isometric contraction); done with flattened, not cupped hand.

B. Nursing care
1. Perform procedure before or 3 hours after meals.
2. Administer bronchodilators about 20 minutes before procedure.
3. Remove all tight/constricting clothing.
4. Have all equipment available (tissues, emesis basin, towel, paper bag).
5. Assist patient to correct prescribed position for postural drainage (patient to assume each postural drainage position for approximately 3–5 minutes).
6. Place towel over area to be percussed.
7. Instruct patient to take several deep breaths.
8. Percuss designated area for approximately 3 minutes during inspiration and expiration.
9. Vibrate same designated area during exhalations of 4–5 deep breaths.
10. Assist patient with coughing when in postural drainage position; some patients may need to sit upright to produce a cough.
11. Repeat the same procedure in all designated positions.
12. After procedure, assist patient to comfortable position and provide good oral hygiene.

Mechanical Ventilation

A. General information
1. Ventilation is performed by mechanical means in individuals who are unable to maintain normal levels of oxygen and carbon dioxide in the blood
2. Indicated in patients with COPD, obesity, neuromuscular disease, severe neurologic depression, thoracic trauma, ARDS; patients who have undergone thoracic or open-heart surgery are likely to be maintained on mechanical ventilation post-op.

B. Types (positive pressure ventilators)
  1. Positive pressure-cycled ventilator: pushes air into the lungs until a predetermined pressure is reached within the tracheobronchial tree; expiration occurs by passive relaxation of the diaphragm.
  2. Volume-cycled ventilator: most popular type for intubated adults and older children; delivers air into the lungs until a certain predetermined tidal volume is reached before terminating inspiration.
  3. Time-cycled ventilator: terminates inspiration after a preset time; tidal volume is regulated by adjusting length of inspiration and flow rate of pressurized gas.
C. Modes of mechanical ventilation
  1. *Assist/control mode:* patient's inspiratory effort triggers ventilator, which then delivers breath; may be set to deliver breath automatically if patient does not trigger it.
  2. *Intermittent mandatory ventilation (IMV):* patient may breathe at own rate. IMV breaths are delivered under positive pressure; however, all other respirations taken by the patient are delivered at ambient pressure and tidal volume is of patient's own determination.
  3. *Positive end expiratory pressure (PEEP):* ventilator delivers additional positive pressure at the end of expiration, which maintains the alveoli in an expanded state.
  4. *Continuous positive airway pressure (CPAP):* achieves the same results as PEEP, except CPAP is used on adult patients who are on a T-piece.
D. Nursing care
  1. Assess for decreased cardiac output and administer appropriate nursing care .
  2. Monitor for positive water balance.
    a. Maintain accurate I&O.
    b. Assess daily weights.
    c. Take PCWP readings as ordered.
    d. Palpate for peripheral edema.
    e. Auscultate chest for altered breath sounds.
  3. Monitor for barotrauma (see Tension Pneumothorax, page 109).
    a. Assess ventilator settings every 4 hours.
    b. Auscultate breath sounds every 2 hours.
    c. Monitor ABGs.
    d. Perform complete pulmonary physical assessment every shift.
  4. Monitor for GI problems (stress ulcer).

Oxygen Therapy

A. Most common therapy for patients with respiratory disease
B. Indications include arterial hypoxemia; COPD; ARDS; tissue, cellular, and circulatory hypoxia.
C. Delivery systems
  1. *Low-flow system:* delivers oxygen at variable liter flows designed to add to patient's inspired air.
    a. *Nasal cannula*
      1) most common mode of oxygen delivery; consists of delivering 100% oxygen through two prongs inserted 1 cm into each nostril; general flow rates of 1–4 liters/minute are used with desired FiO_2 range of 24%–40%.
      2) nursing care
        a) instruct patient to breathe through the nose.
        b) remove cannula and clean nares every 8 hours.
        c) provide mouth care every 2–3 hours.
        d) use gauze pads behind ears to decrease irritation.
        e) assess arterial pO_2 frequently.
    b. *Standard mask*
      1) simple face mask that covers the nose and mouth and provides an additional area for oxygen collection; ranges: 6–12 liters/minute; FiO_2: 40%–65%.
      2) nursing care
        a) instruct patient to breathe through the nose.
        b) remove and clean mask every 2–3 hours.
        c) monitor carefully in patients who are prone to develop obstructed airways.
        d) replace mask with nasal cannula during meals and reposition mask immediately after eating.
    c. *Nonrebreathing mask*
      1) standard mask with a reservoir bag designed to deliver 90%–100% oxygen; a one-way valve between reservoir bag and mask allows the patient to inhale only from the reservoir bag and exhale through separate valves on the side of the mask; ranges: 6–15 liters/minute; FiO_2: 60%–90%.
      2) nursing care
        a) instruct patient to breathe through the nose.
        b) ensure that bag does not collapse completely with each inspiration.
        c) remove and clean mask every 2–3 hours.
  2. *High-flow system:* patient receives entire inspired gas from the apparatus, flow rates must exceed the volume of air required for a person's minute ventilation; *Venturi mask* commonly used
    a. Provides precise delivery of oxygen concentrations of 24%–50%.
    b. Nursing care
      1) provide supplemental oxygen by cannula during meals and other activities where mask interferes.
      2) remove and clean mask every 2–3 hours.

Tracheobronchial Suctioning

A. Suction removal of secretions from the tracheobronchial tree using a sterile catheter inserted into the airway
B. Catheters may be inserted through various routes: nasopharyngeal, oropharyngeal, or via an artificial airway.
C. Purposes
  1. Maintain a patent airway through removal of secretions
  2. Promote adequate exchange of oxygen/carbon dioxide
  3. Substitute for effective coughing
  4. Obtain a specimen for analysis

D. Procedure
   1. Gather suctioning equipment (receptacle for secretions, sterile catheter, sterile gloves and container of sterile normal saline).
   2. Turn vacuum on and test suction system.
   3. Place patient in semi- to high-Fowler's position.
   4. Apply sterile glove, fill sterile cup with solution, and attach sterile catheter to connecting tube.
   5. Increase inspired oxygen concentration to highest point and hyperinflate the lungs before and after each catheter insertion by using self-inflating bag; have patient deep breathe if able.
   6. Use gloved hand to insert catheter.
      a. Oral route
         1) if oral airway in place, slide the catheter alongside it and back to the pharynx; if no oral airway in place, have patient protrude the tongue and guide the catheter into the oropharynx.
         2) insert during inspiration until cough is stimulated or secretions obtained.
      b. Nasal route: advance catheter along the floor of the nares or pass it through an artificial nasal airway until cough is stimulated or secretions obtained.
      c. Artificial airway: insert the catheter into the artificial airway until cough is stimulated or secretions obtained.
   7. Do not cover the thumb control and do not apply suction during insertion of the catheter.
   8. During withdrawal, rotate the catheter while applying intermittent suction.
   9. Whole suctioning procedure including insertion and removal of the catheter should not exceed 10 seconds.
   10. If it is necessary to continue the suctioning process, hyperinflate the lungs, allow the patient to rest briefly, and repeat the process.
   11. Discard catheter, glove, and cup; record amount, color, characteristics of the secretions obtained; note patient's tolerance of procedure.

Tracheostomy Care

A. Performed to avoid bacterial contamination and obstruction of tracheostomy tube; frequency varies depending on amount of secretions
B. Procedure
   1. Explain procedure and provide reassurance to the patient.
   2. If not contraindicated, place patient in semi-Fowler's position to promote lung reexpansion.
   3. Disconnect ventilator or humidification device.
   4. Suction trachea to clear secretions.
   5. Reconnect ventilator or humidifier.
   6. Remove old tracheostomy dressing.
   7. Assemble equipment ("trach care kit").
   8. Set up sterile field and put on sterile glove.
      a. For a single-cannula tube
         1) with sterile gloved hand, wipe patient's neck under trach tube flanges with presoaked sterile sponge.

         2) wipe skin around tracheostomy with a second sponge until cleansed thoroughly (may use wet cotton-tipped applicators to cleanse around stoma).
         3) use each sponge or applicator only once.
         4) allow area to dry and apply a new sterile dressing (free of lint and fibers).
         5) change tracheostomy ties as needed.
      b. For a double-cannula tube
         1) disconnect ventilator or humidification device and unlock the inner cannula of trach tube using ungloved hand.
         2) place inner cannula in basin containing H_2O_2 to remove encrustations.
         3) if patient on a ventilator, insert another inner cannula while old one is being cleaned and reconnect patient to ventilator.
         4) cleanse stomal area and trach tube flanges with presoaked gauze sponges.
         5) clean inner cannula.
         6) remove excess liquid by gentle shaking.
         7) if patient not on a ventilator, gently reinsert inner cannula into tracheostomy tube and lock in place.
         8) allow area to dry, apply dressing and new tracheostomy ties as described above.

EVALUATION

A. Patient expresses reduction in anxiety and fearfulness; relaxed facial expression and body movement.
B. Patient demonstrates normal rate, rhythm, and depth of respiration.
   1. Decreased dyspnea
   2. ABGs within normal limits
   3. Usual or improved breath sounds
C. Patient can use normal voice tone.
D. Patient's weight is within normal limits for age, height, sex, and build; improved anthropometric measurements evidenced.
E. Patient maintains skin integrity; no evidence of redness or skin breakdown.
F. Patient is able to resume ADL without undue fatigue or dyspnea.
G. Patient shows no evidence of ecchymoses, bruises, or joint swelling.
H. Patient expresses relief/control of pain.
   1. Relaxed facial expression
   2. Improved breathing pattern

DISORDERS OF THE RESPIRATORY SYSTEM

Chronic Obstructive Pulmonary Disease (COPD)

Refers to respiratory conditions that produce obstruction of air flow; includes emphysema, bronchitis, bronchiectasis, and asthma.

Emphysema

A. General information
  1. Enlargement and destruction of the alveolar, bronchial, and bronchiolar tissue with resultant loss of recoil, air trapping, thoracic overdistension, sputum accumulation, and loss of diaphragmatic muscle tone
  2. These changes cause a state of carbon dioxide retention, hypoxia, and respiratory acidosis.
  3. Caused by cigarette smoking, infection, inhaled irritants, heredity, allergic factors, aging
B. Assessment findings
  1. Anorexia, fatigue, weight loss
  2. Feeling of breathlessness, cough, sputum production, flaring of the nostrils, use of accessory muscles of respiration, increased rate and depth of breathing, dyspnea
  3. Decreased respiratory excursion, resonance to hyperresonance, decreased breath sounds with prolonged expiration, normal or decreased fremitus
  4. Diagnostic tests: pCO_2 elevated or normal; pO_2 normal or slightly decreased
C. Nursing interventions
  1. Administer medications as ordered.
     a. Bronchodilators: aminophylline, isoproterenol (Isuprel), terbutaline (Brethine), metaproterenol (Alupent), theophylline, isoetharine (Bronkosol); used in treatment of bronchospasm
     b. Antimicrobials: tetracycline, ampicillin to treat bacterial infections
     c. Corticosteroids: prednisone
  2. Facilitate removal of secretions.
     a. Assure fluid intake of at least 3 liters/day.
     b. Provide (and teach patient) chest physical therapy, coughing and deep breathing, and use of hand nebulizers.
     c. Suction as needed.
     d. Provide oral hygiene after expectoration of sputum.
  3. Improve ventilation.
     a. Position patient in semi- or high-Fowler's.
     b. Instruct patient to use diaphragmatic muscle to breathe.
     c. Encourage productive coughing after all treatments (splint abdomen to help produce more expulsive cough).
     d. Employ pursed-lip breathing techniques (prolonged, slow relaxed expiration against pursed lips).
  4. Provide patient teaching and discharge planning concerning

  a. Prevention of recurrent infections
     1) avoid crowds and individuals with known infection.
     2) adhere to high-protein, high-carbohydrate, increased vitamin C diet.
     3) receive immunizations for influenza and pneumonia.
     4) report changes in characteristics and color of sputum immediately.
     5) report worsening of symptoms (increased tightness of chest, fatigue, increased dyspnea).
  b. Control of environment
     1) use home humidifier at 30%–50% humidity.
     2) wear scarf over nose and mouth in cold weather to prevent bronchospasm.
     3) avoid smoking and others who smoke.
     4) avoid abrupt changes in temperature.
  c. Avoidance of inhaled irritants
     1) stay indoors if pollution levels are high.
     2) use air-conditioner with high-efficiency particulate air filter to remove particles from air.
  d. Increasing activity tolerance
     1) start with mild exercises, such as walking, and gradually increase amounts and duration.
     2) use breathing techniques (pursed lip, diaphragmatic) during activities/exercises to control breathing.
     3) have oxygen available as needed to assist with activities.
     4) plan activities that require low amounts of energy.
     5) plan rest periods before and after activities.

Bronchitis

A. General information
  1. Excessive production of mucus in the bronchi with accompanying persistent cough.
  2. Characteristic changes include hypertrophy/hyperplasia of the mucus-secreting glands in the bronchi, decreased ciliary activity, chronic inflammation, and narrowing of the small airways.
  3. Caused by the same factors that cause emphysema
B. Medical management: drug therapy includes bronchodilators, antimicrobials, expectorants (e.g., Robitussin)
C. Assessment findings
  1. Productive (copious) cough, dyspnea on exertion, use of accessory muscles of respiration, scattered rales and rhonchi
  2. Feeling of epigastric fullness, slight cyanosis, distended neck veins, ankle edema
  3. Diagnostic tests: increased pCO_2; decreased pO_2
D. Nursing interventions: same as for Emphysema.

Bronchiectasis

A. General information
  1. Permanent abnormal dilation of the bronchi with destruction of muscular and elastic structures of the bronchial wall

2. Caused by bacterial infection; recurrent lower respiratory tract infections; congenital defects (altered bronchial structures); lung tumors; thick, tenacious secretions
B. Medical management: same as for Emphysema.
C. Assessment findings
   1. Chronic cough with production of mucopurulent sputum, hemoptysis, exertional dyspnea, wheezing
   2. Anorexia, fatigue, weight loss
   3. Diagnostic tests
      a. Bronchoscopy reveals sources and sites of secretions
      b. Possible elevation of WBC
D. Nursing interventions: same as for Emphysema.

Asthma

See page 329.

Pulmonary Tuberculosis

A. General information
   1. Bacterial infectious disease caused by *M. tuberculosis* and spread via airborne droplets when infected persons cough, sneeze, or laugh
   2. Once inhaled, the organisms implant themselves in the lung and begin dividing slowly, causing inflammation, development of the primary tubercle, and eventual caseation and fibrosis.
   3. Infection spreads via the lymph and circulatory systems.
   4. Half of the cases occur in inner city neighborhoods, and incidence is highest in areas with a large population of native Americans. Nonwhites affected four times more often than whites. Men affected more often than women. The greatest number of cases occur in persons age 65 and over. Socially and economically disadvantaged, alcoholic, and malnourished individuals affected more often.
   5. The causative agent, *M. tuberculosis* is an acid-fast bacillus spread via droplet nuclei from infected persons.
B. Assessment findings
   1. Cough (yellow mucoid sputum), dyspnea, hemoptysis, rales (later)
   2. Anorexia, malaise, weight loss, afternoon low-grade fever, pallor, pain, fatigue, night sweats
   3. Diagnostic tests
      a. Chest x-ray indicates presence and extent of disease process, but cannot differentiate active from inactive form
      b. Skin test (PPD) positive; area of induration 10 mm or more in diameter after 48 hours
      c. Sputum positive for acid-fast bacillus (three samples is diagnostic for disease)
      d. Culture positive
      e. WBC and ESR increased
C. Nursing interventions
   1. Administer medications as ordered (see Table 2.20).
   2. Prevent transmission.
      a. Strict isolation not required if patient/family adheres to special respiratory precautions for tuberculosis.

      b. Patient should be in a well-ventilated private room, with the door kept closed at all times.
      c. All visitors and staff should wear masks when in contact with the patient and should discard the used masks before leaving the room; patient should wear a mask when leaving the room for tests.
      d. All specimens should be labelled "AFB precautions."
      e. Handwashing is required after direct contact with the patient or contaminated articles.
   3. Promote adequate nutrition.
      a. Make ongoing assessments of patient's appetite and do kcal counts for 3 days; consult dietician for diet guidelines.
      b. Offer small, frequent feedings and nutritional supplements; assist patient with menu selection stressing balanced nutrition.
      c. Weigh patient at least twice a week.
      d. Encourage activity as tolerated to increase appetite.
   4. Prevent social isolation.
      a. Impart a comfortable, confident attitude when caring for the patient.
      b. Explain the nature of the disease to the patient, family, and visitors in simple terms.
      c. Stress that visits are important, but isolation precautions must be followed.
   5. Vary the patient's routine to prevent boredom.
   6. Discuss the patient's feelings and assess for boredom, depression, anxiety, fatigue, or apathy; provide support and encourage expression of concerns.
   7. Provide patient teaching and discharge planning concerning
      a. Medication regimen: prepare a sheet with each drug name, dosage, time due, and major side effects; stress importance of following medication schedule for prescribed period of time (usually 9 months); include family
      b. Transmission prevention: patient should cover mouth when coughing, expectorate into a tissue and place it in a paper bag; patient should also wash hands after coughing or sneezing; stress importance of plenty of fresh air; include family
      c. Importance of notifying physician at the first sign of persistent cough, fever, or hemoptysis (may indicate recurrence)
      d. Need for follow-up care including physical exam, sputum cultures, and chest x-rays
      e. Availability of community health services
      f. Importance of high-protein, high-carbohydrate diet with inclusion of supplemental vitamins.

Chest Trauma

Fractured Ribs

A. General information
   1. Most common chest injury resulting from blunt trauma
   2. Ribs 4–8 are most commonly fractured because they are least protected by chest muscles. Splintered or displaced

fractured ribs may penetrate the pleura and lungs.

B. Medical management: drug therapy consists of narcotics, intercostal nerve block (injection of intercostal nerves above and below the injury with an anesthetic agent) for pain relief

C. Assessment findings
1. Pain, especially on inspiration
2. Point tenderness and bruising at injury site, splinting with shallow respirations, apprehensiveness
3. Diagnostic tests
   a. Chest x-ray reveals area and degree of fracture
   b. pCO_2 elevated; pO_2 decreased (later)

D. Nursing interventions
1. Provide pain relief/control.
   a. Administer ordered narcotics and analgesics cautiously and monitor effects.
   b. Place patient in semi- or high-Fowler's position to ease pain associated with breathing.
2. Monitor patient closely for complications.
   a. Assess for bloody sputum (indicative of lung penetration).

b. Observe for signs and symptoms of pneumothorax or hemothorax.

Flail Chest

A. General information
1. Fracture of several ribs and resultant instability of the affected chest wall
2. Chest wall is no longer able to provide the bony structure necessary to maintain adequate ventilation; consequently, the flail portion and underlying tissue move paradoxically (in opposition) to the rest of the chest cage and lungs.
3. The flail portion is sucked in on inspiration and bulges out on expiration.
4. Result is hypoxia, hypercarbia, and increased retained secretions.
5. Caused by trauma (sternal rib fracture with possible costochondral separations).

B. Medical management
1. Internal stabilization with a volume-cycled ventilator
2. Drug therapy (narcotics, sedatives)

Table 2.20   Drugs Commonly Used to Treat Tuberculosis

Drug and dosage	Common side effects	Nursing implications
Isoniazid (INH) 10 to 20 mg/kg (up to 300 mg) PO or IM daily, or 15 mg/kg PO or IM twice a week	Peripheral neuritis, a numbness and tingling in hands and feet. Vitamin B_6 (pyridoxine) may be given to prevent or treat this condition. Hepatitis, with the risk increasing with age. Liver enzymes may be routinely monitored in elderly or symptomatic patients. Hyperexcitability may occur with single 300 mg dose.	Tell patient to report signs of neuritis and hepatitis (anorexia, nausea, vomiting, jaundice, malaise, or dark urine). Isoniazid may interfere with phenytoin (Dilantin) metabolism, requiring a lower dose of the TB medication; should be taken on an empty stomach, and the patient should not drink alcohol while on therapy.
Ethambutol (Myambutol) 15 to 25 mg/kg PO daily, or 50 mg/kg PO twice weekly	Optic neuritis, a loss of red-green color discrimination, and decreased visual acuity can occur with dosages of 25 mg/kg. Reversible, if medication discontinued. Skin rash.	Tell patient to notify physician if vision blurs or if unable to see red or green. Use the drug with caution if a visual exam cannot be done and in patients with renal impairment.
Rifampin (Rifadin, Rimactane) 10 to 20 mg/kg (up to 600 mg) PO daily, or 600 mg PO twice a week	Body fluids (urine, tears, saliva, etc.) may turn orange. Hepatitis Flu-like syndrome Purpura (rare)	Tell patients to expect orange-tinged body fluids. Tell patients to report anorexia, nausea, vomiting, jaundice, malaise, or dark urine. Use the drug with caution in cases of liver disease. Rifampin affects the actions of other drugs, including anticoagulants, oral hypoglycemics, corticosteriods, oral contraceptives, and methadone.
Streptomycin 15 to 20 mg/kg (up to 1 gm) IM daily or 25 to 30 mg/kg IM twice a week	Damage to cranial nerve VIII (vestibulocochlear). Damage to the vestibular portion causes dizziness, vertigo, tinnitus, and roaring in ears. Auditory damage causes loss of hearing at high frequency ranges. Renal toxicity.	Baseline renal and audiology studies may be obtained before therapy begins. Tell patient to report any ringing, roaring, or fullness in his ears. Help coordinate outpatient arrangements for IM injections, if necessary.
Pyrazinamide 20 to 40 mg/kg (up to 2 gm) PO daily	Excess uric acid levels, which can cause gout or hepatitis.	Baseline uric acid and liver enzyme levels may be obtained; monitor uric acid and liver enzymes. Instruct patient to report any signs of gout (painful swelling in joints, chills, fever) and hepatitis (anorexia, nausea, vomiting, jaundice, malaise, and dark urine). Use with caution in patients who have liver disease, gout, or renal impairment.

Other drugs used: capreomycin (Capastat), kanamycin (Kantrex), ethionamide (Trecator-SC), para-amino-salicylic acid, and cycloserine (Seromycin).
From Coleman, D., T.B.: The disease that's not dead yet, *RN*, September, 1984, 49–59.

C. Assessment findings
  1. Severe dyspnea; rapid, shallow, grunty breathing; paradoxical chest motion
  2. Cyanosis, possible neck vein distension, tachycardia, hypotension
  3. Diagnostic tests
    a. pO_2 decreased
    b. pCO_2 elevated
    c. pH decreased
D. Nursing interventions
  1. Maintain an open airway: suction secretions/blood from nose, throat, mouth, and via endotracheal tube; note changes in amount, color, characteristics.
  2. Monitor mechanical ventilation (see page 103).
  3. Encourage turning, coughing and deep breathing.
  4. Monitor for signs of shock.

Pneumothorax/Hemothorax

A. General information
  1. Partial or complete collapse of the lung due to an accumulation of air or fluid in the pleural space
  2. Types
    a. *Spontaneous pneumothorax:* the most common type of closed pneumothorax; air accumulates within the pleural space without an obvious cause. Rupture of a small bleb on the visceral pleura most frequently produces this type of pneumothorax.
    b. *Open pneumothorax:* air enters the pleural space through an opening in the chest wall; usually caused by stabbing or gunshot wound.
    c. *Tension pneumothorax:* air enters the pleural space with each inspiration but cannot escape; causes increased intrathoracic pressure and shifting of the mediastinal contents to the unaffected side (mediastinal shift).
    d. *Hemothorax:* accumulation of blood in the pleural space; frequently found with an open pneumothorax resulting in a hemopneumothorax.
B. Assessment findings
  1. Sudden sharp pain in the chest, dyspnea, diminished or absent breath sounds on affected side, decreased respiratory excursion on affected side, hyperresonance on percussion, decreased vocal fremitus, tracheal shift to the opposite side (tension pneumothorax accompanied by mediastinal shift)
  2. Weak, rapid pulse; anxiety; diaphoresis
  3. Diagnostic tests
    a. Chest x-ray reveals area and degree of pneumothorax
    b. pCO_2 elevated
    c. pO_2, pH decreased
C. Nursing interventions
  1. Provide nursing care for the patient with an endotracheal tube: suction secretions, vomitus, blood from nose, mouth, throat, or via endotracheal tube; monitor mechanical ventilation.
  2. Restore/promote adequate respiratory function.

    a. Assist with thoracentesis and provide appropriate nursing care (see page 101).
    b. Assist with insertion of a chest tube to water-seal drainage and provide appropriate nursing care (see page 101).
    c. Continuously evaluate respiratory patterns and report any changes.
  3. Provide relief/control of pain.
    a. Administer narcotics/analgesics/sedatives as ordered and monitor effects.
    b. Position patient in high-Fowler's position.

Atelectasis

A. General information
  1. Collapse of part or all of a lung due to bronchial obstruction
  2. May be caused by intrabronchial obstruction (secretions, tumors, bronchospasm, foreign bodies); extrabronchial compression (tumors, enlarged lymph nodes); or endobronchial disease (bronchogenic carcinoma, inflammatory structures)
B. Assessment findings
  1. Signs and symptoms may be absent depending upon degree of collapse and rapidity with which bronchial obstruction occurs
  2. Dyspnea, decreased breath sounds on affected side, decreased respiratory excursion, dullness to flatness upon percussion over affected area
  3. Cyanosis, tachycardia, tachypnea, elevated temperature, weakness, pain over affected area
  4. Diagnostic tests
    a. Bronchoscopy: may or may not reveal an obstruction
    b. Chest x-ray shows diminished size of affected lung and lack of radiance over atelectic area
    c. pO_2 decreased
C. Nursing interventions (prevention of atelectasis in hospitalized patients is an important nursing responsibility)
  1. Turn and reposition every 1–2 hours while patient is bedridden or obtunded.
  2. Encourage mobility (if permitted).
  3. Promote liquification and removal of secretions.
  4. Avoid administration of large doses of sedatives and opiates that depress respiration and cough reflex.
  5. Prevent abdominal distension.
  6. Administer prophylactic antibiotics as ordered to prevent respiratory infection.

Pleural Effusion

A. General information
  1. Collection of fluid in the pleural space
  2. A symptom, not a disease; may be produced by numerous conditions
  3. Classification
    a. Transudative: accumulation of protein-poor, cell-poor fluid
    b. Suppurative (empyema): accumulation of pus

4. May be found in patients with liver/kidney disease, pneumonia, tuberculosis, lung abscess, bronchial carcinoma, leukemia, trauma, pulmonary edema, systemic infection, disseminated lupus erythematosus, polyarteritis nodosa.

B. Medical management
1. Identification and treatment of the underlying cause
2. Thoracentesis
3. Drug therapy
   a. Antibiotics: either systemic or inserted directly into pleural space
   b. Fibrinolytic enzymes: trypsin, streptokinase-streptodornase to decrease thickness of pus and dissolve fibrin clots
4. Closed chest drainage
5. Surgery: open drainage

C. Assessment findings
1. Dyspnea, dullness over affected area upon percussion, absent or decreased breath sounds over affected area, pleural pain, dry cough, pleural friction rub
2. Pallor, fatigue, fever and night sweats (with empyema)
3. Diagnostic tests
   a. Chest x-ray positive if greater than 250 cc pleural fluid
   b. Pleural biopsy may reveal bronchogenic carcinoma
   c. Thoracentesis may contain blood if cause is cancer, pulmonary infarction, or tuberculosis; positive for specific organism in empyema

D. Nursing interventions: vary depending on etiology
1. Assist with repeated thoracentesis.
2. Administer narcotics/sedatives as ordered to decrease pain.
3. Assist with instillation of medication into pleural space (reposition patient every 15 minutes to distribute the drug within the pleurae).
4. Place patient in high-Fowler's position to promote ventilation.

Pneumonia

A. General information
1. An inflammation of the alveolar spaces of the lung resulting in consolidation of lung tissue as the alveoli fill with exudate
2. The various types of pneumonias are classified according to the offending organism.
3. Bacterial pneumonia accounts for 10% of all hospital admissions; affects infants and elderly most often, and most often occurs in winter and early spring
4. Caused by various organisms: *D. pneumoniae, S. aureus, E. coli, H. influenzae*

B. Assessment findings
1. Cough with greenish to rust-colored sputum production; rapid, shallow respirations with an expiratory grunt; nasal flaring; intercostal rib retraction; use of accessory muscles of respiration; dullness to flatness upon percussion; possible pleural friction rub; high-pitched bronchial breath sounds; rales (early) progressing to coarse (later)
2. Fever, chills, chest pain, weakness, generalized malaise
3. Tachycardia, cyanosis, profuse perspiration, abdominal distension
4. Diagnostic tests
   a. Chest x-ray shows consolidation over affected areas
   b. WBC increased
   c. pO_2 decreased
   d. Sputum specimens reveal particular causative organism

C. Nursing interventions
1. Facilitate adequate ventilation.
   a. Administer oxygen as needed and assess its effectiveness.
   b. Place patient in semi-Fowler's position.
   c. Turn and reposition frequently patients who are immobilized/obtunded.
   d. Administer analgesics as ordered to relieve pain associated with breathing (codeine is drug of choice).
   e. Auscultate breath sounds every 2–4 hours.
   f. Monitor ABGs.
2. Facilitate removal of secretions (general hydration, deep breathing and coughing, tracheobronchial suctioning as needed, expectorants as ordered, aerosol treatments via nebulizer, humidification of inhaled air, chest physical therapy).
3. Observe color, characteristics of sputum and report any changes; encourage patient to perform good oral hygiene after expectoration.
4. Provide adequate rest and relief/control of pain.
   a. Provide bedrest with limited physical activity.
   b. Limit visits and minimize conversations.
   c. Plan for uninterrupted rest periods.
   d. Institute nursing care in blocks to ensure periods of rest.
   e. Maintain pleasant and restful environment.
5. Administer antibiotics as ordered, monitor effects and possible toxicity.
6. Prevent transmission (respiratory isolation may be required for patients with staphylococcal pneumonia).
7. Control fever and chills: monitor temperature and administer antipyretics as ordered, maintain increased fluid intake, provide frequent clothing and linen changes.
8. Provide patient teaching and discharge planning concerning prevention of recurrence
   a. Medication regimen/antibiotic therapy
   b. Need for adequate rest, limited activity, good nutrition with adequate fluid intake and good ventilation
   c. Need to continue deep breathing and coughing for at least 6–8 weeks after discharge
   d. Availability of vaccines (pneumonococcal pneumonia, influenza)
   e. Techniques that prevent transmission (use of tissues when coughing, adequate disposal of secretions)
   f. Avoidance of persons with known respiratory infections
   g. Need to report signs and symptoms of respiratory

infection (persistent or recurrent fever; changes in characteristics, color of sputum; chills; increased pain; difficulty breathing; weight loss; persistent fatigue)

h. Need for follow-up medical care and evaluation.

Bronchogenic Carcinoma

A. General information

1. The majority of primary pulmonary tumors arise from the bronchial epithelium and are therefore referred to as bronchogenic carcinomas.

2. Characteristic pathologic changes include nonspecific inflammation with hypersecretion of mucus, desquamation of cells, hyperplasia and obstruction.

3. Metastasis occurs primarily by direct extension and via the circulatory or lymphatic system.

4. Men over age 40 affected most often; 1 out of every 10 heavy smokers; affects right lung more often than left.

5. Caused by inhaled carcinogens (primarily cigarette smoke but also asbestos, nickel, iron oxides, air silicone pollution; preexisting pulmonary disorders [TB, COPD])

B. Medical management: depends on cell type, stage of disease and condition of patient; may include

1. Radiation therapy

2. Chemotherapy: usually includes cyclophosphamide, methotrexate, vincristine, doxorubicin, and procarbazine; concurrently in some combination

3. Surgery: when entire tumor can be removed

C. Assessment findings

1. Persistent cough (may be productive or blood tinged), chest pain, dyspnea, unilateral wheezing, friction rub, possible unilateral paralysis of the diaphragm

2. Fatigue, anorexia, nausea, vomiting, pallor

3. Diagnostic tests

a. Chest x-ray may show presence of tumor or evidence of metastasis to surrounding structures

b. Sputum for cytology reveals malignant cells

c. Bronchoscopy: biopsy reveals malignancy

d. Thoracentesis: pleural fluid contains malignant cells

e. Biopsy of scalene lymph nodes may reveal metastasis

D. Nursing interventions

1. Provide support and guidance to patient as needed.

2. Provide relief/control of pain.

3. Administer medications as ordered and monitor effects/side effects.

4. Control nausea: administer medications as ordered, provide good oral hygiene, provide small and more frequent feedings.

5. Provide nursing care for a patient with a thoracotomy.

6. Provide patient teaching and discharge planning concerning

a. Disease process, diagnostic and therapeutic interventions

b. Side effects of radiation and chemotherapy

c. Realistic information about prognosis.

Thoracic Surgery

A. General information

1. Types

a. *Exploratory thoracotomy:* anterior or posterolateral incision through the fourth, fifth, sixth, or seventh intercostal spaces to expose and examine the pleura and lung

b. *Lobectomy:* removal of one lobe of a lung; treatment for bronchiectasis, bronchogenic carcinoma, emphysematous blebs, lung abscesses

c. *Pneumonectomy:* removal of an entire lung; most commonly done as treatment for bronchogenic carcinoma

d. *Segmental resection:* removal of one or more segments of lung; most often done as treatment for bronchiectasis

e. *Wedge resection:* removal of lesions that occupy only part of a segment of lung tissue; for excision of small nodules or to obtain a biopsy

2. Nature and extent of disease and condition of patient determine type of pulmonary resection.

B. Nursing interventions: preoperative

1. Provide routine pre-op care.

2. Perform a complete physical assessment of the lungs to obtain baseline data.

3. Explain expected post-op measures: care of incision site, oxygen, suctioning, chest tubes (except if pneumonectomy performed).

4. Teach patient adequate splinting of incision with hands or pillow for turning, coughing, and deep breathing.

5. Demonstrate ROM exercises for affected side.

6. Provide chest physical therapy to help remove secretions.

C. Nursing interventions: postoperative

1. Provide routine post-op care.

2. Promote adequate ventilation.

a. Perform complete physical assessment of lungs and compare with pre-op findings.

b. Auscultate lung fields every 1–2 hours.

c. Encourage turning, coughing and deep breathing every 1–2 hours after pain relief obtained.

d. Perform tracheobronchial suctioning if needed.

e. Assess for proper maintenance of chest drainage system (except after pneumonectomy).

f. Monitor ABGs and report significant changes.

g. Place patient in semi-Fowler's position (if pneumonectomy performed follow surgeon's orders about positioning, often on back or operative side, but not turned to unoperative side).

3. Provide pain relief.

a. Administer narcotics/analgesics prior to turning, coughing, and deep breathing.

b. Assist with splinting while turning, coughing, deep breathing.

4. Provide patient teaching and discharge planning concerning
   a. Need to continue with coughing/deep breathing for 6–8 weeks post-op and to continue ROM exercises
   b. Importance of adequate rest with gradual increases in activity levels
   c. High-protein diet with inclusion of adequate fluids (at least 2 liters/day)
   d. Chest physical therapy
   e. Good oral hygiene
   f. Need to avoid persons with known upper respiratory infections
   g. Adverse signs and symptoms (recurrent fever; anorexia; weight loss; dyspnea; increased pain; difficulty swallowing; shortness of breath; changes in color, characteristics of sputum) and importance of reporting to physician
   h. Avoidance of crowds and poorly ventilated areas.

Adult Respiratory Distress Syndrome (ARDS)

A. General information
   1. A form of pulmonary insufficiency more commonly encountered in adults with no previous lung disorders than in those with existing lung disease
   2. Initial damage to the alveolar-capillary membrane with subsequent leakage of fluid into the interstitial spaces and alveoli, resulting in pulmonary edema and impaired gas exchange
   3. There is cell damage, decreased surfactant production and atelectasis, which in turn produce hypoxemia, decreased compliance, and increased work of breathing.
   4. Predisposing conditions include shock, trauma, infection, fluid overload, aspiration, oxygen toxicity, smoke inhalation, pneumonia, DIC, drug allergies, drug overdoses, neurologic injuries, fat emboli.
   5. Has also been called shock lung.
B. Assessment findings
   1. Dyspnea, cough, tachypnea with intercostal/suprasternal retraction, scattered to diffuse rales/rhonchi
   2. Changes in orientation, tachycardia, cyanosis (rare)
   3. Diagnostic tests
      a. pCO_2 and pO_2 decreased
      b. Hypoxemia
      c. Hgb and Hct possibly decreased
      d. pCO_2 increased in terminal stages
C. Nursing interventions
   1. Promote optimal ventilatory status.
      a. Perform ongoing assessment of lungs with auscultation every 1–2 hours.
      b. Elevate head and chest.
      c. Administer/monitor mechanical ventilation with PEEP.
      d. Assist with chest physical therapy as ordered.
      e. Encourage coughing and deep breathing every hour.
      f. Monitor ABGs and report significant changes.
   2. Promote rest by spacing activities and treatments.
   3. Maintain fluid and electrolyte balance.

Cancer of the Larynx

A. General information
   1. Most common upper respiratory malignancy.
   2. The majority of laryngeal malignancies are squamous cell carcinomas.
   3. Types
      a. Supraglottic (also called extrinsic laryngeal cancer): involves the epiglottis and false cords and is likely to produce no symptoms until advanced stages.
      b. Glottic (also referred to as intrinsic laryngeal cancer): affects the true vocal cords; the most frequently occurring laryngeal cancer and produces early symptoms
   4. Occurs most often in white men in middle or later life
   5. Caused by cigarette smoking, excessive alcohol consumption, chronic laryngitis, vocal abuse, family predisposition to cancer of larynx
B. Medical management
   1. Radiation therapy: may be effective in cases of localized disease, affecting only one vocal cord
   2. Chemotherapy: used as adjuvant therapy to help shrink tumor and eradicate metastases (experimental)
   3. Surgery
      a. Partial laryngectomy: a lesion on the true cord on one side is removed along with adjoining tissue. Useful in early, intrinsic lesions. Patient is able to talk and has a normal airway post-op.
      b. Total laryngectomy (see below)
      c. Radical neck dissection
         1) performed when metastasis from cancer of the larynx is suspected
         2) includes removal of entire larynx, lymph nodes, sternocleidomastoid muscle, internal jugular vein, and spinal accessory nerve
         3) may also involve removal of the mandible, submaxillary gland, part of the thyroid and parathyroid gland
         4) nursing care: same as for Total Laryngectomy, below.
C. Assessment findings
   1. Supraglottic: localized throat pain; burning when drinking hot liquids or orange juice; lump in the neck; eventual dysphagia; dyspnea; weight loss; debility; cough; hemoptysis; muffled voice
   2. Glottic: progressive hoarseness (more than 2-week duration), eventual dyspnea
   3. Enlarged cervical lymph nodes
D. Nursing interventions: provide care for the patient with a laryngectomy.

Total Laryngectomy

A. General information: consists of removal of the entire larynx, hyoid bone, pre-epiglottic space, cricoid cartilage, and 3–4 rings of trachea. The pharyngeal opening to the trachea is closed and remaining trachea brought out to the neck to form a permanent tracheostomy. The result is loss of normal speech and breathing and loss of olfaction.

B. Nursing care: preoperative
1. Provide routine pre-op care.
2. Explain expected procedures after surgery including suctioning, humidification, coughing and deep breathing, IV fluids, nasogastric tube feedings, tracheostomy or laryngectomy tube.
3. Reinforce physician's teaching regarding loss of normal speech, breathing patterns, and sense of smell.
4. Encourage patient/family to talk about fears and hopes following surgery.
5. Introduce patient to changes in modes of communication (esophageal speech, artificial larynx).
6. Establish method of communication to be used immediately post-op (Magic Slate, gestures).

C. Nursing interventions: postoperative
1. Promote optimum ventilatory status.
2. Suction nose frequently because of rhinitis.
3. Assess function of tracheostomy/laryngectomy tube and suction as needed.
4. Promote pain relief.
   a. Elevate head of bed to decrease pressure on suture line.
   b. Administer analgesics as needed and monitor effects.
   c. Assist with moving head and turning by supporting back of neck with hands.
5. Promote wound drainage.
   a. Elevate head of bed to promote lymphatic drainage from head.
   b. Monitor amount, characteristics of drainage.
6. Promote nutrition.
   a. Institute and monitor tube feedings as ordered.
   b. Increase fluid intake as tolerated to improve hydration.
   c. Encourage self-feeding.
   d. Advance to normal diet as soon as patient able to tolerate.
7. Prevent infection.
   a. Assess WBC and report significant increases.
   b. Take temperature every 4 hours.
   c. Maintain sterile technique when suctioning and performing tracheostomy care.
   d. Observe stoma/suture lines for signs of infection
   e. Provide frequent oral hygiene.
   f. Monitor sputum and drainage for changes in color, odor, characteristics.
8. Enhance communication.
   a. Carry out modes of communication determined pre-op.
   b. Assess nonverbal behavior.
   c. Allow patient time to ask questions and do not anticipate answers.
   d. Arrange for volunteer laryngectomee to visit patient and assist with esophageal speech/artificial larynx.
   e. Consult with speech therapist if needed.
   f. Progress to normal diet as soon as possible to regain muscle tone of throat and abdomen.
9. Support patient during adaptation to altered physical status.
   a. Encourage patient to discuss feelings about changes in appearance, body functioning, and life-style; be aware of nonverbal responses to the changes.
   b. Assist to identify and use coping techniques that have been helpful in past.
   c. Suggest flattering clothing styles that don't emphasize chest or neck configuration.
   d. Monitor for and support behaviors indicative of positive adaptation to changes (e.g., interest in appearance).
10. Assess for respiratory complications (dyspnea, cyanosis, tachycardia, tachypnea, restlessness).
11. Provide patient teaching and discharge planning concerning
    a. Tracheostomy/laryngectomy and stomal care
    b. Proper administration of nasogastric tube feedings and maintenance of nasogastric tube (see page 120)
    c. Control of dryness/crusting of tongue by brushing tongue regularly with soft toothbrush and toothpaste and using oral mouthwashes
    d. Need for humidified air at home
    e. Importance of protecting the stoma with a shield or towel while showering, directing shower nozzle away from stoma
    f. Need to use electric razors only for 6 months after surgery as facial area will be numb
    g. Need to lean forward when expectorating secretions and to cover stoma when coughing or sneezing
    h. Snorkle devices to enable swimming (caution is advised since drowning can occur rapidly in these patients)
    i. Need to wear an identification bracelet indicating that patient is a neck breather
    j. Types of stoma guards available
    k. Necessity of installing smoke detectors since sense of smell is lost
    l. Information about prosthetic devices, speech therapy, and reconstructive surgery.

SAMPLE QUESTIONS

Mr. Steven Quick, 17 years old, is admitted to the emergency room after a single vehicle automobile accident. He was not wearing a seat belt and he tells you he was "tossed around" when his car hit a tree. He is very anxious, dyspneic, and in severe pain. The left chest wall moves in during inspiration and balloons out when he exhales.

It is determined that Steven has a flail chest and he is intubated with an endotracheal tube. He is placed on a respirator for mechanical ventilation (control mode, positive pressure).

8. Which physical finding alerts the nurse to an additional problem in respiratory function?
   - 1. Dullness to percussion in the third to fifth intercostal space, midclavicular line
   - 2. Decreased paradoxical motion
   - 3. Louder breath sounds on the right chest
   - 4. pH of 7 in arterial blood gases

9. A chest tube is inserted and connected to water-seal drainage (Pleur-evac). What is the best indicator that the drainage system is functioning correctly?
   - 1. Continuous bubbling in the water-seal chamber
   - 2. Fluctuation in the water-seal (U-tube) chamber
   - 3. Suction tubing attached to a wall unit
   - 4. Vesicular breath sounds throughout the lung fields

The Gastrointestinal System

OVERVIEW OF ANATOMY AND PHYSIOLOGY

The organs of the digestive system are grouped into the alimentary canal (GI tract), consisting of the mouth, esophagus, stomach, and small and large intestine; and the accessory digestive organs, including the liver, pancreas, gallbladder, and ductal system (Figure 2.11). The primary functions of this system are movement of food; digestion; absorption; elimination; and provision of a continuous supply of nutrients, electrolytes, and water.

Mouth

A. Consists of the lips and oral cavity: provides entrance and initial processing for nutrients and sensory data, such as taste, texture, and temperature.

B. Oral cavity contains the teeth, used for mastication, and the tongue, which assists in deglutition, taste sensation, and mastication.

C. The salivary glands, located in the mouth, produce secretions containing ptyalin for starch digestion and mucus for lubrication.

D. The pharynx aids in swallowing and functions in ingestion by providing a route for food to pass from the mouth to the esophagus (see page 98 for further details).

Esophagus

Muscular tube that receives food from the pharynx and propels it into the stomach by peristalsis.

Stomach

A. Located on the left side of the abdominal cavity, occupying the hypochondriac, epigastric, and umbilical regions

B. Stores and mixes food with gastric juices and mucus, producing chemical and mechanical changes in the bolus of food.

   1. The secretion of digestive juices is stimulated by smelling, tasting, and chewing food, which is known as the cephalic phase of digestion.

   2. The gastric phase is stimulated by the presence of food in the stomach; regulated by neural stimulation via the PNS, and hormonal stimulation through secretions of gastrin by the gastric mucosa.

   3. After processing in the stomach the food bolus, called *chyme,* is released into the small intestine through the duodenum.

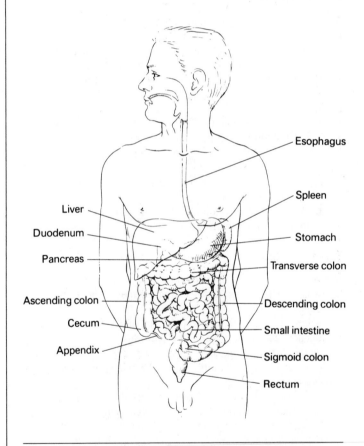

Figure 2.11　Anterior view of the structures in the GI tract.

C. Two sphincters control the rate of food passage
   1. *Cardiac sphincter:* located at the opening between the esophagus and stomach
   2. *Pyloric sphincter:* located between the stomach and duodenum
D. Three anatomic divisions: fundus, body, and antrum
E. Gastric secretions
   1. *Pepsinogen:* secreted by chief cells, located in fundus, aids in protein digestion
   2. *Hydrochloric acid:* secreted by parietal cells, functions in protein digestion, released in response to gastrin
   3. *Intrinsic factor:* secreted by parietal cells, promotes absorption of vitamin B_{12}
   4. Mucoid secretions: coat stomach wall and prevent autodigestion.

Small Intestine

A. Composed of the duodenum, jejunum, and ileum
B. Extends from the pylorus to the *ileocecal valve,* which regulates flow into the large intestine and prevents reflux into the small intestine.
C. Major functions of the small intestine are digestion and absorption of the end products of digestion.
D. Structural features
   1. *Villi* (functional units of the small intestine): fingerlike projections located in the mucous membrane; contain goblet cells that secrete mucus, and absorptive cells that absorb digested foodstuffs.
   2. *Crypts of Lieberkuhn:* produce secretions containing digestive enzymes.
   3. *Brunner's glands:* found in the submucosa of the duodenum, secrete mucus.

Large Intestine

A. Divided into four parts: cecum (with appendix); colon (ascending, transverse, descending, sigmoid); rectum; and anus.
B. Serves as a reservoir for fecal material until defecation occurs; functions to absorb water and electrolytes
C. Microorganisms present in the large intestine are responsible for a small amount of further breakdown and also make some vitamins.
   1. Amino acids are deaminated by bacteria resulting in ammonia, which is converted to urea in the liver.
   2. Bacteria in the large intestine aid in the synthesis of vitamin K and some of the vitamin B groups.
D. Feces (solid waste) leave the body via the rectum and anus.
   1. Anus contains internal sphincter (under involuntary control) and external sphincter (voluntary control)
   2. Fecal matter usually 75% water and 25% solid wastes (roughage, dead bacteria, fat, protein, inorganic matter)

Liver

A. Largest internal organ; located in the right hypochondriac and epigastric regions of the abdomen

B. *Liver lobules:* functional units of the liver, composed of hepatic cells
C. Hepatic sinusoids (capillaries) are lined with Kupffer cells, which carry out the process of phagocytosis.
D. Portal circulation brings blood to the liver from the stomach, spleen, pancreas, and intestines.
E. Functions
   1. Metabolism of fats, carbohydrates, and proteins; oxidizes these nutrients for energy and produces compounds that can be stored.
   2. Production of bile
   3. Conjugation and excretion (in the form of glycogen, fatty acids, minerals, fat-soluble and water-soluble vitamins) of bilirubin.
   4. Storage of vitamins A, D, B_{12}, and iron
   5. Synthesis of coagulation factors
   6. Detoxification of many drugs and conjugation of sex hormones

Biliary System

Consists of the gallbladder and associated ductal system (bile ducts).
A. *Gallbladder:* lies on the under surface of the liver, functions to concentrate and store bile (Figure 2.12).
B. *Ductal system:* provides a route for bile to reach the intestines.
   1. Bile is formed in the liver and excreted into the hepatic duct.
   2. Hepatic duct joins with the cystic duct (which drains the gallbladder) to form the *common bile duct.*
   3. If sphincter of Oddi is relaxed, bile enters the duodenum. If contracted, bile is stored in gallbladder.

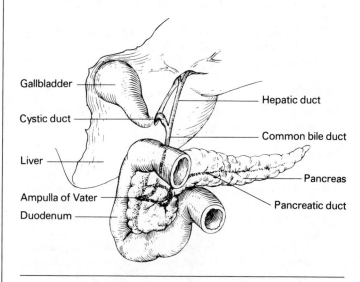

Figure 2.12 Gallbladder and ductal system.

Pancreas

A. Positioned transversely in the upper abdominal cavity.
B. Consists of a head, body, and tail along with a pancreatic duct, which extends along the gland and enters the duodenum via the common bile duct.
C. Has both exocrine and endocrine functions; function in GI system is exocrine.
  1. Exocrine cells in the pancreas secrete trypsinogen and chymotrypsin for protein digestion, amylase to break down starch to dissaccharides, and lipase for fat digestion.
  2. Endocrine function is related to islets of Langerhans (see page 162).

Physiology of Digestion and Absorption

A. Digestion: physical and chemical breakdown of food into absorptive substances
  1. Initiated in the mouth where food mixes with saliva and starch is broken down
  2. Food then passes into the esophagus where it is propelled into the stomach.
  3. In the stomach, food is processed by gastric secretions into a substance called chyme.
  4. In the small intestine, carbohydrates are hydrolyzed to monosaccharides, fats to glycerol, and fatty acids and proteins to amino acids to complete the digestive process.
    a. When chyme enters the duodenum, mucus is secreted to neutralize hydrochloric acid; in response to release of *secretin*, pancreas releases bicarbonate to neutralize acid chyme.
    b. *Cholecystokinin and pancreozymin (CCK-PZ)* are also produced by the duodenal mucosa; stimulate contraction of the gallbladder along with relaxation of the sphincter of Oddi (to allow bile to flow from the common bile duct into the duodenum), and stimulate release of pancreatic enzymes.

ASSESSMENT

Health History

A. Presenting problem
  1. Mouth: symptoms may include dental caries, bleeding gums, dryness or increased salivation, odors, difficulty chewing (note use of dentures)
  2. Ingestion: symptoms may include
    a. Changes in appetite: anorexia or hyperorexia; note food preferences/dislikes
    b. Food intolerances: allergies, fluid, fatty foods
    c. Weight gain/loss: note symptoms/situations that might interfere with appetite (stress, deliberate weight reduction, dental problems); note average weight and percent gain/loss within past 2–9 months.
    d. Dysphagia: note level of sensation where problem occurs, whether it occurs with foods/fluids.
    e. Nausea: note onset and duration, existence of associated symptoms (weakness, headache, vomiting), occurrence before or after meals.
    f. Vomiting: note onset and duration; foods/fluids that can be maintained; associated symptoms (fever, diarrhea).
    g. Regurgitation (reflux): note whether occurs with ingestion of certain foods, any associated symptoms (vomiting), occurrence with certain positions (supine, recumbent).
  3. Digestion/absorption: symptoms may include
    a. Dyspepsia (indigestion): note location of discomfort, whether associated with certain foods, time of day/night of occurrence, associated symptoms (vomiting).
    b. Heartburn (pyrosis): note location, whether pain radiates, whether it occurs before or after meals, time of day when discomfort is most noticeable, foods that aggravate or eliminate symptoms.
    c. Pain: character, frequency, location, duration, distribution, aggravating or alleviating factors.
  4. Bowel habits: symptoms may include
    a. Constipation: note number of stools/day or week, changes in size or color of stool, alterations in food/fluid intake, presence of tenesmus, painful defecation, associated symptoms (abdominal pain, cramps)
    b. Diarrhea: note number of stools/day, consistency, quantity, odor, interference with ADL, associated symptoms (nausea, vomiting, flatus, abdominal distension).
  5. Hepatic/biliary problems: symptoms may include
    a. Jaundice: note location, duration, notable increase/decrease in degree.
    b. Pruritus: note location, distribution, onset.
    c. Urine changes: note color, onset, notable increase or decrease in color change, associated symptoms (pain).
    d. Clay-colored stools: note onset, number/day, associated symptoms (pain, problems with ingestion/digestion).
    e. Increased bleeding: note ecchymoses, purpura, bleeding gums, hematuria.
B. Life-style: eating behaviors (rapid ingestion, skipping meals, snacking), cultural/religious values (vegetarian, kosher foods), ingestion of alcohol, smoking.
C. Use of medications: note use of antacids, antiemetics, antiflatulents, vitamin supplements; aspirin and anti-inflammatory agents.
D. Past medical history: childhood, adult, psychiatric illness; surgery; bleeding disorders; menstrual history; exposure to infectious agents; allergies.

Physical Examination

A. Mouth: inspect/palpate
  1. Outer/inner lips: color, texture, moisture
  2. Buccal mucosa: color, texture, lesions, ulcerations
  3. Teeth/gums: missing teeth, cavities, tenderness, swelling
  4. Tongue: protrusion without deviation, texture, color, moisture

5. Palates (hard and soft): color
B. Abdomen: divided into regions and quadrants (Figure 2.13); note specific location of any abnormality.
   1. Inspect skin: color, scars, striae, pigmentation, lesions, vascularity.
   2. Inspect architecture: contour, symmetry, distension, umbilicus.
   3. Inspect movement: peristalsis, pulsations.
   4. Auscultate peristaltic sounds.
      a. Normal: bubbling, gurgling, 5–30 times/minute
      b. Increased: may indicate diarrhea, gastroenteritis; early intestinal obstruction
      c. Decreased: may indicate constipation, late intestinal obstruction, use of anticholinergics, post-op anesthesia
   5. Auscultate arterial sounds: note presence or absence of bruits in aorta/renal arteries.
   6. Percuss for tenderness/masses; determine distribution of tympany and dullness
      a. Liver span: normal 6–12 cm dullness at the midclavicular line; determine shifting dullness (ascites)
      b. Stomach: normal tympany
      c. Spleen: normal tympany, dullness only if enlarged
      d. Small/large intestine: normal tympany
      e. Bladder: normal tympany, dullness if full
   7. Palpate to depth of 1 cm (light palpation) to determine areas of tenderness, muscle guarding, and masses
   8. Palpate to a depth of 4–8 cm (deep palpation) to identify rigidity, masses, ascites, tenderness, liver margins, spleen

Laboratory/Diagnostic Tests

A. Blood chemistry and electrolyte analysis: albumin, alkaline phosphatase, ammonia, amylase, bilirubin, chloride, LDH, lipase, potassium, SGOT serum glutamic pyruvic transaminase (SGPT), sodium, bromsulphalein (BSP)
   1. Nursing care for BSP test
      a. Instruct patient to fast for 8–12 hours before the test and provide no food during the course of the test; patient may drink water, tea, or black coffee.
      b. Record weight prior to test.
      c. Inform patient that a dye will be injected into the arm slowly and 45 minutes later a blood sample will be drawn from opposite arm.
      d. Observe patient closely for an allergic reaction to the dye.
      e. Eating and drinking can be resumed after blood sample is drawn.
B. Hematologic studies: Hgb and Hct, PT, WBC
C. Serologic studies: carcinoembryonic antigen (CEA), hepatitis-associated antigens
D. Urine studies: amylase, bilirubin
E. Fecal studies: for blood, fat, infectious organisms
   1. A freshly passed, warm stool is the best specimen.
   2. For fat or infectious organisms collect three separate specimens and label day #1, day #2, day #3.
F. Upper GI series (barium swallow)
   1. Fluoroscopic examination of upper GI tract to determine

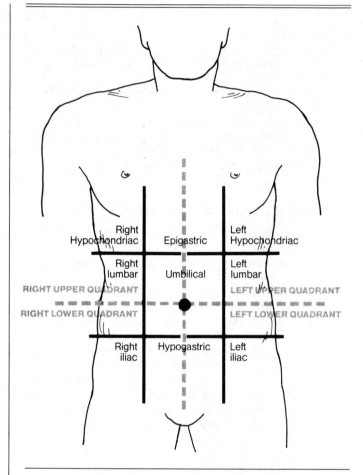

Figure 2.13 Abdominal quadrants (broken lines) and regions (solid lines).

structural problems and gastric emptying time; patient must swallow barium sulfate or other contrast medium; sequential films taken as it moves through the system.
   2. Nursing care: pretest
      a. Keep NPO after midnight or 6–8 hours pretest.
      b. Explain that the barium will taste chalky.
   3. Nursing care: post-test: administer laxatives to enhance elimination of barium and prevent obstruction or impaction.
G. Lower GI series (barium enema)
   1. Barium is instilled into the colon by enema; patient retains the contrast medium while x-rays are taken to identify structural abnormalities of the large intestine or colon.
   2. Nursing care: pretest
      a. Keep NPO for 8 hours pretest.
      b. Give enemas until clear the morning of test.
      c. Administer laxative or suppository.
      d. Explain that cramping may be experienced during the procedure.
   3. Nursing care: post-test: administer laxatives and fluids to assist in expelling barium.

H. Endoscopy (Esophagogastroduodenoscopy)
   1. Direct visualization of the esophagus, stomach, and duodenum by insertion of a lighted fiberscope
   2. Used to observe structures, ulcerations, inflammation, tumors; may include a biopsy
   3. Nursing care: pretest
      a. Keep NPO for 6–8 hours.
      b. Ensure consent form has been signed.
      c. Explain that a local anesthetic will be used to ease discomfort and that speaking during the procedure will not be possible; the patient should expect hoarseness and a sore throat for several days.
   4. Nursing care: post-test
      a. Keep NPO until return of gag reflex.
      b. Assess vital signs and for pain, dysphagia, bleeding.
      c. Administer warm normal saline gargles for relief of sore throat.

I. Colonoscopy
   1. Endoscopic visualization of the large intestine; may include biopsy and removal of foreign substances.
   2. Nursing care: pretest
      a. Keep NPO for 8 hours pre-test.
      b. Administer laxatives for 1-3 days before the exam, and enemas until clear the night before the test.
      c. Ensure a consent form has been signed.
      d. Explain to patient that when the instrument is inserted into the rectum a feeling of pressure might be experienced.
   3. Nursing care: post-test
      a. Observe for rectal bleeding and signs of perforation.
      b. Schedule planned rest periods for the patient.

J. Sigmoidoscopy
   1. Endoscopic visualization of the sigmoid colon
   2. Used to identify inflammation, lesions or remove foreign bodies.
   3. Nursing care: pretest
      a. Offer a light supper and light breakfast.
      b. Do bowel prep.
      c. Explain to patient that the sensation of an urge to defecate or abdominal cramping might be experienced.
   4. Nursing care: post-test: assess for signs of bowel perforation.

K. Gastric analysis
   1. Insertion of a nasogastric tube to examine fasting gastric contents for acidity and volume
   2. Nursing care: pretest
      a. Keep NPO 6–8 hours pretest.
      b. Advise patient about no smoking, anticholinergic medications, antacids for 24 hours prior to test.
      c. Inform patient that tube will be inserted into the stomach via the nose, and instruct to expectorate saliva to prevent buffering of secretions.
   3. Nursing care: post-test: provide frequent mouth care.

L. Oral cholecystogram
   1. Injection of a radiopaque dye and x-ray examination to visualize the gallbladder
   2. Used to determine the gallbladder's ability to concentrate and store the dye and to assess patency of the biliary duct system
   3. Nursing care: pretest
      a. Offer a low-fat meal the evening before the test and black coffee, tea, or water the morning of the exam.
      b. Check for iodine sensitivity and administer dye tablets (Telepaque) as ordered.
   4. Nursing care: post-test: observe for side effects of the dye (nausea, vomiting, diarrhea).

M. Liver biopsy (closed needle)
   1. Invasive procedure where a specially designed needle is inserted into the liver to remove a small piece of tissue for study
   2. Nursing care: pretest
      a. Ensure patient has signed consent form.
      b. Keep NPO 6–8 hours pretest.
      c. Instruct patient to hold breath during the biopsy.
   3. Nursing care: post-test
      a. Assess vital signs every hour for 8–12 hours.
      b. Place patient on right side for a few hours with a pillow against the abdomen to provide pressure on the liver.
      c. Observe puncture site for hemorrhage.
      d. Assess for complications of shock and pneumothorax.

ANALYSIS

Nursing diagnoses for the patient with a disorder of the digestive system may include
A. Actual or potential fluid volume deficit
B. Actual or potential impairment of skin integrity
C. Disturbance in self-concept: body image
D. Alteration in nutrition: less than body requirements
E. Alteration in comfort: pain
F. Alteration in bowel elimination: diarrhea/constipation
G. Noncompliance
H. Potential for injury
I. Impaired physical mobility

PLANNING AND IMPLEMENTATION

Goals

A. Fluid and electrolyte balance will be maintained.
B. Patient's skin integrity will be restored/maintained.
C. Patient will express feelings of self-worth.
D. Patient will verbalize feelings regarding the colostomy/ileostomy.
E. Patient will maintain adequate weight for age, sex, height, and body build.
F. Discomfort from abdominal distension, pruritus, stomatitis, or other irritation of oral mucous membranes will be controlled/relieved.
G. Patient will develop regular bowel habits, decreased frequency of liquid stools, and regular bowel movements.

H. Patient will cooperate with treatment regimen.

I. There will be no evidence of abnormal bleeding.

J. Patient will demonstrate increased strength and endurance and maintenance of an optimal activity level.

Interventions

Enemas

A. General information

1. Instillation of fluid into the rectum, usually for the purpose of stimulating defecation. The various types include
   a. *Cleansing enema* (tap water, normal saline, or soap): used to treat constipation or feces impaction, as bowel cleansing prior to diagnostic procedures or surgery, to help establish regular bowel functions.
   b. *Retention enema* (mineral oil, olive oil, cottonseed oil): usually administered to lubricate or soften a hard fecal mass to facilitate defecation.

B. Nursing care for a cleansing enema

1. Explain procedure and that breathing through the mouth relaxes abdominal musculature and helps to avoid cramps; explain the need to take adequate time to defecate.
2. Assemble equipment: prepare solution and have bedpan, commode, or nearby bathroom ready for use.
3. Position patient and drape adequately.
4. Place waterproof pad under buttocks.
5. Lubricate tube and allow solution to fill the tubing, displacing air.
6. Insert rectal tube, without using force, request that patient take several deep breaths.
7. Administer solution over 5–10 minutes; if cramping occurs slow the speed of instillation.
8. After administration, have the patient retain solution until the urge to defecate becomes strong.
9. Document amount, color, characteristics of stool and patient's reaction during procedure.
10. Assess for dizziness, lightheadedness, abdominal cramps, nausea.

C. Nursing care for a retention enema: same as for a cleansing enema except

1. Oil is used instead of water (comes prepared in commercial kits and is given at body temperature).
2. Administer 150–200 cc of prepared solution.
3. Instruct patient to retain oil for at least 30 minutes in order to take effect.

Gastrostomy

A. General information

1. Insertion of a catheter through an abdominal incision into the stomach where it is secured with sutures
2. Used as an alternative method of feeding, either temporary or permanent, for patients who have problems with swallowing, ingestion, and digestion.

B. Nursing care

1. Maintain skin integrity: inspect and cleanse skin around stoma frequently; keep deep area dry to avoid excoriation.
2. Maintain patency of the gastrostomy tube.
   a. Assess for residual before each feeding (check orders concerning withholding feeding).
   b. Irrigate tube before and after meals.
   c. Measure/record any drainage.
3. Promote adequate nutrition.
   a. Administer feeding with patient in high-Fowler's and keep head of bed elevated for 30 minutes after meals to prevent regurgitation.
   b. Maintain feeding at room temperature.
   c. Ensure that prescribed amount of feeding be given within prescribed amount of time.
   d. Weigh patient daily.
   e. Monitor I&O until feedings are well tolerated.
   f. Allow patient to see, smell, and taste food before meals to stimulate gastric juices.
   g. Monitor for signs of deyhdration.

Nasogastric (NG) Tubes

A. General information

1. Soft rubber or plastic tube inserted through a nostril and into the stomach for gastric decompression, feeding, or obtaining specimens for analysis of stomach contents
2. Types
   a. Levin: single-lumen, nonvented
   b. Salem: a tube within a tube; vented to provide constant inflow of atmospheric air

B. Nursing care

1. Monitor functioning of system and ensure patency of the NG tube: abdominal discomfort/distension, nausea and vomiting, and little or no drainage in collection bottle are all signs that system is not functioning properly.
   a. Assess tube position: aspirate gastric contents to confirm that tube in stomach; inject 10 cc air through tube and auscultate for rapid influx.
   b. Check that tubing is free of kinks; irrigate every 2–4 hours if suction is used and before and after each feeding.
   c. Record amount, color, and odor of drainage.
2. Provide measures to assure maximal comfort.
   a. Apply water-soluble lubricant to lips to prevent dryness.
   b. Keep nares free from secretions.
   c. Provide periodic warm saline gargles to prevent dryness.
   d. Provide frequent mouth care with toothbrush/toothpaste or flavored mouth washes.
   e. If allowed, give patient hard candy or gum to stimulate the flow of saliva and prevent dryness.
   f. Elevate head and chest during and for 1–2 hours after feedings to prevent reflux (most comfortable position when suction is used).
3. Monitor/maintain fluid and electrolyte balance.
   a. Assess for signs of metabolic alkalosis (suctioning causes excessive loss of hydrochloride and potassium).
   b. Administer IV fluids as ordered.

c. If suction used, irrigate NG tube with normal saline to decrease sodium loss.

d. Keep accurate I&O.

e. If suction used provide ice chips sparingly (if allowed) to avoid dilution of electrolytes.

f. Monitor lab values and electrolytes frequently.

Intestinal Tubes

A. General information

1. Tube is inserted via a nostril through the stomach and into the intestine for decompression proximal to an obstruction, relief of an obstruction, decompression of post-op edema at the surgical site.

2. Types

a. Cantor tube: single lumen; instillation of mercury before insertion

b. Miller-Abbott: double lumen; instillation of mercury after insertion

B. Nursing care

1. Facilitate placement of the tube.

a. Position patient in high-Fowler's while tube is being passed from the nose into the stomach; then place patient on right side to aid in advancing the tube from the stomach to duodenum.

b. Continuously monitor tube markings.

c. Tape tube in place only after placement in duodenum is confirmed.

2. Provide measures for maximal comfort, as for NG tube.

EVALUATION

A. Patient's serum electrolytes are within normal limits.

B. Patient's oral intake is adequate; provides increased nutrients in diet.

C. Vital signs are within normal limits.

D. No redness of skin or irritation and breakdown; patient able to describe factors that contribute to skin alterations.

E. Patient actively participates in ADL, treatments, and care; expresses interest in personal well-being.

F. Patient is able to integrate ostomy care into life-style; participates in treatment and self-care activities.

G. Anthropometric measurements are improved.

H. Activity tolerance is increased.

I. Oral intake is increased.

J. Pain is controlled/relieved.

1. Relaxed facial expression

2. Abdominal girth within normal limits; relief of abdominal distension

K. Oral mucosa are pink, smooth, and moist.

L. Patient is adequately hydrated (good skin turgor and mobility).

M. Patient evacuates formed stools on a regular basis with absence of pain.

N. Patient shows no evidence of abnormal bleeding.

1. No ecchymoses, petechiae, bleeding gums, hematemesis, hematuria, or melena

2. No unusual joint swelling

3. Stable Hgb and Hct; vital signs within normal limits

O. Patient has increased activity level within physical limitations.

DISORDERS OF THE GASTROINTESTINAL SYSTEM

Nausea and Vomiting

A. General information

1. *Nausea:* a feeling of discomfort in the epigastrium with a conscious desire to vomit; occurs in association with and prior to vomiting.

2. *Vomiting:* forceful ejection of stomach contents from the upper GI tract. Emetic center in medulla is stimulated (eg, by local irritation of intestine or stomach or disturbance of equilibrium) causing the vomiting reflex.

3. Nausea and vomiting are the two most common manifestations of GI disease.

4. Contributing factors

a. GI disease

b. CNS disorders (meningitis, CNS lesions)

c. Circulatory problems (CHF)

d. Metabolic disorders (uremia)

e. Side effects of certain drugs (chemotherapy, antibiotics)

f. Pain

g. Psychic trauma

h. Response to motion

B. Assessment findings

1. Weakness, fatigue, pallor, possible lethargy

2. Dry mucous membrane and poor skin turgor/mobility (if prolonged with dehydration)

3. Serum sodium, calcium, potassium decreased

4. BUN elevated (if severe vomiting and dehydration)

C. Nursing interventions

1. Maintain NPO until patient able to tolerate oral intake.

2. Administer medications as ordered and monitor effects/side effects.

a. Phenothiazines: chlorpromazine (Thorazine), perphenazine (Trilafon), prochlorperazine (Compazine), trifluoperazine (Stelazine)

b. Antihistamines: benzquinamide (Emete-con), dimenhydrinate (Dramamine), diphenhydramine (Benadryl), hydroxyzine (Atarax, Vistaril), cyclizine (Marezine), meclizine (Antivert), promethazine (Phenergan)

c. Other drugs to help control nausea and vomiting: thiethylperazine (Torecan), trimethobenzamide (Tigan)

3. Notify physician if changes in vomiting pattern.

4. Maintain fluid and electrolyte balance.

a. Administer IV fluids as ordered, keep accurate record of I&O.

b. Record amount/frequency of vomitus.

c. Assess skin tone/turgor for degree of hydration.

d. Monitor laboratory/electrolyte values.

e. Test NG tube drainage or vomitus for blood, bile; monitor pH.
5. Provide measures for maximum comfort.
   a. Institute frequent mouth care with tepid water/saline mouthwashes.
   b. Remove encrustations around nares.
   c. Keep head of bed elevated and avoid sudden changes in position.
   d. Eliminate noxious stimuli from environment.
   e. Keep emesis basin clean.
   f. Maintain quiet environment and avoid unnecessary procedures.
6. When vomiting subsides provide clear fluids (ginger ale, warm tea) in small amounts, gradually introduce solid foods (toast, crackers), and progress to bland foods (baked potato) in small amounts.
7. Provide patient teaching and discharge planning concerning
   a. Avoidance of situations, foods, or liquids that precipitate nausea and vomiting
   b. Need for planned, uninterrupted rest periods
   c. Medication regimen, including side effects
   d. Signs of dehydration
   e. Need for daily weights with frequent anthropometric measurements.

Anorexia/Eating Disorders

See page **503**.

Diarrhea

A. General information
   1. Increase in peristaltic motility producing frequent watery or loosely formed stools. Diarrhea is a symptom of other pathologic processes.
   2. Causes
      a. Chronic bowel disorders
      b. Malabsorption problems
      c. Intestinal infections
      d. Biliary tract disorders
      e. Hyperthyroidism
      f. Saline laxatives
      g. Magnesium-based antacids
      h. Stress
      i. Antibiotics
      j. Neoplasms
      k. Highly seasoned foods
B. Assessment findings
   1. Abdominal cramps/distension, foul-smelling watery stools, increased peristalsis
   2. Anorexia, thirst, tenesmus, anxiety
   3. Decreased potassium and sodium if severe
C. Nursing interventions
   1. Administer antidiarrheals: diphenoxylate with atropine (Lomotil), paregoric, loperamide (Imodium), Kaopectate as ordered; monitor effects.

2. Control fluid/food intake.
   a. Avoid milk and milk products.
   b. Provide liquids with gradual introduction of bland, high-protein, high-calorie, low-fat, low-bulk foods.
3. Monitor and maintain fluid and electrolyte status; record number, characteristics, and amount of each stool.
4. Prevent anal excoriation.
   a. Cleanse rectal area after each bowel movement with mild soap and water and pat dry.
   b. Apply A and D ointment or Desitin to promote healing.
   c. Use a local anesthetic as needed.
5. Provide patient teaching and discharge planning concerning
   a. Medication regimen
   b. Adherence to prescribed diet and avoidance of foods that are known to produce diarrhea
   c. Importance of perineal hygiene and care and daily assessment of skin changes
   d. Importance of good handwashing techniques after each stool
   e. Need to report worsening of symptoms (increased abdominal cramps, increased frequency or amount of stool)
   f. Need to assess daily weights with frequent anthropometric measurements.

Constipation

A. General information
   1. Lengthening of normal (for individual) time period between bowel movements; small volume of dry, hard stool; results from decreased motility of the colon or from retention of feces in the colon or rectum
   2. Causes
      a. Inadequate bulk/liquids in the diet
      b. Lack of physical activity
      c. Retention of barium after radiographic exam
      d. Prolonged use of constipating medications (aluminum-based antacids, anticholinergics, antihistamines, antidepressants, phenothiazines, calcium, iron).
B. Assessment findings
   1. Feeling of abdominal fullness, pressure in the rectum; abdominal distension, dyschezia; increased flatus
   2. Hardened stool upon digital examination
C. Nursing interventions
   1. Promote adequate intake of fluids/foods and dietary modification: increase fluid intake to at least 3000 cc/day; include high-fiber foods in diet.
   2. Administer medications as ordered
      a. Cathartics: milk of magnesia, castor oil, cascara sagrada, senna (Senokot), bisacodyl (Dulcolax), psyllium (Metamucil)
      b. Stool softeners: docusate calcium (Surfak), docusate sodium (Colace)
   3. Prevent accumulation of stool in the colon/rectum.
      a. Instruct patient not to suppress urge to defecate.
      b. Gently massage abdomen to promote stimulation and movement of feces.

4. Provide patient teaching and discharge planning concerning
   a. Need to establish and maintain a regular time to defecate
   b. Diet modification
   c. Medication regimen
   d. Need to assume position of comfort when sitting on toilet.

Stomatitis

See page 36.

Cancer of the Mouth

A. General information
   1. Cancer of the mouth may occur on the lips or within the mouth (tongue, floor of mouth, buccal mucosa, hard/soft palate, pharynx, tonsils).
   2. Most common type of oral tumor is squamous cell carcinoma; most malignancies occur on the lower lip.
   3. More common in men
   4. Caused by
      a. Excessive sun exposure
      b. Tobacco (cigar, pipe, cigarette, snuff)
      c. Excessive alcohol intake
      d. Constant irritation (dental caries)
   5. Early detection is very important; most discovered by dentists in routine checkups.
B. Medical management
   1. Radiation therapy: both primary lesion and affected lymph nodes; radioactive implants
   2. Chemotherapy: sometimes indicated, not used as often as radiation therapy and surgery
   3. Surgery: type depends on location and extent of the tumor.
      a. Mandibulectomy: removal of the mandible
      b. Hemiglossectomy: removal of half the tongue
      c. Glossectomy: removal of the entire tongue
      d. Radical neck dissection
C. Assessment findings
   1. Ulcerations (often painless) on the lip, tongue, or buccal mucosa
   2. Pain or soreness of the tongue upon eating hot or highly seasoned foods
   3. Erythroplakia, leukoplakia
   4. Difficulty chewing/speaking, dysphagia
   5. Positive oral exfoliative cytology
   6. Positive toluidine blue test
D. Nursing interventions
   1. Provide nursing care for the patient receiving radiation therapy
   2. Prepare patient for surgery: in addition to routine pre-op care
      a. Inform patient of expected changes post-op.
      b. Provide explanation of anticipated post-op suctioning, NG tube, drains.
   3. In addition to routine post-op care
      a. Promote drainage.

1) place in side-lying position initially, then Fowler's.
2) suction mouth (except for lip surgery).
3) maintain patency of drainage tubes.
   b. Promote oral hygiene/comfort.
      1) provide mouth irrigations with sterile water, diluted peroxide, normal saline or sodium bicarbonate.
      2) avoid use of commercial mouthwashes, lemon and glycerine swabs.
   c. Monitor/promote optimum nutritional status.
      1) provide tube feedings following a hemiglossectomy.
      2) place oral fluids in back of the throat with an asepto syringe.
      3) provide foods/fluids that are nonirritating and facilitate swallowing (yogurt, puddings).
   d. Monitor for signs and symptoms of facial nerve damage (drooping, uneven smile, circumoral numbness or tingling).

Cancer of the Esophagus

A. General information
   1. Malignant tumors of the esophagus usually appear as ulcerated lesions, most often in middle and lower portions of the esophagus
   2. Penetration of the muscular layers with extension to the outer wall of the esophagus is commonly found. Metastases may cause eventual esophageal obstruction
   3. More common in men than in women (4:1); usually between ages 50–70
   4. Cause unknown; contributing factors include cigarette smoking, excessive alcohol intake, trauma, poor oral hygiene, achalasia, diverticula and lye burns.
B. Medical management
   1. Radiation therapy: used for inoperable tumors, has been found to alleviate symptoms
   2. Chemotherapy: not found effective
   3. Surgery
      a. Esophagectomy: removal of part or all of the esophagus using a Dacron graft to replace the resected portion
      b. Esophagogastrostomy: resection of a portion of the esophagus (usually middle third) and anastomosis of the remaining portion of the stomach
      c. Esophagoenterostomy: resection of portion of the esophagus and anastomosis of a segment of colon to the remaining portion
      d. Palliative gastrostomy: done for the purpose of feeding the patient
C. Assessment findings
   1. Substernal burning after drinking hot fluids
   2. Pain located in the substernal and epigastric areas; usually intensified with swallowing
   3. Weight loss
   4. Barium swallow reveals narrowing of the esophagus at the area of the tumor
   5. Diagnostic test: esophagoscopy with a biopsy reveals malignant cells

D. Nursing interventions
1. Provide nursing care for the patient receiving radiation therapy.
2. Prepare patient for surgery: in addition to routine pre-op care
   a. Provide meticulous oral hygiene including teeth, gums, tongue, and mouth.
   b. Explain that patient may have a chest tube if thoracic approach is used.
   c. Prepare patient for feedings through a gastrostomy.
3. In addition to routine post-op care
   a. Monitor NG tube: expect bloody drainage for approximately 12 hours with gradual change to green then to yellow.
   b. Prevent gastric reflux: place patient in semi-Fowler's position; maintain upright position for 2 hours after meals when patient is able to take fluids/foods orally.
4. Provide emotional support to patient/family; prognosis is grave.
5. Provide patient teaching and discharge planning concerning
   a. Gastrostomy and proper dietary measures
   b. Importance of cessation of smoking and elimination of alcohol consumption
   c. Maintenance of good oral hygiene
   d. Maintenance of a high-calorie, high-protein diet.

Esophageal Varices

See page 134.

Hiatal Hernia

A. General information
1. Sliding hiatal hernia occurs when a portion of the stomach and vagus nerve slide upward into the thorax through an enlarged hiatus in the diaphragm.
2. Result is reflux of gastric juices and inflammation of the lower portion of the esophagus.
3. Occurs more often in women ages 40–70
4. May be caused by congenital weakening of the muscles in the diaphragm around the esophagogastric opening; increased intra-abdominal pressure (obesity, pregnancy, ascites); trauma

B. Medical management
1. Drug therapy: antacids to reduce acidity and relieve discomfort, cholinergics
2. Modification of diet: elimination of spicy foods and caffeine
3. Surgery: reduction of the hiatal hernia via an abdominal or thoracic approach

C. Assessment findings
1. Heartburn, especially after meals, at night or with position changes (particularly recumbent), dysphagia, regurgitation several hours after meals without vomiting
2. Barium swallow displays protrusion of the gastric mucosa through a hiatus
3. Esophagoscopy reveals an incompetent cardiac sphincter

D. Nursing interventions
1. Provide a bland diet with six small feedings/day, as ordered.
2. Administer medications as ordered.
3. Prepare patient for surgery: in addition to routine pre-op care
   a. Inform patient about chest tubes (if thoracic approach to be used).
   b. Provide information regarding NG intubation.
4. In addition to routine post-op care
   a. Decrease/avoid gastric distension.
   b. Promote pulmonary expansion: chest tubes if a thoracic approach; semi-Fowler's position.
5. Provide patient teaching and discharge planning concerning
   a. Modification of diet
   b. Sitting up for meals and 2 hours after meals will help reduce gastric acid reflux
   c. Use of antacids
   d. Eating small, frequent meals slowly to help prevent gastric distension
   e. Need to avoid carbonated beverages and anticholinergic drugs (and OTC medications that contain them)
   f. Avoidance of heavy lifting (to prevent intra-abdominal pressure); bend, kneel, or stoop instead
   g. Importance of treating persistent cough
   h. Adherence to weight-reduction plan if obese.

Gastritis

A. General information
1. An acute inflammatory condition that causes a breakdown of the normal gastric protective barriers with subsequent diffusion of hydrochloric acid into the gastric lumen
2. Results in hemorrhage, ulceration, and adhesions of the gastric mucosa
3. Present in some form (mild to severe) in 50% of all adults
4. Caused by excessive ingestion of certain drugs (salicylates, steroids, Butazolidin), alcohol; food poisoning; large quantities of spicy, irritating foods in diet

B. Assessment findings
1. Anorexia, nausea and vomiting, hematemesis, epigastric fullness/discomfort, epigastric tenderness
2. Decreased Hgb and Hct (if anemic)
3. Endoscopy: inflammation and ulceration of gastric mucosa
4. Gastric analysis: hydrochloric acid usually increased, except in atrophic gastritis

C. Nursing interventions
1. Monitor and maintain fluid and electrolyte balances.
2. Control nausea and vomiting (NPO until able to tolerate foods, then bland diet).
3. Administer medications as ordered: antiemetics, antacids, sedatives.
4. Maintain patency of NG tube.
5. Provide patient teaching and discharge planning concerning avoidance of foods/medications such as coffee, spicy foods, alcohol, salicylates, ibuprofen, steroids.

Peptic Ulcer Disease

Gastric Ulcers

A. General information
1. Ulceration of the mucosal lining of the stomach; most commonly found in the antrum
2. Gastric secretions and stomach emptying rate usually normal
3. Rapid diffusion of gastric acid from the gastric lumen into gastric mucosa, however, causes an inflammatory reaction with tissue breakdown.
4. Also characterized by reflux into the stomach of bile containing duodenal contents.
5. Occurs more often in men, in unskilled laborers, and in lower socioeconomic groups; peak age 40–55 years
6. Caused by smoking, alcohol abuse, emotional tension, and drugs (salicylates, steroids, Butazolidin)

B. Medical management
1. Supportive: rest, bland diet, stress management
2. Drug therapy: antacids, histamine (H_2) receptor antagonists, anticholinergics (see Table 2.21)

Table 2.21 Drug Therapy for Peptic Ulcer

Drug	Action	Side Effects	Nursing Implications
Histamine (H_2) receptor-site antagonists			
Cimetidine (Tagamet)	Inhibits gastric secretion by inhibiting histamine stimulating effect.	Hematopoietic: reversible leukopenia, occasional thrombocytopenia CNS: metabolic encephalopathy, mild restlessness, confusion, hallucinations; agitation, coma Renal: slight increase in creatinine CV: reversible bradycardia GI: transient diarrhea Other: muscle pain, decreased sperm count, impotence, infertility, acnelike rash, gynecomastia Drug interactions: potentiates hypoprothrombinemia in patients taking warfarin (Coumadin)	Instruct patient to take with meals, or, if one higher dose is prescribed, before bedtime. Make periodic evaluations of blood count, renal, and hepatic function. Advise patient to avoid driving and other potentially hazardous activities until reaction to drug is known. Make periodic determination of gastric pH.
Ranitidine (Zantac)	Potent histamine H_2 receptor, site antagonist	Hematopoietic: leukopenia, thrombocytopenia CNS: headache, malaise, dizziness, GI: liver damage, constipation, nausea, abdominal pain Other: rash	Absorption not affected by food. Make periodic evaluations of kidney and liver function. Report severe, persistent headache immediately. Periodic determination of gastric pH.
Antacids			
Aluminum-containing antacids (Amphogel, Rolaids)	Neutralizes gastric acid (increases pH) and provides pain relief.	Constipation, fecal impaction, interfere with anticholinergic absorption, hypophosphatemia, hypercalcemia	Explain that best time to take antacid is after meals. If administered in tablet form, instruct patient to chew thoroughly before swallowing and to follow tablet with ½ glass of water or milk. Note number and consistency of stools.
Magnesium-containing antacids (milk of magnesia)	Neutralizes gastric acid and provides pain relief.	Diarrhea, hypermagnesemia, nausea and vomiting	Explain that best time to take antacid is after meals and at bedtime. Mix suspension with water or follow with sufficient water.
Anticholinergics			
Atropine, dicyclomine (Bentyl), methantheline bromide (Banthine), propantheline bromide (Pro-Banthine), glycopyrrolate (Robinul)	Decreases vagal stimulation of parietal cells; decreases motility and volume of gastric secretions	CNS: headache, insomnia, drowsiness, blurred vision CV: increased pulse, postural blood pressure changes GI: dry mouth, throat; increased thirst; constipation; nausea, paralytic ileus GU: urinary hesitancy; retention, impotence Skin: diaphoresis, urticaria	Advise patient that best time to take is 30 minutes before meals. Antacids may interfere with absorption of anticholinergics. Advise patient to avoid driving and to change positions slowly. Instruct to drink plenty of fluids; suck hard candy to relieve dryness. Assess for abdominal distension. Advise patient to void before each dose. Use cautiously in hot environment.

3. Surgery: various combinations of gastric resections and anastomosis.

C. Assessment findings
1. Pain located in left epigastrium, with possible radiation to the back; usually occurs 1–2 hours after meals
2. Weight loss
3. Hgb and Hct decreased (if anemic)
4. Endoscopy reveals ulceration; differentiates ulcers from gastric cancer
5. Gastric analysis: normal gastric acidity in gastric ulcer, increased in duodenal ulcer
6. Upper GI series: presence of ulcer confirmed

D. Nursing interventions
1. Administer medications as ordered.
2. Provide nursing care for the patient with ulcer surgery.
3. Provide patient teaching and discharge planning concerning
   a. Medication regimen
      1) take medications at prescribed times.
      2) have antacids available at all times.
      3) recognize situations that would increase the need for antacids.
      4) avoid ulcerogenic drugs (salicylates, steroids).
      5) know proper dosage, action, and side effects.
   b. Proper diet
      1) bland diet consisting of six small meals/day.
      2) eat meals slowly.
      3) avoid acid-producing substances (caffeine, alcohol, highly seasoned foods).
      4) avoid stressful situations at mealtime.
      5) plan for rest periods after meals.
      6) avoid late bedtime snacks.
   c. Avoidance of stress-producing situations and development of stress-reduction methods (relaxation techniques, exercises, biofeedback).

Duodenal Ulcers

A. General information
1. Most commonly found in the first 2 cm of the duodenum
2. Occur more frequently than gastric ulcers
3. Characterized by gastric hyperacidity and a significant increased rate of gastric emptying.
4. Occur more often in younger men; more women affected after menopause; peak age 35–45 years
5. Caused by smoking, alcohol abuse, psychologic stress

B. Medical management: same as for gastric ulcers

C. Assessment findings
1. Pain located in midepigastrium and described as burning, cramping; usually occurs 2–4 hours after meals and is relieved by food.
2. Diagnostic tests: same as for Gastric Ulcer.

D. Nursing interventions: same as for Gastric Ulcer.

Ulcer Surgery

A. General information
1. Surgery is performed when peptic ulcer disease does not respond to medical management.
2. Types
   a. *Vagotomy:* severing of part of the vagus nerve innervating the stomach to decrease gastric acid secretion
   b. *Antrectomy:* removal of the antrum of the stomach to eliminate the gastric phase of digestion
   c. *Pyloroplasty:* enlargement of the pyloric sphincter with acceleration of gastric emptying
   d. *Gastroduodenostomy (Billroth I):* removal of the lower portion of the stomach with anastomosis of the remaining portion of the duodenum
   e. *Gastrojejunostomy (Billroth II):* removal of the antrum and distal portion of the stomach and duodenum with anastomosis of the remaining portion of the stomach to the jejunum
   f. *Gastrectomy:* removal of 60%–80% of the stomach
   g. *Esophagojejunostomy (total gastrectomy):* removal of the entire stomach with a loop of jejunum anastomosed to the esophagus
3. Dumping syndrome
   a. Abrupt emptying of stomach contents into the intestine
   b. Common complication of these types of surgery
   c. Associated with the presence of hyperosmolar chyme in the jejunum, which draws fluid by osmosis from the extracellular fluid into the bowel. Decreased plasma volume and distension of the bowel stimulates increased intestinal motility.
   d. Signs and symptoms include weakness, faintness, palpitations, diaphoresis, feeling of fullness or discomfort, nausea and occasionally diarrhea; appear 15–30 minutes after meals and last for 20–60 minutes

B. Nursing interventions: routine preoperative care

C. Nursing interventions: postoperative
1. Provide routine post-op care.
2. Ensure adequate function of NG tube.
   a. Measure drainage accurately to determine necessity for fluid and electrolyte replacement; notify physician if there is no drainage.
   b. Anticipate frank, red bleeding for 12–24 hours.
3. Promote adequate pulmonary ventilation.
   a. Place patient in mid- or high-Fowler's position to promote chest expansion.
   b. Teach patient to splint high upper abdominal incision before turning, coughing, and deep breathing.
4. Promote adequate nutrition.
   a. After removal of NG tube, provide clear liquids with gradual introduction of small amounts of bland food at frequent intervals.
   b. Monitor weight daily.
   c. Assess for regurgitation; if present, instruct patient to eat smaller amounts of food at a slower pace.

5. Provide patient teaching and discharge planning concerning
  a. Gradually increasing food intake until able to tolerate three meals/day
  b. Daily monitoring of weight
  c. Stress-reduction measures
  d. Need to report signs of complications to physician immediately (hematemesis, vomiting, diarrhea, pain, melena, weakness, feeling of abdominal fullness/distension)
  e. Methods of controlling symptoms associated with dumping syndrome
    1) avoidance of concentrated sweets
    2) adherence to six, small, dry, meals/day
    3) maintenance of modified diet
    4) refraining from taking fluids during meals but rather 2 hours after meals
    5) Assuming a recumbent position for $\frac{1}{2}$ hour after meals.

Cancer of the Stomach

A. General information
  1. Most often develops in the the distal third and may spread through the walls of the stomach into adjacent tissues, lymphatics, regional lymph nodes, other abdominal organs, or through the bloodstream to the lungs and bones.
  2. Affects men twice as often as women; more frequent in blacks and Orientals; most commonly occurs between ages 50–70
  3. Causes
    a. Excessive intake of highly salted or smoked foods
    b. Diet low in quantity of vegetables and fruits
    c. Atrophic gastritis
    d. Achlorhydria
B. Medical management
  1. Chemotherapy
  2. Radiation therapy
  3. Treatment for anemia, gastric decompression, nutritional support, fluid and electrolyte maintenance
  4. Surgery: type depends on location and extent of lesion.
    a. Subtotal gastrectomy (Billroth I or II)
    b. Total gastrectomy
C. Assessment findings
  1. Fatigue, weakness, dizziness, shortness of breath, nausea and vomiting, hematemesis, weight loss, indigestion, epigastric fullness, feeling of early satiety when eating, epigastric pain (later)
  2. Pallor, lethargy, poor skin turgor and mobility, palpable epigastric mass
  3. Diagnostic tests
    a. Stool for occult blood positive
    b. CEA positive
    c. Hgb and Hct decreased
    d. SGOT, SGPT, LDH, serum amylase elevated (if liver and pancreatic involvement)
    e. Gastric analysis reveals histologic changes.

D. Nursing interventions
  1. Give consistent nutritional assessment and support.
  2. Provide care for the patient receiving chemotherapy.
  3. Provide care for the patient with gastric surgery (see Ulcer Surgery).

Hernias

A. General information
  1. Protrusion of a viscus from its normal cavity through an abnormal opening/weakened area.
  2. Occurs anywhere but most often in the abdominal cavity
  3. Types
    a. *Reducible*: can be manually placed back into the abdominal cavity.
    b. *Irreducible:* cannot be placed back into the abdominal cavity.
    c. *Inguinal:* occurs when there is weakness in the abdominal wall where the spermatic cord in men and round ligament in women emerge.
    d. *Femoral:* protrusion through the femoral ring; more common in females.
    e. *Incisional:* occurs at the site of a previous surgical incision as a result of inadequate healing postoperatively.
    f. *Umbilical:* most commonly found in children.
    g. *Strangulated:* irreducible, with obstruction to intestinal flow and blood supply.
B. Medical management
  1. Manual reduction, use of a truss (firm support)
  2. Bowel surgery if strangulated
  3. Herniorrhaphy: surgical repair of the hernia by suturing the defect
C. Assessment findings
  1. Vomiting, protrusion of involved area (more obvious after coughing), and discomfort at site of protrusion
  2. Crampy, abdominal pain and abdominal distension (if strangulated with a bowel obstruction)
D. Nursing interventions
  1. Observe patient for complications such as strangulation.
  2. Prepare patient for herniorrhaphy, provide routine pre-op care.
  3. In addition to routine post-op care
    a. Assess for possible distended bladder, particularly with inguinal hernia repair.
    b. Discourage coughing, but deep breathing and turning should be done.
    c. Assist to splint incision when coughing or sneezing.
    d. Apply ice bags to scrotal area (if inguinal repair) to decrease edema.
    e. Scrotal (athletic) support may be ordered in some cases.
  4. Provide patient teaching and discharge planning concerning
    a. Need to avoid strenuous physical activities (e.g., heavy lifting, pulling, pushing) for at least 6 weeks
    b. Need to report any difficulty with urination.

Intestinal Obstructions

A. General information
1. Mechanical intestinal obstruction: physical blockage of the passage of intestinal contents with subsequent distension by fluid and gas; caused by adhesions, hernias, volvulus, intussusception, inflammatory bowel disease, foreign bodies, strictures, neoplasms, fecal impaction
2. *Paralytic ileus (neurogenic or adynamic ileus)*: interference with the nerve supply to the intestine resulting in decreased or absent peristalsis; caused by abdominal surgery, peritonitis, pancreatic toxic conditions, shock, spinal cord injuries, electrolyte imbalances (especially hypokalemia)
3. Vascular obstructions: interference with the blood supply to a portion of the intestine, resulting in ischemia and gangrene of the bowel; caused by an embolus, atherosclerosis

B. Assessment findings
1. Small intestine: nonfecal vomiting; colicky intermittent abdominal pain
2. Large intestine: cramplike abdominal pain, occasional fecal-type vomitus; patient will be unable to pass stools or flatus.
3. Abdominal distension, rigidity, high-pitched bowel sounds above the level of the obstruction, decreased or absent bowel sounds distal to obstruction
4. Diagnostic tests
   a. Flat-plate (x-ray) of the abdomen reveals the presence of gas/fluid
   b. Hct increased
   c. Serum sodium, potassium, chloride decreased
   d. BUN increased

C. Nursing interventions
1. Monitor fluid and electrolyte balance, prevent further imbalance; keep patient NPO and administer IV fluids as ordered.
2. Accurately measure drainage from NG/intestinal tube.
3. Place patient in Fowler's position to alleviate pressure on the diaphragm and encourage nasal breathing to minimize swallowing of air and further abdominal distension.
4. Institute comfort measures associated with NG intubation and intestinal decompression.
5. Prevent complications.
   a. Measure abdominal girth daily to assess for increasing abdominal distension.
   b. Assess for signs and symptoms of peritonitis.
   c. Monitor urinary output.

Chronic Inflammatory Bowel Disorders

Regional Enteritis (Crohn's Disease)

A. General information
1. Chronic inflammatory bowel disease that can affect both the large and small intestine; terminal ileum, cecum, and ascending colon most often affected

2. Characterized by granulomas that may affect all the bowel wall layers with resultant thickening, narrowing, and scarring of the intestinal wall.
3. Both sexes affected equally; more common in the Jewish population; two age peaks: 20–30 years and 40–60 years
4. Cause unknown; contributing factors include food allergies, autoimmune reaction, psychologic disorders

B. Medical management
1. Diet: high calorie, high vitamin, high protein, low residue, milk free; supplementary iron preparations
2. Drug therapy: antimicrobials (especially sulfasalazine) to prevent or control infection, corticosteroids, antidiarrheals, anticholinergics
3. Supplemental parenteral nutrition
4. Surgery: resection of diseased portion of bowel and temporary or permanent ileostomy

C. Assessment findings
1. Right, lower quadrant tenderness and pain; abdominal distension
2. Nausea and vomiting, 3–4 semi-soft stools/day with mucus and pus
3. Decreased skin turgor, dry mucous membranes
4. Increased peristalsis
5. Pallor
6. Diagnostic tests
   a. Hgb and Hct (if anemic) decreased
   b. Sigmoidoscopy negative or reveals scattered ulcers
   c. Barium enema shows narrowing with areas of strictures separated by segments of normal bowel

D. Nursing interventions
1. Provide appropriate nutrition while reducing bowel motility.
   a. Administer/monitor TPN (see page 18).
   b. Provide high-protein, high-calorie, low-residue diet with no milk products (if able to tolerate oral foods/fluids).
   c. Weigh daily, monitor kcal counts, and take periodic anthropometric measurements.
   d. Record number and characteristics of stools daily.
   e. Administer antidiarrheals, antispasmodics and anticholinergics as ordered.
   f. Provide tepid fluids to avoid stimulation of the bowel.
   g. Omit gas-producing foods/fluids from diet.
   h. Administer/monitor enteral tube feedings (see page 18) as ordered.
2. Promote comfort/rest: provide good perineal care with frequent washing and adequate drying after each bowel movement; apply analgesic or protective ointment as needed; provide sitz baths as needed.
3. Provide care for the patient with bowel surgery (see page 129).

Ulcerative Colitis

A. General information
1. Inflammatory disorder of the bowel characterized by inflammation and ulceration that starts in the

rectosigmoid area and spreads upward. The mucosa of the bowel becomes edematous, thickened with eventual scar formation. The colon consequently loses its elasticity and absorptive capabilities.
2. Occurs more often in women and the Jewish population, usually between ages 15–40
3. Cause unknown; contributing factors include autoimmune factors, viral infection, allergies, emotional stress, insecurity

B. Medical management
1. Mild to moderate form
   a. Low-roughage diet with no milk products.
   b. Drug therapy (antimicrobials, corticosteroids, anticholinergics, antidiarrheals, immunosuppressives, hematinic agents.
2. Severe form: patient kept NPO with IVs and electrolyte replacements, NG tube with suction, blood transfusions, surgery.

C. Assessment findings
1. Severe diarrhea (15–20 liquid stools/day containing blood, mucus, and pus); severe tenesmus, weight loss, anorexia, weakness, crampy discomfort
2. Decreased skin turgor, dry mucous membranes
3. Low-grade fever, abdominal tenderness over the colon
4. Diagnostic tests
   a. Sigmoidoscopy reveals mucosa that bleeds easily with ulcer development
   b. Hgb and Hct decreased

D. Nursing interventions: same as for Crohn's Disease.

Diverticulosis/Diverticulitis

A. General information
1. A diverticulum is an outpouching of the intestinal mucosa, most commonly found in the sigmoid colon.
2. *Diverticulosis:* multiple diverticula of the colon
3. *Diverticulitis:* inflammation of the diverticula
4. Men affected more often than women, more common in obese individuals; usually occurs between ages 40–45
5. Caused by stress, congenital weakening of muscular fibers of intestine, and dietary deficiency of roughage and fiber

B. Medical management
1. High residue diet
2. Drug therapy: bulk laxatives, stool softeners, anticholinergics, antibiotics
3. Surgery (rare): resection of diseased portion of colon with temporary colostomy may be indicated

C. Assessment findings
1. Intermittent lower left quadrant pain and tenderness over rectosigmoid area
2. Alternating constipation and diarrhea with blood and mucus
3. Diagnostic tests
   a. Barium enema indicates an inflammatory process
   b. Hgb and Hct decreased (if anemic)

D. Nursing interventions
1. Administer medications as ordered.
2. Provide nursing care for the patient with bowel surgery.
3. Provide patient teaching and discharge planning concerning
   a. Importance of adhering to dietary regimen
   b. Prevention of increased intra-abdominal pressure.
   c. Signs and symptoms of peritonitis and need to notify physician immediately if they occur.

Cancer of the Colon/Rectum

A. General information
1. Adenocarcinoma is the most common type of colon cancer and may spread by direct extension through the walls of the intestine, or through the lymphatic or circulatory system. Metastasis is most often to the liver.
2. Second most common site for cancer in men and women; usually occurs between ages 50–60
3. May be caused by diverticulosis, chronic ulcerative colitis, familial polyposis

B. Medical management: chemotherapy, radiation therapy, bowel surgery

C. Assessment findings
1. Alternating diarrhea/constipation, lower abdominal cramps, abdominal distension
2. Weakness, anorexia, weight loss, pallor, dyspnea
3. Diagnostic tests
   a. Stool for occult blood positive
   b. Hgb and Hct decreased
   c. Sigmoidoscopy reveals a mass
   d. Barium enema shows a colon mass
   e. Digital rectal exam indicates a palpable mass

D. Nursing interventions
1. Administer chemotherapy agents as ordered, provide care for the patient receiving chemotherapy.
2. Provide care for the patient receiving radiation therapy.
3. Provide care for the patient with bowel surgery

Bowel Surgery

A. General information: type of surgery varies depending on location and extent of lesion; may be indicated in Crohn's Disease, ulcerative colitis, intestinal obstructions, colon/rectal cancer.

B. Types: see Table 2.22

C. Nursing interventions common to all bowel surgery
1. In addition to routine pre-op care
   a. Assure adherence to dietary restrictions.
      1) Offer clear liquids only on day before surgery.
      2) Provide high-calorie, low-residue diet 3–5 days before surgery
   b. Assist with bowel preparation.
      1) administer antibiotics 3–5 days pre-op to decrease bacteria in intestine.
      2) administer enemas (possibly with added antibiotics) to further cleanse the bowel.

Table 2.22 Bowel Surgeries

Type	Procedures
Abdominoperineal resection	Distal sigmoid colon, rectum, and anus are removed through a perineal incision and a permanent colostomy is created. Surgery of choice for cancer of the colon/rectum.
Ileostomy	Opening of the ileum onto the abdominal surface; most frequently done for treatment of ulcerative colitis, but may also be done for Crohn's Disease.
Continent ileostomy (Kock's pouch)	An intra-abdominal reservoir with a nipple valve is formed from the distal ileum. The pouch acts as a reservoir for fecal material and is cleaned at regular intervals by insertion of a catheter.
Cecostomy	An opening between the cecum and the abdominal base temporarily diverts the fecal flow to rest the distal portion of the colon after some types of surgery.
Temporary colostomy	Usually located in the ascending or transverse colon; most often done to rest the bowel.
Double-barreled colostomy	The colon is resected and both ends are brought through the abdominal wall creating two stomas, a proximal and a distal; done most often for an obstruction or tumor in the descending or transverse colon.
Loop colostomy	Often a temporary procedure whereby a loop of bowel is brought out above the skin surface and held in place by a glass rod. There is one stoma but two openings, a proximal and a distal.
Permanent colostomy	Consists of a single stoma made when the distal portion of the bowel is removed; most often located in the sigmoid, or descending colon.
Resection with anastomosis	Diseased part of the bowel is removed and remaining portions anastomosed, allowing elimination through the rectum.

    c. Administer vitamins C and K (decreased by bowel cleansing) to prevent post-op complications.
  2. In addition to routine post-op care
    a. Promote elimination.
      1) assess for signs of returning peristalsis.
      2) monitor characteristics of initial stools.
    b. Monitor and maintain fluid and electrolyte balance.
D. Additional nursing interventions specific to abdominoperineal resection
  1. Reinforce and change perineal dressings as needed.
  2. Record type, amount, color of drainage.
  3. Irrigate with normal saline or hydrogen peroxide.
  4. Provide warm sitz baths 4 times/day.
  5. Cover wound with dry dressing and hold in place with T-binder.

E. Additional nursing interventions specific to colostomy
  1. Prevent skin breakdown.
    a. Cleanse skin around stoma with mild soap, water, and pat dry.
    b. Use a skin barrier to protect skin around the stoma.
    c. Assess skin regularly for irritation.
    d. Avoid the use of adhesives on irritated skin.
  2. Control odor, maintain pleasant environment.
    a. Change pouch/seal whenever necessary.
    b. Empty or clean bag frequently, and provide ventilation afterwards; use deodorizer in bag/room if needed
    c. Avoid gas-producing foods.
  3. Promote adequate stomal drainage.
    a. Assess stoma for color and intactness.
    b. Expect mucoid/serosanguinous drainage during the first 24 hours, then liquid-type.
    c. Assess for flatus indicating return of intestinal function.
    d. Monitor for changing consistency of fecal drainage.
  4. Irrigate colostomy as needed.
    a. Position patient on toilet or in high-Fowler's if patient on bedrest.
    b. Fill irrigation bag with desired amount of water (500–1000 cc) and hang bag so the bottom is at shoulder height.
    c. Remove air from tubing and lubricate the tip of the catheter or cone.
    d. Remove old pouch and clean skin and stoma with water.
    e. Gently dilate stoma and insert the irrigation catheter or cone snugly.
    f. Open tubing and allow fluid to enter the bowel.
    g. Remove catheter or cone and allow fecal contents to drain.
    h. Observe and record amount and character of fecal return.
  5. Promote adequate nutrition.
    a. Assess return of peristalsis.
    b. Advance diet as tolerated, add new foods gradually.
    c. Avoid constipating foods.
  6. Provide at least 2500 cc liquid/day.
  7. Encourage patient to discuss concerns and feelings about surgery.
  8. Provide patient teaching and discharge planning concerning
    a. Recognition of complications and need to report immediately
      1) changes in odor, consistency, and color of stools
      2) bleeding from the stoma
      3) persistent constipation or diarrhea.
      4) changes in the contour of the stoma.
      5) persistent leakage around the stoma.
      6) skin irritation despite treatment
    b. Proper procedure for colostomy irrigation.

Peritonitis

A. General information
1. Local or generalized inflammation of part or all of the parietal and visceral surfaces of the abdominal cavity
2. Initial response: edema, vascular congestion, hypermotility of the bowel and outpouring of plasmalike fluid from the extracellular, vascular, and interstitial compartments into the peritoneal space
3. Later response: abdominal distension leading to respiratory compromise, hypovolemia results in decreased urinary output
4. Intestinal motility gradually decreases and progresses to paralytic ileus.
5. Caused by trauma (blunt or penetrating), inflammation (ulcerative colitis, diverticulitis), volvulus, intestinal ischemia, or intestinal obstruction

B. Medical management
1. NPO with fluid replacement
2. Drug therapy: antibiotics to combat infection, analgesics for pain
3. Surgery
   a. *Laporotomy:* opening made through the abdominal wall into the peritoneal cavity to determine the cause of peritonitis
   b. Depending on cause, bowel resection may be necessary

C. Assessment findings
1. Severe abdominal pain, rebound tenderness, muscle rigidity, absent bowel sounds, abdominal distension (particularly if large bowel obstruction)
2. Anorexia, nausea and vomiting
3. Shallow respirations; decreased urinary output; weak, rapid pulse; elevated temperature
4. Diagnostic tests
   a. WBC elevated
   b. Hct elevated (if hemoconcentration)

D. Nursing interventions
1. Assess respiratory status for possible distress.
2. Assess characteristics of abdominal pain and changes over time.
3. Administer medications as ordered.
4. Perform frequent abdominal assessment.
5. Monitor and maintain fluid and electrolyte balance; monitor for signs of septic shock.
6. Maintain patency of NG or intestinal tubes.
7. Place patient in Fowler's position to localize peritoneal contents.
8. Provide routine pre- and post-op care if surgery ordered.

Hemorrhoids

A. General information
1. Congestion and dilation of the veins of the rectum and anus; usually results from impairment of flow of blood through the venous plexus

2. May be internal (above the anal sphincter) or external (outside anal sphincter)
3. Most commonly occur between ages 20–50
4. Predisposing conditions include occupations requiring long periods of standing; increased intra-abdominal pressure caused by prolonged constipation, pregnancy, heavy lifting, obesity, straining at defecation; portal hypertension

B. Medical management
1. Stool softeners, local anesthetics or anti-inflammatory creams
2. Diet modification: high fiber, adequate liquids
3. Hemorrhoidectomy: surgical excision of hemorrhoids indicated when there is prolapse, severe pain, and excessive bleeding

C. Assessment findings
1. Bleeding with defecation, hard stools with streaks of blood
2. Pain with defecation, sitting, or walking
3. Protrusion of external hemorrhoids upon inspection
4. Diagnostic tests
   a. Proctoscopy reveals presence of internal hemorrhoids
   b. Hgb and Hct decreased if bleeding excessive, prolonged

D. Nursing interventions: preoperative
1. Prepare patient for hemorrhoidectomy.
2. In addition to routine pre-op care, provide laxatives/enemas to promote cleansing of the bowel.

E. Nursing interventions: postoperative
1. Provide routine post-op care.
2. Assess for rectal bleeding: inspect rectal area/dressings every 2-3 hours and report significant increases in bloody drainage.
3. Promote comfort.
   a. Assist patient to side-lying or prone position, provide flotation pad when sitting.
   b. Administer analgesics as ordered and monitor effects.
4. Promote elimination: administer stool softeners as ordered and, if possible administer analgesic before first post-op bowel movement.
5. Provide patient teaching and discharge planning concerning
   a. Dietary modifications (high fiber and ingestion of at least 2000 cc/day)
   b. Need to defecate when urge is felt
   c. Use of stool softeners as needed until healing occurs
   d. Sitz baths after each bowel movement for at least 2 weeks after surgery.
   e. Perineal care
   f. Recognition and reporting immediately to physician of the following signs and symptoms
      1) rectal bleeding
      2) continued pain on defecation
      3) puslike drainage from rectal area.

DISORDERS OF THE LIVER

Hepatitis

A. General information

1. Widespread inflammation of the liver tissue with liver cell damage due to hepatic cell degeneration and necrosis; proliferation and enlargement of the Kupffer cells; inflammation of the periportal areas (may cause interruption of bile flow)
2. *Hepatitis A*
   a. Incubation period: 15–45 days
   b. Transmitted by fecal/oral route: often occurs in crowded living conditions; with poor personal hygiene; or from contaminated food, milk, water, or shellfish
3. *Hepatitis B*
   a. Incubation period: 50-180 days
   b. Transmitted by blood and body fluids (saliva, semen, vaginal secretions): often from contaminated needles among IV drug abusers; intimate/sexual contact
4. *Non-A, Non-B hepatitis*
   a. Incubation period: 7–50 days
   b. Transmitted by parenteral route: through blood and blood products, needles, syringes

B. Assessment findings

1. Preicteric stage
   a. Anorexia, nausea and vomiting, fatigue, constipation or diarrhea, weight loss
   b. Right upper quadrant discomfort, hepatomegaly, splenomegaly, lymphadenopathy
2. Icteric stage
   a. Fatigue, weight loss, light-colored stools, dark urine
   b. Continued hepatomegaly with tenderness, lymphadenopathy, splenomegaly
   c. Jaundice, pruritus
3. Posticteric stage
   a. Fatigue, but an increased sense of well-being
   b. Hepatomegaly gradually decreasing
4. Diagnostic tests
   a. All three types of hepatitis
      1) SGPT, SGOT, alkaline phosphatase, bilirubin, ESR: all increased (preicteric)
      2) leukocytes, lymphocytes, neutrophils: all decreased (preicteric)
      3) prolonged PT
   b. Hepatitis A
      1) hepatitis A virus (HAV) in stool before onset of disease
      2) anti-HAV (IgG) appears soon after onset of jaundice; peaks in 1–2 months and persists indefinitely
      3) anti-HAV (IgM): positive in acute infection; lasts 4–6 weeks
   c. Hepatitis B
      1) HBsAg (surface antigen): positive, develops 4–12 weeks after infection
      2) anti-HBsAg: negative in 80% of cases
      3) anti-HBc: associated with infectivity, develops 2–16 weeks after infection

      4) HBeAg: associated with infectivity and disappears before jaundice
      5) anti-HBe: present in carriers, represents low infectivity
   d. Non-A, Non-B: no specific serologic tests

C. Nursing interventions

1. Promote adequate nutrition.
   a. Administer antiemetics as ordered, 30 minutes before meals to decrease occurrence of nausea and vomiting.
   b. Provide small, frequent meals of a high-carbohydrate, moderate- to high-protein, high-vitamin, high-calorie diet.
   c. Avoid very hot or very cold foods.
2. Ensure rest/relaxation: plan schedule for rest and activity periods, organize nursing care to minimize interruption.
3. Monitor/relieve pruritus (see Cirrhosis of the Liver.
4. Administer corticosteroids as ordered.
5. Institute isolation procedures as required; pay special attention to good handwashing technique and adequate sanitation.
6. In hepatitis A administer immune serum globulin (ISG) early to exposed individuals as ordered.
7. In hepatitis B
   a. Screen blood donors for HBsAg.
   b. Use disposable needles and syringes.
   c. Instruct patient/others to avoid sexual intercourse while disease is active.
   d. Administer ISG to exposed individuals as ordered.
   e. Administer hepatitis B immunoglobulin (HBIG) as ordered to provide temporary and passive immunity.
8. In non-A, non-B: use disposable needles and syringes; ensure adequate sanitation.
9. Provide patient teaching and discharge planning concerning
   a. Importance of avoiding alcohol
   b. Avoidance of persons with known infections
   c. Balance of activity and rest periods
   d. Importance of not donating blood
   e. Dietary modifications
   f. Recognition and reporting of signs of inadequate convalescence: anorexia, jaundice, increasing liver tenderness/discomfort
   g. Techniques/importance of good personal hygiene.

Cirrhosis of the Liver

A. General information

1. Chronic, progressive disease characterized by inflammation, fibrosis, and degeneration of the liver parenchymal cells
2. Destroyed liver cells are replaced by scar tissue, resulting in architectural changes and malfunction of the liver.
3. Types
   a. *Laënnec's cirrhosis:* associated with alcohol abuse and malnutrition; characterized by an accumulation of fat in the liver cells progressing to widespread scar formation.

b. *Postnecrotic cirrhosis:* results in severe inflammation with massive necrosis as a complication of viral hepatitis.

c. *Cardiac cirrhosis:* occurs as a consequence of right-sided heart failure; manifested by hepatomegaly with some fibrosis.

d. *Biliary cirrhosis:* associated with biliary obstruction, usually in the common bile duct; results in chronic impairment of bile excretion.

4. Occurs twice as often in men as in women; ages 40–60

B. Assessment findings

1. Fatigue, anorexia, nausea and vomiting, indigestion, weight loss, flatulence, irregular bowel habits

2. Hepatomegaly (early); pain located in the right upper quadrant; atrophy of liver (later); hard, nodular liver upon palpation; increased abdominal girth

3. Changes in mood, alertness, and mental ability; sensory deficits; gynecomastia, decreased axillary and pubic hair in males; amenorrhea in young females

4. Jaundice of the skin, sclera, and mucous membranes; pruritus

5. Easy bruising, spider angiomas, palmar erythema

6. Muscle atrophy

7. Diagnostic tests

a. SGOT, SGPT, LDH, alkaline phosphatase increased

b. Serum bilirubin increased

c. PT prolonged

d. Serum albumin decreased

e. Hgb and Hct decreased

f. BSP increased

C. Nursing interventions

1. Provide sufficient rest and comfort.

a. Provide bedrest with bathroom privileges.

b. Encourage gradual, progressive, increasing activity with planned rest periods.

c. Institute measures to relieve pruritus.

1) do not use soaps and detergents.

2) bathe in tepid water followed by application of an emollient lotion.

3) provide cool, light, nonrestrictive clothing.

4) keep nails short to avoid skin excoriation from scratching.

5) apply cool, moist compresses to pruritic areas.

2. Promote nutritional intake.

a. Encourage small frequent feedings.

b. Promote a high-calorie, low- to moderate-protein, high-carbohydrate, low-fat diet, with supplemental vitamin therapy (vitamins A, B-complex, C, D, K, and folic acid)

3. Prevent infection.

a. Prevent skin breakdown by frequent turning and skin care.

b. Provide reverse isolation for patients with severe leukopenia; pay special attention to handwashing technique.

c. Monitor WBC.

4. Monitor/prevent bleeding.

5. Administer diuretics as ordered.

6. Provide patient teaching and discharge planning concerning

a. Avoidance of agents that may be hepatotoxic (sedatives, opiates, or OTC drugs detoxified by the liver)

b. How to assess for weight gain and increased abdominal girth

c. Avoidance of persons with upper respiratory infections

d. Recognition and reporting of signs of recurring illness (liver tenderness, increased jaundice, increased fatigue, anorexia)

e. Avoidance of all alcohol

f. Avoidance of straining at stool, vigorous blowing of nose and coughing, to decrease the incidence of bleeding.

Ascites

A. General information

1. Accumulation of free fluid in the abdominal cavity

2. Most frequently caused by cirrhotic liver damage, which produces hypoalbuminemia, increased portal venous pressure, and hyperaldosteronism

3. May also be caused by CHF

B. Medical management

1. Supportive: modify diet, bedrest, salt poor albumin

2. Diuretic therapy (see Antihypertensive Drugs, Table 2.18)

3. Surgery

a. *Paracentesis:* insertion of a needle into the peritoneal cavity through the abdomen to remove abnormally large amounts of peritoneal fluid.

1) peritoneal fluid assessed for cell count, specific gravity, protein, and microorganisms.

2) used in patients with acute respiratory or abdominal distress secondary to ascites.

b. *LeVeen shunt (peritoneal-venous shunt):* used in chronic, unmanagable ascites

1) permits continuous reinfusion of ascitic fluid back into the venous system through a silicone catheter with a one-way pressure sensitive valve.

2) one end of the catheter is implanted into the peritoneal cavity and is channeled through the subcutaneous tissue to the superior vena cava where the other end of the catheter is implanted; the valve opens when pressure in the peritoneal cavity is 3–5 cm of water higher than in superior vena cava, thereby allowing ascitic fluid to flow into the venous system.

C. Assessment findings

1. Anorexia, nausea and vomiting, fatigue, weakness, changes in mental functioning

2. Positive fluid wave and shifting dullness on percussion, flat or protruding umbilicus, abdominal distension/taughtness with striae and prominent veins, abdominal pain

3. Peripheral edema, shortness of breath

4. Diagnostic tests
  a. Potassium and serum albumin decreased
  b. PT prolonged
  c. LDH, SGOT, SGPT, BUN, sodium increased
D. Nursing interventions
  1. Monitor nutritional status/provide adequate nutrition with modified diet.
    a. Restrict sodium to 200–500 mg/day.
    b. Restrict fluids to 1000–1500 cc/day.
    c. Promote high-calorie foods/snacks.
  2. Monitor/prevent increasing edema.
    a. Administer diuretics as ordered and monitor for effects.
    b. Measure I&O.
    c. Monitor peripheral pulses.
    d. Measure abdominal girth.
    e. Inspect/palpate extremities, sacrum.
    f. Administer salt-poor albumin to replace vascular volume.
  3. Monitor/promote skin integrity.
    a. Reposition frequently.
    b. Apply lotions to stretched areas.
    c. Assess for redness, breakdown.
  4. Promote comfort: place patient in mid- to high-Fowler's, and reposition frequently.
  5. Provide nursing care for the patient undergoing paracentesis.
    a. Confirm that patient has signed a consent form.
    b. Instruct patient to empty the bladder before the procedure to prevent inadvertent puncture of the bladder during insertion of trocar.
    c. Inform patient that a local anesthetic will be provided to decrease pain.
    d. Place in sitting position to facilitate the flow of fluid by gravity.
    e. Measure abdominal girth and weight before and after the procedure.
    f. Record color, amount, and consistency of fluid withdrawn and patient tolerance during procedure.
    g. Assess insertion site for leakage.
  6. Provide routine pre- and post-op care for the patient with LeVeen shunt.

Esophageal Varices

A. General information
  1. Dilation of the veins of the esophagus, caused by portal hypertension from resistance to normal venous drainage of the liver into the portal vein
  2. This causes blood to be shunted to the esophagogastric veins, resulting in distension, hypertrophy, and increased fragility.
  3. Caused by portal hypertension, which may be secondary to cirrhosis of the liver (alcohol abuse), swallowing poorly masticated food, increased intra-abdominal pressure

B. Medical management
  1. Iced normal saline lavage
  2. Transfusions with fresh whole blood
  3. Vitamin K therapy
  4. Sengstaken-Blakemore tube: a three-lumen tube used to control bleeding by applying pressure on the cardiac portion of the stomach and against bleeding esophageal varices. One lumen serves as NG suction, a second lumen is used to inflate the gastric balloon, the third to inflate the esophageal balloon.
  5. Intra-arterial or IV vasopressin
  6. Surgery for portal hypertension (decompresses esophageal varices and helps to maintain optimal portal perfusion)
    a. Ligation of esophageal and gastric veins to stop acute bleeding
    b. *Portacaval shunt:* end-to-side or side-to-side anastomosis of the portal vein to the inferior vena cava
    c. *Splenorenal shunt:* end-to-side or side-to-side anastomosis of the splenic vein to the left renal vein
    d. *Mesocaval shunt:* end-to-side or use of a graft to anastomose the inferior vena cava to the side of the superior mesenteric vein
C. Assessment findings
  1. Anorexia, nausea and vomiting, hematemesis, fatigue, weakness
  2. Splenomegaly, increased splenic dullness, ascites, caput medusae, peripheral edema, bruits
  3. Diagnostic tests
    a. PT prolonged
    b. Hematest of vomitus positive
    c. Serum albumin, RBC, Hgb, and Hct decreased
    d. LDH, SGOT, SGPT, BUN increased
D. Nursing interventions
  1. Monitor/provide care for patient with Sengstaken-Blakemore tube.
    a. Facilitate placement of the tube: check and lubricate tip and elevate head of bed.
    b. Prevent dislodgment of the tube by placing patient in semi-Fowler's position; maintain traction by securing the tube to a piece of sponge or foam rubber placed on the nose.
    c. Monitor respiratory status; assess for signs of distress and if respiratory distress occurs cut the tubing to deflate the balloons and remove tubing immediately.
    d. Label each lumen to avoid confusion; maintain prescribed amount of pressure on esophageal balloon and deflate balloon as ordered to avoid necrosis.
    e. Observe nares for skin breakdown and provide mouth and nasal care every 1–2 hours (encourage patient to expectorate secretions, suction gently if unable).
  2. Promote comfort: place patient in semi-Fowler's position (if not in shock); provide mouth care.
  3. Monitor for further bleeding and for signs and symptoms of shock; hematest all secretions.
  4. Administer vasopressin as ordered and monitor effects.

5. Provide routine pre- and post-op care if the patient has portasystemic or portacaval shunt.
6. Provide patient teaching and discharge planning concerning
   a. Minimizing esophageal irritation (avoidance of salicylates, alcohol; use of antacids as needed; importance of chewing food thoroughly)
   b. Avoidance of increased abdominal, thoracic, and portal pressure
   c. Recognition and reporting of signs of hemorrhage.

Hepatic Encephalopathy

A. General information
   1. Frequent terminal complication in liver disease
   2. Diseased liver is unable to convert ammonia to urea, so that large quantities remain in the systemic circulation and cross the blood/brain barrier, producing neurologic toxic symptoms.
   3. Caused by cirrhosis, GI hemorrhage, hyperbilirubinemia, transfusions (particularly with stored blood), thiazide diuretics, uremia, dehydration
B. Assessment findings
   1. Early in course of disease; changes in mental functioning (irritability); insomnia, slowed affect; slow slurred speech; impaired judgment; slight tremor; Babinski's reflex, hyperactive reflexes
   2. Progressive disease: asterixis, disorientation, apraxia, tremors, fetor hepaticus, facial grimacing
   3. Late in disease: coma, absent reflexes
   4. Diagnostic tests
      a. Serum ammonia levels increased (particularly later)
      b. PT prolonged
      c. Hgb and Hct decreased
C. Nursing interventions
   1. Conduct ongoing neurologic assessment and report deteriorations.
   2. Restrict protein in diet; provide high carbohydrate intake and vitamin K supplements.
   3. Administer enemas, cathartics, intestinal antibiotics, and lactulose as ordered to reduce ammonia levels.
   4. Protect patient from injury: keep side rails up; provide eye care with use of artificial tears/eye patch.
   5. Avoid administration of drugs detoxified in liver (phenothiazines, gold compounds, methyldopa, acetaminophen).
   6. Maintain patient on bedrest to decrease metabolic demands on liver.

Cancer of the Liver

A. General information
   1. Primary cancer of the liver is extremely rare, but it is a common site for metastasis because of liver's large blood supply and portal drainage. Primary cancers of the colon, rectum, stomach, pancreas, esophagus, breast, lung, and melanomas frequently metastasize to the liver.

2. Enlargement, hemorrhage, and necrosis are common occurrences; primary liver tumors often metastasize to the lung.
3. Higher incidence in men
4. Prognosis poor; disease well advanced before clinical signs evident
B. Medical management
   1. Chemotherapy and radiotherapy (palliative) to decrease tumor size and pain
   2. Resection of liver segment or lobe if tumor is localized
C. Assessment findings
   1. Weakness, anorexia, nausea and vomiting, weight loss, slight increase in temperature
   2. Right upper quadrant discomfort/tenderness, hepatomegaly, blood tinged ascites, friction rub over liver, peripheral edema, jaundice
   3. Diagnostic tests: same as cirrhosis of the liver (page 130) plus
      a. Blood sugar decreased
      b. Alpha fetoprotein increased
      c. Abdominal x-ray, liver scan, liver biopsy all positive
D. Nursing interventions: same as for cirrhosis of the liver plus
   1. Provide emotional support for patient/family regarding poor prognosis.
   2. Provide care of the patient receiving radiation therapy or chemotherapy.
   3. Provide care of patient with abdominal surgery plus
      a. Preoperative
         1) Perform bowel prep to decrease ammonium intoxication.
         2) Administer vitamin K to decrease risk of bleeding.
      b. Postoperative
         1) Administer 10% glucose for first 48 hours to avoid rapid blood sugar drop.
         2) Monitor for hyper/hypoglycemia.
         3) Assess for bleeding (hemorrhage is most threatening complication).
         4) Assess for signs of hepatic encephalopathy.

DISORDERS OF THE GALLBLADDER

Cholecystitis/Cholelithiasis

A. General information
   1. Cholecystitis: acute or chronic inflammation of the gallbladder, most commonly associated with gallstones. Inflammation occurs within the walls of the gallbladder and creates a thickening accompanied by edema. Consequently, there is impaired circulation, ischemia, and eventual necrosis.
   2. Cholelithiasis: formation of gallstones, cholesterol stones most common variety
   3. Most often occur in women after age 40, in postmeno-pausal women on estrogen therapy, in women taking oral contraceptives, and in the obese; Caucasians and native Americans are also more commonly affected.

4. Stone formation may be caused by genetic defect of bile composition, gallbladder/bile stasis, infection.
5. Acute cholecystitis usually follows stone impaction, adhesions; neoplasms may also be implicated.

B. Medical management
1. Supportive treatment: NPO with NG intubation and IV fluids
2. Diet modification with administration of fat-soluble vitamins
3. Drug therapy
   a. Narcotic analgesics (Demerol is drug of choice) for pain
   b. Anticholinergics (atropine) for pain
   c. Antiemetics
4. Surgery: cholecystectomy/choledochostomy

C. Assessment findings
1. Epigastric or right upper quadrant pain, precipitated by a heavy meal or occurring at night
2. Intolerance for fatty foods (nausea, vomiting, sensation of fullness)
3. Pruritus, easy bruising, jaundice, dark amber urine, steatorrhea
4. Diagnostic tests
   a. Direct bilirubin transaminase, alkaline phosphatase, WBC, amylase, lipase: all increased
   b. Oral cholecystogram (gallbladder series): positive for gallstone

D. Nursing interventions
1. Administer pain medications as ordered and monitor for effects.
2. Administer IV fluids as ordered.
3. Provide small, frequent meals of modified diet (if oral intake allowed).
4. Provide care to relieve pruritus.
5. Provide care for the patient with a cholecystectomy or choledochostomy.

Cholecystectomy/Choledochostomy

A. General information
1. Cholecystectomy: removal of the gallbladder with insertion of a T-tube into the common bile duct
2. Choledochostomy: opening of common duct, removal of stone, and insertion of a T-tube

B. Nursing interventions: routine preoperative care

C. Nursing interventions: postoperative
1. Provide routine post-op care.
2. Position patient in semi-Fowler's or side-lying positions; reposition frequently.
3. Splint incision when turning, coughing, and deep breathing.
4. Maintain/monitor functioning of T-tube.
   a. Ensure that T-tube is connected to closed gravity drainage.
   b. Avoid kinks, clamping, or pulling of the tube.
   c. Measure and record drainage every shift.
   d. Expect 300–500 cc bile-colored drainage first 24 hours, then 200 cc/24 hours for 3–4 days.

e. Monitor color of urine and stools (stools will be light colored if bile is flowing through T-tube but normal color should reappear as drainage diminishes).
   f. Assess for signs of peritonitis.
   g. Assess skin around T-tube; cleanse frequently and keep dry.
5. Provide patient teaching and discharge planning concerning
   a. Adherence to dietary restrictions
   b. Resumption of ADL (avoid heavy lifting for at least 6 weeks; resume sexual activity as desired unless ordered otherwise by physician)
   c. Recognition and reporting of signs of complications (fever, jaundice, pain, dark urine, pale stools, pruritus).

Appendicitis

See page **336**.

DISORDERS OF THE PANCREAS

Pancreatitis

A. General information
1. An inflammatory process with varying degrees of pancreatic edema, fat necrosis, or hemorrhage
2. Proteolytic and lipolytic pancreatic enzymes are activated in the pancreas rather than the duodenum, resulting in tissue damage and autodigestion of the pancreas.
3. Occurs most often in the middle aged
4. Caused by alcoholism, biliary tract disease, trauma, viral infection, penetrating duodenal ulcer, abscesses, drugs (steroids, thiazide diuretics and oral contraceptives), metabolic disorders (hyperparathyroidism, hyperlipidemia)

B. Medical management
1. Drug therapy
   a. Analgesics (Demerol) to relieve pain
   b. Smooth-muscle relaxants (papaverine, nitroglycerin) to relieve pain
   c. Anticholinergics (atropine, propantheline bromide [Pro-Banthine]) to decrease pancreatic stimulation
   d. Antacids to decrease pancreatic stimulation
   e. H$_2$ antagonists, vasodilators, calcium gluconate
2. Diet modification
3. Possible NPO
4. Peritoneal lavage
5. Dialysis

C. Assessment findings
1. Pain located in left upper quadrant with radiation to back, flank, or substernal area; may be accompanied by difficulty breathing and is aggravated by eating
2. Vomiting, shallow respirations (with pain), tachycardia, decreased or absent bowel sounds, abdominal tenderness with muscle guarding, positive Grey Turner's spots (ecchymoses on flanks) and positive Cullen's sign (ecchymoses of periumbilical area)

3. Diagnostic tests
   a. Serum amylase and lipase, urinary amylase, blood sugar, lipid levels: all increased
   b. Serum calcium decreased
   c. CT scan shows enlargement of the pancreas
D. Nursing interventions
   1. Administer analgesics, antacids, anticholinergics as ordered, monitor effects.
   2. Withhold food/fluid and eliminate odor and sight of food from environment to decrease pancreatic stimulations.
   3. Maintain NG tube and assess for drainage.
   4. Institute nonpharmacologic measures to decrease pain.
      a. Assist patient to positions of comfort (knee-chest; fetal position).
      b. Teach relaxation techniques and provide a quiet, restful environment.
   5. Provide patient teaching and discharge planning concerning
      a. Dietary regimen when oral intake permitted
         1) high-carbohydrate, high-protein, low-fat diet
         2) eating small, frequent meals instead of three large ones
         3) avoiding caffeine products
         4) eliminating alcohol consumption
         5) maintaining relaxed atmosphere after meals
      b. Recognition and reporting of signs of complications
         1) continued nausea and vomiting
         2) abdominal distension with increasing fullness
         3) persistent weight loss
         4) severe epigastric or back pain
         5) frothy/foul-smelling bowel movements
         6) irritability, confusion, persistent elevation of temperature (2 days).

Cancer of the Pancreas

A. General information
   1. Most pancreatic tumors are adenocarcinomas and half occur in the head of the pancreas
   2. Tumor growth results in common bile duct obstruction with jaundice.
   3. Occurs more often in men and in the Black and Jewish populations; ages 45–65
   4. Contributing factors: chemical carcinogens, cigarette smoking, high-fat diet, diabetes mellitus
   5. Prognosis generally poor
B. Medical management
   1. Radiation therapy
   2. Whipple's procedure (pancreatoduodenectomy): resection of the proximal pancreas, adjoining duodenum, distal portion of the stomach and distal segment of the common bile duct
   3. Drug therapy
      a. Pancreatic enzymes; oral hypoglycemic agents or insulin, bile salts necessary after surgery
      b. Chemotherapy may also be used

C. Assessment findings
   1. Anorexia; rapid, progressive weight loss; dull abdominal pain located in upper abdomen or left hypochondriacal region with radiation to the back, related to eating; jaundice
   2. Diagnostic tests
      a. Increased serum lipase (early)
      b. Increased bilirubin (conjugated)
      c. Increased serum amylase
D. Nursing interventions
   1. See Pancreatitis.
   2. Provide care for the patient receiving radiation therapy or chemotherapy
   3. Routine pre- and post-op care (for patients undergoing Whipple's procedure).
   4. Provide emotional support to patient/family.
   5. Provide patient teaching and discharge planning concerning
      a. Need to eat small frequent meals of a low-fat, high-calorie diet with vitamin supplements.
      b. Importance of adhering to medication regimen after surgery.

SAMPLE QUESTIONS

Mr. Martin Simple is a 23-year-old man with a long history of ulcerative colitis. He is experiencing an exacerbation of the disease and is admitted with severe diarrhea, electrolyte disturbances and severe abdominal pain.

10. Mr. Simple questions the nurse about his prognosis. The best response to this inquiry is
   o 1. Ask your physician.
   o 2. It is rarely fatal.
   o 3. It depends on the form of the disease.
   o 4. Why do you ask?

11. The physician inserts a central venous catheter; the nurse should assist Mr. Simple to assume which of the following positions?
   o 1. Supine
   o 2. Trendelenburg's
   o 3. Reverse Trendelenburg's
   o 4. High-Fowler's

The Genitourinary System

OVERVIEW OF ANATOMY AND PHYSIOLOGY

The genitourinary system includes the kidneys, ureters, urinary bladder, urethra, and the male and female genitalia. This section discusses only the male genitalia; the female reproductive system is covered in Unit 4.

Urinary System

Kidneys

See Figure 2.14.
A. Two bean-shaped organs that lie in the retroperitoneal space on either side of the vertebral column; adrenal glands located on top of each kidney
B. *Renal parenchyma*
  1. Cortex: outermost layer; site of glomeruli and proximal and distal tubules of nephron
  2. Medulla: middle layer; formed by collecting tubules and ducts

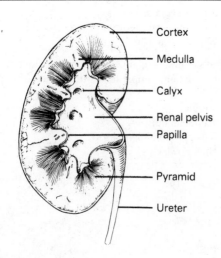

Figure 2.14 Anatomy of the kidney.

Cortex

Medulla

Calyx

Renal pelvis

Papilla

Pyramid

Ureter

C. *Renal sinus and pelvis*
  1. Papillae: projections of renal tissues located at the tips of the renal pyramids
  2. Calices
    a. Minor calix: collects urine flow from collecting duct
    b. Major calix: directs urine from renal sinus to renal pelvis
  3. Urine flows from renal pelvis to ureters
D. *Nephron:* the functional unit of the kidney (Figure 2.15)
  1. Renal corpuscle (vascular system of nephron)
    a. *Bowman's capsule:* a portion of the proximal tubule, surrounds the glomerulus
    b. *Glomerulus:* a capillary network permeable to water, electrolytes, nutrients, and wastes; impermeable to large protein molecules
  2. *Renal tubule:* divided into proximal convoluted tubule, descending loop of Henle, ascending loop of Henle, distal convoluted tubule, and collecting duct

Ureters

A. Two tubes approximately 25–35 cm long
B. Extend from the renal pelvis to the pelvic cavity, where they enter the bladder; convey urine from the kidneys to the bladder
C. Ureterovesical valve prevents backflow of urine into ureters.

Bladder

A. Located behind the symphysis pubis; composed of muscular, elastic tissue that makes it distensible
B. Serves as a reservoir of urine (capable of holding 1000–1800 cc; moderately full bladder usually holds about 500 cc)
C. Internal and external urethral sphincters control the flow of urine; urge to void stimulated by passage of urine past the internal sphincter (involuntary) to the upper part of the urethra. Relaxation of external sphincter (voluntary) produces emptying of the bladder (voiding, micturition).

Urethra

A. A small tube that extends from the bladder to the exterior of the body

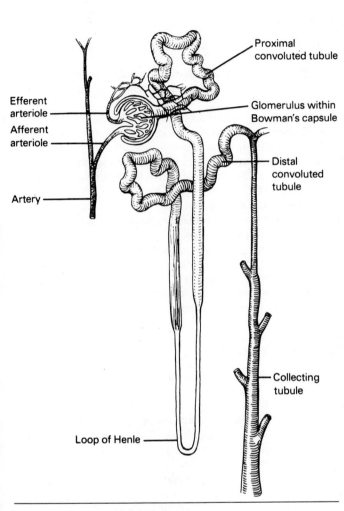

Figure 2.15 The nephron.

a. Requires hydrostatic pressure (supplied by the heart and assisted by vascular resistance [glomerular hydrostatic pressure]) and sufficient circulating volume

b. Pressure in Bowman's capsule opposes hydrostatic pressure and filtration; if glomerular pressure insufficient to force substances out of the blood into the tubules, filtrate formation stops.

2. Glomerular filtration rate (GFR): amount of blood filtrated by the glomeruli in a given time; normal is 125 cc/min

3. Filtrate formed has essentially same composition as blood plasma without the proteins; blood cells and proteins are usually too large to pass the glomerular membrane.

B. Tubular function: the tubules and collecting ducts carry out the functions of reabsorption, secretion, and excretion. Reabsorption of water and electrolytes is controlled by antidiuretic hormone (ADH), released by the pituitary, and aldosterone, secreted by the adrenal glands (see Table 2.24).

1. Proximal convoluted tubule: reabsorption of certain constituents of the glomerular filtrate: 80% of electrolytes and H_2O, all glucose and amino acids and bicarbonate; secretes organic substances and wastes.

2. Loop of Henle: reabsorption of sodium and chloride in the ascending limb; reabsorption of water in the descending limb; concentrates/dilutes urine.

3. Distal convoluted tubule: secretes potassium, hydrogen ions, and ammonia; reabsorbs H_2O (regulated by ADH) and bicarbonate; regulates calcium and phosphate concentrations.

4. Collecting ducts: receive urine from distal convoluted tubules and reabsorb water (regulated by ADH).

C. Normal adult produces 1 liter/day of urine.

Blood Pressure Control

A. Kidneys regulate blood pressure partly through maintenance of volume (formation/excretion of urine).

B. The renin-angiotensin system is the other kidney-controlled mechanism that can contribute to rise in blood pressure. When blood pressure drops, the cells of the glomerulus release renin, which then activates angiotensin to cause vasoconstriction.

Male Reproductive System

See Figure 2.16.

Penis

A. An external structure that serves as a passageway for urine and semen

B. Capable of distension during sexual excitement

C. Distal portion, glans penis, is covered by a prepuce or foreskin that may or may not be removed (circumcised).

Scrotum

A. Saclike structure that hangs from the root of the penis

B. Contains the testes and epididymis, and helps to regulate temperature conducive to sperm production.

B. In females, located behind the symphysis pubis and anterior to the vagina; approximately 3–5 cm long

C. In males, extends the entire length of the penis; approximately 20 cm long

Regulatory Functions of Kidney

Kidneys and urinary system play a major role in maintenance of homeostatic control of the body. Kidneys remove nitrogenous wastes and regulate fluid and electrolyte balance (see page 25) and acid-base balance (see page 26); urine is the end product of these mechanisms.

Formation of Urine

A. Glomerular filtration

1. Ultrafiltration of blood by the glomerulus; beginning of urine formation

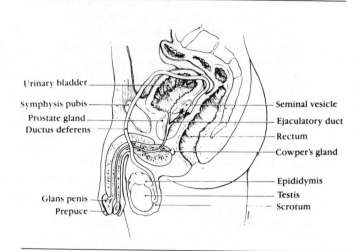

Figure 2.16 The male reproductive tract.
(From "The A&P Workbook," by Elaine Marieb (1988). Courtesy of the Benjamin/Cummings Publishing Company, Inc., Menlo Park, CA.)

Testes

A. Small oval structures suspended in the scrotum
B. Produce sperm (exocrine function) and male hormones (endocrine function, see Table 2.24)

Ductal System

A. *Epididymis:* first part of ductal system
　　1. Soft cordlike structure that lies along the posterolateral surface of each testis
　　2. Head is attached to the top of the testis, tail is continuous with vas deferens; stores spermatozoa while they mature.
B. *Spermatic cord:* consists of vas deferens, arteries, veins, nerves, and lymphatic vessels. Vas deferens joins the duct of the seminal vesicles to become the ejaculatory duct.

Accessory Glands

A. *Prostate:* located below the bladder and in front of the rectum; approximately 4–6 cm long
　　1. Enclosed in firm, fibrous capsule; connected to the urethra and ejaculatory ducts
　　2. Secretes a milky fluid that aids in the passage of spermatozoa and helps keep them viable.
B. *Cowper's glands:* lie on each side of the urethra and just below the prostate; secrete a small amount of lubricating fluid.
C. *Seminal vesicles:* paired structures parallel to the bladder; secrete a portion of the ejaculate and may contribute to nutrition and activation of sperm.

ASSESSMENT

Health History

A. Presenting problem: symptoms may include
　　1. Pain in flank, groin; dysuria
　　2. Changes in urination patterns: frequency, nocturia, hesitancy of stream, urgency, dribbling, incontinence, retention
　　3. Changes in urinary output: polyuria, oliguria, anuria
　　4. Changes in color/consistency of urine: dilute, concentrated, malodorous; hematuria, pyuria
B. Life-style: occupation (type of employment, exposure to chemicals such as carbon tetrachloride, ethylene glycol); level of activity, exercise
C. Nutrition/diet: water, calcium, dairy product intake
D. Past medical history: hypertension, diabetes mellitus, gout, cystitis, kidney infections, connective tissue diseases (systemic lupus erythematosus), infectious diseases, drug use (prescribed/OTC), previous catheterizations, hospitalizations or surgery for renal problems
E. Family history: hypertension, diabetes mellitus, renal disease, gout, connective tissue disorders, urinary tract infections (UTIs), renal calculi

Physical Examination

A. Inspect skin for color, turgor, and mobility; purpuric lesions; integrity.
B. Inspect mouth for color, moisture, odor, ulcerations.
C. Inspect face for edema, particularly periorbital edema.
D. Inspect abdomen and palpate bladder for distension; percuss bladder for tympany or dullness (if full).
E. Inspect extremities for edema.
F. Determine rate, rhythm, and depth of respirations.
G. Inspect muscles for tremors, atrophy.
H. Palpate right and left kidneys for tenderness, pain, enlargement; percuss costovertebral angles for tenderness/pain; fist percuss kidneys for tenderness/pain.
I. Palpate flank area for pain and prostate for size, shape, consistency.
J. Auscultate aorta and renal arteries for bruits.

Laboratory/Diagnostic Tests

A. Urine studies
　　1. Urinalysis: examination to assess the nature of the urine produced
　　　　a. Evaluates color, pH, and specific gravity.
　　　　b. Determines presence of glucose (glycosuria), protein, blood (hematuria), ketones (ketonuria).
　　　　c. Analyzes sediment for cells (presence of WBC called pyuria), casts, bacteria, crystals.
　　2. Urine culture and sensitivity: diagnoses bacterial infections of the urinary tract.
　　3. Residual urine: amount of urine left in bladder after voiding measured via catheter (permanent or temporary) in bladder

4. Creatinine clearance: determines amount of creatinine (waste product of protein breakdown) in the urine over 24 hours, measures overall renal function.

B. Urine collection methods: nursing care
1. Routine urinalysis: wash perineal area if soiled, obtain first voided morning specimen; send to lab immediately (should be examined within 1 hour of voiding).
2. Clean catch (midstream) specimen for urine culture.
    a. Cleanse perineal area.
        1) females: spread labia and cleanse meatus front to back using antiseptic sponges.
        2) males: retract foreskin (if uncircumsized) and cleanse glans with antiseptic sponges.
    b. Have patient initiate urine stream then stop.
    c. Collect specimen in a sterile container.
    d. Have patient complete urination, but not in specimen container.
3. 24-hour specimen (preferred method for creatinine clearance test)
    a. Have patient void and discard specimen; note time.
    b. Collect all subsequent urine specimens for 24 hours.
    c. If specimen is accidently discarded, the test must be restarted.
    d. Record exact start and finish of collection; include date and times.

C. Blood chemistries/electrolytes
1. Bicarbonate
2. BUN: measures renal ability to excrete urea nitrogen
3. Calcium
4. Serum creatinine: specific test for renal disorders; reflects ability of kidneys to excrete creatinine
5. Phosphorus
6. Potassium
7. Sodium

D. KUB/plain film: an abdominal flat plate x-ray showing the kidneys, ureters, and bladder; may identify the number and size of kidneys with tumors, malformations, and calculi

E. Intravenous pyelogram (IVP)
1. Fluoroscopic visualization of the urinary tract after injection with a radiopaque dye
2. Nursing care: pretest
    a. Assess for iodine sensitivity.
    b. Inform patient he will lie on a table throughout procedure.
    c. Administer cathartic or enema the night before.
    d. Keep patient NPO for 8 hours pretest
3. Nursing care: post-test: force fluids.

F. Cystoscopy
1. Use of a light scope (cystoscope) to inspect the bladder
    a. Inserted into the bladder via the urethra
    b. May be used to remove tumors, stones, or other foreign material (use of electrical current to remove tumors is called fulguration); or to implant radium, place catheters in ureters
2. Nursing care: pretest
    a. Explain to patient that procedure will be done under general or local anesthesia.

    b. Confirm consent form is signed.
    c. Administer sedatives 1 hour before test, as ordered.
    d. General anesthesia: keep patient NPO.
    e. Local anesthesia: offer liquid breakfast.
    f. Give enemas as ordered.
3. Nursing care: post-test
    a. Provide warm sitz baths, mild analgesics to relieve discomfort after test.
    b. Monitor I&O and vital signs (especially temperature, as elevation may indicate infection).
    c. Expect mild hematuria at first; urine will be pink-tinged, subsiding over 24–48 hours; monitor for large clots.
    d. Advise patient that burning on urination is normal and will subside.
    e. Force fluids.

ANALYSIS

Nursing diagnoses for the patient with a disorder of the genitourinary system may include
A. Impairment of skin integrity
B. Sexual dysfunction
C. Grieving
D. Alteration in comfort: pain
E. Alteration in fluid volume: excess
F. Fluid volume deficit
G. Alteration in thought processes
H. Potential for injury
I. Disturbance in self-concept: body image, role performance
J. Alteration in oral mucous membranes

PLANNING AND IMPLEMENTATION

Goals

A. Normal skin integrity will be achieved/maintained.
B. Changes in sexual functioning will be accepted.
C. Patient will progress normally through grieving process.
D. Renal colic and pruritus will diminish.
E. Patient will be free from fluid volume excess; will maintain safe, stable potassium and calcium levels.
F. Integrity of oral cavity will be maintained.
G. There will be improvement in thought processes.
H. Patient will be free from unusual bleeding.
I. Patient will adapt to changes in life-style.

Interventions

Urinary Catheterization

A. General information
1. Insertion of a catheter through the external meatus and the urethra into the bladder
2. Purposes include relief from urinary retention, bladder decompression, prevention of bladder obstruction, instillation of medications into the bladder, and splinting the bladder.

B. Nursing care: insertion
  1. Explain procedure to patient and collect necessary equipment (catheter set).
  2. Wash hands and position patient.
  3. Use sterile technique while inserting catheter.
  4. Observe for urine return and obtain specimen.
  5. Connect drainage tubing to catheter (indwelling) and tape.
C. Nursing care: indwelling catheter
  1. Maintain catheter patency: place drainage tubing properly to avoid kinking or pinching.
  2. Observe for signs of obstruction (e.g., decreased urine in collection bag, voiding around the catheter, abdominal discomfort, bladder distension).
  3. Irrigate catheter as necessary.
  4. Insure comfort and safety: relieve bladder spasms by administering B & O suppositories (if ordered); ensure adequate fluid intake and provide perineal care.
  5. Prevent infection: maintain a closed drainage system and prevent backflow of urine by keeping drainage system below level of bladder.
  6. Empty collection bag at least every 8 hours.
  7. Promote acidification of the urine with acid-ash diet and ascorbic acid.
  8. Change catheter/drainage system only when necessary.

Dialysis

A. General information
  1. Removal by artificial means of metabolic wastes, excess electrolytes, and excess fluid from patients with renal failure
  2. Principles
     a. *Diffusion*: movement of particles from an area of high concentration to one of low concentration across a semipermeable membrane
     b. *Osmosis*: movement of water through a semipermeable membrane from an area of lesser concentration of particles to one of greater concentration
B. Purposes
  1. Remove the end products of protein metabolism from blood
  2. Maintain safe levels of electrolytes
  3. Correct acidosis and replenish blood bicarbonate system
  4. Remove excess fluid from the blood
C. Types: hemodialysis and peritoneal dialysis

Hemodialysis

A. General information
  1. Shunting of blood from the patient's vascular system through an artificial dialyzing system, and return of dialyzed blood to the patient's circulation
  2. Dialysis coil acts as the semipermeable membrane; the dialysate is a specially prepared solution.
  3. Access routes
     a. External AV shunt: one cannula inserted into an artery and the other into a vein; both are brought out to the skin surface and connected by a U-shaped shunt.

b. AV fistula: internal anastomosis of an artery to an adjacent vein in a sideways position; fistula is accessed for hemodialysis by venipuncture (average lifetime 3–4 years).
     c. Femoral/subclavian cannulation: insertion of a catheter into one of these large veins for easy access to circulation; procedure is similar to insertion of a CVP line.
B. Nursing care: external AV shunt
  1. Auscultate for a bruit and palpate for a thrill to ensure patency.
  2. Assess for clotting (color change of blood, absence of pulsations in tubing).
  3. Change sterile dressing over shunt daily.
  4. Avoid performing venipuncture, administering IV infusions, giving injections, or taking a blood pressure with a cuff on the shunt arm.
C. Nursing care: AV fistula.
  1. Auscultate for a bruit and palpate for a thrill to ensure patency.
  2. Report bleeding, skin discoloration, drainage, and pain.
  3. Avoid restrictive clothing/dressings over site.
  4. Avoid administration of IV infusions, giving injections, or taking blood pressure with a cuff on the fistula extremity.
D. Nursing care: femoral/subclavian cannulation
  1. Palpate peripheral pulses in cannulized extremity.
  2. Observe for bleeding/hematoma formation.
  3. Position catheter properly to avoid dislodgment during dialysis.
E. Nursing care: before and during hemodialysis
  1. Have patient void.
  2. Chart patient's weight.
  3. Assess vital signs before and every 30 minutes during procedure.
  4. Withhold antihypertensives, sedatives, and vasodilators to prevent hypotensive episode (unless ordered otherwise).
  5. Ensure bedrest with frequent position changes for comfort.
  6. Inform patient that headache and nausea may occur.
  7. Monitor closely for signs of bleeding since blood has been heparinized for procedure.
F. Nursing care: postdialysis
  1. Chart patient's weight.
  2. Assess for complications.
     a. Hypovolemic shock: may occur as a result of rapid removal or ultrafiltration of fluid from the intravascular compartment (see page 28).
     b. Dialysis disequilibrium syndrome (urea is removed more rapidly from the blood than from the brain): assess for nausea, vomiting, elevated blood pressure, disorientation, leg cramps, and peripheral paresthesias.

Peritoneal Dialysis

A. General information: introduction of a specially prepared dialysate solution into the abdominal cavity, where the peritoneum acts as a semipermeable membrane between the dialysate and blood in the abdominal vessels

B. Nursing care
1. Chart patient's weight.
2. Assess vital signs before, every 15 minutes during first exchange, and every hour thereafter.
3. Assemble specially prepared dialysate solution with added medications.
4. Have patient void.
5. Warm dialysate solution to body temperature.
6. Assist physician with trocar insertion.
7. Inflow: allow dialysate to flow unrestricted into peritoneal cavity (10–20 minutes).
8. Dwell: allow fluid to remain in peritoneal cavity for prescribed period (30–45 minutes).
9. Drain: unclamp outflow tube and allow to flow by gravity.
10. Observe characteristics of dialysate outflow.
    a. Normal: clear, pale yellow
    b. Cloudy: infection, peritonitis
    c. Brownish: bowel perforation
    d. Bloody: common during first few exchanges; abnormal if continues
11. Monitor total I&O and maintain records.
12. Assess for complications.
    a. Peritonitis resulting from contamination of solution or tubing during exchange (see page 131).
    b. Respiratory difficulty: may occur from upward displacement of diaphragm due to increased pressure in the peritoneal cavity; assess for signs and symptoms of atelectasis (page 109), pneumonia (page 110), and bronchitis (page 106)
    c. Protein loss: most serum proteins pass through the peritoneal membrane and are lost in the dialysate fluid; monitor serum protein levels closely

EVALUATION

A. Patient is free from skin redness, breakdown.
B. Urine is slightly acidic.
C. Patient maintains sexual relationship with significant other; makes statements indicating identification of self as sexually acceptable.
D. Patient integrates ostomy care into life-style; participates in treatments.
E. Patient expresses pain reduction; has relaxed facial expression and body posture; does not scratch skin.
F. Weight is stable.
G. Intake and output are balanced; patient free from peripheral edema.
H. Patient has normal muscle tone/strength; no paresthesias.
I. Patient is free from nausea, vomiting, cramps; serum potassium and calcium within normal limits.
J. Oral mucosa are pink, moist, and intact; no ulcerations; saliva consistency normal.
K. Patient is oriented to person, place, and time; has improved reasoning ability.
L. Skin and mucous membranes are free from ecchymoses, petechiae; no hematuria, hematemesis, or melena; vital signs within normal limits; adequate Hgb and Hct.
M. Patient integrates treatment regimen into ADL; shows increased interest in appearance; actively participates in treatments.

DISORDERS OF THE GENITOURINARY SYSTEM

Disorders of the Urinary Tract

Cystitis

A. General information
1. Inflammation of the bladder due to bacterial invasion
2. More common in women
3. Predisposing factors include stagnation of urine, obstruction, sexual intercourse, high estrogen levels
B. Assessment
1. Abdominal or flank pain/tenderness, frequency and urgency of urination, pain on voiding, nocturia
2. Fever
3. Diagnostic tests: urine culture and sensitivity reveals specific organism (80% *E. coli*)
C. Nursing interventions
1. Force fluids (3000 cc/day).
2. Provide warm sitz baths for comfort.
3. Assess urine for odor, hematuria, sediment.
4. Administer medications as ordered and monitor effects.
    a. Systemic antibiotics: ampicillin, cephalosporins, aminoglycosides
    b. Sulfonamides: sulfisoxazole (Gantrisin), sulfamethoxazole (Gantanol)
    c. Antibacterials: nitrofurantoin (Macrodantin), methenamine mandelate (Mandelamine), nalidixic acid (NegGram)
5. Provide patient teaching and discharge planning concerning
    a. Importance of adequate hydration
    b. Frequent voiding to avoid stagnation
    c. Proper personal hygiene; women to cleanse from front to back
    d. Voiding after sexual intercourse
    e. Acidification of the urine to decrease bacterial multiplication (acid/ash diet, vitamin C)
    f. Need for follow-up urine cultures.

Bladder Cancer

A. General information
1. Most common site of cancer of the urinary tract
2. Occurs in men 3 times more often than women; peak age 50–70 years
3. Predisposing factors include exposure to chemicals (especially aniline dyes), cigarette smoking, chronic bladder infections

B. Medical management: dependent on the staging of cell type; includes
  1. Radiation therapy, usually in combination with surgery
  2. Chemotherapy: considerable research on both agents and methods of administration
    a. Methods include direct bladder instillations, intra-arterial infusions, IV infusion, oral ingestion
    b. Agents include 5-fluorouracil, methotrexate, bleomycin, mitomycin-C, hydroxyurea, doxorubicin, cyclophosphamide, cisplatin; results variable
  3. Surgery: see Bladder Surgery.
C. Assessment findings
  1. Intermittent painless hematuria, dysuria, frequent urination
  2. Diagnostic tests
    a. Cystoscopy with biopsy reveals malignancy
    b. Cytologic exam of the urine reveals malignant cells
D. Nursing interventions: provide care for the patient receiving radiation therapy or chemotherapy, and for the patient with bladder surgery.

Bladder Surgery

A. General information
  1. *Cystectomy* (removal of the urinary bladder) with one of the various types of urinary diversions is the surgical procedure done for bladder cancer
  2. Types of urinary diversions
    a. *Ureterosigmoidostomy:* ureters are excised from the bladder and implanted into sigmoid colon; urine flows through the colon and is excreted via the rectum
    b. *Ileal conduit:* ureters are implanted into a segment of the ileum that has been resected from the intestinal tract with formation of an abdominal stoma; most common type of urinary diversion
    c. *Cutaneous ureterostomy:* ureters are excised from the bladder and brought through abdominal wall with creation of a stoma
B. Nursing interventions: preoperative
  1. Provide routine pre-op care.
  2. Assess patient's ability to learn prior to starting a teaching program.
  3. Discuss social aspects of living with a stoma (sexuality, changes in body image).
  4. Assess understanding and emotional response of patient/family.
  5. Perform pre-op bowel preparation for procedures involving the ileum or colon.
  6. Inform patient of post-op procedures.
C. Nursing interventions: postoperative
  1. Provide routine post-op care.
  2. Maintain integrity of the stoma.
    a. Monitor for and report signs of impaired stomal healing (pale, dark red, or blue-black color; increased stomal height, edema, bleeding).
    b. Maintain stomal circulation by using properly fitted faceplate.
    c. Monitor for signs and symptoms of stomal obstruction (sudden decrease in urine output, increased abdominal tenderness and distension).
  3. Prevent skin irritation and breakdown.
    a. Inspect skin areas for signs of breakdown daily.
    b. Patch test all adhesives, sprays, and skin barriers before use.
    c. Change appliance only when necessary and when production of urine is slowest (early morning).
    d. Place wick (rolled gauze pad) on stomal opening when appliance is off.
    e. Cleanse peristomal skin with mild soap and water.
    f. Remove alkaline encrustations by applying vinegar and water solution to peristomal area.
    g. Implement measures to maintain urine acidity (acid-ash foods, vitamin C therapy, omission of milk/dairy products).
  4. Provide care for the patient with an NG tube (see page 120); will be in place until bowel motility returns.
  5. Assist patient to identify strengths and qualities that have a positive effect on self-concept.
  6. Provide patient teaching and discharge planning concerning
    a. Maintenance of stomal/peristomal skin integrity
    b. Proper application of appliance
    c. Recommended method of cleaning reusable ostomy equipment (manufacturer's recommendations)
    d. Information regarding prevention of UTIs (adequate fluids; empty pouch when half full; change to bedside collection bag at night)
    e. Control of odor (adequate fluids; avoid foods with strong odor; place small amount of vinegar or deodorizer in pouch)
    f. Reporting signs and symptoms of UTIs (see Cystitis, page 143).

Nephrolithiasis/Urolithiasis

A. General information
  1. Presence of stones anywhere in the urinary tract; frequent composition of stones: calcium, oxalate, and uric acid
  2. Most often occurs in men age 20–55; more common in the summer
  3. Predisposing factors
    a. Diet: large amounts of calcium, oxalate
    b. Increased uric acid levels
    c. Sedentary life-style, immobility
    d. Family history of gout or calculi; hyperparathyroidism
B. Medical management
  1. Surgery
    a. Percutaneous nephrostomy: tube is inserted through skin and underlying tissues into renal pelvis to remove calculi.
    b. Percutaneous nephrostolithotomy: delivers ultrasound waves through a probe placed on the calculus.
  2. Extracorporeal shock-wave lithotripsy: delivers shock waves from outside the body to the stone, causing pulverization.

3. Pain management and diet modification

C. Assessment findings

  1. Abdominal or flank pain; renal colic; hematuria

  2. Cool, moist skin; costovertebral tenderness

  3. Diagnostic tests

    a. KUB: pinpoints location, number, and size of stones

    b. IVP: identifies site of obstruction and presence of nonradiopaque stones

    c. Urinalysis: indicates presence of bacteria, increased protein, increased WBC and RBC

D. Nursing interventions

  1. Strain all urine through gauze to detect stones and crush all clots.

  2. Force fluids (3000–4000 cc/day).

  3. Encourage ambulation to prevent stasis.

  4. Relieve pain by administration of analgesics as ordered and application of moist heat to flank area.

  5. Monitor I&O.

  6. Provide modified diet, depending upon stone consistency.

    a. Calcium stones: limit milk/dairy products; provide acid-ash diet to acidify urine (cranberry or prune juice, meat, eggs, poultry, fish, grapes, whole grains); take vitamin C.

    b. Oxalate stones: avoid excess intake of foods/fluids high in oxalate (tea, chocolate, rhubarb, spinach); maintain alkaline/ash diet to alkalinize urine (milk, vegetables, fruits except prunes, cranberries, and plums).

    c. Uric acid stones: reduce foods high in purine (liver, brains, kidneys, venison, shellfish, meat soups, gravies, legumes); maintain alkaline urine.

  7. Administer allopurinol (Zyloprim) as ordered, to decrease uric acid production.

  8. Provide patient teaching and discharge planning concerning

    a. Prevention of urinary stasis by maintaining increased fluid intake especially in hot weather and during illness; mobility; voiding whenever the urge is felt and at least twice during the night

    b. Adherence to prescribed diet

    c. Need for routine urinalysis (at least every 3–4 months)

    d. Need to recognize and report signs/symptoms of recurrence (hematuria, flank pain).

Pyelonephritis

A. General information

  1. Inflammation of the renal pelvis; may be unilateral or bilateral, acute or chronic

  2. Acute: infection usually ascends from lower urinary tract

  3. Chronic: thought to be a combination of structural alterations along with infection, major cause is ureterovesical reflux, with infected urine backing up into ureters and renal pelvises; result of recurrent infections is eventual renal parenchymal deterioration and possible renal failure

B. Medical management

  1. Acute: antibiotics, antispasmodics, surgical removal of any obstruction

  2. Chronic: antibiotics and urinary antiseptics (sulfanomides, nitrofurantoin); surgical correction of structural abnormality if possible

C. Assessment findings

  1. Acute: fever, chills, nausea and vomiting; severe flank pain or dull ache

  2. Chronic: patient usually unaware of disease; may have bladder irritability, chronic fatigue, or slight dull ache over kidneys; eventually develops hypertension, atrophy of kidneys.

D. Nursing interventions: acute pyelonephritis

  1. Provide adequate comfort and rest.

  2. Monitor I&O.

  3. Administer antibiotics as ordered

  4. Provide patient teaching and discharge planning concerning

    a. Medication regimen

    b. Follow-up cultures

    c. Signs and symptoms of recurrence and need to report.

E. Nursing interventions: chronic pyelonephritis

  1. Administer medications as ordered.

  2. Provide adequate fluid intake and nutrition.

  3. Support patient/family and explain possibility of dialysis, transplant options if significant renal deterioration.

Glomerulonephritis

See page **341**.

Nephrosis

See page **340**.

Acute Renal Failure

A. General information

  1. Sudden inability of the kidneys to regulate fluid and electrolyte balance and remove toxic products from the body

  2. Causes

    a. Prerenal: factors interfering with perfusion and resulting in decreased blood flow and glomerular filtrate, ischemia, and oliguria; include CHF, cardiogenic shock, acute vasoconstriction, hemorrhage, burns, septicemia, hypotension

    b. Intrarenal: conditions that cause damage to the nephrons; include acute tubular necrosis (ATN), endocarditis, diabetes mellitus, malignant hypertension, acute glomerulonephritis, tumors, blood transfusion reactions, hypercalcemia, nephrotoxins (certain antibiotics, x-ray dyes, pesticides, anesthetics)

    c. Postrenal: mechanical obstruction anywhere from the tubules to the urethra; include calculi, BPH, tumors, strictures, blood clots, trauma, anatomic malformation

B. Assessment findings

   a. Oliguric phase (caused by reduction in glomerular filtration rate)

     1) urine output less than 400 cc/24 hours; duration 1–2 weeks

     2) manifested by hyponatremia, hyperkalemia, hyperphosphatemia, hypocalcemia, hypermagnesemia, and metabolic acidosis

     3) diagnostic tests: BUN and creatinine elevated

   b. Diuretic phase (slow, gradual increase in daily urine output)

     1) diuresis may occur (output 3–5 liters/day) due to partially regenerated tubule's inability to concentrate urine

     2) duration: 2–3 weeks; manifested by hyponatremia, hypokalemia and hypovolemia

     3) diagnostic tests: BUN and creatinine elevated

   c. Recovery or convalescent phase: renal function stabilizes with gradual improvement over next 3–12 months

C. Nursing interventions

   1. Monitor/maintain fluid and electrolyte balance.

     a. Obtain baseline data on usual appearance and amount of patient's urine.

     b. Measure I&O every hour; note excessive losses.

     c. Administer IV fluids and electrolyte supplements as ordered.

     d. Weigh daily and report gains.

     e. Monitor lab values; assess/treat fluid and electroylyte and acid-base imbalances as needed (see Tables 2.6 and 2.7).

   2. Monitor alteration in fluid volume.

     a. Monitor vital signs, PA, PCWP, CVP as needed.

     b. Weigh patient daily.

     c. Maintain strict I&O records.

     d. Assess every hour for hypervolemia; provide nursing care as needed.

       1) maintain adequate ventilation.

       2) decrease fluid intake as ordered.

       3) administer diuretics, cardiac glycosides, and antihypertensives as ordered; monitor effects.

     e. Assess every hour for hypovolemia; replace fluids as ordered.

     f. Monitor ECG and auscultate heart as needed.

     g. Check urine, serum osmolality/osmolarity and urine specific gravity as ordered.

   3. Promote optimal nutritional status.

     a. Weigh daily.

     b. Maintain strict I&O.

     c. Administer TPN as ordered.

     d. With enteral feedings, check for residual and notify physician if residual volume increases.

     e. Restrict protein intake.

   4. Prevent complications from impaired mobility (pulmonary embolism, skin breakdown, contractures,

atelectasis; see Table 2.23).

   5. Prevent fever/infection.

     a. Take rectal temperature and obtain orders for cooling blanket/antipyretics as needed.

     b. Assess for signs of infection.

     c. Use strict aseptic technique for wound and catheter care.

   6. Support patient/family and reduce/relieve anxiety.

     a. Explain pathophysiology and relationship to symptoms.

     b. Explain all procedures and answer all questions in easy-to-understand terms.

     c. Refer to counseling services as needed.

   7. Provide care for the patient receiving dialysis if used.

   8. Provide patient teaching and discharge planning concerning

     a. Adherence to prescribed dietary regime

     b. Signs and symptoms of recurrent renal disease

     c. Importance of planned rest periods

     d. Use of prescribed drugs only

     e. Signs and symptoms of UTI or respiratory infection, need to report to physician immediately.

Chronic Renal Failure

A. General information

   1. Progressive, irreversible destruction of the kidneys that continues until nephrons are replaced by scar tissue; loss of renal function gradual

   2. Predisposing factors: recurrent infections, exacerbations of nephritis, urinary tract obstructions, diabetes mellitus, hypertension

B. Medical management

   1. Diet restrictions

   2. Multivitamins

   3. Hematinics

   4. Aluminum-hydroxide gels

   5. Antihypertensives

C. Assessment findings

   1. Nausea, vomiting; diarrhea or constipation; decreased urinary output; dyspnea

   2. Stomatitis, hypotension (early), hypertension (later), lethargy, convulsions, memory impairment, pericardial friction rub, CHF

   3. Diagnostic tests: urinalysis

     a. Protein, sodium, and WBC elevated

     b. Specific gravity, platelets, and calcium decreased

D. Nursing interventions

   1. Prevent neurologic complications.

     a. Assess every hour for signs of uremia (fatigue, loss of appetite, decreased urine output, apathy, confusion, elevated blood pressure, edema of face and feet, itchy skin, restlessness, seizures).

     b. Assess for changes in mental functioning.

     c. Orient confused patient to time, place, date, and persons; institute safety measures to protect patient from falling out of bed.

d. Monitor serum electrolytes, BUN, and creatinine as ordered.
2. Promote optimal GI function.
  a. Assess/provide care for stomatitis
  b. Monitor nausea, vomiting, anorexia; administer antiemetics as ordered.
  c. Assess for signs of GI bleeding.
3. Monitor/prevent alteration in fluid and electrolyte balance.
4. Assess for hyperphosphatemia (paresthesias, muscle cramps, seizures, abnormal reflexes), and administer aluminum hydroxide gels (Amphojel, AlternaGEL) as ordered.
5. Promote maintenance of skin integrity.
  a. Assess/provide care for pruritus.
  b. Assess for uremic frost (urea crystallization on the skin) and bathe in plain water.
6. Monitor for bleeding complications, prevent injury to patient.
  a. Monitor Hgb, Hct, platelets, RBC.
  b. Hematest all secretions.
  c. Administer hematinics (folic acid) as ordered.
  d. Avoid IM injections.
7. Promote/maintain maximal cardiovascular function.
  a. Monitor blood pressure and report significant changes.
  b. Auscultate for pericardial friction rub.
  c. Perform circulation checks routinely.
  d. Administer diuretics as ordered and monitor output.
  e. Modify digitalis dose as ordered (digitalis is excreted in kidneys).
8. Provide care for patient receiving dialysis.

Kidney Transplantation

A. General information
  1. Transplantation of a kidney from a donor to recipient to prolong the lives of persons with renal failure
  2. Sources of donor selection
    a. Living relative with compatible serum and tissue studies, free from systemic infection, and emotionally stable
    b. Cadavers with good serum and tissue crossmatching; free from renal disease, neoplasms, and sepsis; absence of ischemia/trauma.
B. Nursing interventions: preoperative
  1. Provide routine pre-op care.
  2. Discuss the possibility of post-op dialysis/immunosuppressive drug therapy with patient and family.
C. Nursing interventions: postoperative
  1. Provide routine post-op care.
  2. Monitor fluid and electrolyte balance carefully.
    a. Monitor I&O hourly and adjust IV fluid administration accordingly.
    b. Anticipate possible massive diuresis.
  3. Encourage frequent and early ambulation.

4. Monitor vital signs, especially temperature; report significant changes.
5. Provide mouth care and nystatin (Mycostatin) mouth washes for candidiasis.
6. Administer immunosuppressive agents as ordered.
  a. Azathioprine (Imuran): assess for manifestations of anemia, leukopenia, thrombocytopenia, oral lesions.
  b. Cyclophosphamide (Cytoxan): assess for alopecia, hypertension, kidney/liver toxicity, leukopenia.
  c. Antilymphocytic globulin (ALG), antithymocytic globulin (ATG): assess for fever, chills, anaphylactic shock, hypertension, rash, headache.
  d. Corticosteroids (prednisone, methylprednisolone sodium succinate [Solu-Medrol]): assess for peptic ulcer and GI bleeding, sodium/water retention, muscle weakness, delayed healing, mood alterations, hyperglycemia, acne.
7. Assess for signs of acute rejection.
  a. Occurs 4 days to 4 months after transplant.
  b. Signs include decreased urinary output, fever, pain/tenderness over transplant site, edema, sudden weight gain, increasing blood pressure, generalized malaise, rise in serum creatinine, and decrease in creatinine clearance.
8. Provide patient teaching and discharge planning concerning
  a. Medication regimen: names, dosages, frequency, and side effects
  b. Signs and symptoms of rejection and the need to report immediately
  c. Dietary restrictions: restricted sodium and calories, increased protein
  d. Daily weights
  e. Frequent medical follow-up with lab studies
  f. Avoidance of crowds/people with known infections.

Nephrectomy

A. General information
  1. Surgical removal of an entire kidney
  2. Indications include renal tumor, massive trauma, removal for a donor, polycystic kidneys
B. Nursing interventions: preoperative care
  1. Provide routine pre-op care.
  2. Ensure adequate fluid intake.
  3. Assess electrolyte values and correct any imbalances before surgery.
  4. Avoid nephrotoxic agents in any diagnostic tests.
  5. Advise patient to expect flank pain after surgery if retroperitoneal approach (flank incision) is used.
  6. Explain that patient will have chest tube if a thoracic approach is used.
C. Nursing interventions: postoperative
  1. Provide routine post-op care.
  2. Assess urine output every hour; should be 30–50 cc/hour.

3. Observe urinary drainage on dressing and estimate amount.
4. Weigh daily.
5. Maintain adequate functioning of chest drainage system; ensure adequate oxygenation and prevent pulmonary complications.
6. Administer analgesics as ordered.
7. Encourage early ambulation.
8. Teach patient to splint incision while turning, coughing, deep breathing.
9. Provide patient teaching and discharge planning concerning
   a. Prevention of urinary stasis
   b. Maintenance of acidic urine
   c. Avoidance of activities that might cause trauma to the remaining kidney (contact sports, horseback riding)
   d. No lifting heavy objects for at least 6 months
   e. Need to report unexplained weight gain, decreased urine output, flank pain on unoperative side, hematuria
   f. Need to notify physician if cold or other infection present for more than 3 days
   g. Medication regimen and avoidance of OTC drugs that may be nephrotoxic (except with physician approval).

Disorders of the Male Reproductive System

Epididymitis

A. General information
   1. Inflammation of epididymis, one of the most common intrascrotal infections
   2. May be sexually transmitted, usually caused by *N. gonorrhoeae, C. trachomatis;* also caused by GU instrumentation, urinary reflux
B. Assessment findings
   1. Sudden scrotal pain, scrotal edema, tenderness over the spermatic cord
   2. Diagnostic test: urine culture reveals specific organism
C. Nursing interventions
   1. Administer antibiotics and analgesics as ordered.
   2. Provide bedrest with elevation of the scrotum.
   3. Apply ice packs to scrotal area to decrease edema.

Prostatitis

A. General information
   1. Inflammatory condition that affects the prostate gland
   2. Several forms: acute bacterial prostatitis, chronic bacterial prostatitis, or abacterial chronic prostatitis
   3. Acute and chronic bacterial prostatitis usually caused by *E. coli, N. gonorrhoeae, Enterobacter* or *Proteus* species, and group D streptococci
   4. Most important predisposing factor: lower UTIs

B. Assessment findings
   1. Acute: fever, chills, dysuria, urethral discharge, prostatic tenderness, copious purulent urethral discharge upon palpation
   2. Chronic: backache; perineal pain; mild dysuria; frequency; enlarged, firm, and slightly tender prostate upon palpation
   3. Diagnostic tests
      a. WBC elevated
      b. Bacteria in initial urinalysis specimens
C. Nursing interventions
   1. Administer antibiotics, analgesics, and stool softeners as ordered.
   2. Provide increased fluid intake.
   3. Provide sitz baths/rest to relieve discomfort.
   4. Provide patient teaching and discharge planning concerning
      a. Importance of maintaining adequate hydration
      b. Antibiotic therapy regimen (may need to remain on medication for several months)
      c. Activities that drain the prostate (masturbation, sexual intercourse, prostatic massage).

Benign Prostatic Hypertrophy (BPH)

A. General information
   1. Mild to moderate glandular enlargement, hyperplasia, and overgrowth of the smooth muscles and connective tissue
   2. As the gland enlarges, it compresses the urethra resulting in urinary retention.
   3. Most common problem of the male reproductive system; occurs in 50% of men over age 50; 75% of men over age 75
   4. Cause unknown; may be related to hormonal mechanism
B. Assessment findings
   1. Nocturia, frequency, decreased force and amount of urinary stream, hesitancy (more difficult to start voiding), hematuria
   2. Enlargement of prostate gland upon palpation by digital rectal exam
   3. Diagnostic tests
      a. Urinalysis: alkalinity increased; specific gravity normal or elevated
      b. BUN and creatinine elevated (if longstanding BPH)
      c. Cystoscopy reveals enlargement of gland and obstruction to urine flow
C. Nursing interventions
   1. Administer antibiotics as ordered.
   2. Force fluids.
   3. Provide care for the catheterized patient.
   4. Provide care for the patient with prostatic surgery (below).

Cancer of the Prostate

A. General information
   1. Second most common site of cancer in men
   2. Usually an adenocarcinoma; growth related to the presence of androgens
   3. Spreads from the prostate to the seminal vesicles, urethral mucosa, bladder wall, external sphincter, and lymphatic system
   4. Highest incidence is in black men age 60 or over
   5. Cause unknown
B. Medical management
   1. Drug therapy: estrogens, chemotherapeutic agents
   2. Radiation therapy
   3. Surgery: radical prostatectomy
C. Assessment findings: same as for BPH above but diagnostic test results are
   1. Elevated acid phosphatase (distant metastasis) and alkaline phosphatase (bone metastasis)
   2. Bone scan: abnormal in metastatic areas
D. Nursing interventions
   1. Administer medications as ordered and provide care for the patient receiving chemotherapy.
   2. Provide care for the patient receiving radiation therapy.
   3. Provide care for the patient with a prostatectomy.

Prostatic Surgery

A. General information
   1. Indicated for benign prostatic hypertrophy and prostatic cancer.
   2. Types
      a. *Transurethral resection (TUR):* insertion of a resectoscope into the urethra to excise prostatic tissue; good for poor surgical risks, does not require an incision; most common type of surgery for BPH
      b. *Suprapubic prostatectomy:* the prostate is approached by a low abdominal incision into the bladder to the anterior aspect of the prostate; for large tumors obstructing the urethra
      c. *Retropubic prostatectomy:* to remove a large mass high in the pelvic area; involves a low midline incision below the bladder and into the prostatic capsule
      d. *Perineal prostatectomy:* often used for prostatic cancer; the incision is made through the perineum, which facilitates radical surgery if a malignancy is found.
B. Nursing interventions: preoperative
   1. Provide routine pre-op care.
   2. Institute and maintain urinary drainage.
   3. Force fluids; administer antibiotics, acid-ash diet to eradicate UTI.
   4. Reinforce what surgeon has told patient/family regarding effects of surgery on sexual function.

C. Nursing interventions: postoperative
   1. Provide routine post-op care.
   2. Ensure patency of 3-way Foley.
   3. Monitor continuous bladder irrigations with sterile saline solution (removes clotted blood from bladder), and control rate to keep urine light pink changing to clear.
   4. Expect hematuria for 2–3 days.
   5. Irrigate catheter with normal saline as ordered.
   6. Control/treat bladder spasms; encourage short, frequent walks; decrease rate of continuous bladder irrigations (if urine is not red and is without clots); administer anticholinergics (propantheline bromide [Pro-Banthine]) or antispasmodics (B & O suppositories) as ordered.
   7. Prevent hemorrhage: administer stool softeners to discourage straining at stool; avoid rectal temperatures and enemas; monitor Hgb and Hct.
   8. Report bright red, thick blood in the catheter; persistent clots, persistent drainage on dressings.
   9. Provide for bladder retraining after Foley removal.
      a. Instruct patient to perform perineal exercises (stopping and starting stream during voiding; pressing buttocks together then relaxing muscles) to improve sphincter control.
      b. Limit liquid intake in evening.
      c. Restrict caffeine-containing beverages.
      d. Withhold anticholinergics and antispasmodics (these drugs relax bladder and increase chance of incontinence) if permitted.
   10. Provide patient teaching and discharge planning concerning
      a. Continued increased fluid intake
      b. Signs of UTI and need to report them
      c. Continued perineal exercises
      d. Avoidance of heavy lifting, straining during defecation, and prolonged travel (at least 8–12 weeks)
      e. Measures that promote urinary continence
      f. Possible impotence (more common after perineal resection)
         1) discuss ways of expressing sexuality (massage, cuddling)
         2) suggest alternative methods of sexual gratification and use of assistive aids
         3) discuss possibility of penile prosthesis with physician
      g. Need for annual and self-exams.

SAMPLE QUESTIONS

Mr. Dan Doad, 55, is hospitalized for bladder cancer. He is scheduled for ileal loop surgery to create a urostomy.

12. Which information is MOST important for the nurse to include in a teaching plan for Mr. Doad when learning to change his urostomy appliance?
    o 1. Change the appliance before going to bed
    o 2. Cut the wafer 1/2 inch larger than the stoma
    o 3. Cleanse the peristomal skin with soap and water.
    o 4. Use firm pressure to attach the wafer to the skin

13. Which nursing intervention best prevents urinary tract infections in Mr. Doad ?
    o 1. Allowing the bag to fill completely
    o 2. Attaching a larger bag at night
    o 3. Restricting fluids to less than 1000 cc daily
    o 4. Changing the appliance every 8 hours

The Musculoskeletal System

OVERVIEW OF ANATOMY AND PHYSIOLOGY

The musculoskeletal system consists of the bones, muscles, joints, cartilage, tendons, ligaments, and bursae. Its major function is to provide a structural framework for the body and to provide a means for movement.

Bones

A. Functions
1. Provide support to skeletal framework
2. Assist in movement by acting as levers for muscles
3. Protect vital organs and soft tissues
4. Manufacture of RBCs in the red bone marrow (hematopoiesis)
5. Provide site for storage of calcium and phosphorus

B. Types of bones
1. Long: central shaft (diaphysis) made of compact bone and two ends (epiphyses) composed of cancellous bone (e.g., femur and humerus)
2. Short: cancellous bone covered by thin layer of compact bone (e.g., carpals and tarsals)
3. Flat: two layers of compact bones separated by a layer of cancellous bone (e.g., skull and ribs)
4. Irregular: sizes and shapes vary (e.g., vertebrae and mandible)

Joints

A. Articulation of bones occurs at joints; movable joints provide stabilization and permit a variety of movements

B. Classification (according to degree of movement)
1. Synarthroses: immovable joints
2. Amphiarthroses: partially movable joints
3. Diarthroses (synovial): freely movable joints
   a. Have a joint cavity (synovial cavity) between the articulating bone surfaces
   b. Articular cartilage covers the ends of the bones
   c. A fibrous capsule encloses the joint
   d. Capsule is lined with synovial membrane that secretes synovial fluid to lubricate the joint and reduce friction.

Muscles

A. Functions
1. Provide shape to the body
2. Protect the bones
3. Maintain posture
4. Cause movement of body parts by contraction

B. Types of muscles
1. *Cardiac:* involuntary; found only in heart
2. *Smooth:* involuntary; found in walls of hollow structures (e.g., intestines)
3. *Striated (skeletal):* voluntary

C. Characteristics of skeletal muscles
1. Muscles are attached to the skeleton at the point of origin and to bones at the point of insertion.
2. Have properties of contraction and extension, as well as elasticity, to permit isotonic (shortening and thickening of the muscle) and isometric (increased muscle tension) movement.
3. Contraction is innervated by nerve stimulation.

Cartilage

A. A form of connective tissue
B. Major functions are to cushion bony prominences and offer protection where resiliency is required.

Tendons and Ligaments

A. Composed of dense, fibrous connective tissue
B. Functions
1. Ligaments attach bone to bone
2. Tendons attach muscle to bone

ASSESSMENT

Health History

A. Presenting problem
1. Muscles: symptoms may include pain, cramping, weakness
2. Bones and joints: symptoms may include stiffness, swelling, pain, redness, heat, limitation of movement

B. Life-style: usual patterns of activity and exercise (limitations in ADL, use of assistive devices such as canes or walkers), nutrition (obesity) and diet, occupation (sedentary, heavy lifting, or pushing)

C. Use of medications: drugs taken for musculoskeletal problems

D. Past medical history: congenital defects, trauma, inflammations, fractures, back pain

E. Family history: arthritis, gout

Physical Examination

A. Inspect for overall body build, posture, and gait.

B. Inspect and palpate joints for swelling, deformity, masses, movement, tenderness, crepitations.

C. Inspect and palpate muscles for size, symmetry, tone, strength.

Laboratory/Diagnostic Tests

A. Hematologic studies
1. Muscle enzymes: CPK, aldolase, SGOT
2. ESR
3. Rheumatoid factor
4. Complement fixation
5. Lupus erythematosus cells (LE prep)
6. Antinuclear antibodies (ANA)
7. Anti-DNA
8. C-reactive protein
9. Uric acid

B. X-rays: detect injury to or tumors of bone or soft tissue

C. Bone scan
1. Measures radioactivity in bones 2 hours after IV injection of a radioisotope; detects bone tumors, osteomyelitis.
2. Nursing care
   a. Have patient void immediately before the procedure.
   b. Explain that patient must remain still during the scan itself.

D. Arthroscopy
1. Insertion of fiberoptic endoscope (arthroscope) into a joint to visualize it, perform biopsies, or remove loose bodies from the joint
2. Performed in OR using aseptic technique
3. Nursing care
   a. Maintain pressure dressing for 24 hours.
   b. Advise patient to limit activity for several days.

E. Arthrocentesis: insertion of a needle into the joint to aspirate synovial fluid for diagnostic purposes or to remove excess fluid

F. Myelography
1. Lumbar puncture used to withdraw a small amount of CSF, which is replaced with a radiopaque dye; used to detect tumors or herniated intravertebral discs
2. Nursing care: pretest
   a. Keep NPO after liquid breakfast.
   b. Check for iodine allergy.
   c. Confirm that consent form has been signed and explain procedure to patient.

3. Nursing care: post-test (see also Lumbar Puncture, page 46)
   a. If oil-based dye (e.g., Pantopaque) was used, keep patient flat for 12 hours.
   b. If water-based dye (e.g., Amipaque) was used
      1) elevate head of bed 30°–45° to prevent upward displacement of dye, which may cause meningeal irritation and possibly seizures.
      2) institute seizure precautions and do not administer any phenothiazine drugs to patient.

G. Electromyography
1. Measures and records activity of contracting muscles in response to electrical stimulation; helps differentiate muscle disease from motor neuron dysfunction
2. Nursing care: explain procedure to the patient and advise that some discomfort may occur due to needle insertion.

ANALYSIS

Nursing diagnoses for patients with disorders of the musculoskeletal system may include
A. Impaired physical mobility
B. Alteration in comfort: pain
C. Self-care deficit
D. Potential for injury
E. Knowledge deficit
F. Disturbance in self-concept: body image, self-esteem, role performance

PLANNING AND IMPLEMENTATION

Goals

A. Patient will attain optimum level of mobility.
B. Patient will achieve maximum comfort level.
C. Patient will perform self-care activities to the best degree possible.
D. Patient will be free from injury.
E. Patient will demonstrate knowledge concerning disease process, prescribed medications, and treatment and prevention of complications.
F. Patient will adapt to alterations in body image and role performance; increased self-esteem.

Interventions

Preventing Complications of Immobility

See Table 2.23.

Range-of-Motion (ROM) Exercises

A. Movement of joint through its full ROM to prevent contractures and increase or maintain muscle tone/strength
B. Types
1. Active: carried out by patient; increases and maintains muscle tone; maintains joint mobility

2. Passive: carried out by nurse without assistance from patient; maintains joint mobility only; body part not to be moved beyond its existing ROM
3. Active assistive: patient moves body part as far as possible and nurse completes remainder of movement
4. Active resistive: contraction of muscles against an opposing force; increases muscle size and strength

Isometric Exercises

A. Active exercise through contraction/relaxation of muscle; no joint movement; length of muscle does not change.
B. Patient increases tension in muscle for several seconds and then relaxes.
C. Maintains muscle strength and size.

Assistive Devices for Walking

A. *Cane*
1. Types: single, straight-legged cane; tripod cane; quad cane
2. Nursing care: teach patient to hold cane in hand opposite affected extremity, and to advance cane at the same time the affected leg is moved forward.

B. *Walker*
1. Mechanical device with four legs for support
2. Nursing care: teach patient to hold upper bars of walker at each side, then to move the walker forward and step into it.
C. *Crutches:* teaching the patient proper use of crutches is an important nursing responsibility.
1. Assure proper length.
   a. When patient assumes erect position the top of crutch is 2 inches below the axilla, and the tip of each crutch is 6 inches in front and to the side of the feet.
   b. Patient's elbows should be slightly flexed when hand is on hand grip.
   c. Weight should not be borne by the axillae.
2. Crutch gaits
   a. Four-point gait: used when weight bearing is allowed on both extremities
      1) advance right crutch.
      2) step forward with left foot.
      3) advance left crutch.
      4) step forward with right foot.
   b. Two-point gait: typical walking pattern, an acceleration of four-point gait

---

Table 2.23   Preventing Complications of Immobility

System	Complication	Nursing Intervention
Cardiovascular	Orthostatic hypotension Deep vein thrombosis and pulmonary embolism Increased workload on heart	Active or passive ROM exercises Isometric exercises of the legs Frequent turning Slow mobilization No pillows behind knees Antiembolism stockings
Respiratory	Decreased chest expansion Accumulation of secretions in respiratory tract	Frequent turning Encourage frequent coughing and deep breathing
Integumentary	Breakdown of skin integrity (abrasions, decubitus ulcers) caused by friction, pressure or shearing forces	Frequent turning and repositioning Regular inspection of skin for signs of pressure Gentle massage of skin, especially over bony prominences
Gastrointestinal	Constipation	Frequent movement and turning in bed Increase in fluid intake Adequate dietary intake with increase in high-fiber foods Use of stool softeners/laxatives as ordered
Musculoskeletal	Atrophy and weakness of muscles Contractures Demineralization of bone (osteoporosis)	Active and passive ROM and isometric exercises Encourage participation in ADL as much as possible Proper positioning and repositioning of joints
Urinary	Increased calcium from bone destruction (calculi formation) Increased urine pH (alkaline) Stasis of urine in kidney and bladder Urinary infection	Increase in fluid intake Decrease in calcium intake, especially milk and milk products Use of acid-ash foods Use of commode if possible
Neurologic	Sensory deprivation and isolation	Frequent contact by staff Orienting measures (clock, calendar) Diversional activities (television, radio, hobbies) Inclusion of patient in decision-making activities

1) step forward moving both right crutch and left leg simultaneously.
2) step forward moving both left crutch and right leg simultaneously.

c. Three-point gait: used when weight bearing is permitted on one extremity only
  1) advance both crutches and affected extremity several inches, maintaining good balance.
  2) advance the unaffected leg to the crutches, supporting the weight of the body on the hands.
d. Swing-to gait: used for patients with paralysis of both lower extremities who are unable to lift feet from floor
  1) both crutches are placed forward.
  2) patient swings forward to the crutches.
e. Swing-through gait: same indications as for swing-to gait
  1) both crutches are placed forward.
  2) patient swings body through the crutches.

Care of the Patient with a Cast

A. Cast drying
  1. Use palms of hands, not finger tips, to support cast when moving patient.
  2. Support cast on pillows along length of cast until dry (usually 24 hours).
  3. Turn patient every 2 hours to reduce pressure and promote drying.
  4. Do not cover the cast until it is dry (may use fan to facilitate drying).
  5. Do not use heat lamp or hair dryer on plaster cast.
B. Assessment
  1. Perform neurovascular checks to area distal to cast.
    a. Report absent or diminished pulse, cyanosis or blanching, coldness, lack of sensation, inability to move fingers or toes, excessive swelling.
    b. Report complaints of burning, tingling, or numbness.
  2. Note any odor from the cast that may indicate infection.
  3. Note any bleeding on cast in a surgical patient.
  4. Check for "hot spots" that may indicate inflammation under cast.
C. General care
  1. "Petal" cast edges with strips of adhesive tape or moleskin to prevent irritation.
  2. Prevent complications of immobility.
  3. Administer pain medications as ordered; instruct patient to report if pain unrelieved by medication or if any new pain appears.
D. Provide patient teaching and discharge planning concerning
  1. Isometic and ROM exercises as appropriate
  2. Reinforcement of instructions given on crutch walking
  3. Never getting cast wet or inserting foreign bodies under cast
  4. If a cast that has previously dried and hardened does become wet, may use hair dryer over wet spot for "quick dry" of stain
  5. Recognition and reporting of signs of impaired circulation or of infection.

Care of the Patient in Traction

A. A pulling force exerted on bones to reduce and/or immobilize fractures, reduce muscle spasm, correct or prevent deformities
B. Types
  1. Skin traction: weights are attached to a moleskin or adhesive strip secured by elastic bandage, or other special device (e.g., foam rubber boot) used to cover the affected limb.
    a. *Buck's extension*
      1) exerts straight pull on affected extremity
      2) generally used to temporarily immobilize the leg in a patient with a fractured hip
      3) shock blocks at the foot of the bed produce counter traction and prevent the patient from sliding down in bed
    b. *Russell traction*
      1) knee is suspended in a sling attached to a rope and pulley on a Balkan frame, creating upward pull from the knee; weights are attached to foot of bed (as in Buck's extension) creating a horizontal force exerted on the tibia and fibula
      2) generally used to stabilize fractures of the femoral shaft while patient is awaiting surgery
      3) elevating foot of bed slightly provides countertraction
      4) head of bed should remain flat
      5) foot of bed usually elevated by shock blocks to provide counter traction
    c. *Cervical traction*
      1) cervical head halter attached to weights that hang over head of bed
      2) used for soft tissue damage or degenerative disc disease of cervical spine to reduce muscle spasm and maintain alignment
      3) usually intermittent traction
      4) elevate head of bed to provide countertraction
    d. *Pelvic traction*
      1) pelvic girdle with extension straps attached to ropes and weights
      2) used for low back pain to reduce muscle spasm and maintain alignment
      3) usually intermittent traction
      4) patient in semi-Fowler's position with knee gatched
      5) secure pelvic girdle around iliac crests
  2. Skeletal traction: traction applied directly to the bones using pins, wires, or tongs (e.g., Crutchfield tongs) that are surgically inserted; used for fractured femur, tibia, humerus, cervical spine
  3. Balanced suspension traction: produced by a counterforce other than the patient's weight; extremity floats or balances in the traction apparatus; patient may change position without disturbing the line of traction
  4. *Thomas splint and Pearson attachment* (usually used with skeletal traction in fractures of the femur)
    a. Hip should be flexed at 20°
    b. Use footplate to prevent footdrop.

C. Nursing care
   1. Check traction apparatus frequently to assure that
      a. Ropes are aligned and weights hanging freely.
      b. Bed is in proper position.
      c. Line of traction is with the long axis of the bone.
   2. Maintain patient in proper alignment.
      a. Align in center of bed.
      b. Do not rest affected limb against foot of bed.
   3. Perform neurovascular checks to affected extremity.
   4. Observe for and prevent foot drop.
      a. Provide footplate.
      b. Encourage dorsiflexion exercises.
   5. Observe for and prevent thrombophlebitis (especially in Russell traction due to pressure on popliteal space).
   6. Observe for and prevent skin irritation and breakdown (especially over bony prominences and traction application sites).
      a. Russell traction: check popliteal area frequently and pad the sling with felt covered by stockinette or ABDs.
      b. Thomas splint: pad top of splint with same material as in Russell traction.
      c. Cervical traction: pad chin area and protect ears.
   7. Provide pin care for patients in skeletal traction.
      a. Usually consists of cleansing and applying antibiotic ointment, but individual agency policies may vary.
      b. Observe for any redness, drainage, odor.
   8. Assist with ADL; provide overhead trapeze to facilitate moving, using bedpan, etc.
   9. Prevent complications of immobility.
   10. Encourage active ROM exercises to unaffected extremities.
   11. Check carefully for orders about turning.
      a. Buck's extension: patient may turn to unaffected side (place pillows between legs before turning).
      b. Russell traction and balanced suspension traction: patient may turn slightly from side to side without turning body below the waist.

EVALUATION

A. Optimum level of mobility is attained.
B. Pain is relieved or is more manageable.
C. Patient performs self-care at optimum level.
D. Injuries are prevented.
E. Patient demonstrates knowledge of disease process, uses prescribed medications and treatments correctly, and reports complications.
F. Patient successfully adjusts to alterations in body image and role performance and exhibits increased self-esteem.

DISORDERS OF THE MUSCULOSKELETAL SYSTEM

Rheumatoid Arthritis (RA)

A. General information
   1. Chronic systemic disease characterized by inflammatory changes in joints and related structures
   2. Occurs in women more often than men (3:1); peak incidence between ages 35–45
   3. Cause unknown, but may be an autoimmune process; genetic factors may also play a role.
   4. Predisposing factors include fatigue, cold, emotional stress, infection.
   5. Joint distribution is symmetric (bilateral); most commonly affects smaller peripheral joints of hands and also commonly involves wrists, elbows, shoulders, knees, hips, ankles, and jaw.
   6. If unarrested, affected joints progress through four stages of deterioration: synovitis, pannus formation, fibrous ankylosis, and bony ankylosis.
B. Medical management
   1. Drug therapy
      a. Aspirin: mainstay of treatment, has both analgesic and anti-inflammatory effect.
      b. Nonsteroidal anti-inflammatory drugs (NSAIDs): indomethacin (Indocin), phenylbutazone (Butazolidin); newer agents include ibuprofen (Motrin), fenoprofen (Nalfon), naproxen (Naprosyn), sulindac (Clinoril); act by blocking local inflammatory mediators to reduce pain and inflammation.
      c. Gold compounds (chrysotherapy)
         1) injectable form: sodium thiomalate (Myochrysine), aurothioglucose (Solganal); given IM once a week; take 3–6 months to become effective; side effects include proteinuria, mouth ulcers, skin rash, aplastic anemia; monitor blood studies and urinalysis frequently.
         2) oral form: auranofin (Ridaura); smaller doses are effective; take 3–6 months to become effective; diarrhea also a side effect with oral form; blood and urine studies should also be monitored.
      d. Corticosteroids
         1) intra-articular injections temporarily suppress inflammation in specific joints.
         2) systemic administration used only when patient does not respond to less potent anti-inflammatory drugs.
   2. Physical therapy to minimize joint deformities
   3. Surgery to remove severely damaged joints (e.g., total hip replacement)
C. Assessment findings
   1. Fatigue, anorexia, malaise, weight loss, slight elevation in temperature
   2. Joints are painful, warm, swollen, limited in motion, stiff in morning and after periods of inactivity, and may show crippling deformity in long-standing disease.

3. Muscle weakness secondary to inactivity
4. History of remissions and exacerbations
5. Some patients have additional extra-articular manifestations: subcutaneous nodules; eye, vascular, lung, or cardiac problems.
6. Diagnostic tests
   a. X-rays show various stages of joint disease
   b. CBC: anemia is common
   c. ESR elevated
   d. Rheumatoid factor positive
   e. ANA may be positive
   f. C-reactive protein elevated

D. Nursing interventions
1. Assess joints for pain, swelling, tenderness, limitation of motion.
2. Promote maintenance of joint mobility and muscle strength.
   a. Perform ROM exercises several times a day; use of heat prior to exercise may decrease discomfort; stop exercise at the point of pain.
   b. Use isometric or other exercise to strengthen muscles.
3. Change position frequently; alternate sitting, standing, lying.
4. Promote comfort and relief/control of pain.
   a. Ensure balance between activity and rest.
   b. Provide 1–2 scheduled rest periods throughout day.
   c. Rest and support inflamed joints; if splints used, remove 1–2 times/day for gentle ROM exercises.
5. Ensure bedrest if ordered for acute exacerbations.
   a. Provide firm mattress.
   b. Maintain proper body alignment.
   c. Have patient lie prone for $\frac{1}{2}$ hour twice a day.
   d. Avoid pillows under knees.
   e. Keep joints mainly in extension, not flexion.
   f. Prevent complications of immobility.
6. Provide heat treatments (warm bath, shower, or whirlpool; warm, moist compresses; paraffin dips) as ordered.
   a. May be more effective in chronic pain.
   b. Reduce stiffness, pain, and muscle spasm.
7. Provide cold treatments as ordered; most effective during acute episodes.
8. Provide psychologic support and encourage patient to express feelings.
9. Assist patient in setting realistic goals; focus on patient strengths.
10. Provide patient teaching and discharge planning concerning
    a. Use of prescribed medications and side effects
    b. Self-help devices to assist in ADL and to increase independence
    c. Importance of maintaining a balance between activity and rest
    d. Energy conservation methods
    e. Performance of ROM, isometric, and prescribed exercises
    f. Maintenance of well-balanced diet

g. Application of resting splints as ordered
h. Avoidance of undue physical or emotional stress
i. Importance of follow-up care.

Osteoarthritis

A. General information
1. Chronic, nonsystemic disorder of joints characterized by degeneration of articular cartilage
2. Women and men affected equally; incidence increases with age
3. Cause unknown; most important factor in development is aging (wear and tear on joints), others include obesity, joint trauma.
4. Weight bearing joints (spine, knees, hips) and terminal interphalangeal joints of fingers most commonly affected

B. Assessment findings
1. Pain (aggravated by use and relieved by rest) and stiffness of joints
2. Heberden's nodes: bony overgrowths at terminal interphalangeal joints
3. Decreased ROM, possible crepitation
4. Diagnostic tests
   a. X-rays show joint deformity as disease progresses
   b. ESR may be slightly elevated when disease is inflammatory

C. Nursing interventions
1. Assess joints for pain and ROM.
2. Relieve strain and prevent further trauma to joints.
   a. Encourage rest periods throughout day.
   b. Use cane or walker when indicated.
   c. Ensure proper posture and body mechanics.
   d. Promote weight reduction if obese.
   e. Avoid excessive weight bearing activities and continuous standing.
3. Maintain joint mobility and muscle strength.
   a. Provide ROM and isometic exercises.
   b. Ensure proper body alignment.
   c. Change patient's position frequently.
4. Promote comfort/relief of pain.
   a. Administer medications as ordered: aspirin and NSAIDs most commonly used; intra-articular injections of corticosteroids relieve pain and improve mobility.
   b. Apply heat as ordered (e.g., warm baths, compresses, hot packs) or ice to reduce pain.
5. Prepare patient for joint replacement surgery if necessary.
6. Provide patient teaching and discharge planning concerning
   a. Use of prescribed medications and side effects
   b. Importance of rest periods
   c. Measures to relieve strain on joints
   d. ROM and isometric exercises
   e. Maintenance of a well-balanced diet
   f. Use of heat/ice as ordered.

Gout

A. General information
1. A disorder of purine metabolism; causes high levels of uric acid in the blood and the precipitation of urate crystals in the joints
2. Inflammation of the joints caused by deposition of urate crystals in articular tissue.
3. Occurs most often in males
4. Familial tendency

B. Medical management
1. Drug therapy
   a. Acute attack: Colchicine IV or PO (discontinue if diarrhea occurs); NSAIDs such as indomethacin (Indocin), naproxen (Naprosyn), phenylbutazone (Butazolidin)
   b. Prevention of attacks
      1) uricosuric agents (probenecid [Benemid], sulfinpyrazone [Anturane]) increase renal excretion of uric acid
      2) allopurinal (Zyloprim) inhibits uric acid formation
2. Low-purine diet may be recommended
3. Joint rest and protection
4. Heat or cold therapy

C. Assessment finding
1. Joint pain, redness, heat, swelling; joints of foot (especially great toe) and ankle most commonly affected (acute gouty arthritis stage)
2. Headache, malaise, anorexia
3. Tachycardia; fever; tophi in outer ear, hands, and feet (chronic tophaceous stage)
4. Diagnostic test: uric acid elevated

D. Nursing interventions
1. Assess joints for pain, motion, appearance.
2. Provide bedrest and joint immobilization as ordered.
3. Administer antigout medications as ordered.
4. Administer analgesics for pain as ordered.
5. Increase fluid intake to 2000–3000 cc/day to prevent formation of renal calculi.
6. Apply local heat or cold as ordered.
7. Apply bed cradle to keep pressure of sheets off joints.
8. Provide patient teaching and discharge planning concerning
   a. Medications and their side effects
   b. Modifications for low-purine diet: avoidance of shellfish, liver, kidney, brains, sweetbreads, sardines, anchovies
   c. Limitation of alcohol use
   d. Increase in fluid intake
   e. Weight reduction if necessary
   f. Importance of regular exercise

Systemic Lupus Erythematosus (SLE)

A. General information
1. Chronic connective tissue disease involving multiple organ systems
2. Occurs most frequently in young women
3. Cause unknown; immune, genetic, and viral factors have all been suggested.
4. Pathophysiology
   a. A defect in body's immunologic mechanisms produces autoantibodies in the serum directed against components of the patient's own cell nuclei.
   b. Affects cells throughout the body resulting in involvement of many organs, including joints, skin, kidney, CNS, and cardiopulmonary system.

B. Medical management
1. Drug therapy
   a. Aspirin and NSAIDs to relieve mild symptoms such as fever and arthritis
   b. Corticosteroids to suppress the inflammatory response in acute exacerbations or severe disease
   c. Immunosuppressive agents such as azathioprine (Imuran), cyclophosphamide (Cytoxan) to suppress the immune response when patient unresponsive to more conservative therapy
2. Plasmapheresis (plasma exchange)
3. Supportive therapy as organ systems become involved

C. Assessment findings
1. Fatigue, fever, anorexia, weight loss, malaise, history of remissions and exacerbations
2. Joint pain, morning stiffness
3. Skin lesions
   a. Erythematous rash on face, neck, or extremities may occur
   b. Butterfly rash over bridge of nose and cheeks
   c. Photosensitivity with rash in areas exposed to sun
4. Oral or nasopharyngeal ulcerations
5. Alopecia
6. Renal system involvement (proteinuria, hematuria, renal failure)
7. CNS involvement (peripheral neuritis, seizures, organic brain syndrome, psychosis)
8. Cardiopulmonary system involvement (pericarditis, pleurisy)
9. Increased susceptibility to infection
10. Diagnostic tests
    a. ESR elevated
    b. CBC: anemia; WBC and platelet counts decreased
    c. ANA positive
    d. LE prep positive
    e. Anti-DNA positive
    f. Chronic false positive test for syphilis

D. Nursing interventions
1. Assess symptoms to determine systems involved.
2. Monitor vital signs, I&O, daily weights.
3. Administer medications as ordered.
4. Institute seizure precautions and safety measures with CNS involvement.
5. Provide psychologic support to patient/family.
6. Provide patient teaching and discharge planning concerning

a. Disease process and relationship to symptoms
b. Medication regimen and side effects
c. Importance of adequate rest
d. Use of daily heat and exercises as prescribed for arthritis
e. Need to avoid physical or emotional stress
f. Maintenance of a well-balanced diet
g. Need to avoid direct exposure to sunlight (wear hat and other protective clothing)
h. Need to avoid exposure to persons with infections
i. Importance of regular medical follow-up
j. Availability of community agencies.

Osteomyelitis

A. General information
1. Infection of the bone and surrounding soft tissues, most commonly caused by *S. aureus*
2. Infection may reach bone through open wound (compound fracture or surgery), through the blood stream, or by direct extension from infected adjacent structures.
3. Infections can be acute or chronic; both cause bone destruction.
B. Assessment findings
1. Malaise, fever
2. Pain and tenderness of bone, redness and swelling over bone, difficulty with weight bearing; drainage from wound site may be present
3. Diagnostic tests
a. CBC: WBC elevated
b. Blood cultures may be positive
c. ESR may be elevated
C. Nursing interventions
1. Administer analgesics and antibiotics as ordered.
2. Use sterile technique during dressing changes.
3. Maintain proper body alignment and change position frequently to prevent deformities.
4. Provide immobilization of affected part as ordered.
5. Provide psychologic support and diversional activities (depression may result from prolonged hospitalization).
6. Prepare patient for surgery if indicated.
a. Incision and drainage of bone abscess
b. Sequestrectomy: removal of dead, infected bone and cartilage
c. Bone grafting after repeated infections
7. Provide patient teaching and discharge planning concerning
a. Use of prescribed oral antibiotic therapy and side effects
b. Importance of recognizing and reporting signs of complications (deformity, fracture) or recurrence.

Fractures

A. General information
1. A break in the continuity of bone, usually caused by trauma

2. Pathologic fractures: spontaneous bone break, found in certain diseases or conditions (osteoporosis, osteomyelitis, multiple myeloma, bone tumors)
3. Types
a. Complete: separation of bone into two parts
1) transverse
2) oblique
3) spiral
b. Incomplete (partial): fracture does not go all the way through the bone, only part of the bone is broken.
c. Comminuted: bone is broken or splintered into pieces.
d. Closed or simple: bone is broken without break in skin.
e. Open or compound: break in skin with or without protrusion of bone.
B. Medical management
1. Traction
2. Reduction
a. Closed reduction through manual manipulation followed by application of cast
b. Open reduction
3. Application of a cast
C. Assessment findings
1. Pain, aggravated by motion; tenderness
2. Loss of motion; edema, crepitus, ecchymosis
3. Diagnostic test: x-ray reveals break in bone
D. Nursing interventions
1. Provide emergency care of fractures
2. Perform neurovascular checks on affected extremity.
3. Observe for signs of fat emboli especially in the patient with multiple long-bone fractures.
4. Encourage diet high in protein and vitamins to promote healing.
5. Encourage fluids to prevent constipation, renal calculi, and UTIs.
6. Provide care for the patient in traction, with a cast, or with open reduction.
7. Provide patient teaching and discharge planning concerning
a. Cast care if indicated
b. Crutch walking (page 153) if necessary
c. Signs of complications and need to report them.

Open Reduction and Internal Fixation

A. General information
1. Open reduction of fractures requires surgery to realign bones; may include internal fixation with pins, screws, wires, plates, rods or nails
2. Indications include
a. Compound fractures
b. Fractures accompanied by serious neurovascular injuries
c. Fractures with widely separated fragments
d. Comminuted fractures
e. Fractures of the femur
f. Fractures of joints

B. Nursing interventions: preoperative
  1. Provide routine pre-op care.
  2. Provide meticulous skin preparation to prevent infection.
C. Nursing interventions: postoperative
  1. Provide routine post-op care.
  2. Maintain affected limb in proper alignment.
  3. Perform neurovascular checks to affected extremity.
  4. Observe for post-op infection.

Fractured Hip

A. General information
  1. Fracture of the head, neck (intracapsular fracture) or trochanteric area (extracapsular fracture) of the femur
  2. Occurs most often in elderly women
  3. Predisposing factors include osteoporosis and degenerative changes of bone.
B. Medical management
  1. Buck's or Russell traction as temporary measures to maintain alignment of affected limb and reduce the pain of muscle spasm
  2. Surgery
     a. Open reduction and internal fixation with pins, nails, and/or plates
     b. Hemiarthroplasty: insertion of prosthesis (e.g., Austin-Moore) to replace head of femur
C. Assessment findings
  1. Pain in affected limb
  2. Affected limb appears shorter, external rotation
  3. Diagnostic test: x-ray reveals hip fracture
D. Nursing interventions
  1. Provide general care for the patient with a fracture.
  2. Provide care for the patient with Buck's or Russell traction (page 154).
  3. Monitor for disorientation and confusion in the elderly patient; reorient frequently and provide safety measures.
  4. Perform neurovascular checks to affected extremity.
  5. Prevent complications of immobility.
  6. Encourage use of trapeze to facilitate movement.
  7. Administer analgesics as ordered for pain.
  8. In addition to routine care for the patient with open reduction and internal fixation
     a. Check dressings for bleeding, drainage, infection: empty Hemovac and note output; keep compressed to facilitate drainage.
     b. Assess patient's LOC.
     c. Reorient the confused patient frequently.
     d. Avoid oversedating the elderly patient.
     e. Turn patient every 2 hours.
     f. Turn to unoperative side only.
     g. Place 2 pillows between legs while turning and when lying on side.
     h. Institute measures to prevent thrombus formation.
        1) apply elastic stockings.
        2) encourage dorsiflexion of foot.
        3) administer anticoagulants such as aspirin if ordered.
     i. Encourage quadripceps setting and gluteal setting exercises when allowed.
     j. Observe for adequate bowel and bladder function.
     k. Assist patient in getting out of bed, usually on first or second post-op day.
     l. Pivot or lift into chair as ordered.
     m. Avoid weight bearing until allowed.
  9. Provide care for the patient with a hip prosthesis if necessary (similar to care for patient with total hip replacement).

Total Hip Replacement

A. General information
  1. Replacement of both acetabulum and head of femur with prostheses
  2. Indications
     a. Rheumatoid arthritis or osteoarthritis causing severe disability and intolerable pain
     b. Fractured hip with nonunion
B. Nursing interventions
  1. Provide routine pre-op care.
  2. In addition to routine post-op care
     a. Maintain abduction of affected limb at all times with abductor splint or 2 pillows between legs.
     b. Prevent external rotation (may vary depending on surgeon) by placing trochanter rolls along leg.
     c. Prevent hip flexion.
        1) keep head of bed flat if ordered.
        2) may raise bed to 20°–30° for meals if allowed.
     d. Turn only to unoperative side if ordered; use abductor splint or 2 pillows between knees while turning and when lying on side.
     e. Assist patient in getting out of bed when ordered.
        1) time varies with surgeon, usually 2–4 days post-op.
        2) avoid weight bearing until allowed.
        3) avoid adduction and hip flexion; do not use low chair.
  3. Provide patient teaching and discharge planning concerning
     a. Prevention of adduction of affected limb and hip flexion
        1) do not cross legs.
        2) use raised toilet set.
        3) do not bend down to put on shoes or socks.
        4) do not sit in low chairs.
     b. Signs of wound infection
     c. Exercise program as ordered
     d. Partial weight bearing only until full weight bearing allowed.

Herniated Nucleus Pulposus (HNP)

A. General information
  1. Protrusion of nucleus pulposus (central part of intervertebral disc) into spinal canal causing compression of spinal nerve roots

2. Occurs more often in men
3. Herniation most commonly occurs at the fourth and fifth intervertebral spaces in the lumbar region
4. Predisposing factors include heavy lifting or pulling and trauma.

B. Medical management
   1. Conservative treatment
      a. Bedrest
      b. Traction
         1) lumbosacral disc: pelvic traction
         2) cervical disc: cervical traction
      c. Drug therapy
         1) anti-inflammatory agents
         2) muscle relaxants
         3) analgesics
      d. Local application of heat and diathermy
      e. Corset for lumbosacral disc
      f. Cervical collar for cervical disc
      g. Epidural injections of corticosteroids
   2. Surgery
      a. Laminectomy with or without spinal fusion
      b. Chemonucleolysis
         1) injection of chymopapain (derivative of papaya plant) into disc to reduce size and pressure on affected nerve root
         2) used as alternative to laminectomy in selected cases

C. Assessment findings
   1. Lumbosacral disc
      a. Back pain radiating across buttock and down leg (along sciatic nerve)
      b. Weakness of leg and foot on affected side
      c. Numbness and tingling in toes and foot
      d. Positive straight-leg-raise test: pain on raising leg
      e. Depressed or absent Achilles reflex
      f. Muscle spasm in lumbar region
   2. Cervical disc
      a. Shoulder pain radiating down arm to hand
      b. Weakness of affected upper extremity
      c. Paresthesias and sensory disturbances
   3. Diagnostic tests: myelogram localizes site of herniation

D. Nursing interventions
   1. Ensure bedrest on a firm mattress with bed board.
   2. Assist patient in applying pelvic or cervical traction as ordered.
   3. Maintain proper body alignment.
   4. Administer medications as ordered.
   5. Prevent complications of immobility.
   6. Provide additional comfort measures to relieve pain
   7. Provide pre-op care for patient receiving chemonucleolysis.
      a. Administer cimetidine (Tagamet) and diphenhydramine HCl (Benadryl) every 6 hours as ordered to reduce possibility of allergic reaction.
      b. Possibly administer corticosteroids before procedure.
   8. Provide post-op care for patient receiving chemonucleolysis.
      a. Observe for anaphylaxis.
      b. Observe for less serious allergic reaction (e.g., rash, itching, rhinitis, difficulty in breathing).
      c. Monitor for neurologic deficits (numbness or tingling in extremities or inability to void).
   9. Provide patient teaching and discharge planning concerning
      a. Back strengthening exercises as prescribed
      b. Maintenance of good posture
      c. Use of proper body mechanics, how to lift heavy objects correctly
         1) maintain straight spine.
         2) flex knees and hips while stooping.
         3) keep load close to body.
      d. Prescribed medications and side effects
      e. Proper application of corset or cervical collar
      f. Weight reduction if needed.

Laminectomy

A. General information
   1. Surgical excision of part of posterior arch of vertebrae and removal of protruded disc
   2. Indications
      a. Most commonly used for herniated nucleus pulposus not responsive to conservative therapy or with evidence of decreasing sensory or motor status
      b. Also indicated for spinal decompression as with spinal cord injury, to remove fragments of broken bone, or to remove spinal neoplasm or abscess
   3. Spinal fusion may be done at the same time if spine is unstable.

B. Nursing interventions: preoperative
   1. Provide routine pre-op care.
   2. Teach patient log rolling (turning body as a unit while maintaining alignment of spinal column) and use of bedpan.

C. Nursing interventions: postoperative
   1. Provide routine post-op care.
   2. Position patient as ordered.
      a. Lower spinal surgery: generally flat
      b. Cervical spinal surgery: slight elevation of head of bed
   3. Maintain proper body alignment; with cervical spinal surgery avoid neck flexion and apply cervical collar as ordered.
   4. Turn patient every 2 hours.
      a. Use log rolling technique and turning sheet.
      b. Place pillows between legs while on side.
   5. Assess for complications.
      a. Monitor sensory and motor status every 2–4 hours.
      b. With cervical spinal surgery patient may have difficulty swallowing and coughing.
         1) monitor for respiratory distress.
         2) keep suction and tracheostomy set available.

6. Check dressings for hemorrhage, CSF leakage, infection.
7. Promote comfort.
   a. Administer analgesics as ordered.
   b. Provide additional comfort measures and positioning.
8. Assess for adequate bladder and bowel function.
   a. Monitor every 2–4 hours for bladder distension.
   b. Assess bowel sounds.
   c. Prevent constipation.
9. Prevent complications of immobility.
10. Assist with ambulation.
    a. Usually out of bed day after surgery.
    b. Apply brace or corset if ordered.
    c. If patient allowed to sit, use straight-back chair and keep feet flat on floor.
D. Provide patient teaching and discharge planning concerning
   1. Wound care
   2. Maintenance of good posture and proper body mechanics
   3. Activity level as ordered
   4. Recognition and reporting of signs of complications such as wound infection, sensory or motor deficits.

Spinal Fusion

A. General information
   1. Fusion of spinous processes with bone graft from iliac crest to provide stabilization of spine
   2. Performed in conjunction with laminectomy
B. Nursing interventions
   1. Provide pre-op care as for laminectomy.
   2. In addition to post-op care for laminectomy
      a. Position patient correctly.
         1) lower spinal fusion: keep bed flat for first 12 hours, then may elevate head of bed 20°–30°, keep off back for first 48 hours.
         2) cervical spinal fusion: elevate head of bed slightly.
      b. Assist with ambulation.
         1) time varies with surgeon and extent of fusion.
         2) usually out of bed 3–4 days post-op.
         3) apply brace before getting patient out of bed.
         4) apply special cervical collar for cervical spinal fusion.
      c. Promote comfort: patient may experience considerable pain from graft site.
   3. In addition to patient teaching and discharge planning for laminectomy, advise patient that
      a. Brace will be needed for 4 months and lighter corset for 1 year after surgery.
      b. It takes 1 year until graft becomes stable.
      c. No bending, lifting, stooping, or sitting for prolonged periods for 4 months.
      d. Walking without excessive tiring is healthful exercise.
      e. Diet modification will help prevent weight gain resulting from decreased activity.

Harrington Rod Insertion

See page **347**.

Amputation of a Limb

See page 84.

SAMPLE QUESTIONS

Mrs. Diana Fox has been diagnosed with rheumatoid arthritis for the past eight years. Her condition is deteriorating despite conservative treatment, and intramuscular gold is prescribed by the physician.

14. When teaching Mrs. Fox about gold (chrysotherapy), it is important that the nurse emphasize
    o 1. Cushing's syndrome is common.
    o 2. improvement may not occur for 3–6 months.
    o 3. side effects are rare.
    o 4. the need to take this drug daily.

15. During the physical examination of Mrs. Fox, the nurse should expect to find
    o 1. asymmetric joint involvement.
    o 2. Heberden's nodes.
    o 3. obesity.
    o 4. small joint involvement.

The Endocrine System

OVERVIEW OF ANATOMY AND PHYSIOLOGY

The endocrine system is composed of an interrelated complex of glands (pituitary, adrenals, thyroid, parathyroids, islets of Langerhans of the pancreas, ovaries, and testes) that secrete a variety of hormones directly into the bloodstream. Its major function, together with the nervous system, is to regulate body functions.

Hormone Regulation

A. *Hormones:* chemical substances that act as messengers to specific cells and organs (target organs), stimulating and inhibiting various processes; two major categories
   1. Local: hormones with specific effect in the area of secretion (e.g., secretin, cholecystokinin-pancreozymin [CCK-PZ])
   2. General: hormones transported in the blood to distant sites where they exert their effect (e.g., cortisol)
B. *Negative feedback mechanisms:* major means of regulating hormone levels
   1. Decreased concentration of a circulating hormone triggers production of a stimulating hormone from the pituitary gland; this hormone in turn stimulates its target organ to produce hormones.
   2. Increased concentration of a hormone inhibits production of the stimulating hormone, resulting in decreased secretion of the target organ hormone.
C. Some hormones are controlled by changing blood levels of specific substances (e.g., calcium, glucose).
D. Certain hormones (e.g., cortisol or female reproductive hormones) follow rhythmic patterns of secretion.
E. Autonomic and CNS control (pituitary-hypothalamic axis): hypothalamus controls release of the hormones of the anterior pituitary gland through *releasing and inhibiting factors* that stimulate or inhibit hormone secretion.

Structure and Function of Endocrine Glands

See Table 2.24.

Pituitary Gland (Hypophysis)

A. Located in sella turcica at the base of the brain
B. "Master gland" of the body, composed of three lobes
   1. Anterior lobe (adenohypophysis)
      a. Secretes tropic hormones (hormones that stimulate target glands to produce their hormone): adrenocorticotropic hormone (ACTH), thyroid-stimulating hormone (TSH), follicle-stimulating hormone (FSH), luteinizing hormone (LH)
      b. Also secretes hormones that have direct effect on tissues: somatotropic or growth hormone, prolactin
      c. Regulated by hypothalamic releasing and inhibiting factors and by negative feedback system
   2. Posterior lobe (neurohypophysis): does not produce hormones; stores and releases antidiuretic hormone (ADH) and oxytocin, produced by the hypothalamus
   3. Intermediate lobe: secretes melanocyte-stimulating hormone (MSH)

Adrenal Glands

A. Two small glands, one above each kidney
B. Consist of two sections
   1. Adrenal cortex (outer portion): produces mineralocorticoids, glucocorticoids, sex hormones
   2. Adrenal medulla (inner portion): produces epinephrine, norepinephrine

Thyroid Gland

A. Located in anterior portion of the neck
B. Consists of two lobes connected by a narrow isthmus
C. Produces thyroxine (T_4), triiodothyronine (T_3), thyrocalcitonin

Parathyroid Glands

A. Four small glands located in pairs behind the thyroid gland
B. Produce parathormone (PTH)

Pancreas

A. Located behind the stomach

B. Has both endocrine and exocrine functions (see page 117 for further information about the exocrine function of the pancreas)

C. Islets of Langerhans (alpha and beta cells) involved in endocrine function

   1. Beta cells: produce insulin

   2. Alpha cells: produce glucagon

Gonads

A. Ovaries: located in pelvic cavity, produce estrogen and progesterone

B. Testes: located in scrotum, produce testosterone

ASSESSMENT

Health History

A. Presenting problem: symptoms may include

   1. Change in appearance: hair, nails, skin (change in texture or pigmentation); change in size, shape, or symmetry of head, neck, face, eyes, or tongue

   2. Change in energy level

   3. Temperature intolerance

   4. Development of abnormal secondary sexual characteristics; change in sexual function

   5. Change in emotional state, thought pattern, or intellectual functioning

Table 2.24   Hormone Functions

Endocrine Gland	Hormones	Functions
Pituitary		
Anterior lobe	TSH	Stimulates thyroid gland to release thyroid hormones.
	ACTH	Stimulates adrenal cortex to produce and release adrenocorticoids.
	FSH, LH	Stimulate growth, maturation, and function of primary and secondary sex organs.
	GH or somatotropin	Stimulates growth of body tissues and bones.
	Prolactin or LTH	Stimulates development of mammary glands and lactation.
Posterior lobe	ADH	Regulates water metabolism; released during stress or in response to an increase in plasma osmolality to stimulate reabsorption of water and decrease urine output.
	Oxytocin	Stimulates uterine contractions during delivery and the release of milk in lactation.
Intermediate lobe	MSH	Affects skin pigmentation.
Adrenal		
Adrenal cortex	Mineralocorticoids (e.g., aldosterone)	Regulate fluid and electrolyte balance; stimulate reabsorption of sodium, chloride, and water; stimulate potassium excretion.
	Glucocorticoids (e.g., cortisol, corticosterone)	Increase blood glucose levels by increasing rate of glyconeogenesis; increase protein catabolism, increase mobilization of fatty acids; promote sodium and water retention; anti-inflammatory effect; aid body in coping with stress.
	Sex hormones (androgens, estrogen, progesterone)	Influence development of secondary sex characteristics.
Adrenal medulla	Epinephrine, norepinephrine	Function in acute stress; increase heart rate, blood pressure; dilate bronchioles; convert glycogen to glucose when needed by muscles for energy.
Thyroid	T_3, T_4	Regulate metabolic rate; carbohydrate, fat, and protein metabolism; aid in regulating physical and mental growth and development.
	Thyrocalcitonin	Lowers serum calcium by increasing bone deposition.
Parathyroid	PTH	Regulates serum calcium and phosphate levels.
Pancreas (Islets of Langerhans)		
Beta cells	Insulin	Allows glucose to diffuse across cell membrane; converts glucose to glycogen.
Alpha cells	Glucagon	Increases blood glucose by causing glyconeogenesis and glycogenolysis in the liver; secreted in response to low blood sugar.
Ovaries	Estrogen, progesterone	Development of secondary sex characteristics in the female, maturation of sex organs, sexual functioning, maintenance of pregnancy.
Testes	Testosterone	Development of secondary sex characteristics in the male, maturation of sex organs, sexual functioning.

6. Signs of increased activity of sympathetic nervous system (e.g., nervousness, palpitations, tremors, sweating)

7. Change in bowel habits, appetite, or weight; excessive hunger or thirst

8. Change in urinary pattern

B. Life-style: any increased stress

C. Past medical history: growth and development (any delayed or excessive growth); diabetes, thyroid disease, hypertension, obesity, infertility

D. Family history: endocrine diseases, growth problems, obesity, mental illness

Physical Examination

A. Check height, weight, body stature, and body proportions.

B. Observe distribution of muscle mass, fat distribution, any muscle wasting.

C. Inspect for hair growth and distribution.

D. Check condition and pigmentation of skin; presence of striae.

E. Inspect eyes for any bulging.

F. Observe for enlargement in neck area and quality of voice.

G. Observe development of secondary sex characteristics.

H. Palpate thryoid gland (normally cannot be palpated): note size, shape, symmetry, any tenderness, presence of any lumps or nodules.

Laboratory/Diagnostic Tests

A variety of tests may be performed to measure the amounts of hormones present in the serum or urine in assessing pituitary, adrenal, and parathyroid functions; these tests will be referred to when appropriate under specific disorders of the endocrine system.

Thyroid Function

A. Serum studies: nonfasting blood studies (no special preparation necessary)
1. Serum T_4 level: measures total serum level of thyroxine
2. Serum T_3 level: measures serum triiodothyronine level
3. TSH: measurement differentiates primary from secondary hypothyroidism

B. Radioactive iodine uptake (RAIU)
1. Administration of ^{123}I or ^{131}I orally; measurement by a counter of the amount of radioactive iodine taken up by the gland after 24 hours
2. Performed to determine thyroid function; increased uptake indicates hyperactivity; minimal uptake may indicate hypothyroidism
3. Nursing care
   a. Take thorough history; thyroid medication must be discontinued 7–10 days prior to test; medications containing iodine, cough preparations, excess intake of iodine-rich foods, and tests using iodine (e.g., IVP) can invalidate this test.
   b. Assure patient that no radiation precautions are necessary.

C. Thyroid scan
1. Administration of radioactive isotope (orally or IV) and visualization by a scanner of the distribution of radioactivity in the gland
2. Performed to determine location, size, shape, and anatomic function of thyroid gland; identifies areas of increased or decreased uptake; valuable in evaluating thyroid nodules
3. Nursing care: same as RAIU

Pancreatic Function

A. Fasting blood sugar: measures serum glucose levels; patient fasts from midnight before the test

B. 2-hour postprandial blood sugar: measurement of blood glucose 2 hours after a meal is ingested
1. Fast from midnight before test
2. Patient eats a meal consisting of at least 75 gm carbohydrate or ingests 100 gm glucose
3. Blood drawn 2 hours after the meal

C. Oral glucose tolerance test: most specific and sensitive test for diabetes mellitus
1. Fast from midnight before test
2. Patient ingests 100 gm glucose; blood sugars are drawn at 30 and 60 minutes and then hourly for 3–5 hours; urine specimens may also be collected
3. Diet for 3 days prior to test should include 200 gm carbohydrate and at least 1500 kcal/day
4. During test, assess the patient for reactions such as dizziness, sweating. and weakness

ANALYSIS

Nursing diagnoses for the patient with a disorder of the endocrine system may include

A. Alteration in nutrition: less than/more than body requirements

B. Alteration in comfort: pain

C. Impairment of skin integrity

D. Potential for injury

E. Sleep pattern disturbance

F. Alteration in tissue perfusion: peripheral

G. Alteration in pattern of urinary elmination

H. Fluid volume deficit

I. Fluid volume excess

J. Alteration in cardiac output: decreased

K. Alteration in thought processes

L. Disturbance in self-concept: body image, role performance

M. Ineffective individual coping

N. Sexual dysfunction

O. Knowledge deficit

P. Noncompliance

PLANNING AND IMPLEMENTATION

Goals

A. Patient will regain optimal nutritional status.
B. Patient will attain maximal comfort level.
C. Optimum skin integrity will be maintained.
D. Patient will be free from injury.
E. Rest and activity will be balanced.
F. Peripheral circulation will be improved.
G. Patient will have adequate urinary elimination and fluid volume.
H. Patient will maintain adequate cardiac output.
I. Patient will be oriented to optimal level.
J. Patient will adapt to altered body image and loss of function; will have increased self-esteem.
K. Patient will use positive coping behaviors in dealing with the effects of acute or chronic illness.
L. Patient will regain optimum sexual health.
M. Patient will state understanding of disease process, prescribed medications and treatments, and possible complications.
N. Patient will increase compliance with treatment plan.

Interventions

Care of the Patient on Corticosteroid Therapy

A. General information
  1. Types of preparations include cortisone, hydrocortisone, prednisone, dexamethasone (Decadron)
  2. Indications
    a. Replacement therapy in primary and secondary adrenocortical insufficiency
    b. Symptomatic treatment for anti-inflammatory effect of numerous inflammatory, allergic, or immunoreactive disorders (e.g., arthritis, SLE, bronchial asthma, skin diseases, ocular disorders, allergic diseases, inflammatory bowel disorders, cerebral edema and increased ICP, shock, nephrotic syndrome, malignancies, myasthenia gravis, multiple sclerosis)
  3. Common side effects: salt and water retention, sweating, increased appetite
  4. Adverse reactions
    a. Cardiovascular: hypertension, CHF
    b. GI: peptic ulcer, ulcerative esophagitis
    c. Integumentary: petechiae, ecchymoses, purpura, hirsutism, acne, thinning of skin, striae, redistribution of body fat in subcutaneous tissue, abnormal pigmentation, poor wound healing
    d. Endocrine: impaired glucose metabolism, hyperglycemia, menstrual dysfunction, growth retardation
    e. Musculoskeletal: muscle weakness, osteoporosis
    f. Neurologic: personality changes, headache, syncope, vertigo, irritability, insomnia, seizures
    g. Ophthalmologic: cataract formation, glaucoma
    h. Other: hypokalemia, thrombophlebitis, masking of signs of infection, increased susceptibility to infection
    i. Sudden withdrawal may precipitate acute adrenal insufficiency.
B. Nursing care
  1. Administer with food or milk; instruct patient to report gastric distress (antacids may be necessary).
  2. Give in a single daily dose, preferably before 9 A.M. (corticosteroids suppress adrenal function least when given in early morning, the time of maximal adrenocortical activity).
  3. Instruct patient to avoid infections and to report immediately if one is suspected.
  4. Instruct patient never to withdraw the drug abruptly, as this may cause acute adrenal insufficiency.
  5. Observe patient for any mental changes (e.g., irritability, mood swings, euphoria, depression).
  6. Alert women that menstrual irregularity may develop.
  7. Monitor blood pressure, I&O, weight, blood glucose, and serum potassium.
  8. Advise patients to restrict salt intake.
  9. Encourage intake of foods high in potassium.

EVALUATION

A. Patient maintains normal weight; no evidence of malnutrition.
B. Pain is reduced or is more manageable.
C. Skin is intact and free from irritation.
D. Patient is free from injuries.
E. Patient maintains normal balance between rest and activity.
F. Patient has improved peripheral circulation.
  1. Warm, pink skin
  2. Adequate capillary refill
  3. Presence of pulses
  4. Normal sensation and movement
G. Patient has adequate patterns of urinary elimination.
H. Blood pressure and urine output are within normal limits; no signs of dehydration.
I. Peripheral edema is reduced.
J. Vital signs return to normal levels.
K. Orientation to time, place, and person; able to evaluate reality.
L. Patient uses effective coping behaviors to successfully adapt to effects of illness, changes in body image, and loss of function.
M. Patient demonstrates increased self-esteem.
N. Patient verbalizes satisfying sexual activity/expression.
O. Patient demonstrates and uses knowledge of disease process, prescribed medications and treatments; reports any complications.
P. Patient shows compliance with treatment plan.

DISORDERS OF THE ENDOCRINE SYSTEM

Specific Disorders of the Pituitary Gland

Hypopituitarism

A. General information
   1. Hypofunction of the anterior pituitary gland resulting in deficiencies of both the hormones secreted by the anterior pituitary gland and those secreted by the target glands
   2. May be caused by tumor, trauma, surgical removal, or irradiation of the gland; or may be congenital (pituitary dwarfism, see page 351)

B. Medical management: specific treatment depends on cause
   1. Tumor: surgical removal or irradiation of the gland
   2. Regardless of cause, treatment will include replacement of hormones: corticosteroids, thyroid hormone, sex hormones, gonadotropins (may be used to restore fertility).

C. Assessment findings
   1. Tumor: bitemporal hemianopia, headache
   2. Varying signs of hormonal disturbances, depending on which hormones are being undersecreted (e.g., menstrual dysfunction, hypothyroidism, adrenal insufficiency)
   3. Retardation of growth if condition occurs before epiphyseal closure
   4. Diagnostic tests
      a. Skull x-ray, CT scan may reveal pituitary tumor
      b. Plasma hormone levels may be decreased depending on specific hormones undersecreted

D. Nursing interventions
   1. Provide care for the patient undergoing hypophysectomy or radiation therapy if indicated.
   2. Provide patient teaching and discharge planning concerning
      a. Hormone replacement therapy
      b. Importance of follow-up care.

Hyperpituitarism

A. General information
   1. Hyperfunction of the anterior pituitary gland resulting in oversecretion of one or more of the anterior pituitary hormones
   2. Overproduction of the growth hormone produces acromegaly in adults and gigantism in children (if hypersecretion occurs before epiphyseal closure); see page 351
   3. Usually caused by a benign pituitary adenoma

B. Medical management: surgical removal or irradiation of the gland

C. Assessment findings
   1. Tumor: bitemporal hemianopia; headache
   2. Hormonal disturbances depending on which hormones are being excreted in excess
   3. Acromegaly caused by oversecretion of growth hormones: transverse enlargement of bones, especially noticeable in skull and in bones of hands and feet; features become coarse and heavy; lips become heavier; tongue enlarged

   4. Diagnostic tests
      a. Skull x-ray, CT scan reveal pituitary tumor
      b. Plasma hormone levels reveal increased growth hormone, oversecretion of other hormones

D. Nursing interventions
   1. Monitor for hyperglycemia and cardiovascular problems, (hypertension, angina, CHF) and modify care accordingly.
   2. Provide psychologic support and acceptance for alterations in body image.
   3. Provide care for the patient undergoing hypophysectomy or radiation therapy if indicated.

Hypophysectomy

A. General information
   1. Partial or complete removal of the pituitary gland
   2. Indications: pituitary tumors, diabetic retinopathy, metastatic cancer of the breast or prostate, which may be endocrine dependent
   3. Surgical approaches
      a. Craniotomy: usually transfrontal
      b. Transphenoidal: incision made in inner aspect of upper lip and gingiva; sella turcica is entered through the floor of the nose and sphenoid sinuses
      c. Cryohypophysectomy: destruction of the gland using extreme cold

B. Nursing care
   1. In addition to pre-op care of the craniotomy patient (page 58), explain post-op expectations.
   2. In addition to post-op care of the craniotomy patient, observe for signs of target gland deficiencies (diabetes insipidus, adrenal insufficiency, hypothyroidism) due to total removal of the gland or to post-op edema.
      a. Perform hourly urine outputs and specific gravities; alert physician if urine output is greater than 800–900 cc/2 hours or if specific gravity is less than 1.004.
      b. Administer cortisone replacement as ordered.
   3. If transphenoidal approach used
      a. Elevate the head of the bed to 30° to decrease headache and pressure on the sella turcica.
      b. Administer mild analgesics for headache as ordered.
      c. Observe for and prevent CSF leak from surgical site.
         1) discourage vigorous coughing, sneezing, straining at stool.
         2) observe for clear drainage from nose or post-nasal drip (constant swallowing); check drainage for glucose; positive results indicate that drainage is CSF.
         3) if leakage does occur
            a) elevate head of bed and call the physician.
            b) most leaks will resolve in 72 hours with bedrest and elevation.
            c) may do daily spinal taps to decrease CSF pressure.
            d) administer antibiotics as ordered to prevent meningitis.

4. Provide patient teaching and discharge planning concerning
   a. Hormone therapy
     1) if gland is completely removed, patient will have permanent diabetes insipidus (see below)
     2) cortisone and thyroid hormone replacement
     3) replacement of sex hormones
       a) testosterone: may be given for impotence in men
       b) estrogen: may be given for atrophy of the vaginal mucosa in women
       c) human pituitary gonadotropins: may restore fertility in some women
   b. Need for lifelong follow-up and hormone replacement
   c. Need to wear Medic-Alert bracelet
   d. If transphenoidal approach was used
     1) avoid bending and straining at stool for 2 months post-op.
     2) no toothbrushing until sutures are removed and incision heals (about 10 days)

Diabetes Insipidus

A. General information
   1. Hypofunction of the posterior pituitary gland resulting in deficiency of ADH
   2. Characterized by excessive thirst and urination
   3. Caused by tumor, trauma, inflammation, pituitary surgery
B. Assessment findings
   1. Polydipsia (excessive thirst) and severe polyuria with low specific gravity
   2. Fatigue, muscle weakness, irritability, weight loss, signs of dehydration
   3. Tachycardia, eventual shock if fluids not replaced
   4. Diagnostic tests
     a. Urine specific gravity less than 1.004
     b. Water deprivation test reveals inability to concentrate urine
C. Nursing interventions
   1. Maintain fluid and electrolyte balance.
     a. Keep accurate I&O.
     b. Weigh daily.
     c. Administer IV/oral fluids as ordered to replace fluid losses.
   2. Monitor vital signs and observe for signs of dehydration and hypovolemia.
   3. Administer hormone replacement as ordered
     a. Vasopressin (Pitressin) and vasopressin tannate (Pitressin tannate in oil): given by IM injection
       1) warm to body temperature before giving.
       2) shake tannate suspension to ensure uniform dispersion.
     b. Lypressin (Diapid): nasal spray
   4. Provide patient teaching and discharge planning concerning
     a. Lifelong hormone replacement; lypressin as needed to control polyuria and polydipsia
     b. Need to wear Medic-Alert bracelet.

Disorders of the Adrenal Gland

Addison's Disease

A. General information
   1. Primary adrenocortical insufficiency; hypofunction of the adrenal cortex causes decreased secretion of the mineralocorticoids, glucocorticoids, and sex hormones
   2. Relatively rare disease caused by
     a. Idiopathic atrophy of the adrenal cortex possibly due to an autoimmune process
     b. Destruction of the gland secondary to tuberculosis or fungal infection
B. Assessment findings
   1. Fatigue, muscle weakness
   2. Anorexia, nausea, vomiting, abdominal pain, weight loss
   3. History of frequent hypoglycemic reactions
   4. Hypotension, weak pulse
   5. Bronzelike pigmentation of the skin
   6. Decreased capacity to deal with stress
   7. Diagnostic tests: low cortisol levels, hyponatremia, hyperkalemia
C. Nursing interventions
   1. Administer hormone replacement therapy as ordered.
     a. Glucocorticoids (cortisone, hydrocortisone): to simulate diurnal rhythm of cortisol release, give 2/3 of dose in early morning and 1/3 of dose in afternoon
     b. Mineralocorticoids: fludrocortisone acetate (Florinef)
   2. Monitor vital signs.
   3. Decrease stress in the environment.
   4. Prevent exposure to infection.
   5. Provide rest periods; prevent fatigue.
   6. Monitor I&O.
   7. Weight daily.
   8. Provide small, frequent feedings of diet high in carbohydrates, sodium, and protein to prevent hypoglycemia, hyponatremia and provide proper nutrition.
   9. Provide patient teaching and discharge planning concerning
     a. Disease process; signs of adrenal insufficiency
     b. Use of prescribed medications for lifelong replacement therapy; never omit medications
     c. Need to avoid stress, trauma, and infections, and to notify physician if these occur as medication dosage may need to be adjusted
     d. Stress management techniques
     e. Diet modification (high in protein, carbohydrates, and sodium)
     f. Use of salt tablets (if prescribed) or ingestion of salty foods (potato chips) if experiencing increased sweating
     g. Importance of alternating regular exercise with rest periods
     h. Avoidance of strenuous exercise especially in hot weather.

Addisonian Crisis

A. General information
   1. Severe exacerbation of Addison's disease caused by acute adrenal insufficiency
   2. Precipitating factors
      a. Strenuous activity, infection, trauma, stress, failure to take prescribed medications
      b. Iatrogenic: surgery on pituitary or adrenal glands, rapid withdrawal of exogenous steroids in a patient on long-term steroid therapy
B. Assessment findings: severe generalized muscle weakness, severe hypotension, hypovolemia, shock (vascular collapse)
C. Nursing interventions
   1. Administer IV fluids (5% dextrose in saline, plasma) as ordered to treat vascular collapse.
   2. Administer IV glucocorticoids (hydrocortisone [Solu-Cortef]) and vasopressors as ordered.
   3. If crisis precipitated by infection, administer antibiotics as ordered.
   4. Maintain strict bedrest and eliminate all forms of stressful stimuli.
   5. Monitor vital signs, I&O, daily weights.
   6. Protect patient from infection.
   7. Provide patient teaching and discharge planning: same as for Addison's disease.

Cushing's Syndrome

A. General information
   1. Condition resulting from excessive secretion of corticosteroids, particularly the glucocorticoid cortisol
   2. Occurs most frequently in females between ages 30–60
   3. Primary Cushing's syndrome: caused by adrenocortical tumors or hyperplasia
   4. Secondary Cushing's syndrome (also called Cushing's disease): caused by functioning pituitary or nonpituitary neoplasm secreting ACTH, causing increased secretion of glucocorticoids
   5. Iatrogenic: caused by prolonged use of corticosteroids
B. Assessment findings
   1. Muscle weakness, fatigue, obese trunk with thin arms and legs, muscle wasting
   2. Irritability, depression, frequent mood swings
   3. Moon face, buffalo hump, pendulous abdomen
   4. Purple striae on trunk, acne, thin skin
   5. Signs of masculinization in women; menstrual dysfunction, decreased libido
   6. Osteoporosis, decreased resistance to infection
   7. Hypertension, edema
   8. Diagnostic tests: cortisol levels increased, slight hypernatremia, hypokalemia, hyperglycemia
C. Nursing interventions
   1. Maintain muscle tone.
      a. Provide ROM exercises.
      b. Assist with ambulation.
   2. Prevent accidents or falls and provide adequate rest.
   3. Protect patient from exposure to infection.
   4. Maintain skin integrity.
      a. Provide meticulous skin care.
      b. Prevent tearing of skin: use paper tape if necessary.
   5. Minimize stress in the environment.
   6. Monitor vital signs; observe for hypertension, edema.
   7. Measure I&O and daily weights.
   8. Provide diet low in calories, sodium and high in protein, potassium, calcium, and vitamin D.
   9. Monitor urine for glucose and acetone; administer insulin if ordered.
   10. Provide psychologic support and acceptance.
   11. Prepare patient for hypophysectomy or radiation if condition is caused by a pituitary tumor.
   12. Prepare patient for an adrenalectomy if condition is caused by an adrenal tumor or hyperplasia.
   13. Provide patient teaching and discharge planning concerning
      a. Diet modifications
      b. Importance of adequate rest
      c. Need to avoid stress and infection
      d. Change in medication regimen (alternate day therapy or reduced dosage) if cause of the condition is prolonged corticosteroid therapy.

Primary Aldosteronism (Conn's Syndrome)

A. General information
   1. Excessive aldosterone secretion from the adrenal cortex
   2. Seen more frequently in women, usually between ages 30–50
   3. Caused by tumor or hyperplasia of adrenal gland
B. Assessment findings
   1. Headache, hypertension
   2. Muscle weakness, polyuria, polydipsia, metabolic alkalosis, cardiac arrhythmias (due to hypokalemia)
   3. Diagnostic tests
      a. Serum potassium decreased, alkalosis
      b. Urinary aldosterone levels elevated
C. Nursing interventions
   1. Monitor vital signs, I&O, daily weights.
   2. Maintain sodium restriction as ordered.
   3. Administer spironolactone (Aldactone) and potassium supplements as ordered.
   4. Prepare the patient for an adrenelectomy (page 169) if indicated.
   5. Provide patient teaching and discharge planning concerning
      a. Use and side effects of medication if the patient is being maintained on spironolactone therapy
      b. Signs and symptoms of hypo/hyperaldosteronism
      c. Need for frequent blood pressure checks and follow-up care.

Pheochromocytoma

A. General information
   1. Functioning tumor of the adrenal medulla that secretes excessive amounts of epinephrine and norepinephrine

2. Occurs most commonly between ages 40–60
3. May be hereditary in some cases
B. Assessment findings
   1. Severe headache, apprehension, palpitations, profuse sweating, nausea
   2. Hypertension, tachycardia, vomiting, hyperglycemia, dilation of pupils, cold extremities
   3. Diagnostic tests
      a. Increased plasma levels of catecholamines; elevated blood sugar; glycosuria
      b. Elevated urinary catecholamines and urinary vanillylmandelic acid (VMA) levels
      c. Presence of tumor on x-ray
C. Nursing interventions
   1. Monitor vital signs, especially blood pressure.
   2. Administer medications as ordered to control hypertension.
   3. Promote rest; decrease stressful stimuli.
   4. Monitor urine tests for glucose and acetone.
   5. Provide high-calorie, well-balanced diet; avoid stimulants such as coffee, tea.
   6. Provide care for the patient with an adrenalectomy (see below) as ordered; observe postadrenelectomy patient carefully for shock.
   7. Provide patient teaching and discharge planning: same as for adrenalectomy.

Adrenalectomy

A. General information
   1. Removal of one or both adrenal glands
   2. Indications
      a. Tumors of adrenal cortex (Cushing's syndrome, hyperaldosteronism) or medulla (pheochromocytoma)
      b. Metastatic cancer of the breast or prostate
B. Nursing interventions: preoperative
   1. Provide routine pre-op care.
   2. Correct metabolic/cardiovascular problems.
      a. Pheochromocytoma: stabilize blood pressure.
      b. Cushing's syndrome: treat hyperglycemia and protein deficits.
      c. Primary hyperaldosteronism: treat hypertension and hypokalemia.
   3. Administer glucocorticoid preparation on the morning of surgery as ordered to prevent acute adrenal insufficiency.
C. Nursing interventions: postoperative
   1. Provide routine post-op care.
   2. Observe for hemorrhage and shock.
      a. Monitor vital signs, I&O.
      b. Administer IV therapy and vasopressors as ordered.
   3. Prevent infections (suppression of immune system makes patients especially susceptible).
      a. Encourage coughing and deep breathing to prevent respiratory infection.
      b. Use meticulous aseptic technique during dressing changes.
   4. Administer cortisone or hydrocortisone as ordered to maintain cortisol levels.

5. Provide general care for the patient with abdominal surgery.
D. Provide patient teaching and discharge planning concerning
   1. Self-administration of replacement hormones
      a. Bilateral adrenalectomy: lifelong replacement of glucocorticoids and mineralocorticoids
      b. Unilateral adrenalectomy: replacement therapy for 6–12 months until the remaining adrenal gland begins to function normally
   2. Signs and symptoms of adrenal insufficiency
   3. Importance of follow-up care.

Specific Disorders of the Thyroid Gland

Simple Goiter

A. General information
   1. Enlargement of the thyroid gland not caused by inflammation or neoplasm
   2. Types
      a. Endemic: caused by nutritional iodine deficiency, most common in the "goiter belt" (midwest, northwest, and Great Lakes region); occurs most frequently during adolescence and pregnancy
      b. Sporadic: caused by
         1) ingestion of large amounts of goitrogenic foods (contain agents that decrease thyroxine production): e.g., cabbage, soybeans, rutabagas, peanuts, peaches, peas, strawberries, spinach, radishes
         2) use of goitrogenic drugs: propylthiouracil, large doses of iodine, phenylbutazone, para-amino salicylic acid, cobalt, lithium
         3) genetic defects that prevent synthesis of thyroid hormone
   3. Low levels of thyroid hormone stimulate increased secretion of TSH by pituitary; under TSH stimulation the thyroid increases in size to compensate and produces more thyroid hormone.
B. Medical management
   1. Drug therapy
      a. Hormone replacement with levothyroxine (Synthroid) (T_4), dessicated thyroid, or liothyronine (Cytomel) (T_3)
      b. Small doses of iodine (Lugol's or potassium iodide solution) for goiter resulting from iodine deficiency
   2. Avoidance of goitrogenic foods or drugs in sporadic goiter
   3. Surgery: subtotal thyroidectomy (if goiter is large) to relieve pressure symptoms and for cosmetic reasons
C. Assessment findings
   1. Dysphagia, enlarged thyroid, respiratory distress
   2. Diagnostic tests
      a. Serum T_4 level low-normal or normal
      b. RAIU uptake normal or increased
D. Nursing interventions
   1. Administer replacement therapy as ordered.

2. Provide care for patient with subtotal thyroidectomy (page 171) if indicated.
3. Provide patient teaching and discharge planning concerning
   a. Use of iodized salt in preventing and treating endemic goiter
   b. Thyroid hormone replacement.

Hypothyroidism (Myxedema)

A. General information
   1. Slowing of metabolic processes caused by hypofunction of the thyroid gland with decreased thyroid hormone secretion; causes myxedema in adults and cretinism in children (see page **351**).
   2. Occurs more often in women between ages 30–60
   3. Primary hypothyroidism: atrophy of the gland possibly caused by an autoimmune process
   4. Secondary hypothyroidism: caused by decreased stimulation from pituitary TSH
   5. Iatrogenic: surgical removal of the gland or overtreatment of hyperthyroidism with drugs or radioactive iodine
   6. In severe or untreated cases, *myxedema coma* may occur
      a. Characterized by intensification of signs and symptoms of hypothyroidism and neurologic impairment leading to coma
      b. Mortality rate high; prompt recognition and treatment essential
      c. Precipitating factors: failure to take prescribed medications; infection; trauma; exposure to cold; use of sedatives, narcotics, or anesthetics
B. Medical management
   1. Drug therapy: levothyroxine (Synthroid), thyroglobulin (Proloid), desiccated thyroid, liothyronine (Cytomel)
   2. Myxedema coma is a medical emergency.
      a. IV thyroid hormones
      b. Correction of hypothermia
      c. Maintenance of vital functions
      d. Treatment of precipitating causes
C. Assessment findings
   1. Fatigue; lethargy; slowed mental processes; dull look; slow, clumsy movements
   2. Anorexia, weight gain, constipation
   3. Intolerance to cold; dry, scaly skin; dry, sparse hair; brittle nails
   4. Menstrual irregularities; generalized interstitial nonpitting edema
   5. Bradycardia, cardiac complications (CAD, angina pectoris, MI, CHF)
   6. Increased sensitivity to sedatives, narcotics, and anesthetics
   7. Exaggeration of these findings in myxedema coma: weakness, lethargy, syncope, bradycardia, hypotension, hypoventilation, subnormal body temperature

8. Diagnostic tests
   a. Serum T_3 and T_4 level low
   b. Serum cholesterol level elevated
   c. RAIU decreased
D. Nursing interventions
   1. Monitor vital signs, I&O, daily weights; observe for edema and signs of cardiovascular complications.
   2. Administer thyroid hormone replacement therapy as ordered and monitor effects.
      a. Observe for signs of thyrotoxicosis (tachycardia, palpitations, nausea, vomiting, diarrhea, sweating, tremors, agitation, dyspnea).
      b. Increase dosage gradually, especially in patients with cardiac complications.
   3. Provide a comfortable, warm environment.
   4. Provide a low-calorie diet.
   5. Avoid the use of sedatives; reduce the dose of any sedative, narcotic, or anesthetic agent by half as ordered.
   6. Institute measures to prevent skin breakdown.
   7. Provide increased fluids and foods high in roughage to prevent constipation; administer stool softeners as ordered.
   8. Observe for signs of myxedema coma; provide appropriate nursing care.
      a. Administer medications as ordered.
      b. Maintain vital functions: correct hypothermia, maintain adequate ventilation.
   9. Provide patient teaching and discharge planning concerning
      a. Thyroid hormone replacement
         1) take daily dose in the morning to prevent insomnia.
         2) self-monitor for signs of thyrotoxicosis.
      b. Importance of regular follow-up care
      c. Need for additional protection in cold weather
      d. Measures to prevent constipation.

Hyperthyroidism (Grave's Disease)

A. General information
   1. Secretion of excessive amounts of thyroid hormone in the blood causes an increase in metabolic processes
   2. Overactivity and changes in the thyroid gland may be present
   3. Most often seen in women between ages 30–50
   4. Cause unknown, but may be an autoimmune process
   5. Symptomatic hyperthyroidism may also be called thyrotoxicosis.
B. Medical management
   1. Drug therapy
      a. Antithyroid drugs (propylthiouracil and methimazole [Tapazole]): block synthesis of thyroid hormone; toxic effects include agranulocytosis
      b. Adrenergic blocking agents (commonly propanolol [Inderal]): used to decrease sympathetic activity and alleviate symptoms such as tachycardia

2. Radioactive iodine therapy
   a. Radioactive isotope of iodine (e.g., ^{131}I) given to destroy the thyroid gland, thereby decreasing production of thyroid hormone
   b. Used in middle-aged or older patients who are resistant to, or develop toxicity from, drug therapy
   c. Hypothyroidism is a potential complication.
3. Surgery: thyroidectomy performed in younger patients for whom drug therapy has not been effective

C. Assessment findings
1. Irritability, agitation, restlessness, hyperactive movements, tremor, sweating, insomnia
2. Increased appetite, hyperphagia, weight loss, diarrhea, intolerance to heat
3. Exophthalmos (protrusion of the eyeballs), goiter
4. Warm, smooth skin; fine, soft hair; pliable nails
5. Tachycardia, increased systolic blood pressure, palpitations
6. Diagnostic tests
   a. Serum T_3 and T_4 levels elevated
   b. RAIU increased

D. Nursing interventions
1. Monitor vital signs, daily weights.
2. Administer antithyroid medications as ordered.
3. Provide for periods of uninterrupted rest.
   a. Assign to a private room away from excessive activity.
   b. Administer medications to promote sleep as ordered.
4. Provide a cool environment.
5. Minimize stress in the environment.
6. Encourage quiet, relaxing diversional activities.
7. Provide a diet high in carbohydrates, protein, calories, vitamins, and minerals with supplemental feedings in between meals and at bedtime; omit stimulants.
8. Observe for and prevent complications.
   a. Exophthalmos: protect eyes with dark glasses and artificial tears as ordered.
   b. Thyroid storm: see below.
9. Provide patient teaching and discharge planning concerning
   a. Need to recognize and report signs and symptoms of agranulocytosis (fever, sore throat, skin rash) if taking antithyroid drugs
   b. Signs and symptoms of hyper/hypothyroidism.

Thyroid Storm

A. General information
1. Uncontrolled and potentially life-threatening hyperthyroidism caused by sudden and excessive release of thyroid hormone into the blood stream
2. Precipitating factors: stress, infection, unprepared thyroid surgery
3. Now quite rare

B. Assessment findings
1. Apprehension, restlessness

2. Extremely high temperature (up to 106°F [40.7°C]), tachycardia, CHF, respiratory distress, delirium, coma
C. Nursing interventions (see also Hyperthermia)
1. Maintain a patent airway and adequate ventilation; administer oxygen as ordered.
2. Administer IV therapy as ordered.
3. Administer medications as ordered: antithyroid drugs, corticosteroids, sedatives, cardiac drugs.

Thyroidectomy

A. General information
1. Partial or total removal of the thyroid gland
2. Indications
   a. Subtotal thyroidectomy: hyperthyroidism
   b. Total thyroidectomy: thyroid cancer
B. Nursing interventions: preoperative
1. Ensure that the patient is adequately prepared for surgery.
   a. Cardiac status is stable.
   b. Weight and nutritional status are normal.
2. Administer antithyroid drugs as ordered, to suppress the production and secretion of thyroid hormone and to prevent thyroid storm.
3. Administer iodine preparations (Lugol's or potassium iodide solution) to reduce the size and vascularity of the gland and prevent hemorrhage.
C. Nursing interventions: postoperative
1. Monitor vital signs and I&O.
2. Check dressings for signs of hemorrhage; check for wetness behind neck.
3. Place patient in semi-Fowler's position and support head with pillows.
4. Observe for respiratory distress secondary to hemorrhage, edema of the glottis, laryngeal nerve damage, or tetany; keep tracheostomy set, oxygen, and suction nearby.
5. Assess for signs of tetany due to hypocalcemia secondary to accidental removal of parathyroid glands; keep calcium gluconate available (see Hypoparathyroidism, page 172).
6. Encourage the patient to rest voice.
   a. Some hoarseness is common
   b. Check every 30–60 minutes for extreme hoarseness or any accompanying respiratory distress.
7. Observe for thyroid storm due to release of excessive amounts of thyroid hormone during surgery.
8. Administer IV fluids as ordered until the patient is tolerating fluids by mouth.
9. Administer analgesics as ordered for incisional pain.
10. Relieve discomfort from sore throat.
    a. Cool mist humidifier to thin secretions.
    b. Administer analgesic throat lozenges before meals and PRN as ordered.
    c. Encourage fluids.
11. Encourage coughing and deep breathing every hour.

12. Assist the patient with ambulation: instruct the patient to place hands behind neck to decrease stress on suture line.
13. Provide patient teaching and discharge planning concerning
    a. Signs and symptoms of hypo/hyperthyroidism
    b. Self-administration of thyroid hormones if total thyroidectomy performed
    c. Application of lubricant to the incision once sutures are removed
    d. Performance of ROM neck exercises 3–4 times a day
    e. Importance of regular follow-up care.

Specific Disorders of the Parathyroid Glands

Hypoparathyroidism

A. General information
1. Disorder characterized by hypocalcemia resulting from a deficiency of parathormone (PTH) production
2. May be hereditary, idiopathic, or caused by accidental damage to or removal of parathyroid glands during thyroidectomy

B. Assessment findings
1. Acute hypocalcemia (tetany)
    a. Tingling of fingers and around lips, painful muscle spasms, dysphagia, laryngospasm, seizures, cardiac arrhythmias
    b. Chvostek's sign: sharp tapping over facial nerve causes twitching of mouth, nose, and eye
    c. Trousseau's sign: carpopedal spasm induced by application of blood pressure cuff for 3 minutes
2. Chronic hypocalcemia
    a. Fatigue, weakness, muscle cramps
    b. Personality changes, irritability, memory impairment
    c. Dry, scaly skin; hair loss; loss of tooth enamel
    d. Tremor, cardiac arrhythmias, cataract formation
    e. Diagnostic tests
        1) serum calcium levels decreased
        2) serum phosphate levels elevated
        3) skeletal x-rays reveal increased bone density

C. Nursing interventions
1. Administer calcium gluconate by slow IV drip as ordered for acute hypocalcemia.
2. Administer medications for chronic hypocalcemia.
    a. Oral calcium preparations: calcium gluconate, lactate, carbonate (Os-Cal)
    b. Large doses of vitamin D (Calciferol) to help absorption of calcium
    c. Aluminum hydroxide gel (Amphogel) or aluminum carbonate gel, basic (Basaljel) to decrease phosphate levels
3. Institute seizure and safety precautions.
4. Provide quiet environment free from excessive stimuli.
5. Monitor for signs of hoarseness or stridor; check for Chvostek's and Trousseau's signs.
6. Keep emergency equipment (tracheostomy set, injectable calcium gluconate) at bedside.

7. For tetany or generalized muscle cramps, may use rebreathing bag to produce mild respiratory acidosis.
8. Monitor serum calcium and phosphate levels.
9. Provide high-calcium, low-phosphorus diet.
10. Provide patient teaching and discharge planning concerning
    a. Medication regimen; oral calcium preparations and vitamin D to be taken with meals to increase absorption
    b. Need to recognize and report signs and symptoms of hypo/hypercalcemia
    c. Importance of follow-up care with periodic serum calcium levels.

Hyperparathyroidism

A. General information
1. Increased secretion of PTH that results in an altered state of calcium, phosphate, and bone metabolism
2. Most commonly affects women between ages 35–65
3. Primary hyperparathyroidism: caused by tumor or hyperplasia of parathyroid glands
4. Secondary hyperparathyroidism: caused by vitamin D deficiency, malabsorption, chronic renal failure

B. Assessment findings
1. Bone pain (especially at back), bone demineralization, pathologic fractures
2. Renal colic, kidney stones, polyuria, polydipsia
3. Anorexia, nausea, vomiting, gastric ulcers, constipation
4. Muscle weakness, fatigue
5. Irritability, personality changes, depression
6. Cardiac arrhythmias, hypertension
7. Diagnostic tests
    a. Serum calcium levels elevated
    b. Serum phosphate levels decreased
    c. Skeletal x-rays reveal bone demineralization

C. Nursing interventions
1. Administer IV infusions of normal saline solution and give diuretics as ordered; monitor I&O and observe for fluid overload and electrolyte imbalances.
2. Assist patient with self-care: provide careful handling, moving, and ambulation to prevent pathologic fractures.
3. Monitor vital signs; report irregularities.
4. Force fluids; provide acid-ash juices.
5. Strain urine for stones.
6. Provide low-calcium, high-phosphorus diet.
7. Provide care for the patient undergoing parathyroidectomy (see Thyroidectomy, page 171).
8. Provide patient teaching and discharge planning concerning
    a. Need to engage in progressive ambulatory activities
    b. Increased intake of fluids
    c. Use of calcium preparations and importance of high-calcium diet following a parathyroidectomy

Specific Disorders of the Pancreas

Diabetes Mellitus

A. General information
1. Hyperglycemia resulting from absolute or relative lack of insulin
2. Chronic, systemic disease characterized by disorders in the metabolism of carbohydrate, fat, and protein; eventually produces structural abnormalities in various tissues and organs
3. Most common endocrine problem; affects over 10 million people in the U.S.
4. Exact etiology unknown; predisposing factors include heredity, autoimmunity, and/or viruses, as well as other factors such as obesity and stress
5. Types
   a. Type I (insulin-dependent diabetes mellitus [IDDM])
   1) secondary to destruction of beta cells in the pancreas resulting in little or no insulin production
   2) usually occurs in children (see page 330) or in nonobese adults
   b. Type II (non-insulin-dependent diabetes mellitus [NIDDM])
   1) secondary to alterations in insulin receptors on cell membrane causing resistance to insulin
   2) usually occurs in obese adults
   c. Diabetes may also be secondary to other conditions such as pancreatic disease, Cushing's syndrome; use of certain drugs (steroids, thiazide diuretics, oral contraceptives)
6. Pathophysiology
   a. Lack of insulin causes hyperglycemia (insulin is necessary for the transport of glucose across the cell membrane).

b. Hyperglycemia leads to osmotic diuresis as large amounts of glucose pass through the kidney; results in polyuria and glycosuria.
c. Diuresis leads to cellular dehydration and fluid and electrolyte depletion causing polydipsia (excessive thirst).
d. Polyphagia (hunger and increased appetite) results from cellular starvation.
e. The body turns to fats and protein for energy; but in the absence of glucose in the cell, fats cannot be completely metabolized and ketones (intermediate products of fat metabolism) are produced.
f. This leads to ketonemia, ketonuria (contributes to osmotic diuresis), and metabolic acidosis (ketones are acid bodies).
g. Ketones act as CNS depressants and can cause coma.
h. Excess loss of fluids and electrolytes leads to hypovolemia, hypotension, renal failure, and decreased blood flow to the brain resulting in coma and death unless treated.
7. Acute complications of diabetes include diabetic ketoacidosis (page 175), insulin reaction (page 176), hyperglycemic hyperosmolar nonketotic coma (page 176).

B. Medical management
1. Strict diet modification and regulation (see Exchange Lists, Appendix 1)
   a. Used with insulin therapy in Type I
   b. May be used alone or in combination with oral hypoglycemic agents in Type II; occasionally used with insulin, although Type II not insulin dependent
2. Drug therapy
   a. Insulin: used for Type I diabetes (also occasionally used in Type II diabetes)
   1) types (Table 2.25)

Table 2.25 Characteristics of Insulin Preparations

| Drug | Synonym | Appearance | Action in Hours | | | Compatible Mixed with |
			Onset	Peak	Duration	
Rapid Acting						
Insulin injection	Regular insulin	Clear	½–1	2–4	6–8	All insulin preparations
Insulin, zinc suspension, prompt	Semilente insulin	Cloudy	½–1	4–6	12–16	Lente preparations
Intermediate acting						
Isophane insulin injection	NPH insulin	Cloudy	1–1½	8–12	18–24	Regular insulin injection
Insulin zinc suspension	Lente insulin	Cloudy	1–1½	8–12	18–24	Regular insulin and Semilente preparations
Long acting						
Insulin zinc suspension, extended	Ultralente insulin	Cloudy	4–8	16–20	30–36	Regular insulin and Semilente preparations
Protamine zinc insulin suspension	Protamine zinc insulin (PZI)	Cloudy	4–8	14–20	30–36	Regular insulin injection

Table 2.26   Oral Hypoglycemic Agents

Drug	Dosage (mg/day)	Onset of Action (Hours)	Duration of Action (Hours)
First generation sulfonylureas			
Acetohexamide (Dymelor)	250–1500	½	12–24
Chlorpropamide (Diabinese)	100–500	1	24–72
Tolazamide (Tolinase)	100–1000	4–6	14–24
Tolbutamide (Orinase)	250–2000	½	6–12
Second generation sulfonylureas			
Glipizide (Glucotrol)	2.5–40	1–1½	16–24
Glyburide (DiaBeta, Micronase)	1.25–20	2–4	24

    a) short acting: used in treating ketoacidosis; during surgery, infection, trauma; management of poorly controlled diabetes; to supplement longer-acting insulins
    b) intermediate: used for maintenance therapy
    c) long acting: used for maintenance therapy in patients who experience hyperglycemia during the night with intermediate acting insulin
   2) various preparations of short-, intermediate-, and long-acting insulins are available; they differ as to their origin (beef, pork, purified pork, and human).
   3) purified or human insulins are used for patients who develop local or systemic reactions or severe lipodystrophies with other insulin preparations.
  b. Oral hypoglycemic agents (Table 2.26)
   1) used for Type II diabetics who are not controlled by diet and exercise
   2) increase the ability of islet cells of the pancreas to secrete insulin; may have some effect on cell receptors to decrease resistance to insulin
 3. Exercise: helpful adjunct to therapy as exercise decreases the body's need for insulin.
C. Assessment findings
 1. All types: polyuria, polydipsia, polyphagia, fatigue, blurred vision, susceptibility to infection
 2. Type I: anorexia, nausea, vomiting, weight loss
 3. Type II: obesity; frequently no other symptoms
 4. Diagnostic tests
  a. Fasting blood sugar, 2-hour postprandial blood sugar, and oral glucose tolerance test all elevated
  b. Urine tests
   1) Clinitest, Testape: positive for glucose
   2) Acetest, Ketostix: may be positive for acetone
D. Nursing interventions
 1. Administer insulin or oral hypoglycemic agents as ordered; monitor for hypoglycemia, especially during

period of drug's peak action.
 2. Provide special diet as ordered.
  a. Ensure that the patient is eating all meals.
  b. If all food is not ingested, provide appropriate substitutes according to the exchange lists or give measured amount of orange juice to substitute for left-over food; provide snack later in the day.
 3. Monitor urine sugar and acetone (second voided specimen).
 4. Perform fingersticks to check blood glucose levels as ordered.
 5. Observe for signs of hypo/hyperglycemia.
 6. Provide meticulous skin care and prevent injury.
 7. Maintain I&O; weigh daily.
 8. Provide emotional support; assist patient in adapting to change in life-style and body image.
 9. Observe for chronic complications and plan care accordingly.
  a. Atherosclerosis: leads to coronary artery disease, MI, CVA, and peripheral vascular disease.
  b. Microangiopathy: most commonly affects eyes and kidneys.
  c. Kidney disease
   1) recurrent pyelonephritis
   2) diabetic nephropathy
  d. Ocular disorders
   1) premature cataracts
   2) diabetic retinopathy
  e. Peripheral neuropathy
   1) affects peripheral and autonomic nervous systems.
   2) causes diarrhea, constipation, neurogenic bladder, impotence, decreased sweating.
 10. Provide patient teaching and discharge planning concerning
  a. Disease process
  b. Diet

1) patient should be able to plan meals using exchange lists before discharge.

2) emphasize importance of regularity of meals; never skip meals.

c. Insulin

1) how to draw up into syringe

a) use insulin at room temperature.

b) gently roll vial between palms of hands.

c) draw up insulin using sterile technique.

d) if mixing insulins, draw up clear insulin before cloudy insulin.

2) injection technique

a) systematically rotate sites to prevent lipodystrophy (hypertrophy or atrophy of tissue).

b) insert needle at a 90° angle.

3) may store current vial of insulin at room temperature; refrigerate extra supplies.

4) provide many opportunities for return demonstration.

d. Oral hypoglycemic agents

1) stress importance of taking the drug regularly.

2) avoid alcohol intake since a disulfiram (Antabuse)-like reaction may occur.

e. Urine testing

1) perform tests before meals and at bedtime.

2) use second voided specimen.

3) be consistent in brand of urine test used.

4) report results in percentages.

5) report to physician if results are greater than 1%, especially if experiencing symptoms of hyperglycemia.

f. General care

1) perform good oral hygiene and have regular dental exams.

2) have regular eye exams.

3) care for "sick days" (e.g., cold or flu)

a) do not omit insulin or oral hypoglycemic agents since infection causes increased blood sugar.

b) if nausea or vomiting occurs, sip clear liquids (provide patient with information on acceptable clear liquid diet).

c) test urine for sugar and acetone at least 4 times a day.

d) notify physician if necessary.

g. Foot care

1) wash feet with mild soap and water and pat dry.

2) apply lanolin to feet to prevent drying and cracking.

3) cut toenails straight across.

4) avoid constricting garments such as garters.

5) wear clean, absorbent socks (cotton or wool).

6) purchase properly fitting shoes and break new shoes in gradually.

7) never go barefoot.

8) inspect feet daily and notify physician if cuts, blisters, or breaks in skin occur.

h. Exercise

1) undertake regular exercise; avoid sporadic, vigorous exercise.

2) food intake may need to be increased before exercising.

3) exercise is best performed after meals when the blood sugar is rising.

i. Complications

1) learn to recognize signs and symptoms of hypo/hyperglycemia.

2) eat candy or drink orange juice with sugar added for insulin reaction (hypoglycemia).

j. Need to wear a Medic-Alert bracelet.

Ketoacidosis (DKA)

A. General information

1. Acute complication of diabetes mellitus characterized by hyperglycemia and accumulation of ketones in the body; causes metabolic acidosis

2. Occurs in insulin-dependent diabetics

3. Precipitating factors: undiagnosed diabetes, neglect of treatment; infection, cardiovascular disorder; other physical or emotional stress

4. Onset slow, may be hours to days

B. Assessment findings

1. Polydipsia, polyphagia, polyuria

2. Nausea, vomiting, abdominal pain

2. Skin warm, dry, and flushed

3. Dry mucous membranes; soft eyeballs

4. Kussmaul's respirations or tachypnea; acetone breath

5. Alterations in LOC

6. Hypotension, tachycardia

7. Diagnostic tests

a. Serum glucose and ketones elevated

b. BUN, creatinine, Hct elevated (due to dehydration)

c. Serum sodium decreased, potassium (may be normal or elevated at first)

d. ABGs: metabolic acidosis with compensatory respiratory alkalosis

C. Nursing interventions

1. Maintain a patent airway.

2. Maintain fluid and electrolyte balance.

a. Administer IV therapy as ordered.

1) normal saline (0.9% NaCl), then hypotonic (0.45% NaCl) sodium chloride

2) when blood sugar drops to 250 mg/dl, may add 5% dextrose to IV.

3) potassium will be added when the urine output is adequate.

b. Observe for fluid and electrolyte imbalances, especially fluid overload, hypokalemia, and hyperkalemia.

3. Administer insulin as ordered.

a. Regular insulin IV (drip or push) and/or subcutaneously (SC).

b. If given IV drip, give with small amounts of albumin since insulin adheres to IV tubing.

   c. Monitor blood sugar levels frequently.

4. Monitor urine for sugar and acetone frequently.

5. Check urine output every hour.

6. Monitor vital signs.

7. Assist patient with self-care.

8. Provide care for the unconscious patient if in a coma (page 47).

9. Discuss with patient the reasons ketosis developed and provide additional diabetic teaching if indicated.

Insulin Reaction/Hypoglycemia

A. General information

   1. Abnormally low blood sugar, usually below 50 mg/dl

   2. Usually caused by insulin overdosage, too little food, nutritional and fluid imbalances from nausea and vomiting, excessive exercise

   3. Onset rapid; may develop in minutes to hours

B. Assessment findings

   1. Headache, dizziness, difficulty problem solving, restlessness, hunger, visual disturbances

   2. Slurred speech; alterations in gait; decreasing LOC; pallor; cold, clammy skin; diaphoresis

   3. Diagnostic test: serum glucose level 50–60 mg/dl or lower

C. Nursing interventions

   1. Administer oral sugar in the form of candy or orange juice with sugar added if the patient is alert.

   2. If the patient is unconscious, administer 20–50 cc 50% dextrose IV push, or 1 mg glucagon IM, IV, or SC, as ordered.

   3. Explore with patient reasons for hypoglycemia and provide additional diabetic teaching as indicated

Hyperglycemic Hyperosmolar Nonketotic Coma (HHNK)

A. General information

   1. Complication of diabetes, characterized by hyperglycemia and a hyperosmolar state without ketosis

   2. Occurs in non-insulin-dependent diabetics or nondiabetic persons (typically elderly patients)

   3. Precipitating factors: undiagnosed diabetes; infections or other stress; certain medications (e.g., dilantin, thiazide diuretics); dialysis; hyperalimentation; major burns; pancreatic disease

B. Assessment findings

   1. Similar to ketoacidosis but without Kussmaul respirations and acetone breath

   2. Laboratory tests

      a. Blood glucose level extremely elevated

      b. BUN, creatinine, Hct elevated (due to dehydration)

      c. Urine positive for glucose

C. Nursing interventions: treatment and nursing care is similar to DKA, excluding measures to treat ketosis and metabolic acidosis.

SAMPLE QUESTIONS

Mrs. Annette Duprey, 57 years old, was admitted to the hospital for uncontrolled diabetes. Lab studies reveal a fasting blood sugar of 310. Her admission diagnosis is Type I diabetes mellitus.

16. Mrs. Duprey needs to understand that the type of diabetes that she has

   ○ 1. is associated with the destruction of beta cells.

   ○ 2. usually causes complete fat metabolism.

   ○ 3. often occurs in obese individuals.

   ○ 4. is rarely controlled.

17. Mrs. Duprey asks why she must mix two insulins. The nurse explains that regular insulin is added to NPH to ensure

   ○ 1. immediate onset of the regular insulin.

   ○ 2. onset of the regular insulin within 2 hours.

   ○ 3. a peak action of the NPH insulin at 2 hours.

   ○ 4. a total duration of action of 24 hours.

The Integumentary System

OVERVIEW OF ANATOMY AND PHYSIOLOGY

The integumentary system consists of the skin and its appendages, such as hair, nails, and various glands. The integumenary system not only provides a barrier against the external environment, it also plays a role in maintenance of the body's internal environment.

Skin

A. Functions
   1. Protection: barrier to noxious agents (microorganisms, parasites, chemical substances) and to loss of water and electrolytes
   2. Thermoregulation: radiant cooling, evaporation
   3. Sensory perception: touch, temperature, pressure, pain
   4. Metabolism: excretion of water and sodium, production of vitamin D, wound repair

B. Layers
   1. *Epidermis*
      a. The avascular outermost layer
      b. Stratified into several layers
      c. Composed mainly of keratinocytes and melanocytes
         1) keratinocytes produce *keratin*, responsible for formation of hair and nails
         2) melanocytes produce *melanin*, a pigment that gives color to skin and hair
      d. Appendages (hair and nails, eccrine sweat glands, sebaceous glands, apocrine sweat glands) all derived from epidermis
   2. *Dermis:* layer beneath the epidermis composed of connective tissue that contains lymphatics, nerves, and blood vessels; elasticity of skin results from presence of collagen, elastin, and reticular fibers in the dermis, which also nourish the epidermis
   3. *Subcutaneous layer:* layer beneath the dermis composed of loose connective tissue and fat cells; stores fat; important in temperature regulation

Hair

A. Covers most of the body surface (except palms of hands, soles of feet, lips, nipples, and parts of external genitalia)
B. *Hair follicles:* tube-like structures, derived from epidermis, from which hair grows
C. Hair functions as protection from external elements and from trauma.
D. Hair growth is controlled by hormonal influences and by blood supply.
E. Loss of body hair is called *alopecia*.

Nails

A. Dense layer of flat, dead, cells; filled with keratin
B. Systemic illnesses may be reflected by changes in the nail or its bed; common changes include
   1. *Clubbing:* enlargement of fingers and toes, nail becomes convex; caused by chronic pulmonary or cardiovascular disease
   2. *Beau's line:* transverse groove caused by temporary halt in nail growth because of systemic disorder

Glands

A. *Eccrine sweat glands:* located all over the body; participate in heat regulation
B. *Apocrine sweat glands:* odiferous glands, found primarily in axillary, nipple, anal, and pubic areas; bacterial decomposition of excretions causes body odor.
C. *Sebaceous glands:* oil glands, located all over the body except for palms of hands and soles of feet (abundant on face, scalp, upper chest, and back); produce *sebum.*

ASSESSMENT

Health History

A. Presenting problem: symptoms may include changes in color or texture of skin, hair, nails; pruritus; infections; tumors; lesions; dermatitis; ecchymoses; rashes; dryness

B. Life-style: hygienic practices (skin-cleansing measures, use of cosmetics [type, brand names]); skin exposure (duration of exposure to sun, irritants [occupational] cold weather)

C. Nutrition/diet: intake of vitamins, essential nutrients, water; food allergies

D. Use of medications: steroids, vitamin use, hormones, antibiotics, chemotherapeutic agents

E. Past medical history: renal, hepatic, or collagen diseases; trauma or surgery; food, drug, or contact allergies

F. Family history: diabetes mellitus, allergic disorders, blood dyscrasias, specific dermatologic problems, cancer

Physical Examination

A. Color: note areas of uniform color; pigmentation; redness, jaundice, cyanosis.

B. Vascular changes
   1. Purpuric lesions: note ecchymoses, petechiae.
   2. Vascular lesions: note angiomas, hemangiomas, venous stars.

C. Lesions: note color, type (see page 179), size, distribution, location, consistency, grouping (annular, circular, linear, or clustered).

D. Edema: differentiate pitting from nonpitting.

E. Moisture content: note dryness, clamminess.

F. Temperature: note whether increased or decreased, distribution of temperature changes.

G. Texture: note smoothness, coarseness.

H. Mobility/turgor: note whether increased or decreased.

Laboratory/Diagnostic Studies

A. Blood chemistry/electrolytes: calcium, chloride, magnesium, potassium, sodium

B. Hematologic studies: Hbg, Hct, RBC, WBC

C. Biopsy
   1. Removal of a small piece of skin for examination to determine diagnosis
   2. Nursing care: instruct patient to keep biopsied area dry until healing occurs.

D. Skin testing
   1. Administration of allergens or antigens on the surface of or into the dermis to determine hypersensitivity
   2. Three types: patch, scratch, and intradermal

ANALYSIS

Nursing diagnoses for patients with a disorder of the integumentary system may include

A. Alteration in comfort: pain

B. Impairment of skin integrity

C. Alteration in nutrition: less than body requirements

D. Alteration in tissue perfusion

E. Alteration in respiratory function: ineffective breathing pattern

F. Disturbance in self-concept: body image

PLANNING AND IMPLEMENTATION

Goals

A. Patient will have decreased pain.

B. Burn, graft, and skin lesions will heal.

C. Patient will maintain adequate nutritional status.

D. Patient will maintain adequate tissue perfusion.

E. Patient will maintain adequate respiratory function.

F. Patient will adapt to changes in appearance.

Interventions

Skin Grafts

A. Replacement of damaged skin with healthy skin to provide protection of underlying structures or to reconstruct areas for cosmetic or functional purposes

B. Graft sources
   1. *Autograft:* patient's own skin
   2. *Isograft:* skin from a genetically identical person (identical twin)
   3. *Homograft or allograft:* cadaver of same species
   4. *Heterograft or xenograft:* skin from another species (such as a porcine graft)
   5. *Human amniotic membrane*

C. Nursing care: preoperative
   1. Donor site: cleanse with antiseptic soap the night before and morning of surgery as ordered.
   2. Recipient site: apply warm compresses and topical antibiotics as ordered.

D. Nursing care: postoperative
   1. Donor site
      a. Keep area covered for 24–48 hours.
      b. Use bed cradle to prevent pressure and provide greater air circulation
      c. Outer dressing may be removed 24–72 hours postsurgery; maintain fine mesh gauze (innermost dressing) until it falls off spontaneously.
      d. Trim loose edges of gauze as it loosens with healing.
      e. Administer analgesics as ordered (more painful than recipient site).
   2. Recipient site
      a. Elevate site when possible.
      b. Protect from pressure (use bed cradle).
      c. Apply warm compresses as ordered.
      d. Assess for hematoma, fluid accumulation under graft.
      e. Monitor circulation distal to graft.
   3. Provide emotional support and monitor behavioral adjustments; refer for counseling if needed.

E. Provide patient teaching and discharge planning concerning
   1. Applying lubricating lotion to maintain moisture on surfaces of healed graft for at least 6–12 months
   2. Protecting grafted skin from direct sunlight for at least 6 months
   3. Protecting graft from physical injury

4. Need to report changes in graft (fluid accumulation, pain, hematoma)
5. Possible alteration in pigmentation and hair growth; ability to sweat lost in most grafts
6. Sensations may or may not return.

EVALUATION

A. Patient verbalizes pain relief, has relaxed facial expression.
B. Patient has decreased redness, discharge, and discomfort; presence of granulation tissue in healing wounds.
C. Serum proteins and cholesterol are normal; weight returns to pre-burn level; patient has usual strength and activity.
D. Skin is warm and has usual color.
   1. Pedal pulses palpable
   2. Capillary refill less than 3 seconds
   3. Blood pressure and pulse within normal limits
E. Patient has normal rate, rhythm, and depth of respirations, improved breath sounds and arterial blood gases.
F. Patient participates actively in ADL and social activities; shows active interest in personal appearance.

DISORDERS OF THE INTEGUMENTARY SYSTEM

Primary Lesions of the Skin

A. *Macule:* a flat, circumscribed area of color change in the skin without surface elevation, up to 2 cm in diameter
B. *Papule:* a circumscribed solid and elevated lesion, up to 1 cm in size
C. *Nodule:* a solid, elevated lesion extending deeper into the dermis, 1–2 cm in diameter
D. *Wheal:* a slightly irregular, transient superficial elevation of the skin with a palpable margin (e.g., hive)
E. *Vesicle:* circumscribed elevated lesion filled with serous fluid, less than 1 cm in diameter
F. *Bulla:* a vesicle larger than 1 cm in diameter
G. *Pustule:* a vesicle or bulla containing purulent exudate

Contact Dermatitis

A. General information
   1. An irritation of the skin from a specific substance or from a hypersensitivity immune reaction from contact with a specific antigen
   2. Caused by irritants (mechanical, chemical, biologic); allergens
B. Assessment findings
   1. Pruritus
   2. Erythema; localized edema; vesicles (oozing, crusting, and scaling [later])
   3. Diagnostic test: skin testing reveals hypersensitivity to specific antigen
C. Nursing interventions

1. Promote healing of lesions with application of wet dressings of Burrow's solution for 20 minutes 4 times a day.
2. Provide relief from pruritus (see Cirrhosis of the Liver, page 132).
3. Administer topical steroids and antibiotics as ordered.
4. Provide patient teaching and discharge planning concerning
   a. Avoidance of causative agent
   b. Preventing skin dryness
      1) use mild soaps (Ivory).
      2) soak in plain water for 20–30 minutes.
      3) apply prescribed steroid cream immmediately after bath.
      4) avoid extremes of heat and cold.
   c. Allowing crusts and scales to drop off skin naturally as healing occurs
   d. Avoidance of wool, nylon, or fur fibers on sensitive skin
   e. Need to use gloves if handling irritant or allergenic substances.

Psoriasis

A. General information
   1. Chronic type of dermatitis that involves accelerated turnover rate of the epidermal cells
   2. Predisposing factors include stress, trauma, infection; changes in climate may produce exacerbations; familial predisposition to the disease
B. Medical management
   1. Topical corticosteroids
   2. Coal tar preparations
   3. Ultraviolet light
   4. Antimetabolites (methotrexate)
C. Assessment findings
   1. Mild pruritus
   2. Sharply circumscribed scaling placques that are mostly present on the scalp, elbows, and knees; yellow discoloration of nails
D. Nursing interventions
   1. Apply occlusive wraps over prescribed topical steroids.
   2. Protect areas treated with coal tar preparations from direct sunlight for 24 hours.
   3. Administer methotrexate as ordered, assess for side effects.
   4. Provide patient teaching and discharge planning concerning
      a. Feelings about changes in appearance of skin (encourage patient to cover arms and legs with clothing if sensitive about appearance)
      b. Importance of adhering to prescribed treatment and avoidance of commercially advertised products.

Acne

See page 355.

Pediculosis

See page 354.

Skin Cancer

A. General information
  1. Types of skin cancers
     a. *Basal cell epithelioma:* most common type of skin cancer; locally invasive and rarely metastasizes; most frequently located between the hairline and upper lip
     b. *Squamous cell carcinoma (epidermoid):* grows more rapidly than basal cell carcinoma and can metastasize; frequently seen on mucous membranes, lower lip, neck, and dorsum of the hands
     c. *Malignant melanoma:* least frequent of skin cancers, but most serious; capable of invasion and metastasis to other organs
  2. Precancerous lesions
     a. *Leukoplakia:* white, shiny patches in the mouth and on the lip
     b. *Nevi (moles):* junctional nevus may become malignant (signs include a color change to black, bleeding and irritation); compound and dermal nevi unlikely to become cancerous
     c. *Senile keratoses:* brown, scalelike spots on older individuals
  3. Contributing factors include hereditary predisposition (fair, blue-eyed people; redheads and blondes); irritation (chemicals or ultraviolet rays)
  4. Occurs more often in those with outdoor occupations who are exposed to more sunlight.
B. Medical management: varies depending on type of cancer; surgical excision with or without radiation therapy most common; chemotherapy and immunotherapy for melanoma
C. Assessment findings: characteristics depend on specific type of lesion; biopsy reveals malignant cells
D. Nursing interventions: provide patient teaching concerning
  1. Limitation of contact with chemical irritants
  2. Protection against ultraviolet radiation from sun
     a. Wear thin layer of clothing.
     b. Use sun block or lotion containing para-amino benzoic acid (PABA).
  3. Need to report lesions that change characteristics and/or those that do not heal.

Herpes Zoster (Shingles)

A. General information
  1. Acute viral infection of the nervous system
  2. The virus causes an inflammatory reaction in isolated spinal and cranial sensory ganglia and the posterior gray matter of the spinal cord.
  3. Contagious to anyone who has not had varicella or who is immunosuppressed
  4. Caused by activation of latent varicella-zoster virus
B. Medical management
  1. Analgesics

  2. Corticosteroids
  3. Acetic acid compresses
C. Assessment findings
  1. Neuralgic pain, malaise, itching, burning
  2. Cluster of skin vesicles along course of peripheral sensory nerves, usually unilateral and primarily on trunk, thorax, or face
D. Nursing interventions
  1. Apply acetic acid compresses or white petrolatum to lesions.
  2. Administer medications as ordered.
     a. Analgesics for pain
     b. Systemic corticosteroids: monitor for side effects of steroid therapy (see page 165).

Herpes Simplex Virus, Type I

A. General information
  1. Causes cold sores or fever blisters, canker sores, and herpetic whitlow
  2. Common disorder, frequently seen in women
  3. Primary infection occurs in children, recurrences in adults
  4. Self-limiting virus
B. Assessment findings: clusters of vesicles, may ulcerate or crust; burning, itching, tingling; usually appears on lip or cheek
C. Nursing interventions: keep lesions dry; apply topical antibiotics or anesthetic as ordered.

Burns

A. Types
  1. Thermal: most common type; caused by flame, flash, scalding, and contact (hot metals, grease)
  2. Smoke inhalation: occurs when smoke (particulate products of a fire, gases, and superheated air) causes respiratory tissue damage
  3. Chemical: caused by tissue contact, ingestion or inhalation of acids, alkalies, or vesicants
  4. Electrical: injury occurs from direct damage to nerves and vessels when an electric current passes through the body.
B. Classification
  1. *Partial thickness*
     a. Superficial (first degree)
        1) depth: epidermis only
        2) causes: sunburn, splashes of hot liquid
        3) sensation: painful
        4) characteristics: erythema, blanching on pressure, no vesicles
     b. Deep (second degree)
        1) depth: epidermis and dermis
        2) causes: flash, scalding, or flame burn
        3) sensation: very painful
        4) characteristics: fluid-filled vesicles; red, shiny, wet after vesicles rupture
  2. *Full thickness* (third and fourth degree)
     a. Depth: all skin layers and nerve endings; may involve muscles, tendons, and bones

    b. Causes: flame, chemicals, scalding, electric current

    c. Sensation: little or no pain

    d. Characteristics: wound is dry, white, leathery, or hard

C. Medical managaement

    1. Supportive therapy: fluid management (IVs), catheterization

    2. Wound care: tubbing, debridement (enzymatic or surgical)

    3. Drug therapy

        a. Topical antibiotics: mafenide (Sulfamylon), silver sulfadiazine (Silvadene), silver nitrate, povidone-iodine (Betadine) solution

        b. Systemic antibiotics: gentamicin

        c. Tetanus toxoid or hyperimmune human tetanus globulin (burn wound good medium for anaerobic growth)

        d. Analgesics

    4. Surgery: excision and grafting

D. Assessment

    1. Extent of burn injury by rule of nines: head and neck (9%); each arm (9%), each leg (18%), trunk (36%), genitalia (1%)

    2. Severity of burn

        a. Major: partial thickness greater than 25%; full thickness greater than or equal to l0%

        b. Moderate: partial thickness 15%–25%; full thickness less than 10%

        c. Minor: partial thickness less than 15%; full thickness less than 2%

E. Stages

    1. *Emergent phase*

        a. Remove person from source of burn.

            1) thermal: smother burn beginning with the head.

            2) smoke inhalation: ensure patent airway.

            3) chemical: remove clothing that contains chemical; lavage area with copious amounts of water.

            4) electrical: note victim position, identify entry/exit routes, maintain airway.

        b. Wrap in dry, clean sheet or blanket to prevent further contamination of wound and provide warmth.

        c. Assess how and when burn occurred.

        d. Provide IV route if possible.

        e. Transport immediately.

    2. *Shock phase* (first 24–48 hours)

        a. Plasma to interstitial fluid shift causing hypovolemia; fluid also moves to areas that normally have little or no fluid (third-spacing).

        b. Assessment findings

            1) dehydration, decreased blood pressure, elevated pulse, decreased urine output, thirst

            2) diagnostic tests: hyperkalemia, hyponatremia, elevated Hct, metabolic acidosis

    3. *Fluid remobilization or diuretic phase* (2–5 days post-burn)

        a. Interstitial fluid returns to the vascular compartment.

        b. Assessment findings

            1) elevated blood pressure, increased urine output

            2) diagnostic tests: hypokalemia, hyponatremia, metabolic acidosis

    4. *Convalescent phase*

        a. Starts when diuresis is completed and wound healing and coverage begin.

        b. Assessment findings

            1) dry, waxy-white appearance of full thickness burn changing to dark brown; wet, shiny and serous exudate in partial thickness

            2) diagnostic test: hyponatremia

F. Nursing interventions

    1. Provide relief/control of pain.

        a. Administer morphine sulfate IV and monitor vital signs closely.

        b. Administer analgesics/narcotics 30 minutes before wound care.

        c. Position burned areas in proper alignment.

    2. Monitor alterations in fluid and electrolyte balance.

        a. Assess for fluid shifts and electrolyte alterations (see Table 2.6, page 24).

        b. Monitor Foley catheter output hourly (30 cc/hour desired).

        c. Weigh daily.

        d. Monitor circulation status regularly.

        e. Administer/monitor crystalloids/colloids/H_2O solutions.

    3. Promote maximal nutritional status.

        a. Monitor tube feedings/TPN if ordered.

        b. When oral intake permitted, provide high-calorie, high-protein, high-carbohydrate diet, with vitamin and mineral supplements.

        c. Serve small portions.

        d. Schedule wound care and other treatments at least 1 hour before meals.

    4. Prevent wound infection.

        a. Place patient in controlled sterile environment.

        b. Use hydrotherapy for no more than 30 minutes.

        c. Observe wound for separation of eschar and cellulitis.

        d. Apply mafenide (Sulfamylon) as ordered.

            1) administer analgesics 30 minutes before application.

            2) monitor acid-base status and renal function studies.

            3) provide daily tubbing for removal of previously applied cream.

        e. Apply silver sulfadiazine (Silvadene) as ordered.

            1) administer analgesics 30 minutes before application.

            2) observe for and report hypersensitivity reactions (rash, itching, burning sensation in unburned areas).

            3) store drug away from heat.

        f. Apply silver nitrate as ordered.

            1) handle carefully; solution leaves a gray or black stain on skin, clothing, and utensils.

            2) administer analgesic before application.

            3) keep dressings wet with solution; dryness increases the concentration and causes precipitation of silver salts in the wound.

        g. Apply povidone-iodine (Betadine) solution as ordered.

1) administer analgesics before application.
2) assess for metabolic acidosis/renal function studies.
h. Administer gentamicin as ordered: assess vestibular/auditory and renal functions at regular intervals.

5. Prevent GI complications.
  a. Assess for signs and symptoms of paralytic ileus.
  b. Assist with insertion of NG tube to prevent/control Curling's/stress ulcer; monitor patency/drainage.
  c. Administer prophylactic antacids through NG tube and/or IV cimetidine (to prevent gastric pH of less than 5).
  d. Monitor bowel sounds.
  e. Test stools for occult blood.

6. Provide patient teaching and discharge planning concerning
  a. Care of healed burn wound
    1) assess daily for changes.
    2) wash hands frequently during dressing change.
    3) wash area with prescribed solution or mild soap and rinse well with H_2O; dry with clean towel.
    4) apply sterile dressing.
  b. Prevention of injury to burn wound
    1) avoid trauma to area.
    2) avoid use of fabric softeners or harsh detergents (might cause irritation).
    3) avoid constrictive clothing over burn wound.
  c. Adherence to prescribed diet
  d. Importance of reporting formation of blisters, opening of healed area, increased or foul-smelling drainage from wound, other signs of infection.
  e. Methods of coping and resocialization.

SAMPLE QUESTIONS

Mr. Simon Wells, 37 years old, is seen in the outpatient clinic for treatment of psoriasis.

18. The nurse should anticipate which of the following findings in Mr. Wells?
    o 1. Intense pain
    o 2. Discoloured nails
    o 3. Abdominal lesions
    o 4. Hyperpigmented skin

19. The physician prescribes coal tar preparations as part of the treatment plan. The nurse should include which statement in her teaching plan for Mr. Wells?
    o 1. Avoid sunlight immediately after the treatment.
    o 2. Ingest the coal tar with liberal amounts of water.
    o 3. Eat a high-carbohydrate diet.
    o 4. Restrict activity for 24 hours.

UNIT 2: Reprints

Are you ready for this bedside emergency?

This first installment in a new series deals with wound dehiscence and evisceration—potentially fatal postop complications. Learn what fast actions to take and which patients are at risk.

By Sandy L. Sarsany, RN, CCRN

Rachel Andrews, 61 years old, seemed to be making an uneventful recovery from emergency surgery to relieve a bowel obstruction. During the evening of her fifth postop day, however, she felt something pop when she coughed. She called for her nurse to check her incision.

The first thing the nurse noticed was a serosanguineous or reddish-yellow stain spreading across the front of her patient's gown. When she lifted the gown, her fear was confirmed—Mrs. Andrews had a complete wound dehiscence. The peritoneal and fascial edges of her incision had split open.

Mrs. Andrews was now at risk for evisceration—the protrusion of the intestines through the open abdominal wound. Though rare, this very serious complication can lead to infection, shock, and sometimes, even death.

Although wound dehiscence and evisceration can happen anytime

THE AUTHOR, a flight nurse at University Hospital in Cleveland, wrote this article while working as a critical care instructor at Trumbull Memorial Hospital in Warren, Ohio.

Produced by Mary-Beth Moriarty, RN, CCRN

after surgery, they most frequently occur five to eight days postop. You're not likely to see complete wound dehiscence or evisceration very often—for every 200 patients who have surgery, only one or two develop these complications. Certain patients are more at risk because of their age, nutritional status, and medical history. (See page 34 for details.)

If faced with this emergency, would you know what to do? Compare your response with that of Mrs. Andrews' nurse.

Keep the patient calm to prevent evisceration

The nurse called for help but remained with Mrs. Andrews. Although dehiscence seldom causes pain, it is a frightening experience. The nurse explained what had happened, reassured Mrs. Andrews that her surgeon would be in to see her soon, and prepared her for the possibility of additional surgery.

She asked Mrs. Andrews to stay quiet. Any sudden strain—even a cough or a sneeze—can increase in-

tra-abdominal pressure and cause evisceration. To relax abdominal muscles and lessen intra-abdominal pressure, the nurse placed Mrs. Andrews in semi-Fowler's position with her knees slightly bent.

As the nurse started to apply sterile gauze dressings to the edges of the wound and a binder for added support, Mrs. Andrews coughed. The nurse immediately placed her gloved hands on either side of the wound to provide support. Despite her efforts, several small loops of bowel could now be seen in the wound.

The nurse did not try to push the intestines back into the abdomen. Instead, she covered the exposed bowel with sterile gauze. To keep the intestinal mucosa moist and to prevent infection, she wet the dressings with sterile saline and covered them with sterile towels.

Coping with a crisis takes a team effort

In the midst of this, a second nurse had responded and was handling other essential tasks. She alerted

Identifying patients at risk for dehiscence

Postop wound dehiscence is rare, but certain conditions that can delay healing put some patients at greater risk than others. Here are the factors to consider:

▶ Age. Dehiscence occurs most often in the elderly. Patients over 45 are four times more likely to develop wound separation.

▶ Medication. Steroids such as hydrocortisone and prednisone interfere with the body's metabolism and therefore delay wound-healing.

▶ Malnutrition. A lack of protein and vitamins, especially vitamin C, impairs collagen production, making wounds less able to withstand tension. Conditions that will influence a patient's nutritional status—anemia, cancer, dia-

betes, liver or kidney disease, and GI surgery—increase a patient's risks for malnutrition and wound dehiscence.

▶ Infection. Enzymes produced by bacteria can damage tissues.

▶ Smoking. Peripheral vasoconstriction decreases blood supply and oxygen delivery to the wound. Coughing—a common problem for smokers—will increase the intra-abdominal pressure. That, in turn, increases tension on the wound.

▶ Wound location. A vertical abdominal incision is more likely to disrupt nerves and blood vessels, and, therefore, more likely to eviscerate. Vertical sutures create a greater pull on abdominal muscles, making a wound separation more likely.

---

the head nurse to the emergency and then brought needed supplies to the room.

The second nurse started monitoring Mrs. Andrews' vital signs. She watched for changes in heart rate and blood pressure that could signal the onset of shock. She inserted an IV line for the infusion of blood and fluids during surgery.

She made sure a nasogastric tube and suction equipment were on hand in case the surgeon wished to insert the tube before taking Mrs. Andrews to the OR. The nurse did not attempt to insert the NG tube before the physician arrived. Doing so could have caused Mrs. Andrews

to cough, which would have increased the evisceration.

Moving Mrs. Andrews onto a stretcher would have placed further strain on her wound, so the two nurses helped transport the patient to the OR in her bed.

In the OR, the surgeon returned the bowel to its correct postion and closed the wound with retention sutures. This type of suture passes through all layers of the abdominal wall, reducing the chance of recurrent dehiscence. If the exposed bowel had been edematous or the wound infected, the surgeon might have closed the fascia but left the remaining layers open with sterile

packing in place until the edema or infection cleared.

Take steps to prevent recurrent dehiscence

When Mrs. Andrews came back from surgery, the nurse monitored her vital signs, respiratory status, and urine output—all part of a standard postop assessment.

The nurse inspected the wound at least every two hours. She looked for signs of infection, wound separation, and edema, especially around the retention sutures. The nurse gave Mrs. Andrews IV antibiotics as ordered to prevent infection. She documented and reported any changes to the doctor immediately. She also checked for abdominal distention and made sure the NG tube was draining properly.

Mrs. Andrews was given pain medication as needed. The nurse showed Mrs. Andrews how to use a pillow and her hands to support her incision when she coughed.

Mrs. Andrews made a slow but steady recovery from her second surgery. The edges of her wound did separate. But this problem was quickly reported to the surgeon. He closed the edges with Steri-Strips and the wound healed completely. Her nurse's quick response in an emergency and the careful follow-up care helped Mrs. Andrews avoid the serious complications often associated with wound dehiscence and evisceration. ■

Morphine: The benefits are worth the risks

Though morphine can control cancer pain, many doctors and nurses hesitate to use it because of its side effects. Here's what you need to know to give this drug, derived from the opium poppy, safely and effectively.

By Susan J. Brown,
RN, MSN, OCN

Morphine is the most feared of all narcotic analgesics. It has acquired this unfortunate reputation because of one particular side effect—respiratory depression—and its potential for abuse and addiction.

To avoid these problems, physicians often prescribe ineffective amounts of morphine and some nurses administer these doses less frequently than prescribed, causing patients to suffer needlessly. Their pain could be relieved safely with morphine if doctors and nurses knew more about the drug than just its reputation.

Pain is an excruciatingly personal experience. Unrelieved, it can become the focal point of a patient's life—nothing else will matter. The kind of pain control that you can sometimes get only with morphine allows a patient to reclaim his humanity and get on with the business of living.

While nurses don't prescribe morphine, we do play an important role in administering it and evaluating its effectiveness. By knowing why morphine works, how to administer it effectively, and when to be concerned about its side effects, we can help our patients achieve better pain control.

Why morphine relieves pain

A chemical derivative of opium, morphine binds at specific sites—the opioid receptors, which are located primarily in the brain and spinal cord. The binding process alters the biochemical reactions that occur in response to pain, interfering with the conduction of painful stimuli and raising the body's pain threshold.

Morphine also produces changes in a patient's emotional status—a patient taking the drug doesn't perceive pain as being severe. This unique ability to create indifference to pain makes morphine—and other drugs like it—a very powerful analgesic.

How to administer morphine effectively

The route of administration, the dose, and the time interval between doses can all influence morphine's ability to control pain. The drug can be administered several ways—by mouth, by intramuscular or subcutaneous injection, and by intermittent or continuous epidural, intrathecal, intravenous, or subcutaneous infusion. It can even be given as a rectal suppository.

The route selected depends on the severity of pain, the previous use of analgesics, the patient's ability to swallow, the presence or absence of nausea, vomiting, or a low platelet count, and the availability of muscle mass or venous access.

The more direct the delivery route, the smaller the dose of morphine required. When the drug is given intrathecally, for example, minute doses—0.2 to 1 mg—can control pain for up to 24 hours. That's because the drug, when injected into cerebrospinal fluid, bypasses the bloodstream and travels directly to the opioid receptors.

When morphine is absorbed into the bloodstream from the gastroin-

THE AUTHOR, an oncology clinical nurse specialist, is assistant director of oncology at St. Francis Medical Center in Trenton, N.J.

Produced by Mary-Beth Moriarty, RN, CCRN

testinal tract—as it would be if the drug were given orally—it travels first to the liver, where it's metabolized. This means up to 50% of the morphine may be inactivated before it reaches the rest of the body—the so-called "first pass effect." Thus higher doses are needed when morphine is given orally.

Delays affect pain control

No matter what the delivery route or how large the dose, morphine must be administered when it's needed for effective pain control. Delays can increase a patient's anxiety, and that in turn can increase his pain.

Around-the-clock adminstration is more effective than prn administration. This method not only eliminates delays but also helps maintain a constant serum level of the drug, leading to better pain control. Studies have shown, moreover, that patients who receive morphine on a regular schedule use smaller amounts while experiencing greater pain relief.

To avoid an accidental overdose, it's important to know how long the effects of morphine last—the duration of action—with each of the various routes of adminstration. For example, a single dose of intrathecal morphine can be effective for as long as 24 hours. But when the drug is given intravenously, a dose may be effective for no more than two to four hours.

Some patients are started on morphine because other analgesics have not relieved their pain. In that case, you can use an equianalgesic chart to determine how much

How to use an equianalgesic chart

To change the route of administration or to switch to a different pain medication altogether, you can use an equianalgesic chart to determine the correct dose. While nurses do not prescribe such changes, knowing equivalent doses can help you evaluate a patient's response to a change in medication.

Assume your patient has been receiving meperidine 75 mg IM but is being switched to morphine. By using an equianalgesic chart like the one shown below, you'd see that 10 mg would be the equivalent dose of IM morphine. If your patient had been getting 10 mg of morphine IM, the chart would tell you that the equivalent oral dose would be 60 mg.

The doses shown here come from an equianalgesic chart prepared by the Sloan-Kettering Institute for Cancer Research.

Generic name (trade name)	Intramuscular dose (mg)	Oral dose (mg)
Morphine sulfate	10	60
Anileridine (Leritine)	30	50
Codeine	130	200
Hydromorphone (Dilaudid)	1.5	7.5
Levorphanol (Levo-Dromoran)	2	4
Meperidine (Demerol)	75	300
Methadone (Dolophine)	10	20
Oxycodone	—	30
Oxymorphone (Numorphan)	1	—
Pentazocine (Talwin)	60	180

morphine will be needed to equal the dose of the drug they had been receiving. One such chart is shown above.

The initial dose of morphine for such patients is usually greater than the equianalgesic dose. Once the patient's pain is under control, you can cut back on subsequent doses.

When to look for respiratory depression

The rule of thumb when working with morphine is to give no more than necessary to relieve pain. Since the response to morphine will vary with each patient, you'll need to assess each individual for pain and adjust the dose of morphine to meet his needs. You'll also need to

How much morphine does that patient need?

The amount of morphine required for adequate pain control will vary with each patient. While there is no clearcut way to determine how much morphine a patient needs, these guidelines will be helpful when therapy begins.

Route	Dose	Duration	Special concerns
Oral	Solutions: 10 mg/5 cc 20 mg/5 cc 20 mg/1 cc	4 to 6 hours	Dilute in juice before administering.
	Short-acting tablets: 15 mg 30 mg	4 to 6 hours	Can be crushed and mixed with food if the patient has trouble swallowing. Prn doses should be prescribed to relieve breakthrough pain.
	Sustained-release tablets: 30 mg	8 to 12 hours	Pain should be well controlled with short-acting morphine before using these tablets. Do not crush them. Do not give them more often than every 8 hours.
Rectal	Suppository: 5 mg 10 mg 20 mg	4 to 6 hours for single dose	
Injection	Subcutaneous: 5 to 20 mg based on 10 mg/70 kg	4 to 6 hours for single dose	Risk of respiratory side effects may last as long as 90 minutes after an injection. May be given as a continuous infusion.
	Intramuscular: Same dosage as subcutaneous route	4 to 6 hours	Risk of respiratory depression lasts up to 30 minutes after injection.
	Intravenous: Initial dose 2 to 10 mg/70 kg, then adjust to individual response. For continuous drip, mix 125 mg or 250 mg MS in 250 cc D_5W for a concentration of 0.5 to 1.0 mg/cc. Use a loading dose 1 mg to 5 mg prior to starting drip.	2 to 4 hours/ one dose	Dilute prior to injecting. To calculate drip rate, divide daily total dose by 24. If infusion infiltrates, restart drip at lower rate to prevent overdose until morphine in infiltrated tissue is absorbed. Risk of side effects is greatest 15 to 30 minutes after injection. Bolus injection rate is 1 mg/minute.
	Epidural: Initial dose 5 mg. Repeat doses 1 to 2 mg prn. Continuous drip 2 to 4 mg/24 hours. Maximum dose 10 mg/24 hours.	24 hours	Use only preservative-free preparations. Have naloxone and emergency equipment on hand in case of respiratory depression.
	Intrathecal: 0.2 mg to 1.0 mg	24 hours	Follow the same precautions as for epidural route. Not recommended for long-term use.

watch for side effects—especially respiratory depression.

Normally, an increase in carbon dioxide in the blood stimulates the respiratory center in the brain to increase the rate of breathing. Morphine depresses this response. The drug also depresses activity in the medullary and pontine centers that control the rhythm of breathing. The net result is a decrease in the rate and depth of respirations. Breathing can become irregular or periodic, and respiratory arrest can occur.

The risk of respiratory depression is greatest immediately after the first dose, when you give the drug intrathecally or epidurally, and when there's a change in the dose or route of administration.

Medication reverses morphine's effects

If respiratory depression does occur, mechanical ventilation may be required to support the patient until the effects of the drug wear off. Naloxone hydrocholoride (Narcan) 0.4 mg may be given intravenously to reverse the effects of morphine. The patient will still need close observation after naloxone is given, however. This drug's duration of action is shorter than morphine's, and additional doses may be needed to prevent respiratory depression from recurring.

If you must give naloxone to combat respiratory side effects, keep in mind that it also reverses pain control. The patient is able to breathe better, but he may also be in a great deal of pain. And, since naloxone also works at the opioid receptor sites, subsequent doses of pain medication may be less effective until all of the naloxone has

My wish for Willie

A widow shares how it feels when the health-care team is afraid to give morphine.
By Linda Henson

As my beloved husband lay dying of cancer, I had only one wish—that he would die in peace, free from the pain that wracked his body whenever his pain medication wore off.

My wish was not granted, however. Willie Henson died in excruciating pain. He should not have had to die that way.

Although the surgeons removed the cancer from Willie's colon, it had already spread. After months

THE AUTHOR is pursuing a bachelor's degree in nursing at Michigan State University.

Produced by Mary-Beth Moriarty, RN, CCRN

of chemotherapy treatments, his doctors decided the prognosis was hopeless, and Willie's comfort became their first priority. Morphine was prescribed to ease his pain. It did—until the day when he needed it most.

"They won't give him his shot!"

The day Willie died our 17-year-old daughter, Bobbi, and my closest friend stayed with him for a few hours while I ran some necessary errands. When I returned to my husband's hospital room, I found Bobbi frightened and upset: "Mom,

Dad's hurting and they won't give him his shot!"

I looked at Willie. He was moaning and thrashing about, obviously in severe pain. No wonder. The morphine he had been receiving every two hours was three hours overdue.

I immediately spoke to Willie's nurse. She checked his vital signs and left the room. When half an hour passed and she still hadn't returned, it dawned on me that she was trying to avoid giving Willie any morphine. I sought out another nurse. Reluctantly, she gave Willie a shot.

been eliminated from the patient's body.

Other side effects cause discomfort

Respiratory depression isn't the only side effect you'll see with morphine. While side effects such as nausea, vomiting, and postural hypotension aren't as serious as respiratory depression, they can interfere with a patient's comfort and pain relief. The other side effects include:

Nausea and vomiting. Morphine stimulates the area of the brain that controls vomiting. Ambulation has been found to increase nausea and vomiting, which means that patients should avoid walking or moving about immediately after receiving their medication. Antiemetics can help prevent this side effect.

Postural hypotension. Peripheral blood vessels dilate in response to morphine. When this happens, less blood returns to the central circulation, resulting in postural hypotension. Patients can compensate by moving slowly when they change position. To give the body time to adjust, tell them to sit up for a few moments before they stand up or start to walk.

Urinary retention. An increase in tone in the bladder muscles also occurs with morphine. Patients can experience urgency and urinary retention—a side effect that tends to be most common in patients who are receiving intrathecal or epidural morphine. Careful monitoring of fluid intake and output will help identify the problem. Intermittent or even continuous bladder catheterization may be necessary if retention occurs.

Flushed skin. Morphine stimu-

By then Willie was in so much pain that the morphine didn't help for very long. Within two hours, he was again twisting and thrashing about. Loud moans communicated his agony.

I sought out his nurse again and asked her to give him another shot. She refused. Willie's vital signs were weak, she explained, and she was afraid the morphine would depress his respirations.

I tried to reason with with her. I pointed out that Willie was dying—all anyone could do for him now was to make him more comfortable. His doctor, I reminded her, had ordered the morphine just for that purpose.

"It could be me who goes to jail"

I was stunned by her response: "If I give him a shot and it kills him, it wouldn't be the doctor or you who gets in trouble. It could be me who goes to jail."

I continued to beg for Willie's medication. At last, the nurse called a resident. She examined the chart and gave Willie a shot of morphine. It helped, but only for a little while. Later, I found out why—the house doctor had given Willie only half the prescribed dose.

In desperation, I called Willie's private physician. He spoke to Willie's nurse. Although the shots of morphine resumed, the cycle of pain control had been broken.

A few hours later, my husband died, still in excruciating pain. He had suffered unnecessarily not because his pain was intractable, but because his nurse was afraid.

Knowing why she acted as she did hasn't helped me accept Willie's agony. Even though I've come to terms with my grief, one question still haunts me: Why did my husband have to die in so much pain?

After Willie's death, I enrolled in a nursing program at a local university. Through my studies and conversations with nurses and doctors, I've come to realize that there's no simple answer to my question.

All of us—nurses, doctors, pharmacists, patients, and legislators—must work together to eradicate these fears. We must become more familiar with different methods of pain control. We must work for laws that will protect the rights of patients and caregivers as well.

My hope now is that as a nurse, I will be able to act in my patient's best interest without fear of legal repercussions. My wish is that I will never again witness the unnecessary pain and suffering that my husband was forced to endure.

lates the release of histamine. This causes flushed skin, increased perspiration, and itching. Release of histamine can also cause bronchospasm. While this side effect does not occur very commonly, it can be a particular problem if the patient has a history of asthma or other respiratory disease.

Mood changes. Some patients receiving morphine may experience lethargy, sleepiness, and a reduced ability to concentrate because the drug decreases activity in the cortex, reticular formation and limbic systems, and the brain stem. These patients may also experience mood changes ranging from apathy to euphoria.

Constipation— a common problem

Constipation is frequently a problem for patients on morphine. That's because the drug decreases peristalsis—the rhythmic contractions that move the contents of the bowel through the intestines.

A bowel regimen that includes plenty of fluids, stool softeners, drugs that stimulate peristalsis, and laxatives can help patients avoid this problem. If constipation does occur, the patient can usually get relief from suppositories and enemas.

If these measures don't work, ask the physician if you can give your patient 0.4 mg of naloxone mixed in orange juice. When taken orally, naloxone counteracts the effects of morphine in the gastrointestinal tract. Because oral naloxone is not well absorbed, the systemic effects of morphine are not reversed. Thus, naloxone relieves constipation, but without any loss of pain relief.

Still, this remedy should be tried only when all other measures fail.

One dose of the mixture should be all a patient needs to relieve constipation. The other measures—*not* repeated oral doses of naloxone— should then be used to prevent the problem from recurring.

Most of the side effects of morphine—constipation is an exception—diminish as the patient's body adapts to the drug. Unfortunately, the body also develops a tolerance to the drug's analgesic effects. This means that larger and larger doses of morphine are required to produce the same degree of pain control.

Tolerance doesn't equal addiction

Don't confuse tolerance or physical dependence with addiction. They are not different words that mean the same thing.

Patients who develop a tolerance to morphine are not addicted to the drug. They simply require larger doses of morphine to relieve their pain because their bodies have become accustomed to the drug's analgesic effects.

A patient has developed a physical dependence on morphine if physical symptoms such as chills, nausea, abdominal cramps, and irritability occur when the drug is abruptly discontinued. As the patient's body readjusts to functioning without morphine, the symptoms will disappear.

Both tolerance and physical dependence are *involuntary* physiologic reactions—patients cannot control their development. Addiction, on the other hand, involves the *voluntary* use of a drug—in this case morphine—for its psychological effects.

Counting minutes until the next dose

Many nurses incorrectly believe that patients who watch the clock, counting the minutes until their next dose of morphine, are becoming addicted. Patients who complain of pain even when receiving high doses of the drug are also suspect. A more likely explanation for such behavior is inadequate pain relief because of tolerance or an increase in pain as the patient's disease progresses.

Making a patient wait for his next dose of morphine will not "spare" him from becoming addicted. Such action will only increase his pain and decrease the effectiveness of the drug when he finally receives it.

Patients who receive morphine continuously for pain control may well develop tolerance or physical dependence. It's very unlikely that they will become addicted, however. One study indicates that fewer than 1% of all patients who received morphine became psychologically dependent.

Morphine is not a wonder drug. But when used with knowledge and skill, it can offer what may be the only hope of relief to many patients with intractable pain and provide them with the comfort and dignity they deserve. ■

BIBLIOGRAPHY Anderson, J.L. Nursing management of the cancer patient in pain: A review of the literature. *Cancer Nursing* 1:33, 1982. Burns, N. *Nursing and Cancer*. Philadelphia: W.B. Saunders Company, 1982. Donovan, M. and Girton, S. *Cancer Care Nursing* (2nd ed.). Norwalk, Conn.: Appleton-Century-Crofts, 1984. Donovan, M. Cancer pain: you can help! *Nurs. Clin. North Am.* 17:713, December 1982. McCaffrey, M. *Nursing Management of the Paitent With Pain* (2nd ed.). Philadelphia: J.B. Lippincott Company, 1979. Payne, R. and Foley, K. Advances in the treatment of cancer pain. *Cancer Treatment Reports* 68:173, 1984. Reiche, S.D. Choice of a strong analgesic for cancer patients. *Cancer Nursing* 1:67, 1982. Schwartz, T. Prolonged regional analgesia with morphine-epidurally. *RN* 5:32, May 1982. Spencer, R.T. et al. *Clincial Pharmacology and Nursing Management* (2nd ed.). Philadelphia: J.B. Lippincott Company, 1986. Stewart, S. Controlling pain with epidural narcotics: nursing implications. *Critical Care Nurse* 6:50, March 1986.

Coping with infections that AIDS patients develop

Here's a rundown on the diseases you're likely to encounter, and the measures you should take to protect yourself against each of those diseases, when a patient's HIV infection becomes AIDS.

By Peter Ungvarski, RN,C

Nursing a person who has AIDS means you must be concerned with the human immunodeficiency virus infection *and* at least one other disease.

HIV destroys the immune cells, eventually leaving the patient vulnerable to many pathogens that healthy immune systems reject or keep from reaching clinically significant levels. Only when the patient develops one of these opportunistic diseases—so-called because they take advantage of the host's compromised immunity—does he or she receive a definite diagnosis of AIDS.

For some 60% of patients, *Pneumocystis carinii* pneumonia is the opportunistic infection that marks the progression of HIV infection to AIDS. Another quarter of AIDS

THE AUTHOR, a Clinical Nurse Specialist in HIV infection, works for the Visiting Nurse Service of New York. He is completing his master's degree at Hunter College, New York.

Produced by David Anderson

diagnoses are made when patients with HIV infection develop one of the other protozoal, fungal, viral, or bacterial infections described in the chart that begins on the next page. In some 10% of cases, the initial opportunistic complication is a cancer—usually Kaposi's sarcoma. Whatever opportunistic disease occurs at the onset of AIDS, however, most patients will eventually experience problems with multiple organisms and pathologies.

Besides being the most prevalent, *Pneumocystis carinii* pneumonia is typical of AIDS-related infections. It's caused by a protozoan that is present in air, water, and soil, as well as in and on human beings and animals. So it's largely unavoidable. Your AIDS patient with acute PCP or other opportunistic infection will probably have a severe case, requiring aggressive treatment involving some drug toxicity. If he fails to respond, you

should consider the possibility of concurrent infection. If he recovers, he'll be highly vulnerable to repeat episodes, and may need to take medications for the rest of his life to prevent them.

Standard treatment for HIV infection is zidovudine (Retrovir). The chart describes the standard treatment for the most common AIDS-related opportunistic infections. Tear it out and use it to plan your nursing care for the patient with AIDS.

Protecting yourself from infection

Whenever a patient has an infectious disease—whether it be AIDS or not—you must plan his care with consideration to your own protection as well. The Centers for Disease Control recommends a three-level approach—general infection control routines, universal blood and body fluid precautions, and disease specific measures—to protect caregivers from AIDS and AIDS-related infections. Some other infection control experts see a potentially dangerous loophole in the CDC guidelines, however, and recommend an alternative approach called Body Systems Isolation.

General infection control routines help to prevent your hands from collecting and perhaps passing on to other patients opportunistic and other organisms—such as *Candida albicans* and cytomegalovirus—that a patient may be harboring. Wash your hands frequently. Wear latex or vinyl gloves whenever you anticipate touching potentially infectious body areas or secretions. Gloves are especially important if your hands have cuts, scratches, or any other breaks.

Universal blood and body fluid precautions protect you from HIV and hepatitis B, which are primarily blood-borne pathogens. Wear gloves, gown or apron, protective eyewear, and mask as necessary to shield mucous membranes and non-intact skin from any contact with blood. Shield yourself, too, from contact with semen, vaginal secretions, or synovial, pleural, peritoneal, pericardial, cerebrospinal, or amniotic fluid. Utilize gloves, gown or apron, and whatever other barriers are necessary to avoid secretions and excretions when they contain visible blood. Also, adhere strictly the CDC safety guidelines when you're handling needles and sharps. Be sure to leave used needles attached to syringes and drop them into a puncture-proof container. Don't recap, bend, or break a used needle.

The most common opportunistic diseases

This list tells you how to care for patients with the AIDS-related opportunistic infections seen most often in the U.S. A patient's lifestyle and area of residence influence the specific disease he or she is most likely to develop. For example, male homosexuals are more likely to develop herpes simplex infection than IV drug abusers, and histoplasmosis is most common in the South Central and Middle Central states.

Disease and Pathogen	Sites of Infection
Pneumocystis carinii pneumonia (PCP) *Pneumocystis carinii*, a protozoan found in air, water, soil, carried by domestic animals, and possibly latent in most people.	Lungs; sometimes spreads to the spleen, lymph nodes, and blood.
Toxoplasmosis *Toxoplasma gondii*, a protozoan found in air, water, soil, and in some cats and other animals. Most often acquired by ingestion of uncooked infected lamb or pork, unpasteurized dairy products, raw eggs, or vegetables. Mothers can give it to unborn children. Other human-human transmission does not occur.	Produces lesions in the central nervous system; may also involve the heart and lungs.
Cryptosporidiosis *Cryptosporidium*, a protozoan primarily acquired through oral contact with feces of an infected animal, or oral sexual contact with an infected person.	Gastrointestinal tract.
Isosporiasis *Isospora belli*, a protozoan primarily acquired through eating uncooked beef or pork, or through oral sexual contact with an infected person.	Gastrointestinal tract.
Mycobacterium avium-intracellulare (MAI) infection *Mycobacterium avium-intracellulare*, a bacterium found in soil, water, animals, eggs and unpasteurized dairy products, and other foods. MAI infection is atypical and non-communicable.	Disseminated.

Symptoms	Medications and side effects	Disease-specific precautions
Fever, cough, shortness of breath, chills, chest pain, sputum production in late disease.	**Trimethoprim-sulfamethoxazole (Bactrim, Septra):** skin rash, itching, Stevens-Johnson syndrome, extreme fatigue, dysphagia, fever, leukopenia, sore throat, thrombocytopenia, hepatitis, hematuria, diarrhea, dizziness, headache, anorexia, nausea, vomiting. **IM or IV pentamidine isethionate (Pentam 300):** azotemia, serum creatinine elevations, pain and induration at intramuscular sites, abscess or necrosis at injection sites, elevated liver function tests, leukopenia, nausea, vomiting, hypotension, syncope, blood sugar imbalances. **Aerosolized pentamidine isethionate:** investigational. **Dapsone:** nausea, vomiting, abdominal pain, vertigo, blurred vision, tinnitus, insomnia, fever, headache, phototoxicity, lupus, anemia. **Sulfadoxine-pyrimethamine (Fansidar):** allergic skin reactions, nausea and vomiting, glossitis, stomatitis, headache, peripheral neuritis, mental depression, fatigue, weakness.	None.
Fever, chills, headache, visual disturbances, lethargy, confusion, hemiparesis, seizures.	**Sulfadiazine:** same as Trimethoprim-sulfamethoxazole. **Pyrimethamine (Daraprim):** anorexia, vomiting, megaloblastic anemia, leukopenia, thrombocytopenia, glossitis.	None.
Copious diarrhea, abdominal pain, anorexia, nausea, vomiting, dehydration, weight loss, weakness, fever.	**Spiramycin:** nausea, vomiting, diarrhea, abdominal pain, acute colitis. **Eflornithine (Ornidyl):** investigational.	Gloves and gown/apron when handling feces. Private room when patient has poor hygiene.
Diarrhea, abdominal pain, nausea, vomiting, anorexia, weight loss, weakness, fever.	**Trimethoprim-sulfamethoxazole:** *see under Pneumocystis carinii.*	Gloves and gown/apron when handling feces. Private room when patient has poor hygiene.
Fever, malaise, night sweats, anorexia, diarrhea, weight loss.	**Isoniazid (INH):** paresthesia and peripheral neuropathy, elevated liver function test values, anorexia, nausea, vomiting, fatigue, malaise, weakness. **Rifabutin (Ansamycin):** hepatotoxicity, neutropenia, nausea, vomiting, diarrhea, skin rash, itching. **Clofazimine (Lamprene):** reddish-brown discoloration of skin, conjunctiva, sweat, hair, urine, and feces; abdominal pain, diarrhea.	Gloves and gown/apron when handling wound drainage. *Continued on next page . . .*

196

Disease-specific infection control measures are added as necessary to protect against transmissible AIDS-related pathogens. While
some of these pathogens can be
transmitted to healthy individuals
through contact with feces and other secretions, most of them cannot
penetrate competent immune systems and therefore require no extra precautions.

Because many patients are more
than likely to have multiple illnesses, some of the experts fear that
the CDC's recommendations may
leave nurses vulnerable to infection
by pathogens that have not yet
been diagnosed. They advocate a
single comprehensive system of
self-protection for nurses to use
with all patients:

Body systems isolation (BSI)
includes general and universal precautions in addition to every measure that's appropriate whenever a
patient has HIV and opportunistic
infection. In practice this amounts
mainly to using protective wear to
avoid exposure to feces or other secretions, whether or not they contain visible blood. Because BSI
precautions are uniform for all patients, regardless of diagnosis,
these safeguards protect the patient against HIV, opportunistic infections, and other transmissible
pathogens even before they are
recognized.

Understanding the appropriate
infection control routines—also described in the chart—only enhances
the quality of the care you give
your patients who have AIDS. And
the good care that you deliver today can lead to even better care tomorrow. We are beginning to make

Disease and Pathogen	Sites of Infection
Mycobacterium avium-intracellulare (MAI) infection *Continued from previous page*	
Candidiasis *Candida albicans,* a fungus that inhabits the oropharynx, vagina, large intestine, and skin, causing no harm as long as immunity remains undamaged. May occur as a secondary infection in conjunction with herpes simplex virus lesions.	Anywhere skin or mucous membrane is damaged, including IV therapy and pressure monitoring sites, etc.
Cryptococcosis *Cryptococcus neoformans,* a fungus found in air, water, soil; contained in pigeon droppings, and found on window ledges and nesting places, raw fruits, and vegetables. Acquired by inhalation.	Central nervous system, lungs; can be disseminated.
Histoplasmosis *Histoplasma capsulatum,* a fungus released into the atmosphere from bird and bat droppings, acquired by inhalation. Commonest in Middle and South Central United States.	Disseminated.
Cytomegalovirus (CMV) Cytomegalovirus, an organism found in saliva, semen, cervical secretions, urine, feces, blood, breast milk; it causes problems only when immunity is compromised.	Disseminated.
Herpes simplex virus (HSV) infection Herpes simplex virus 1 is spread by contact with infected oral secretions. Herpes simplex virus 2 is spread by contact with infected genital secretions. Patient can spread either variety by touching lesions, then touching other body parts.	Mouth, perianal area; can be disseminated.
Progressive multifocal leukoencephalopathy (PML) J.C. virus, transmission routes unclear.	Brain.

Symptoms	Medications and side effects	Disease-specific precautions
	Ethambutol (Myambutol): reversible blurring of vision, anaphylaxis, skin irritation, nausea, vomiting, fever, malaise, headache, confusion. **Cycloserine (Seromycin):** convulsions, drowsiness, headache, tremor, other central nervous system disturbances. **Ethionamide (Trecator-SC):** nausea, vomiting, peripheral and optic neuritis, mental depression, postural hypotension, skin rash. **Rifampin (Rifadin, Rimactane):** urine discoloration, heartburn, nausea, vomiting, abdominal cramps, headache, drowsiness, fatigue. **Streptomycin:** nausea, vomiting, vertigo, numbness of the face, rash, fever, itching, elevated white cell count.	
Thrush, esophagitis, perianal irritation, vaginitis, proctitis, inflammation around fingernails; can be disseminated.	**Clotrimazole (Mycelex):** abdominal pain, diarrhea, nausea, vomiting. **Nystatin (Mycostatin, Nilstat, Nystex):** diarrhea, nausea, vomiting, stomach pain. **Ketoconazole (Nizoral):** hepatitis, gynecomastia, nausea, vomiting, decreased libido, diarrhea, dizziness, drowsiness, photophobia, skin rash, itching, sleepiness. **Amphotericin B (Fungizone):** *see below.*	None.
Altered cognition, low grade fever, headache, nausea, vomiting, meningeal signs.	**Amphotericin B (Fungizone):** fever, chills, nausea, anorexia, pain at infusion site, anemia, renal failure with altered urination rate. **Flucytosine (Ancobon, 5-FC):** skin rash, lowered white and red cell counts, confusion, hallucinations, diarrhea, nausea, vomiting, dizziness, drowsiness, headache.	None.
Fever, chills, cough, muscle aches, headache, abdominal pain.	**Amphotericin B:** *see under Cryptococcosis.* **Ketoconazole:** *see under Candidiasis.*	None.
Fever, profound fatigue, muscle and joint aches, night sweats, impaired vision, cough, dyspnea, abdominal pain, diarrhea.	**Gancyclovir (DHPG):** leukopenia, bone marrow depression, elevated liver enzymes, edema, nausea, muscle aches, headache, anorexia, disorientation, rash, phlebitis.	Private room if the patient has enteritis and poor hygiene. Gloves and gown/apron for handling excretions and secretions if soiling is likely.
Painful burning, itching vesicular lesions; sometimes colitis, pericarditis, esophagitis, pneumonia.	**Acyclovir (Zovirax):** skin rash, diarrhea, light-headedness, headache, nausea, vomiting, thirst, fatigue.	Gloves and gown/apron for handling secretions from lesions. Private room if disseminated or severe.
Impaired speech, vision, and thought; ataxia and limb weakness. Advanced disease can cause profound dementia.	No known effective treatment.	None.

progress against AIDS-related opportunistic infections. *Pneumocystis* pneumonia, for example, is now diagnosed sooner and treated more successfully than seven years ago. Patients survive longer, and there is even hope that prophylactic treatment with aerosolized pentamidine will eliminate this deadly disease. ■

BIBLIOGRAPHY Armstrong, D. Opportunistic infections in the acquired immune deficiency syndrome. *Semin. Oncol.* 14:40, 1987. Braude, A.I. (ed). *Infectious Diseases and Medical Microbiology.* Philadelphia: W.B. Saunders, 1986. Centers for Disease Control. Update: Universal precautions for prevention of transmission of human immunodeficiency virus, hepatitis B virus, and other blood-borne pathogens in health-care settings. *MMWR* 37:377, 1988. Jacobs, K.S. and Piano, M.R. The clinical picture of AIDS: underlying pathological processes. In *The Person With AIDS: Nursing Perspectives*, Durham, J.D. and Cohen, L. (eds.). New York: Springer, 1987. Kaplan, L.D., Wofsy, C.B., et al. Treatment of patients with acquired immunodeficiency syndrome and associated manifestations. *JAMA* 257:1367, March 13, 1987. Lynch, P., Jackson, M.M., et al. Rethinking the role of isolation practices in the prevention of nosocomial infections. *Ann. Int. Med.* 107:243, Sept. 1987. Masur, H., Kovacs, J.A., et al. Infectious complications of AIDS. In *AIDS: Etiology, Diagnosis, Treatment & Prevention*, DeVita, V.T., Hellman, S., et al (eds.). Philadelphia: Lippincott, 1985. Rothenberg, R., Woefel, M., et al. Survival with acquired immunodeficiency syndrome: experience with 5833 cases in New York City. *N. Engl. J. Med.* 317:1297, Nov. 19, 1987.

Helping an MS patient live a better life

Using a motorized wheelchair is just one way the author copes with multiple sclerosis. Here she shares ways nurses can make life easier for patients while medicine searches for cause and cure.
By Jacqueline Mayer Ferguson, RN, MS

For those of us who have it, multiple sclerosis might better be named "the disease of many losses." Some are nearly imperceptible, others demand that we reorder our lives. The disease commonly causes reduced coordination, weakness, fatigue, numbness, visual disruption, loss of bladder control, and mental changes. Potentially, it may manifest in as many ways as the central nervous system has functions.

The 250,000 people—two-thirds of them women—in the United States who have MS find that it progresses unpredictably. Some 20% have benign MS, with mild and infrequent attacks. Another 25% have exacerbating/remitting disease, with occasional attacks and some permanent residual symptoms. The 40% of patients with chronic/relapsing disease retain more impairments after attacks, gradually experiencing moderate or severe disability. The remaining 15% have chronic progressive disease, where each new loss is a permanent one.

To help the MS patient live as fully as possible, you must know the facts of the disease, respond resourcefully to a wide variety of needs, and relate with compassion.

Diagnosing MS can be complicated

MS strikes between the ages of 20 and 50. Typically, the patient seeks out a doctor because she's experiencing abnormal burning or prickling sensations, numbness, or eye abnormalities such as optic neuritis or diplopia. Other early symptoms include problems with bowel and bladder, or gait.

The neurologist takes an exhaustive history, looking for evidence that the patient has had two or more distinct neurological symptoms at separate times. This is typical of MS, which affects different locations in the central nervous system, usually in an exacerbating and remitting fashion.

Next, the neurologist assesses for motor changes such as abnormal reflexes, ataxia, muscle weakness, or other clear indications of neurological abnormality.

A lumbar puncture is often ordered. Spinal fluid usually shows increases and abnormalities of immunoglobulin G when MS is present. At times evoked potential tests are ordered as well. These procedures measure the speed of cerebral nerve transmissions when the brain is stimulated by light, sound, or touch. They may be slowed down by MS.

The diagnostic workup may include CT scans or MRI studies of the central nervous system. They may show scars—which are called "plaques"—in the white matter. Plaques are produced in the course of demyelination—the stripping of myelin, a fatty substance that surrounds nerve fibers and facilitates conduction of impulses. Demyelination, the major pathological process of MS, is the cause of the patient's symptoms and impairments.

Almost all signs and symptoms of MS may be produced by other diseases, such as brain tumors or infarcts. That's why the final step in

THE AUTHOR was a counselor at the U.S. Merchant Marine Academy at Kings Point, New York, when this article was written. She is currently president of the multiple sclerosis club, a self-help group, at North Shore University Hospital in North Shore, Long Island.

Produced by David Anderson

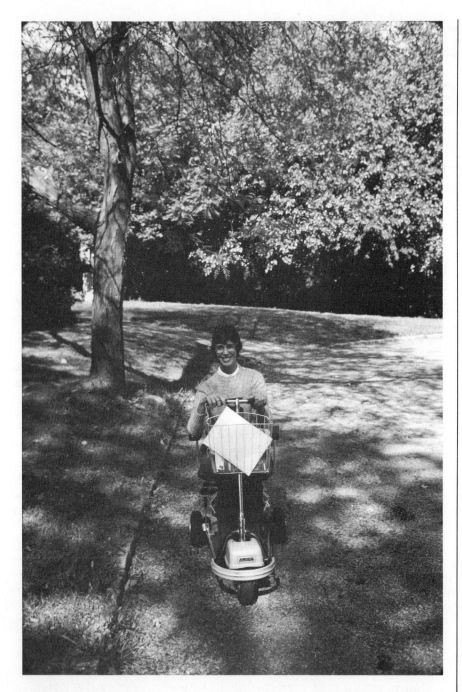

the diagnosis is a decision that MS is the best explanation for all of the patient's problems taken together.

My own diagnosis of MS is described on page 26.

Nursing care for MS patients

There is no known cure for MS. Care focuses on symptomatic relief, keeping the patient active for as long as possible, and preventing complications.

Whether the MS patient is mildly or severely disabled, some principles of care remain constant. She should:

▶ Maintain a balanced diet and exercise program.

▶ Be cautious about temperature extremes. Very hot or cold weather—even a warm bath—may temporarily worsen established symptoms or bring on new ones.

▶ Manage stress, which can also worsen symptoms temporarily.

▶ Pace activities and plan frequent rest periods to prevent excessive fatigue, a major problem in MS.

When the patient has reduced mobility

The care plan also addresses disabilities, especially loss of mobility and coordination.

Encourage the patient with impaired mobility to exercise daily to maintain muscle tone and prevent contractures. Call in a physical therapist to help tailor an exercise program. For the home, suggest grab bars in the bathroom, left- and right-handed banisters on stairways, or a stairway lift. Eventually, many patients need canes, Canadian crutches, or wheelchairs. In one large survey, some 50% of patients who'd had multiple sclerosis for 12 years or more needed assistance to get around.

Your patient may complain that her hand begins to tremble whenever she tries to do manual tasks—a symptom known as "intention tremor." She can reduce the tremor by steadying her hand against a fixed object, and minimize its inconvenience by simplifying certain tasks. Advise her to use Velcro fasteners, for instance, instead of buttons, shoelaces, or hooks and eyes.

Spasticity, a frequent problem of MS patients, can usually be relieved with baclofen (Lioresal). This medication may prove to be a mixed blessing. When the spasticity is relieved, her legs may be

The mystery of MS

What causes multiple sclerosis, and how does it develop? Although the picture is far from complete, most experts believe that MS is an autoimmune disease. Diseases of this type—such as rheumatoid arthritis—occur when the patient's immune system turns against his own healthy cells. As evidence that this happens in MS, doctors point to the demyelination plaques that form on the patient's white matter. They contain large numbers of macrophages and T_4 lymphocytes and produce antibody.

MS may be touched off by an infection. According to this theory, some infectious agent stimulates the immune system to attack central nervous system myelin. Physicians believe that several viruses—possibly including canine distemper, measles, and herpes simplex—may trigger multiple sclerosis in this way.

MS may begin in childhood or adolescence. This conclusion is drawn from epidemiological analysis that shows a person's risk of developing MS depends partly on where he lives up to age 15. An individual who spends those years in a cold climate is more likely to develop MS than one who spends them in warmth.

There are genetic factors. MS is more common among people of European ancestry than other white racial groups, and twice as common among whites as among blacks. It is rare among the Chinese and Japanese, unknown among Gypsies, Yakuts, Bantus, Hutterites, and American Indians. Parents, siblings, and children of a person with MS are some 12 to 20 times more likely to develop the disease than an unrelated person from the same ethnic group living in the same climate. Recent immunological techniques have shown that inheriting certain tissue types—HLA-3, B-7, and DR-2—doubles or quadruples a person's risk of MS.

Current medical treatments for MS reflect the idea that MS is an autoimmune disease:

▶ ACTH and other corticosteroids are standard treatment to resolve acute exacerbations quickly. They suppress the immune system and reduce inflammation, yet they do not affect the long-term course of multiple sclerosis.

▶ Other immunosuppressant medications may slow the long-term progress of MS. Of these drugs, cyclophosphamide (Cytoxan) has so far produced the best results—seeming to stabilize most patients for six to 24 months. Cop-1—a genetically engineered immune substance—recently yielded encouraging results when tested on a small number of patients with mild, exacerbating/remitting disease. Monoclonal antibody is also in early testing stages.

▶ Physicians are encouraged by results with total lymphoid irradiation—alone or used with corticosteroids—to suppress the patient's immune system. Total lymphoid irradiation seems to slow progression for 12 to 24 months. Plasmapheresis is sometimes used to the same purpose, but is probably impractical for general use.

While some of these approaches help and others are promising, the way to a truly effective treatment for MS remains a mystery for the present.

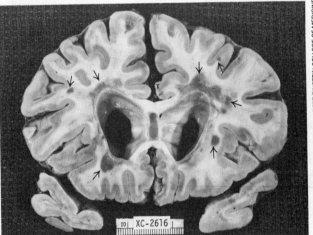

COURTESY OF DR. CEDRIC S. RAINE, ALBERT EINSTEIN COLLEGE OF MEDICINE

The arrows in the photo above point to demyelination plaques in the brain of an MS patient. The plaques appear as gray areas in the white matter. Scarring and the loss of myelin, which makes the white matter white, give the plaques their gray, glassy appearance.

wobbly or they may not support her at all.

Closely monitor the skin of patients who are immobilized, have decreased cutaneous sensation, or are incontinent. Prevent sores by keeping skin clean and dry. Position the patient so that her weight is not concentrated on her heels, sacrum, or other pressure areas. Turn her frequently.

Help the bedridden patient to cough and deep breathe often, and have her turn her body from side to side q2h.

Avoid giving liquids to the patient who has difficulty swallowing, because they can easily be aspirated. Instead, offer ice chips, fruit ices, or gelatin desserts to supply fluids. Eventually, a few patients lose their gag reflex and need tube or gastrostomy feedings.

How to help with elimination problems

Most MS patients experience bladder retention, urgency, nocturia, hesitancy, incontinence, or some combination of these conditions. Your patient's problem may be due to one of three types of neurogenic bladder.

Failure-to-empty bladders are best controlled with intermittent self-catheterization. Teach the patient to use this technique as often as the physician orders—at least four times daily. Advise her that frequent and complete emptying of the bladder helps prevent urinary tract infection. Also, an overloaded bladder can cause urinary reflux leading to serious kidney infections. If the patient and family members are unable to manage

catheterization, the physician may order an indwelling catheter.

Failure-to-store bladders usually respond to anticholinergic medications such as oxybutyrin chloride (Ditropan) or propantheline (Probanthine). Imipramine (Tofranil), an antidepressant, also promotes urinary retention and fights depression, a common problem, as well.

Mixed bladder, the most common problem, combines a hyperactive bladder muscle with a urinary sphincter that contracts when it should relax. The result is unpredictable voiding. Treatment with self-catheterization and anticholinergics usually restores control.

The patient with a neurogenic bladder is particularly prone to urinary tract infections. To help prevent them, urge plenty of fluids.

Due to decreased sensation, the MS patient may not experience the most familiar symptoms of bladder infection: pain and urination on voiding. Teach her to watch for other signs: increased frequency, urgency, incontinence, change in the odor or cloudiness of urine. She should see a doctor if she develops chills, fever, or flank pain. These may indicate pyelonephritis or other more advanced infections.

Some patients with neurogenic bladders become constipated because they limit fluid intake in order to avoid incontinence. This distress usually disappears when the bladder control is established and adequate fluid intake—2 qts/day—is resumed.

The patient may develop constipation that is specifically due to MS. Initiate a bowel training pro-

gram—high roughage diet, plenty of fluids and prune juice at the same time every day. She may also require a stool softener or glycerin suppository.

Counsel the patient to make the best of life

Many of the MS patient's losses require extensive continuous adjustment. You can help by listening to the patient and referring her to a specialist when necessary.

Many patients, for example, experience loss of orgasm or impotence. This may be reversible if it's due to fatigue, depression, or drugs such as anticholinergics or lioresal. It may be irreversible if it's due to demyelination.

If sexual losses are permanent, encourage the patient to discuss her feelings and to rethink her sexuality and relationships. Point out that affection, embracing, touching, feeling, caressing, and physical intimacy may still continue. Urge honest, caring discussions between patients and sexual partners.

Your patient may develop cognitive problems due to MS or depression. Patients sometimes lose some eye-hand coordination and visual skills so that driving and reading, for example, become difficult. If short-term memory is affected, advise the patient to carry a pad to jot down reminders.

When MS attacks the frontal lobe of the brain, the patient may develop sudden mood swings and outbursts. Don't take it personally. Afterwards, discuss the problem with the patient and suggest that she learn to use imagery or another calming technique when she feels on the verge of going out of control.

Depression, anger, and frustration are natural responses to the losses and uncertainty MS brings. Your care, concern, and supportive listening can do much to help control these emotions. To relieve depression, some patients take imipramine or other antidepressants. To help the patient deal with the uncertainty of the future, encourage her to take one day at a time.

For additional information and contacts that may greatly help you and your patient, contact the National Multiple Sclerosis Society at (800) 624-8236, or write to them at 205 East 42nd Street, New York, N.Y., 10017. A local chapter may be listed in your phone book.

For me, one quote about MS has been an inspiration. "I cannot cure your disease, but it may run a benign course. In any event, I will try to help you, because much can be done to make life easier for you."

These words are used by Danish physician Tore Broman when he tells patients that they have MS. Nurses who adopt his attitude will aid their patients immeasurably. ■

BIBLIOGRAPHY Blaivas, J.G. Management of bladder dysfunction in multiple sclerosis. *Neurology* 30(7):12, July 1980. Bornstein, M., et al. A preliminary trial of Cop 1 in exacerbating-remitting multiple sclerosis. *N. Engl. J. Med.* 317:408, Aug. 13, 1987. Giesser, B. Multiple sclerosis: current concepts in management. *Drugs* 29(1):88, Jan. 1985. International Federation of Multiple Sclerosis Societies. *Therapeutic Claims in Multiple Sclerosis.* New York: National Multiple Sclerosis Society, 1986. Kimberg, I. *Moving with Multiple Sclerosis.* New York: National Multiple Sclerosis Society, 1985. Kurtzke, T. Epidemiologic contributions to multiple sclerosis: an overview. *Neurology* 30(7):61, July 1980. Scheinberg, L.C., ed. *Multiple Sclerosis: A Guide for Patients and Their Families.* New York: Raven Press, 1983. Tragott, U. Relevance of white blood cells in multiple sclerosis. *MS Quarterly Report* 5(3):29, July 1986. Waksman, B. Causes and cure of multiple sclerosis: basic scientific research. *Paraplegia News* 38(8):31, Aug. 1984.

MS—a personal story

What's one sure way to learn about a disease? Get it!

My earliest awareness of a definite MS symptom occurred around 1971. I was teaching my two boys to play tennis. When they overshot the ball, I found that I couldn't run backwards to get it.

I made a differential diagnosis for myself—pernicious anemia, tertiary syphilis, brain tumor, multiple sclerosis. And then, because I couldn't face the possibilities, I made a conscious decision to forget the incident.

In retrospect, I think I knew it was MS. I had other disquieting symptoms. My bladder was undependable. I experienced urgency, frequency, nocturia, and occasional incontinence. I was also credéing my bladder—pushing in behind my suprapubic bone to complete voiding. I told myself I had a cystocele, but I really knew better.

My vision blurred from time to time.

My arms and legs lost strength. Working part time as a visiting nurse, I began to find it increasingly difficult to pull my patients up in bed. I told myself the problem was motivational—that I just did not want to give bedside care anymore. I decided to go back to school to get my bachelors and then my masters degrees.

I was in graduate school studying the central nervous system and also working part time in the college infirmary, when I lost pain and temperature sensation on the right side of my body. There was no longer any denying that something was wrong. I went to see a neurologist. He told me he thought I might have MS, and to come back if new symptoms appeared.

In search of an explanation that I could more easily accept, I told myself I was an "anxiety neurotic" and I began psychotherapy. Although I wasn't really neurotic, I certainly was anxious, becoming exponentially more so each time a new symptom appeared.

My moment of truth finally came in 1978. I had a major exacerbation of symptoms—vertigo with severe vomiting, followed by diplopia, tremor of both hands, ataxia, unsteady gait, and pins and needles sensation in my hands and feet. A friend drove me to the neurologist's office. The doctor listened to my complaints and then did a quick neurological examination. When he scratched the bottom of my feet, my toes flared up and out in the classically abnormal Babinski response. When I saw it I screamed. He said, "I'm sorry, Jackie. You have multiple sclerosis."

The wall of denial came tumbling down.

The diagnosis of multiple sclerosis can be devastating, and some patients never learn to live with it. I experienced a reactive depression. I lost my appetite—and about

50 pounds—and slept most of the time. When I was awake I was usually crying.

Every day new symptoms appeared. My husband and I knew we had to tell our boys. We waited until I was in remission, so that they could see that there would be good times as well as bad. Telling our children was enormously difficult, on each of us, on all of us.

I continued working as long as I could, in order to have enough years of service to qualify for permanent major medical insurance. Toward the end, my husband came to the office and helped with tasks I could no longer manage.

Housebound, I began to reorganize my life, preparing for the worst while hoping for the best.

Eventually I obtained an almost-complete remission.

I returned to school and finished my masters degree as a Nurse Practitioner in Mental Health Care. After graduation, I persuaded the administration to create a counseling position for me in the college infirmary. Switching from clinical nurse to counselor removed the need for strength and agility—which I no longer have.

My disease has at present converted from "chronic/remitting" to "chronic progressive." Adjusting to it is a constant, ongoing challenge. My husband and our boys give me strength when my own runs down.

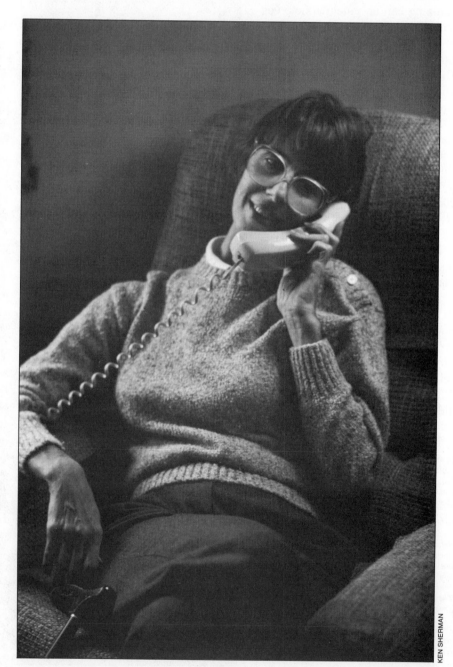

KEN SHERMAN

Stroke:
How to contain the damage

When your patient suffers a stroke, you'll find yourself in a race
to keep him alive and prevent the neurological damage from spreading.
This first of two articles tells you how you can help stabilize
the patient during the acute phase of the stroke.

By Rebecca Gary, RN, MSN, Betty Jax Jermier, RN, MSN,
and April Hickey, RN, MSN

A severe stroke leaves its victim poised on the verge of total disability and death. To pull him back from the brink, you must contain his spreading neurological damage and restore hemodynamic stability. Only then can you turn your attention to helping him take the first crucial steps on the long road to rehabilitation.

In this article, you'll learn what you can do to help bring your patient through the initial crisis. Next month we'll talk about how to deal with the neurological impairments a stroke can leave behind.

How and why
strokes happen

Strokes occur when rupture or obstruction of an artery sharply reduces blood supply to a portion of the brain. Strokes caused by bleeding are called hemorrhagic strokes.

THE AUTHORS: Ms. Gary is a clinical instructor at the King Khalid Eye Specialist Hospital in Riyadh, Saudi Arabia. Ms. Jermier is a clinical educator at Shands Hospital at the University of Florida at Gainesville. Ms. Hickey is a staff nurse in the ICU at Good Samaritan Hospital in Dayton, Ohio.

Produced by David Anderson

Those that are caused by obstruction of an artery are called ischemic strokes.

Hemorrhagic strokes usually result from rupture of aneurysms related to high blood pressure or atherosclerotic disease. They announce themselves by a terrible headache, confusion, nausea, and vomiting. If the patient has suffered a subarachnoid hemorrhage, he'll probably also have rigidity of the neck, photophobia, and a low-grade fever. The victim of an intracerebral hemorrhage usually undergoes rapid neurological deterioration. He's commonly lethargic on admission to the hospital and slowly progresses into coma over the next few days.

Hemorrhagic strokes prove fatal 50% to 90% of the time, depending on the magnitude and location of the bleeding.

Ischemic strokes are more common and more survivable. They generally result from atherosclerotic disease or embolisms. Such strokes often follow transient isch-

emic attacks by 30 days or less. A TIA consists of self-limited symptoms of impending arterial occlusion such as double vision or loss of vision, numbness in the hands or arms, vertigo, and falling. TIA symptoms resolve completely within 24 hours.

Other factors that can precipitate strokes include myocardial infarction, cardiac dysrhythmias, trauma, exercise, hypotension, hypoxia, meningitis, hypoglycemia, and the use of anticoagulant drugs.

Recognizing
stroke patterns

Strokes produce two distinct patterns of neurological impairment. Taken together, they point to the area that's lost its blood supply.

One pattern reflects which artery has been affected. As brain tissue served by the artery loses its oxygen supply, it ceases to function and the patient loses those capacities governed by it. Thus, a stroke affecting a right or left carotid or cerebral artery can render the victim blind, paralyzed, or without feeling on the opposite side of his body. Confusion and speech disturbances also occur.

Aphasia generally indicates that the left side of the brain has been damaged, since most people have their word and language centers on that side.

The situation is more dangerous when the basilar artery becomes blocked or interrupted, cutting off the oxygen supply to the posterior brain. Then you'll see dizziness, numbness (usually of the face), double vision, defects in one or both visual fields, loss of control over the muscles of speech, or a staggering gait and other coordination problems.

The second pattern of impairments, associated with increased intracranial pressure, indicates how far forward (rostral) or back (caudal) the damage is. Generally, the farther back the damage, the lower the patient's level of consciousness, the more fundamental the physiological processes affected, and the worse the prognosis. The chart on the opposite page lists the neurological consequences of increased ICP in all major areas of the brain.

Immediate care of the stroke patient
Depending on the extent of oxygen deprivation, tissues die and the patient's impairments become permanent within hours or days. Therefore, immediate stroke treatment aims to restore circulation to the patient's brain as quickly as possible. Meanwhile, you must try to keep the patient from developing complications.

First, make sure your patient has a clear, functioning airway. Patients whose respiratory centers have been damaged may need to be intubated.

Next, assess the patient's hemodynamic status. You may find practically any normal or abnormal pattern, depending on the location and extent of stroke damage. For instance, brain stem hemorrhages may drastically raise or lower blood pressure. Cerebral ischemia may give rise to a pattern of widening pulse pressure and decreased heart rate caused by increased intracranial pressure.

If your patient's blood pressure is high, elevate his head at least 30°. This will reduce intracranial pressure and reduce the tendency to hemorrhage. If blood pressure is low, lay the patient flat to increase cerebral perfusion. The physician will probably order antihypertensives or volume expanders, whichever is appropriate, to lower or raise the patient's blood pressure into a normal or slightly above-normal range.

Once you've checked the airway and circulation, assess your patient's neurological status beginning with his level of consciousness. If you're unfamiliar with the terminology for LOC or neurological deficits, describe the abnormalities you see in your own words. Take careful note of the type, location, and degree of any deficits. Besides giving you clues to the location and severity of the stroke, this initial assessment will form the basis for assessing your patient's subsequent progress.

Take a medical history as soon as you can. Be sure to ask about the risk factors listed on page 40. The history will help you determine the etiology of the stroke and warn you of related health problems that could complicate treatment and nursing care.

Strokes can cause seizures, especially in their early stages. Seizures greatly endanger patients by further reducing circulation to the brain. Therefore, you will give most patients anticonvulsant medication—usually phenytoin sodium (Dilantin), sometimes phenobarbital—right away. If your patient does have a seizure, record its onset, duration, intensity, and the effect it has on his level of consciousness.

Unless the patient's symptoms are very minor, he will also be given steroids and possibly dehydrating agents such as mannitol or urea to reduce cerebral edema. Edema can cause permanent brain damage by compressing tissues and vessels.

Medical therapy for ischemic strokes
Physicians use medical or surgical means to restore blood flow through stroke-damaged vessels or to encourage collateral circulation. The methods that are used to treat ischemic and hemorrhagic strokes differ significantly.

Ischemic strokes are usually treated medically. The choice of medications depends on the duration and severity of the stroke.

Patients with mild symptoms of brief duration receive aspirin or dipyridamole (Persantine), drugs that impede platelet aggregation.

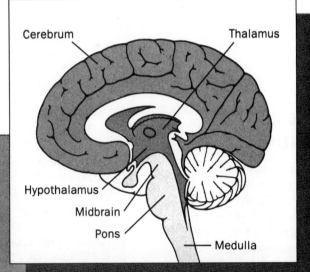

KATHY MITCHELL GREY

Where is ICP building up?

The nature and severity of the neurological damage your stroke patient suffers depends in part on where intracranial pressure builds up in his brain. Generally, the farther back toward the brainstem the buildup occurs, the worse the damage and prognosis. The chart below summarizes the neurological impact of elevated ICP on the major areas of the brain.

Affected area	Neurological effects of elevated ICP				
	Level of consciousness	Papillary response	Doll's eye movement	Respiratory pattern	Motor activity
Cerebrum	Confusion, inappropriate thought processes	Normal	Present	Eupnea (normal)	Normal
Diencephalon (thalamus and hypothalamus)	Lethargy/stupor	Small (2-3 mm) and reactive	Present	Eupnea to Cheyne-Stokes (alternating hyperpnea and apnea)	Gegenhalten posture/ decorticate
Brainstem Midbrain	Semi-coma/ coma	Midposition (3-5 mm) and non-reactive	Impaired	Cheyne-Stokes to central neurogenic breathing (prolonged hyperpnea)	Decorticate/ decerebrate
Pons	Coma	Pinpoint and non-reactive	Impaired	Apneustic (pauses at ends of inspiration and expiration)	Decerebrate
Medulla	Coma	Midposition fixed or dilated	Absent	Ataxic (irregular pattern)	Flaccid

These agents slow clotting in the cerebral blood vessels, giving the blood's natural fibrinolytic factors time to break down obstructions that have already formed.

When your patient is on dipyridamole, give 50 mg to 75 mg tid as ordered an hour or more before meals. This drug can cause headache, dizziness, and nausea. It can also exacerbate hypotension.

The patient's symptoms may resolve within 24 hours, before ischemia has caused permanent tissue death. If they do, the patient's experience is classified as a transient ischemic attack.

Patients whose symptoms are more severe and longer lasting receive anticoagulation therapy with IV heparin. Anticoagulation is also attempted whenever the patient's stroke results from embolism, regardless of the severity of the symptoms. The physician aims for a heparin dose that will lengthen the PTT to between 1.5 and two times normal. After a loading dose of 5,000 to 10,000 units you'll infuse 700 to 1,200 units an hour as ordered, depending on the PTT.

Don't give heparin through a piggyback because some other drugs

Risk factors for stroke

For Ischemic strokes
Coronary artery disease
Peripheral vascular disease
Elevated blood lipids
Hematocrit above 55%
Cigarette smoking
Vasculitis

For hemorrhagic strokes
Black race
Use of oral contraceptives

For all strokes
Hypertension
Advanced age
Diabetes
Obesity
Excessive use of alcohol

negate its effect. Check for signs of bleeding with daily guaiac stool and hematuria tests. Check PTT at least once a day. Take measures to keep your patient from bleeding—have him use soft tooth wipes rather than a toothbrush, for example.

Once the patient's symptoms stop evolving, the doctor will substitute Coumadin for the heparin.

To compensate for reduced cerebral perfusion, you'll give oxygen. You'll also give medications to keep blood pressure near normal.

Chances are that your patient's treatment won't immediately halt the progress of ischemia in his brain. Ischemia can continue to spread for as long as two weeks, during which time your neurological assessments will show a gradual worsening of symptoms. Symp-

toms will then stabilize and may even improve.

Even after two weeks, the patient may recover completely. This occurs when collateral circulation makes up the oxygen deficit to tissues before necrosis occurs. The patient's experience is then classified as a reversible ischemic neurological deficit, or RIND.

If, however, the patient's stroke leaves him with fixed deficits—functions lost forever because brain tissue has died from lack of oxygen—he's suffered a completed stroke.

When the treatment for ischemia is surgery

The physician may resort to surgery to remove a thrombotic or stenotic lesion that has caused—or is threatening to cause—an ischemic stroke.

If the lesion lies in a vessel outside the cranial vault, he'll probably choose carotid endarterectomy. This procedure cleans atherosclerotic plaque from the vessel walls.

If the lesion lies inside the cranial vault, extracranial-intracranial arterial bypass is appropriate. One common type of EIAB brings the superficial temporal artery of the scalp in through the skull and grafts it to the intracranial middle cerebral artery at a point distal to the blockage. The temporal artery then supplies blood to the cerebral artery, making up the flow that was lost due to the blockage.

Before your patient goes to surgery, tell him what dressings, catheters, and other equipment to expect when he wakes. Prepare him to find his head shaved. Advise him

to ask for pain medication as soon as he begins to hurt.

Preview postop routines for your patient before he goes to surgery. Emphasize the need to cough and deep breathe hourly. Tell him that he'll walk, if he's able, on the morning after surgery. He'll start returning to a normal diet as soon as you hear normal bowel sounds.

Steps to prevent postop complications

After surgery, your main concern will be to keep the newly opened or bypass vessel patent. You'll want to keep your patient's head elevated 30° in a midline position without flexion or hyperextension. Palpate his temporal and carotid pulses lightly q4h. Observe for hematoma formation at the operative site. After an endarterectomy, watch for edema of the neck that might signal arterial blockage or bleeding.

Assess your patient hourly for neurological signs of cerebral ischemia, watching especially for return of his preoperative symptoms.

The patient's blood pressure may fluctuate as a result of manipulation of his carotid sinus during surgery or a sympathetic response to stress. These conditions will correct themselves, usually within 24 hours. Meanwhile the doctor may order fluid replacement for hypotension that could cause ischemia.

A chronic hypertensive patient will resume his usual antihypertensive medication after surgery to help prevent further arterial damage or rupturing the inter-arterial graft if he's had an EIAB.

If your patient has had an EIAB, you have to keep pressure off his operative side to prevent arterial occlusion. Tell him not to lie on that side. Keep his head dressings loose. If he wears glasses, remove the bow (the sidepiece that goes over the ear) on the operative side.

Care of the patient with hemorrhage

Treatment of hemorrhagic stroke depends primarily on the location of the hemorrhage.

An intracerebral hemorrhage is usually treated medically. Your patient will receive antihypertensive medication, probably IV nitroprusside, to bring his blood pressure down. This goal must be pursued slowly and cautiously and the effects of therapy monitored closely. Too great a drop in blood pressure can increase ischemia by reducing cerebral perfusion.

If the patient's ICP is elevated, you must take measures to decrease it. These may include hyperventilation and administration of drugs such as mannitol, decadron, urea, and maybe a phenobarbital drip.

A clot that forms to seal an artery, thereby stopping hemorrhage, must be protected. To prevent rebleeding, monitor your patient's blood pressure closely and warn him not to perform the Valsalva maneuver. Aminocaproic acid (Amicar) reduces the threat of clot lysis by promoting formation of scar tissue.

The doctor may decide to treat intracerebral hemorrhage surgically if the symptoms are very severe. Many such hemorrhages are inoperable, however, because the surgeon can't reach the site without

---

Diagnostic tests for stroke patients

The physician will order certain diagnostic tests to help him learn more about the patient's stroke and determine the appropriate treatment. Here are the major tests and the nursing measures you must take to protect your patient from complications.

CT scan. Stroke patients undergo a CT scan to aid in determining the location of a stroke and to look for cerebral edema. Make sure beforehand that your patient has no allergy to iodine or shellfish, which would put him at risk for a reaction to the dye that's used for the CT scan.

Once the CT scan has been done, the patient may undergo implantation of a ventriculostomy catheter, which you'll use to monitor his ICP in the days to come.

Lumbar puncture. The physician will perform this procedure for a patient who has, or may have, suffered a hemorrhagic stroke. Clear cerebrospinal fluid indicates that there is intracerebral bleeding. Bloody CSF may mean that a vessel is broken in the subarachnoid space, probably due to an aneurysm.

Lumbar puncture is contraindicated for patients with very elevated ICP because it can provoke fatal brain herniation. Keep your patient flat on his back for six to eight hours after a puncture—longer if he develops a headache. Check the puncture site frequently for signs of CSF leak. Medicate your patient for any nausea and vomiting. Push fluids.

Angiogram. If the patient's symptoms and history suggest hemorrhagic stroke, the physician may order an angiogram to determine the exact condition of the affected artery. He'll also order the test for a patient who has suffered an ischemic stroke severe enough to warrant surgery. The test shows him what part of the artery to operate on.

Prior to the angiogram, find out whether the patient has allergies to iodine or shellfish, which could cause a reaction to the dye. Since vasospasm and stroke can complicate this procedure, make frequent checks of your patient's vital signs, neurological status, and pedal and groin pulses during and after the angiogram. To prevent hematoma, avoid flexion of the groin at the puncture site for eight to 12 hours after the test. Check the puncture site frequently for bleeding.

In addition to the foregoing procedures, the physician will probably order blood to be drawn for a renal profile and glucose test. These tests rule out electrolyte and metabolic imbalances that might cause symptoms mimicking stroke.

---

precipitating further neurological damage or death.

Subarachnoid hemorrhages are usually treated surgically. The surgeon clips the aneurysm or repairs the arterio-venous malformation that's causing it.

The physician generally delays surgery for intracerebral or sub-

arachnoid hemorrhage until four to 10 days after the onset of the bleed. This allows time for the vasospasm that follows the rupture of a vessel to subside. To alleviate vasospasm, it may be necessary to administer fluids, oxygen, and calcium channel blocking drugs.

The most common complications

of corrective surgery for hemorrhage are renewed vasospasm, rebleeding, ischemia, and hydrocephalus. Hydrocephalus may resolve spontaneously as the body reabsorbs blood. However, if it doesn't, the surgeon must take the patient back to the OR to insert a ventriculostomy or a permanent ventricular-peritoneal shunt for drainage.

Thanks to doctors' improved understanding of the causes of strokes, stroke patients have better prospects now than they did as recently as five years ago. However, most still incur some permanent neurological damage. Dealing with that damage is the subject of next month's installment, "Stroke: How to start the long road back." ■

BIBLIOGRAPHY Buonanno, F. and Toole, J. Management of patients with established ("completed") cerebral infarction. *Stroke*, 12(1):7, January 1981. Caronna, J. and Levy, D. Clinical predictors of outcome in ischemic stroke. *Neurologic Clinics*, February 1983. Hoff, J. Surgical frontiers in stroke management. *Clin. Neurosurg.* 29:534, 1982. Russell, R. Pathogenesis of transient ischemic attacks. *Neurologic Clinics*, February 1983. Yatsu, F. Acute medical therapies of strokes. *Clin. Neurosurg*, 29:524, 1982. Zarins, C. et al. Increased cerebral blood flow after external carotid artery revascularization. *Surgery*, 89(6):730, June 1981.

Spinal cord injury: Nursing the patient toward a new life

A patient who's sustained an injury to the spinal cord will need most of your time, but the satisfaction you'll get from supporting him through a drastic change will be a handsome reward.

By June Hart Romeo, BSN, BSEd, MAEd

All nursing forces must mobilize immediately when the emergency department calls to say they'll be sending up a patient with a spinal cord injury. This patient will need close, intense supervision, so the first thing you do is call a brief staff conference to reassign your other patients.

Next, you will need to requisition one of the specialized beds that allow you to reposition the patient without moving the spinal cord.

You'll also have to decide where to put the patient and his bed. A private room is best. You'll need plenty of space to work around all four sides of the big bed, and you may need to fit suction and other equipment in the room, too. Furthermore, the frequent comings

THE AUTHOR: Ms. Romeo is clinical instructor in the neurological intensive care unit at Cleveland Clinic Foundation, Cleveland.

Produced by David Anderson

and goings involved in caring for a spinal injury would unduly disturb other patients.

How to handle the patient's arrival

The patient should arrive strapped supine to a backboard, with his head and neck stabilized between IV bags or sandbags. A nurse from the emergency department will accompany him. She'll describe the history of his injury and his condition after stabilization in the ED.

Introduce yourself to the patient, make eye contact, and touch him reassuringly. Quickly assess him for any breathing difficulties, bleeding, and changing level of consciousness. Tell him you'll sit down and answer all his questions as soon as you get him settled in his room.

Enlist the help of several other nurses to transfer the patient to his specialized bed. Logroll him carefully, making sure to keep the injured spine from flexing. Fasten the appropriate straps to keep him secure, and make sure that any tubes and catheters are working.

Planning surgery and stabilizing the spine

The doctor will schedule surgery quickly if X-rays show bone fragments or foreign objects threatening the spinal cord. Otherwise he may wait until acute tissue swelling subsides—usually within a week—and then perform surgery to permanently stabilize the damaged segment. The most common procedures are vertebral fusion, laminectomy, and implantation of wires or Harrington rods.

Pending surgery, an unstable cervical spine requires traction to keep it extended and stationary. The easiest traction equipment, Gardner-Wells tongs, can be attached at the bedside. The main alternative, Crutchfield tongs, are usually attached in the OR, occasionally at the bedside.*

Prior to attachment, patches of hair are shaved where the screws will go. The patient usually receives local anesthetic and an anti-anxiety agent such as diazepam (Valium). He'll feel pressure, but not pain. Talk him through the experience. Emphasize that there's no danger of the screws penetrating to his brain.

The patient will probably receive IV corticosteroids to reduce cord edema. He'll also have an X-ray every three days or so to check swelling, and to make sure bone splinters haven't moved closer to the spinal cord.

Spinal injuries are often stable enough not to require surgery. The patient must still be kept immobile, however, during the early stages of healing.

The patient who has a stable injury of the cervical spine may wear a Halo brace for six to eight weeks. The Halo keeps the spine extended and aligned while allowing the patient to get out of bed and walk. Wrenches that unfasten the vent in the vest should be taped to it so that they're immediately at hand if CPR is necessary.

Assist the patient the first few times he gets up. He's likely to experience orthostatic hypotension, so have him rise slowly and rest sitting on the side of the bed for a few minutes before standing. Caution the patient with a Halo brace that its unaccustomed weight may upset

*For a complete discussion of traction and traction devices, see "Nursing the patient in traction," in the Jan. 1988 issue and "Special care for skeletal traction," in the Feb. 1988 issue.

his balance. (It should go without saying that patients should not be pulled into a sitting position by the brace, but unfortunately, it happens rather commonly.)

Patients with stable injuries to the thoracic or lumbar spine may wear leather belt-type braces once they're allowed out of bed.

When the patient is immobilized and stabilized, complications become your central concern. The most common problems result from spinal shock—which will occur an hour or so after cord injury and usually lasts about three weeks—and immobility.

After spinal shock resolves, however, as many as half of all patients who have a spinal cord injury are at risk of developing autonomic hyperreflexia. This complication—which is also known as autonomic dysreflexia, paroxysmal hypertension, autonomic spasticity, and mass-reflex phenomenon—is considered a medical emergency.

Hyperreflexia demands quick action

Autonomic hyperreflexia is a sympathetic overresponse to a mild stimulus. Symptoms include throbbing headache, blurred vision, nasal congestion, nausea, sweating below the level of the cord injury, bradycardia, and gooseflesh. The patient's systolic blood pressure may rise to 300 mm Hg or more.

This syndrome usually develops when the cord has been completely transected above the level of T6. It rarely occurs after incomplete injuries. You're most likely to see autonomic hyperreflexia during the early rehabilitation phase after spinal

shock has resolved.

The patient will very likely suffer a stroke and die unless you rapidly control his blood pressure. Here's what to do:

Sit the patient upright to lower intracranial blood pressure.

Call for help, but don't leave the patient.

Look for the stimulus. It's most often a kinked catheter, full bladder, or pain, but can be something as mild as a breeze or pressure against the skin. Another possible cause, fecal impaction, is best checked by a doctor, since digital examination of the anal area can provoke the condition you want to reverse. Once you find the cause, removing it will usually resolve the episode.

Reassure the patient by telling him what's happening and what you're doing to help.

Check the blood pressure at two to three minute intervals until it stabilizes.

If the stimulus cannot be found or removed a ganglionic blocking agent such as Hyperstat or Apresoline may be ordered by IV push. You should keep these drugs on hand whenever you're caring for a patient who's at risk of developing autonomic hyperreflexia.

A few patients develop hyperreflexia for the first time after being discharged, up to a year after the injury. Once a patient has a first episode of hyperreflexia, he's at increased risk for others, and may continue to have them throughout life. Train all spinal injury patients and their families to recognize the symptoms and search out the potential causes.

The right bed can make a big difference

One nurse can provide complete care of the spinal injury patient on a Roto Rest bed. A system of adjustable arms, clamps, and pads makes immobilization and traction simple. A motor rocks the bed from side to side, promoting pulmonary and venous drainage. Gentle and continuous motion, together with an easy-to-clean mattress pad that eliminates the need for sheets, greatly reduce the risk of pressure sores. Trap doors give access to the patient's back for skin care. Under the bed are holders for bedpans and X-ray plates.

Two or more nurses are needed to care for the patient on a CircOlectric bed. A motor that the patient can control drives him around a circular track, from supine to upright to prone position, and back again. This prevents complications of immobility, but the patient may slip and become wedged between the frames if he's not strapped in tightly enough. An extra frame must be placed over the patient to keep him from falling whenever he's put into either a full-standing or prone position.

The Stryker bed involves sandwiching the patient between two frames, with all the inconvenience that involves for the patient and nurse. This bed turns the patient around a smaller axis than the CircOlectric—from supine to side-lying to prone and back. It must be turned manually, which means that the patient must call a nurse when he wants to change position.

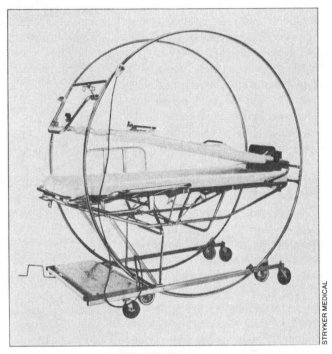

The CircOlectric bed

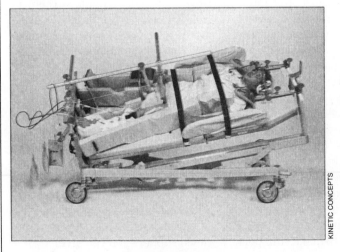

The Roto Rest bed

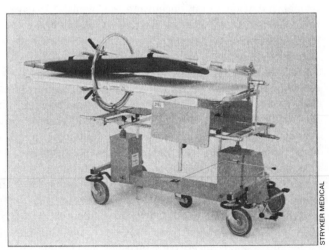

The Stryker bed

Prevent complications of bladder and bowel

The flaccidity and arreflexia of the bladder that results from spinal shock can lead to urinary retention and overflow incontinence. If you use an indwelling catheter to control the flow of urine, be sure to keep the system closed so that bacteria don't get in. If you perform intermittent catheterization, do so every four to six hours. Some patients can regain bladder control with retraining when spinal shock resolves, and some will have to learn self-catheterization.

Spinal shock paralyzes the bowel, too. To prevent impactions, administer soapsuds enemas every three days. When shock begins to resolve, stimulate bowel function with stool softeners, abdominal massage, or suppositories. A comprehensive bowel retraining program is described on the next page.

Assist the patient in regaining maximum bladder and bowel control by encouraging fluid intake and proper nutrition. Your encouragement plays a major role in the patient's success in retraining.

Prevent complications caused by immobility

Secretions pool in the lungs of the immobilized patient. They'll cause respiratory problems if he doesn't bring them up. Have him cough and deep breathe hourly. Turn him every two hours. Auscultate his lungs once each shift. Should you hear any rasping, wheezing, or decreased breath sounds, you may have him use an incentive spirometer. Chest physiotherapy also helps clear lungs. Some patients with high cervical injuries need

---

Bowel retraining: an early goal in rehabilitation

A bowel retraining program is a vital first step in promoting independence, bolstering self-image, and motivating the patient for further rehabilitation.

Start by checking the patient's nutrition. He must eat an adequate number of calories and drink sufficient fluids for bowel retraining to succeed. Roughage helps regulate movements.

Schedule bowel stimulation at the same time every day. Try to make the time consistent with the patient's pre-injury bowel habits. You'll get the best results if attempts at defecation follow a meal by about 30 minutes. That's because a powerful duodenocolonic push occurs then.

When the time comes, clear any impaction from the bowel. Position the patient on a bedside commode or toilet. If the patient is confined to bed and must use a bedpan, pay close attention to proper positioning and skin care.

Insert a bisacodyl (Dulcolax) or glycerin suppository high up in the rectum. Let the patient rest for about 20 minutes. Massage his abdomen from right to left and down, to stimulate the large intestine.

If the patient doesn't defecate within an hour, gently stimulate the anal sphincter with your finger two or three times. If this doesn't bring results, end the routine for the day. Tell the patient to call for assistance, however, if he feels stirrings: Some people take as long as three hours to react to suppositories.

Once the patient's bowels begin to move, you may want to switch over to an every-other-day or every-third-day schedule according to the patient's pre-injury frequency. In general, modify the program as needed for the patient's convenience.

---

ventilator care because the intercostal or phrenic nerve impulses that drive breathing are disrupted.

Skin breakdown and decubiti are a danger. If your patient is not on a kinetic therapeutic bed, you need to reposition him every hour or two. Keep the skin dry. Don't, however, use rings or donuts that are supposed to protect against pressure sores by reducing the weight load on the coccyx: Nursing research has shown them to be counterproductive.

Monitor food intake and major electrolyte levels to make sure poor nutrition doesn't compromise tissue repair. Many patients have poor appetites. Company at meal times can help stimulate them to eat. Encourage the family to bring familiar foods, china, and good silver from home. Some patients, of course, need to be fed.

Help the patient cope emotionally

The patient with a spinal injury comes to you with his life broken into pieces—how many, he doesn't yet know. Overwhelmed by dismay and uncertainty, he may either withdraw or be angry and hostile. In either case, he needs all the emotional support you can give.

Identify yourself each time you come into the patient's room. Announce every intervention before performing it. In this way you'll give him a sense of structure and the knowledge that caring professionals are doing everything that can be done. Make yourself available to answer all his questions.

Give the patient prism glasses while he's supine. They'll enable him to watch television, see visitors, and follow some of the activity around him. Prism glasses blur vision, however, and some patients become disoriented from wearing them too much.

Suggest ways for the patient to occupy himself. Listening to music is one obvious example. Some public libraries lend books recorded on cassette tape.

If none of this helps your patient accept his new condition, respect his attitude.

Preparing the patient for discharge

The patient may be able to sit up in a wheelchair or ambulate anywhere from 12 hours to a week after sur-

gery, depending on the injury and the procedure performed. These advances will be delayed, of course, until spinal shock resolves. They may never occur if cord damage is too severe.

Begin planning for discharge as soon as the patient's condition begins to stabilize. Help him look ahead to how he will live with his new limitations. Encourage realistic hopes that some abilities will return. This will blunt the shattering impact that may occur when the full extent of the changes in his life becomes clear. If his disability is severe, he may find his employability as well as his role in the family drastically changed. Occupational therapy and psychiatric counseling can ease this transition.

You also need to let the patient discuss concerns about sexuality. Depending on the level of the spinal lesion, the patient's ability to have intercourse may be preserved or permanently impaired. You may reassure all patients, however,

that no matter what their disabilities may be, they're still capable of sexual expression. Offer to refer them to counseling for help in this difficult area.

Some patients must wear a Halo or other brace at home for many weeks. Show family members how to care for the brace and the skin beneath it. Teach the patient who will be bedridden how to use a mirror to monitor his skin condition. He'll probably also need a home care nurse.

Your patient may go to a rehabilitation facility before returning home. He may, indeed, spend the rest of his life in a long-term care facility. Whatever his fate, he'll remember your dedication to bringing him through a deep crisis. ∎

BIBLIOGRAPHY Hickey, J.V. *The clinical practice of neurologial and neurosurgical nursing* (2nd ed.). Philadelphia, J.B. Lippincott, 1986. Larrabee, J.H. The person with spinal cord injury: physical care during early recovery. *Am. J. Nurs.* 77:1320, 1977. Rudy, E.B. *Advanced neurological and neurosurgical nursing.* St. Louis: C.V. Mosby, 1984. Youmans, J.R. *Neurological surgery* (vol. 5). Philadelphia: W.B. Saunders, 1983.

Chest pain: Your response to a classic warning

Angina is a signal that the heart has been pushed to its limit. Understanding why pain occurs and how it's treated will give you the confidence you need to help your patient through it.

By Virginia L. Thompson, RN, CCRN

"I shouldn't have eaten so fast," Mr. Howell groaned. "It gave me a lot of gas."

I turned off his call light and looked at him thoughtfully. "You hurt? Where?"

He was leaning forward in bed and rubbing his chest just below the sternum.

"Are you sure it's not chest pain?" I asked.

"No," he insisted. "Absolutely not. I just ate too much."

I gave him the antacid he requested and waited a minute, tidying the room and checking his IVs.

Mr. Howell had been admitted with chest pain to the coronary care unit three days before. When a cardiac catheterization showed narrowing and near-occlusion of two coronary arteries, his cardiologist recommended bypass sur-

THE AUTHOR is a CCU staff nurse at South Miami Hospital in Florida.

Produced by Karin L. Emra, RN, BSN

gery. Cardiac isoenzyme levels were slightly elevated, but did not reflect infarction, and continuous nitroglycerin and heparin drips were ordered to manage the ischemia. Surgery was delayed until Mr. Howell had time to stabilize.

"Is the pain easing?" I asked.

"Not yet," said Mr. Howell. He was still leaning forward. I turned on his oxygen and gently put the nasal cannula on his face, then checked his vital signs. His blood pressure was a little higher than his admission baseline. I watched his cardiac monitor for rate and rhythm changes, and set up and ran a 12-lead ECG.

"I'm feeling it more up here now," he said, rubbing his sternum. "Maybe it's chest pain after all."

I increased his nitro drip, following the physician's order for titration, and rechecked his blood pressure. Now and then I patted him on

the arm—to reassure him while satisfying myself that he wasn't perspiring.

"How's your pain?" I asked.

"A little better, but now it's going into my left shoulder and arm."

I increased his nitro drip another 5 mcg/min increment.

"It's beginning to go away now," he said almost immediately. "It feels so much better already."

I took his BP again and found the systolic only 10 mm/Hg lower than his baseline value. His color was good. With the pain resolved, I left the nitro drip at the new level, documented the event, and added the 12-lead ECG strip to his chart, comparing it to previous tracings. Then I called his cardiologist to report the episode.

Angina: A message from the heart

Mr. Howell's angina is a symptom that his heart muscle is starved for oxygen. It's similar to the pain that runners feel when their leg muscles become hypoxic. When the myocardium's oxygen needs aren't met, its metabolism changes, causing the release of lactic acid and toxins. With ischemia, cell membrane permeability is increased as well. Substances released from the cells and the metabolic changes stimulate nerve endings near the heart, causing pain. The heart muscle itself cannot send out such a message since it lacks afferent pain fibers.

People experience angina in different ways—as severe indigestion or burning, heaviness, ache, or squeezing or crushing pressure. One patient likened it to an elephant standing on his chest. As he said this, he placed a clenched fist over his sternum—a classic sign of angina.

The pain is usually felt behind the sternum and may radiate to the neck, throat, jaw, shoulders, or arms (usually the left arm). A sense of anxiety and doom is common.

It's common, too, for a patient to fear he's having a myocardial infarction. Angina is certainly a sign that the heart is in trouble, but most anginal discomfort responds promptly to rest and medication. Limiting the duration of the oxygen shortage can prevent permanent damage to the heart.

In most patients, the cause of angina is atherosclerosis. Fibrous plaque builds up on the inner walls of the arteries, narrowing the lumen and reducing blood flow. Research is revealing coincident clot formation to be a significant, contributing factor.

Despite the narrowing, enough

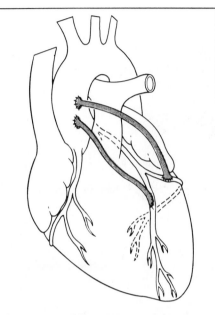

In double bypass surgery, two sections of saphenous or mammary vessel are grafted from the aorta to points below the blockage in the clogged arteries.

BETH ANNE WILLERT

oxygen may reach the myocardium for normal needs. But when exertion, emotional stress, a heavy meal, or even exposure to cold or hot, humid weather increases its work, more oxygen is needed. If coronary arteries cannot deliver enough blood, myocardial ischemia and angina result.

Other conditions can also affect the heart's blood and oxygen supply and demand, causing angina. These include dysrhythmias, coronary artery spasm, valvular stenosis, left ventricular hypertrophy, hyperthyroidism, systemic hypertension, anemia, and hypoxia.

Distinguish among the types of angina

With stable angina—also called effort or chronic angina—a patient can usually predict the level of exertion that will cause an ischemic attack. Rest and sublingual nitroglycerin usually bring relief in three to five minutes.

Unstable angina is less predictable and more serious. Sometimes called pre-infarction angina, it may appear suddenly or develop gradually in a patient who has had mild, stable angina for years. Stable angina is reclassified as unstable when it becomes more intense and frequent, lasts longer, and is brought on by less exertion or occurs at complete rest.

For either classification, an ECG taken during discomfort reveals ST-T wave abnormalities that return to normal when the episode resolves, reflecting ischemia without transmural infarction. Though the transient ST segment depression and T wave inversion or elevation may assist with diagnosis, conditions other than ischemia can cause such abnormalities.

A third type of angina, variant or Prinzmetal's, results from vasospasm rather than atherosclerosis, although atherosclerosis may also be present. Usually not affected by exertion, it often occurs at rest, most commonly in the early part of the day. If prolonged, the constricting spasm of a coronary artery can lead to necrosis of cardiac tissue and acute MI, just as occlusion can.

Variant angina is rare and can be difficult to diagnose. An ECG or angiogram may appear normal unless the artery goes into spasm during testing. With spasm, the ECG shows ST segment elevation with an upright or inverted T wave,

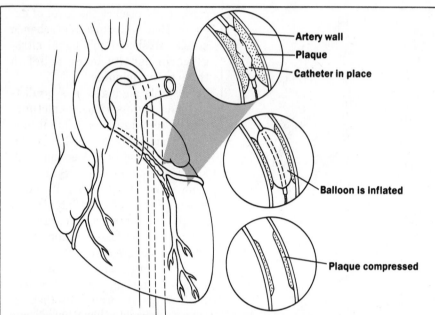

Artery wall
Plaque
Catheter in place

Balloon is inflated

Plaque compressed

In percutaneous transluminal coronary angioplasty, a balloon-tipped catheter is threaded to the blockage. When the balloon is inflated it compresses the plaque permitting adequate blood flow. Angioplasty is usually limited to patients with blockage in the proximal portion of a single artery.

which mimics the change during acute MI. When the anginal episode is over, the segments return to the patient's normal pattern.

An essential part of a differential diagnosis for angina is a complete and accurate history of symptoms and, in the case of coronary artery disease, the patient's risk factors. These include a family history, being male, hypertensive, obese, a smoker, and having diabetes, hyperlipidemia, stress, and a sedentary lifestyle.

Non-invasive procedures that will help determine the cause and extent of the problem causing the angina include ECG, echocardiogram, chest X-ray, treadmill stress test with or without thallium scintigraphy, nuclear isotope imaging, and serum levels of lipoproteins,

cardiac enzymes, and arterial blood gases.

Cardiac catheterization and angiography often follow, to find out exactly where vital arteries are narrowed or blocked. This lets the doctor decide whether bypass surgery, percutaneous transluminal coronary angioplasty (PTCA), or a change in medication is most likely to help the patient.

Know the meds and what they do
Several classes of drugs are available to increase blood and oxygen supply or decrease myocardial oxygen demand.

Nitrates—usually nitroglycerin or isosorbide dinitrate—are prescribed most frequently. These vasodilators relax smooth muscle in

the capillaries and cause peripheral dilation. That reduces venous return to the heart, decreasing the amount of blood in the ventricle at the end of diastole (preload). Because nitrates dilate arterioles as well as capillaries, they also reduce the resistance the heart must overcome to pump blood out of the ventricle during systole (afterload). These actions reduce the heart's work load.

Nitroglycerin comes in different forms. Many patients take it sublingually, by spray or tablet, to relieve symptoms or prophylactically before exertion. For steady administration there are capsules or tablets, ointments, and transdermal patches. Patients like Mr. Howell, who have been hospitalized for unstable angina, may be given the drug intravenously by infusion pump.

Nitroglycerin preparations for parenteral use require dilution in dextrose 5% in water or sodium chloride 0.9%. Preparations will vary in concentration and volume, therefore manufacturer's recommendations need to be followed faithfully. Use glass bottles and tubing that isn't made of polyvinyl chloride (PVC), which readily absorbs nitroglycerin.

Before an infusion begins, the patient should have an indwelling systemic arterial catheter—or at least a portable, oscillometric blood pressure device—in place for constant monitoring of systolic, diastolic, and mean arterial blood pressures and heart rate. Titrate IV nitroglycerin carefully, increasing the dose by 5 mcg/min every three to five minutes. If blood pressure and pain don't respond by 20

Angina: Teaching for discharge

Patients with angina need to learn why it occurs and what they can do to control it. Elizabeth DiGiacomo-Geffers, RN, MPH, CNAA, CEN, regional director of ambulatory nursing for FHP in Fountain Valley, Calif., provides a teaching plan:

To keep your teaching at an appropriate level begin by asking the patient to tell you what he already knows about angina. Be especially sensitive to his emotional readiness to learn. A patient who has negative feelings—denial, anger, or fear, for example—may require additional time to process new information. Acknowledge such emotions and pace your teaching accordingly. Your patient's anxiety should lessen considerably as he comes to understand his condition and how to successfully live with it.

Have the patient describe how he feels during an angina attack and identify activities that usually provoke one. Explain why the pain occurs and how it can be prevented. Here are some key points to include:

▶ Any physical exertion will increase the heart's demand for oxygen. That means the patient should avoid certain activities such as heavy lifting or isometric exercises and pace himself during other types of exercise—climbing stairs or walking long distances, for example. He should take nitroglycerin prophylactically before sex and any other activity that's known to bring on angina.

▶ Emotionally stressful situations should be avoided, whenever possible, because both heart rate and blood pressure can be affected. For instance, he may be able to revise his work schedule to avoid rush-hour traffic. He should also learn relaxation techniques and the art of delegating responsibility to others.

▶ A heavy meal will increase the heart's work load. Encourage lighter meals, eaten at a leisurely pace and then followed by an hour of rest or quiet activities.

▶ Temperature extremes may make the heart work harder. In cold weather the patient should dress warmly, wear a scarf over his mouth, and walk slowly. When it's hot, he should take on fewer activities and limit time spent outside.

▶ Nicotine gum, nasal decongestants, and "diet pills" can elevate heart rate and blood pressure and should be avoided.

▶ Constipation can cause straining during bowel movements. Encourage regular, paced exercise such as walking. Suggest the use of stool softeners, a diet rich in fiber, and adequate fluid intake.

Teach your patient the risk factors for atherosclerosis if this is the cause of his angina, and discuss how to modify those that apply to him. If there are several of them, beware of overwhelming him. An obese smoker with high cholesterol, a 60-hour work week, and a sedentary lifestyle isn't likely to think he can mend all his ways immediately. Help him establish priorities and choose a place to begin changing his habits.

Discuss his heart medications with him—exactly what they do, how and when to take them, and all the possible side effects. Write this information down and give it to him to take home for reference.

Tell him to carry nitroglycerin with him at all times, in its original vial and tightly capped. Tablets should be discarded six months after the vial has been opened for the first time. If the tablet doesn't tingle or feel warm when placed under the tongue, then it's no longer effective and the vial should be replaced.

Explain what to do when angina strikes. The patient should stop whatever he's doing, sit or lie down, and place a nitroglycerin tablet under his tongue. If relief doesn't come within five minutes, he should take another tablet, wait five minutes, and repeat the nitro one more time if he's still uncomfortable.

If pain continues after he's taken three nitro tablets, he should have someone drive him to the nearest emergency room or call for an ambulance. Emphasize that he shouldn't drive himself. He should also seek emergency assistance if his angina increases in severity or frequency or occurs when he's at rest. Such changes might indicate a heart attack.

Always try to make your teaching sessions a family affair. Their involvement, understanding, and support are important to the patient's successful rehabilitation.

mcg/min, the doctor may increase the increments to 10 mcg/min and later 20 mcg/min. When the blood pressure begins to drop, the increments should be reduced and intervals lengthened. Titration continues cautiously until pain is relieved or blood pressure drops below an acceptable level. That level depends on the patient's baseline, but a general rule is to stop at a systolic of 100. The patient may get a headache as the dosage increases. Give acetaminophen.

Beta-adrenergic blockers like

propranolol (Inderal) are frequently prescribed in conjunction with nitrates. These agents further reduce the myocardium's oxygen consumption by blocking the catecholamine-induced increases in heart rate, systolic blood pressure, and also the rate and force of cardiac contractions.

While effective for effort angina, beta blockers worsen variant angina caused by spasm.

Calcium channel blockers, in combined therapy with nitrates, relieve variant angina. They are also used to treat stable and unstable angina, given in addition to nitrates and cautiously with beta blockers.

Nifedipine (Adalat, Procardia), verapamil hydrochloride (Calan, Isoptin), and diltiazem hydrochloride (Cardizem) increase coronary blood flow. Verapamil and diltiazem decrease cardiac contractility, heart rate, and the demand for oxygen. Nifedipine, on the other hand, raises the heart rate while acting as a strong vasodilator, increasing coronary perfusion and lowering blood pressure.

Most patients take nifedipine capsules orally, but you can also administer the drug sublingually to relieve acute angina. Simply puncture a capsule with a sterile #18 needle and squeeze the liquid under the patient's tongue. Sublingual medications act rapidly, so be prepared to monitor the patient's blood pressure.*

Anticoagulants, antiplatelet drugs, and fibrolytic agents are

*For more on the nitrates, beta blockers, and calcium channel blockers, see "The nurse's guide to cardiovascular drugs" in the Aug. and Sept. 1988 issues of **RN**.

considered for therapy because of their effective action against thrombus formation.

Because blood clots can form easily in a compromised artery and may occlude it completely, Mr. Howell's physician ordered a heparin drip.

Narcotic analgesics like morphine sulfate are given during an ischemic attack to ease pain and anxiety. They act as vasodilators as well. Avoid intramuscular injections, since many cardiac enzyme levels will increase with muscular injury.

Invasive procedures to correct blood flow

Patients like Mr. Howell, who have many or severe bouts of angina, marginally controlled by drugs, need aggressive treatment to improve blood supply to the myocardium.

Coronary artery bypass grafting (CABG) is performed to bypass stenosis or occlusion in one or more arteries. The cardiologist uses segments of the patient's internal mammary artery or saphenous vein to connect the aorta to the coronary artery at a point below the blockage.

Percutaneous transluminal coronary angioplasty (PTCA), an invasive, non-surgical alternative is usually limited to patients with blockage in the proximal portion of a single artery. Complications during or after PTCA may need emergency bypass surgery, so the patient must be suitable for CABG.

During PTCA, the cardiologist, aided by fluoroscopy, passes a fine, balloon-tipped catheter through an artery in the arm or leg, up into the aorta, and on into the coronary artery. When the catheter reaches

the blockage, he inflates the balloon, compressing the plaque and dilating the vessel.

Research with laser angioplasty shows promise.

Helping your patient through the pain

When your patient has an angina attack, persuade him to sit down and rest. Get a 12-lead ECG (especially for a newly admitted patient or one with known unstable angina), give nitroglycerin, and take vital signs. If oxygen has been ordered, make certain he uses it. The angina may resolve with rest and nitroglycerin. Be sure to document the episode and your actions in your nurse's notes and notify the physician.

If the nitroglycerin does not bring relief, an infarction may be impending or already in progress. Signal for assistance and get a message to the physician stat. Be on the lookout for dyspnea, diaphoresis, hypotension, and pallor or cyanosis.

If the patient's nervous and talks, gently remind him that he's using oxygen his heart needs, and that the pain will go away more quickly if he remains quiet. Reassure him.

Remember that cardiac patients frequently deny their disease. Like Mr. Howell, they would prefer to attribute their pain to a recent meal, an overdue bowel movement . . . anything else except the heart.

Once a patient accepts the fact that his pain is, indeed, angina, he becomes fearful that he's having a heart attack. It's extremely important to remain with him and support him until after the pain is gone.

Your calm, matter-of-fact, take-charge attitude will help reduce anxiety, fear, and pain. Dim the lights, turn off the television, and explain to your patient you'll remain with him until he is comfortable and at ease. Your presence

and caring is certain to make a real difference. ∎

BIBLIOGRAPHY Alspach, J.G. and Williams, S., eds. *Core Curriculum For Critical Care Nursing* (3rd ed.). Philadelphia: W.B. Saunders Company, 1985. American Heart Association: 1988 Heart Facts. Dallas, Texas, 1988. Muller, E., Zoltan, G.T., et al. Nifedipine and conventional therapy for unstable angina pectoris: a randomized, double-bind comparison. *Circulation* 69:728, 1984. Schlant, R.C. and Hurst, J.W. *Handbook of the Heart.* New York: McGraw-Hill Book Company, 1988. Solomon, J. *Introduction to Cardiovascular Nursing.* Baltimore: Williams and Wilkins, 1988. Talkington, S. and Raterink, G., eds. *Every Nurse's Guide to Cardiovascular Care.* New York: John Wiley & Sons, 1987. Understanding Angina. Videotape produced by The American Heart Association, Dallas, Texas, 1984. Vinsant, M.D. and Spence, J.I. *A Common Sense Approach To Coronary Care* (3rd ed.). St. Louis: C.V. Mosby, 1981.

What you need to know about today's pacemakers

Rapid advances in pacemaker technology can mean changes in the care you give pacemaker patients. Here's an overview of current—and future—pacemaker models, indications for their use, and complications you'll need to watch out for.

By Linda Porterfield RN, BSN, and James G. Porterfield, MD

Matthew Aldrich, a 68-year-old cardiac patient, had a permanent pacemaker implanted three days ago. Normally, such a patient would be getting ready for discharge, but Mr. Aldrich has developed signs of an infection at the implantation site. His physician decides to keep him in the hospital to continue his IV antibiotic therapy and to monitor his condition, and he's assigned to your med/surg unit.

You realize that you don't remember very much about pacemakers. That means you'll need to get some up-to-date information about these devices. In addition, you'll need to find out why Mr. Aldrich needed a pacemaker and how to tell if it's working properly. Last, but certainly not least, you'll

THE AUTHORS: Linda Porterfield is a PhD candidate in pharmacology and works in the cardiovascular research lab at the University of Tennessee. James G. Porterfield is a cardiologist with the Cardiology Group of Memphis and a clinical instructor in medicine at the University of Tennessee.

need to know how to get your patient ready to go home with his new pacemaker.

The new look in pacemakers

A pacemaker is a battery-powered pulse generator with a wire lead that attaches to the heart. Epicardial leads attach to the outer surface of the heart. More common are endocardial leads, which are placed inside the heart.

To position an endocardial lead, the cardiologist inserts the wire lead into the cephalic, subclavian, or external jugular vein. From there, he threads it into the right ventricle, monitoring placement with fluoroscopic X-ray equipment. At the tip of the lead are small tines that hook onto the inside surface of the heart. They secure the lead until fibrosis further stabilizes it.

Once the lead is in place, the physician connects it to the pulse gen-

erator. He then makes a small incision and implants the generator just under the skin—usually in the upper chest or abdomen.

Today's pulse generators are about $2\frac{1}{2}$ inches long, $1\frac{1}{2}$ inches wide, and $\frac{1}{2}$ inch thick, which means they're smaller and easier to implant than earlier models. Usually only local anesthesia is required.

When pacemakers work only on demand

Demand pacemakers—the most common type implanted today—operate only when needed. They sense the intrinsic or natural heart rate in the chamber where the lead is located.

If the heart's natural rate falls below the preset pacemaker rate, the pulse generator delivers timed electrical impulses. These impulses stimulate the heart to contract, thereby maintaining an adequate rate and cardiac output. If the heart's natural rate is faster than the preset rate, the device delivers no impulses.

Newer pacemakers can be reprogrammed from an outside signal. Thus the physician can change the rate, stimulus strength and duration, and sensing level without removing and re-inserting the pulse generator. This spares the patient from further surgery.

The new pacemakers also have batteries that last longer, so they don't have to be changed as often as those in previous models.

Who needs a pacemaker?

Last year more than 100,000 patients received implanted cardiac pacemakers. Like Mr. Aldrich, most of these were over age 65. Many have sick sinus syndrome—a dysfunction in which the SA node generates or conducts impulses slowly and irregularly or not at all. Some patients have partial or complete blockage elsewhere in the conduction system—the AV node is the most common—that can lead to syncope, confusion, or congestive heart failure. Atrial fibrillation with a slow ventricular response and hypersensitive carotid sinus syndrome are two other conditions that require a cardiac pacemaker implant.

Preop care and teaching

As you review his chart, you discover that Mr. Aldrich needed a pacemaker because he had sick sinus syndrome with increasingly frequent episodes of syncope during the past year.

The preop care Mr. Aldrich received before the implantation was similar to that given to any pacemaker patient—a history and physical exam, chest X-ray, and blood tests. To determine if he might react to medication, anesthesia, or—in rare instances—the materials in the pacemaker, his nurse also asked if he had any allergies.

Throughout Mr. Aldrich's preop teaching sessions, his nurse reviewed the basic anatomy and physiology of the heart. She also showed him a demonstration model of a pacemaker and gave him a booklet containing specific information about the pacemaker he would receive.

The nurse told Mr. Aldrich he would be awake for the surgery and might feel some discomfort. She explained that it would consist of a small—about two inches long—incision, which would be done under a local anesthetic. The total time away from his unit, he was told, would be about two hours.

Mr. Alrich was NPO before the implant to decrease the risk of vomiting, and he was given an antibiotic to decrease the risk of infection. An ECG machine continuously monitored his heart rate.

Watch for these postop problems

When Mr. Aldrich returned to his room, his nurses checked his dressing for signs of bleeding. They also checked his vital signs, observed the cardiac monitor for any signs of pacemaker malfunction, and placed ECG strips on his chart at specified intervals to document proper pacemaker function. The type of pace-

maker Mr. Aldrich received and the settings were recorded on his chart.

Mr. Aldrich showed no signs of pacemaker malfunction. He was out of bed and walking the day after the procedure. He resumed his normal diet and medications.

On his third postop day, however, Mr. Aldrich developed a fever and some redness at the implantation site. That's when he was transferred to your unit for further antibiotic therapy.

Is that pacemaker working properly?

In addition to keeping an eye on Mr. Aldrich for more signs of infection, you'll make sure the pacemaker is functioning the way it's supposed to.

Look for "pacemaker spikes" on the ECG. These spikes mean that the pacemaker is delivering electrical impulses. Because Mr. Alrich has a demand pacemaker, the spikes should appear only when his spontaneous heart rate falls below the preset pacemaker rate.

If his heart rate slows and no pacemaker spikes appear, the device is not functioning properly. The cause might be a dislodged lead, an incorrect sensitivity setting, or electrical interference. In any case, the physician should be notified immediately.

Be sure to notify the physician, too, if the spikes appear at an inappropriate time during the cardiac cycle. If the pacemaker fires during the T wave, the stimulus can cause ventricular tachycardia or fibrillation—both life-threatening arrhythmias. Watch for premature

Current terminology and future technology

A three-letter code has been developed for describing permanent pacemakers. The first letter indicates which heart chamber is paced: A = atrium, V = ventricle, D = dual or both chambers. The second letter identifies which chamber is sensed: A = atrium, V = ventricle, D = dual (both chambers), O = neither chamber. The third letter indicates the pacemaker's response: I = inhibited, T = triggered, D = dual (both functions).

Thus, the VVI pacemaker paces the ventricle, senses in the ventricle, and is inhibited by a spontaneously conducted electrical impulse. This is the most common type of pacemaker.

The new DDD pacemaker is capable of pacing and sensing in both chambers. It can be inhibited when it senses spontaneous electrical activity, or triggered when it doesn't. Although this pacemaker requires the implanting of two leads—one in the atrium and one in the ventricle—it can mimic normal heart function by sequentially sensing and pacing both chambers, depending on the patient's need.

Two other new features are rate-responsiveness and self-correction.

A rate-responsive pacemaker can sense changes in the patient's activity and translate those changes to a new pacing rate. If the patient is jogging, for example, the pacing rate will change to reflect the increase in activity.

A self-correcting pacemaker will be able to sense a problem such as loss of capture and reprogram itself to solve the problem.

ventricular contractions, which can be caused by irritation from a "floppy" electrode.

If the ECG does not show a QRS complex following the pacemaker spike, you have "loss of capture." This means the electrical impulse from the pacemaker is not strong enough to stimulate a contraction. Common causes of this problem in the early postop period are an electrode tip that's out of position or damage to the wire lead. Later on, a weak battery may be the cause.

Notify the physician if you see loss of capture. The more the patient depends on the pacemaker to maintain an adequate heart rate and rhythm, the more serious the problem.

Palpitations, dizziness, or syncope, which can be caused by any of the problems already mentioned, should also be reported. Reprogramming the pulse generator may correct some of these problems. If the trouble is a displaced lead, however, additional surgery might be necessary.

You should also report dyspnea, chest pain, a heart rate below the preset rate, and prolonged irregularities. These might indicate rare complications such as embolism, ventricular perforation, constrictive pericarditis, or pacemaker-generated arrhythmias.

Prepare the patient for going home

Mr. Aldrich's pacemaker continues to function properly. His suture line at the implantation site is still red, but his temperature is now normal. His physician plans to discharge him in two days.

To help Mr. Aldrich and his family adjust to living with a pacemaker, you'll want to cover these points in your discharge teaching:

Activities and exercise. Review the instructions Mr. Aldrich received from his physician about when to resume driving, work, exercise, and sexual relations. Most patients are told to avoid contact sports, but they're allowed to resume most other activities about four weeks after pacemaker insertion. By this time, fibrosis holds the lead in place, and the pacemaker pocket has healed.

Incision site. Tell the patient to wear loose clothing over the chest until the incision site heals. Tell him to report any signs of infection—warmth, redness, swelling, or drainage at the insertion site. Erosion—puckering or indented areas in the skin—could indicate an allergic reaction to the pulse generator, and should also be reported.

Diet and medication. Since having a pacemaker does not affect a patient's diet, you can assure Mr. Aldrich that he can continue to eat as he did before his hospitalization.

Even with the pacemaker he may still require certain cardiac medications—nitrates or calcium channnel blockers, for example. Remind him to take all medications as directed.

Identification card. Remember to give Mr. Aldrich a pacemaker identification card and tell him to carry it at all times. The card should say who manufactured the pacemaker and describe its settings and programmable functions.

It should also give the name and telephone number of the patient's physician and the hospital where the pacemaker was implanted.

Suggest that Mr. Aldrich make a copy of the card and keep it at home; this will simplify replacement in case the original is lost or stolen. Also suggest that he wear a Medic Alert tag, which is more easily noticed in an emergency than a wallet card.

Battery life. The lithium iodide battery that powers the pulse generator usually lasts six to 12 years. As the battery runs down, the electrical impulses may deviate from the preset rate. To detect this or related problems, tell Mr. Aldrich to check his radial pulse for one minute every day. If his pulse is slower than the preset rate, he should suspect a problem and notify his physician.

Electrical devices. Present day pacemakers are usually well shielded against electrical interference from radios, TVs, microwave ovens, and other household appliances. But large engines, telephone transformers, or certain anti-theft alarm systems have intense magnetic fields that can temporarily disrupt pacemaker function.

If this happens, the patient might experience palpitations. If he suspects electrical interference, he should immediately turn off the offending appliance. If that's not possible, he should stay at least five feet away from the device.

Telephone monitoring. Checking pacemaker function can be difficult for a homebound patient or one who lives far from his physician. Such a patient can buy or lease a

ECG changes that point to pacemaker malfunction

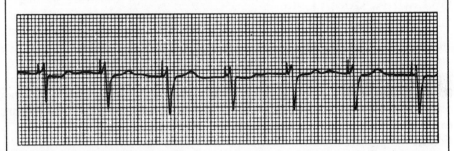

ECG tracings are used to identify normal pacemaker activity. The ECG strip above illustrates normal function for a VVI pacemaker—each pacer spike is followed by a QRS complex.

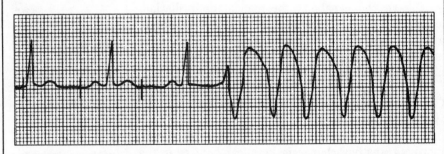

This tracing shows a malfunction in pacemaker sensing. The pacemaker is not inhibited by the heart's own activity. It fires during the T wave which results in ventricular tachycardia.

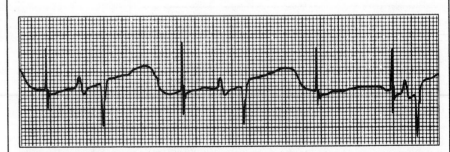

Failure to capture occurs when the heart doesn't respond to pacemaker stimulation. As shown above, there is no cardiac activity—in this case QRS complexes—after the pacer spikes.

A guide to external pacing

By Paul R. Cooper, RN

Just as there have been dramatic improvements in permanent implanted pacemakers, there have also been improvements in temporary external pacemakers. In the past, the only ways to guarantee adequate current conduction for external pacing were painful or time consuming. Pacing needles were positioned under the skin in the patient's chest, or the physician had to fix the electrodes in a telephone handset and hold it against the patient's chest.

Today's external pacing units have large electrode surfaces that are saturated with a conductive gel and attached to the patient's chest. The most sophisticated units have the capability for manual defibrillation, automatic sensing, variable rates, variable voltage, and ECG monitoring. Many of the new units also have indicator lights to show when they're pacing and when battery power is low.

The life-saving role of electric current

External pacing systems, which are also called non-invasive transthoracic pacemakers, can be used in the emergency treatment of severe bradycardia. These pacemakers have been successful in the treatment of third-degree AV block, for example, but not for asystole—cardiac standstill.

THE AUTHOR is a staff nurse in the emergency department at A.O. Fox Hospital in Oneonta, N.Y.

An external pacing system is used for the hour or so that it might take to transport a patient or to treat a temporary condition. It can also be used while physicians are waiting to insert temporary or permanent electrode catheters.

To accomplish external pacing, one large electrode is applied to the patient's chest and another to his back. The electrical current of 50 to 200 milliamps will seem strong compared to voltages of 0.5 to 20 milliamps typically used for internal pacing. But the higher current is needed because more muscle and bone tissue stands be-

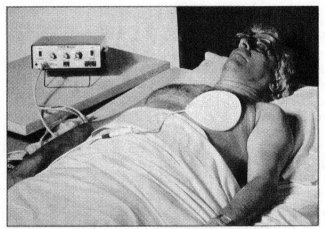

Dry the skin on the patient's left anterior chest. Place a self-adhesive electrode over the patient's heart, with the center of the electrode between his fourth and fifth ribs.

small device—it's about the size of a transistor radio—that transmits a single-lead ECG by telephone to a monitoring service. If there are any abnormalities, the patient and his doctor are notified. The cost of the equipment and the phone calls are usually covered by insurance.

When you've dealt with these

points, Mr. Aldrich will be off to a good start. And you'll have the satisfaction of knowing that you both have a better understanding of pacemaker technology. ■

BIBLIOGRAPHY Conklin, E.F. et al. Does your patient need a pacemaker? *Patient Care* 19:95, June 1985. Famularom M.A. and Kennedy H.L.

Ambulatory electrocardiology in the assessment of pacemaker function. *Am. Heart J.* 104:1086, 1982. O'Neill M.J. and Davis D. Pacemakers in noncardiac surgery. *Surg. Clinics of N.A.* 63:1102, 1983. Phibbs, B. and Marriott, H.J.L. Complications of permanent transvenous pacing. *New Eng. J. Med.* 312:1428, 1985. Pierson, M.A. and Boosinger, J.K. Follow-up of cardiac pacemaker recipients: A pilot study. *Heart Lung* 13:431, 1984. Shively B. and Goldschlager N. Progress in cardiac pacing. *Arch. Intern. Med.* 145:2238, 1985.

tween the electrode and the heart. You can touch the patient without getting a shock as long as both electrodes are firmly in place.

This life-saving procedure can be carried out for up to an hour and a half, but after that it should be replaced by a more reliable pacing system such as a temporary or permanent catheter electrode.

If you're interested in doing a feature-by-feature comparison of external pacemakers, you can contact the Emergency Care Research Institute, a nonprofit organization that lists characteristics for nine current models. The ECRI address is 5200 Butler Pike, Plymouth Meeting, Pa. 19462. The telephone number is (215) 825-6000.

Effective pacing step by step

Begin by telling the patient that you're going to attach a device that will help his heart maintain a better rate. Explain that the device may cause discomfort, but assure him that he'll get a sedative. Then proceed with the steps illustrated in the photos below.

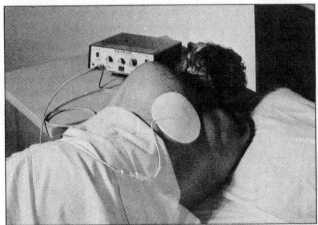

Turn the patient onto his right side. After drying the skin on the left side of his back, place a self-adhesive electrode between his shoulder blades and slightly to the left of midline. If the patient isn't able to turn, place one electrode on each side of his chest at the fourth intercostal space in the midaxillary line. This placement, however, is less efficient and sometimes causes more pain.

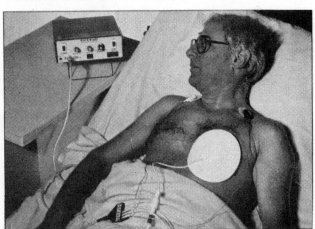

Position the patient on his back again and place ECG monitoring electrodes just above the patient's clavicles. So placed, they'll be out of the way in case the patient needs to be defibrillated. Now you're ready to begin pacing. The physician will determine the amount of current to be delivered. It will be as low as possible but high enough to produce a femoral pulse with each surge of current. Check the patient's heart rate and rhythm, blood pressure, respirations, and femoral pulse every five to 15 minutes.

Why deep vein thrombosis is so dangerous

Even the treatment of this disease can be dangerous. Only when you fully realize the hazards can you confront them with confidence.
By Beth Ellen McMahan, RN, BSN, MSN

Last month Jerry Taylor was flying home from a business trip when his left calf began to ache. When he consulted a physician, the doctor took one look at Jerry's leg and admitted him to the hospital.

Why was the doctor so concerned? Because he thought Jerry might have deep vein thrombosis—one or more clots in the deep veins of his calf.

Although similar to superficial thrombosis, deep vein thrombosis is more difficult to diagnose and far more dangerous. It can all too easily cause pulmonary embolism, a condition that accounts for up to a third of all hospital deaths. Moreover, the anticoagulants used to treat deep vein thrombosis can cause serious bleeding. Thus the cure can be almost as dangerous as the disease.

Caring for the patient with deep vein thrombosis is a two-stage process. When he's first admitted, you'll need to tell him about the problem and what to expect from the various tests he'll undergo. If

THE AUTHOR is a cardiovascular clinical nursing specialist at Mount Auburn Hospital in Cambridge, Mass.

Produced by Estelle Beaumont, RN, MS

the diagnosis is confirmed, you'll have to be constantly on guard to ensure that the therapy is carefully regulated.

Causes and contributing factors

Deep vein thrombosis can be caused by injury, immunological response, sickle cell anemia, or polycythemia vera. In Jerry's case the cause wasn't known, but he had at least two contributing factors. He was past middle age, and, as a passenger in a plane, he had been immobilized for several hours. Other contributing factors include previous thrombosis, congestive heart failure, surgery, childbirth, shock, estrogen therapy, and advanced cancer.

Though clots can form in the arms or even the central venous system, most deep vein thrombosis occurs in the calves or thighs. Like Jerry, most patients have leg pain as their sole symptom. Some however, have pain only when the foot is dorsiflexed—Homan's sign—or no pain at all.

When admitting a patient with suspected deep vein thrombosis,

put him in bed immediately. Then assess his symptoms as follows:
► Inspect his legs for prominent veins, stretched or shiny skin, red or blue skin discoloration, and swelling. You'll most likely see swelling behind the knees and around the ankles.
► Measure and record the circumference of the calf to evaluate the degree of swelling. Lightly mark the skin over the shin bone with a felt tip marker so that subsequent measurements can be made at the same place. If you must lift the patient's leg, use the palms of your hands rather than your fingertips to avoid causing him any more pain or dislodging a clot.
► Test for temperature variations. Simultaneously put one hand on each ankle, then on each calf, knee, and thigh, comparing the temperature of the painful leg with the normal one. A warm leg can indicate a vein blockage; a cold leg, an arterial blockage. Before you make this comparison, make sure the patient hasn't had an ice bag or hot water bottle on his leg in the last 10 minutes. You'll find it easier to make temperature comparisons if you

wash your hands in cold water and dry them thoroughly before you start.

The importance of diagnostic tests

Because leg pain and other symptoms can be caused by a torn muscle or arterial thrombosis, other tests are needed to confirm deep vein thrombosis. The most common procedures used to pinpoint the condition include Doppler ultrasound, impedance plethysmography, and venography.

Doppler ultrasound is a non-invasive test that can be done in the patient's room, either by a physician or a specially trained nurse or technician. The ultrasound probe is placed over the patient's femoral, iliac, or popliteal veins to listen for changes in blood velocity. The sound changes if blood flow is slowed or stopped by a clot.

When explaining the procedure to the patient, reassure him that he won't be stuck with any needles. Also tell him that a clear jelly-like substance will be applied to his skin to help transmit sound better.

Impedance plethysmography is another non-invasive test. Usually done in the patient's room or in a vascular testing laboratory, it detects changes in blood volume.

Electrodes attached to a recording instrument that measures electrical resistance are placed on the patient's calf. The examiner fits a blood pressure cuff around the patient's thigh and inflates it enough to block venous outflow but still permit arterial inflow. When maximum venous capacity is reached—usually in 45 to 120 seconds—the

---

Pulmonary embolism: Preparing for the worst

When a thrombus breaks free from a venous wall and travels through the right side of the heart to the lungs, the effect can be minor to severe, depending on the size and location of the clot.

A massive embolus blocking a major lung artery can cause poor ventilation and perfusion leading to hypoxia, a rapid increase in lung pressure, and right ventricular workload. Soon afterwards comes right ventricular failure—cor pulmonale—decreased cardiac output, and death.

Symptoms of pulmonary embolism include profound dyspnea, chest pain, cyanosis, low blood pressure, weak and rapid pulse, coughing, bloody sputum, and cool, clammy extremities. Additional symptoms might include fear, enlarged neck veins, pleural friction rub, and a galloping heart rhythm.

Notify the physician immediately if the patient has any of these symptoms. The physician may order diagnostic tests such as a chest X-ray, lung scan, arterial blood gases, or a pulmonary angiogram. The angiogram is the most definitive test but also the most dangerous. Injecting the X-ray dye can cause allergic reactions or cardiac arrhythmias.

For therapy, the physician usually prescribes streptokinase or urokinase to dissolve the clot or sometimes heparin to keep more clots from forming.

Until the physician arrives, try to relieve difficult breathing by raising the head of the bed and giving oxygen. Help insert an endotracheal tube if necessary. Check vital signs frequently, and hook an ECG monitor to the patient if possible.

---

cuff is released. The rate of venous outflow will be measured on the recording device. If an obstruction exists, the graph will show a much more gradual return to baseline than the normal three seconds.

To improve diagnostic accuracy, many physicians will order both an ultrasound test and an impedance plethysmography.

Venography is an invasive test that's done in the X-ray department. The doctor injects a dye into the leg veins, takes X-rays, and examines them for evidence of a blockage. It's a more definitive test for diagnosing deep vein thrombosis, but can also be more dangerous. Many doctors order

this test only if ultrasound and plethysmography equipment aren't available or if results of those tests are inconclusive.

Be sure to ask your patient if he has ever had an allergic reaction to X-ray dye. If so, alert the doctor.

Starting the patient on anticoagulants

The twin goal of treating deep vein thrombosis is to prevent venous insufficiency and pulmonary embolism. Anticoagulants can accomplish both goals. But bear in mind that these drugs can also cause serious bleeding. If the patient is allergic to anticoagulants or has a

The do's and don'ts of anticoagulant therapy

Teach your patient about anticoagulants early. He needs to see the importance of complying with his medication regimen, keeping appointments for lab tests, and monitoring for signs of bleeding.

In addition, he should know why he's taking his medication. Explain that it will keep new clots from forming but won't dissolve existing clots.

Remind the patient to take his medication at the same time each day, and to take exactly the amount prescribed. This will keep serum anticoagulant levels within a narrow therapeutic range.

Warn him to check with his physician before beginning or discontinuing any medication, including over-the-counter medications. Drugs as commonplace as antacids, antihistamines, and vitamin C can decrease the effect of warfarin. Similarly, alcohol, antibiotics, and ibuprofen, among others, can increase the effect.

Encourage the patient to wear a Medic Alert bracelet or tag to let emergency personnel know that he's taking anticoagulants.

Stress the urgency of reporting signs of bleeding to the physician, including blood in the urine or stool, unusual bleeding from the nose, gums, or skin, severe headache, stomach or joint pain, and any bleeding that doesn't stop within 10 minutes. Have him use an electric razor and keep his nails clipped to avoid accidental cuts. To avoid trauma, warn him not to participate in contact sports.

bleeding disorder, severe hypertension, or ulcerative colitis, anticoagulants are contraindicated.

Usually the first anticoagulant to be prescribed will be IV heparin, a fast-acting drug that suppresses clot formation by inhibiting conversion of prothrombin to thrombin and fibrinogen to fibrin.

Heparin can be given subcutaneously or intravenously. If given IV, it can be via intermittent injections using a heparin lock or continuous infusion using a pump or controller.

Many doctors prefer the continuous method because it helps ensure consistent delivery and can decrease the risk of bleeding. Keep in mind, though, that heparin doesn't dissolve clots that already exist. It just keeps new clots from forming.

Continuous therapy usually begins with 5,000 units given as a bolus. That's followed with an infusion at a rate of about 1,000 units per hour. The exact dose depends on the patient's weight and partial thromboplastin times. When you calculate the drip rate for the infusion, check with the pharmacist to confirm that it's correct.

Remember, however, that other drugs the patient may be taking can interfere with heparin's effects. Digitalis, tetracyclines, nicotine, and antihistamines, for instance, can decrease the effects. Aspirin, dextran, ibuprofen, indomethacin, hydroxychloroquine, and dipyridamole increase it. If the patient is taking any of these, alert the doctor so he can either stop them or adjust the anticoagulant dosage.

Heparin therapy is usually continued for seven to 10 days. The patient will be started on an oral anticoagulant, warfarin (Coumadin), during the last three to four days of heparin therapy. It takes that long for the warfarin to begin affecting the prothrombin time.

Like heparin, warfarin prolongs clotting time, but by a different method. It prevents vitamin K from synthesizing clotting factors formed in the liver.

Be alert for side effects

When giving anticoagulants, watch for bleeding from the patient's nose, incisions, IV sites, and gums. Also watch for more subtle signs of bleeding: black tarry stools, red urine, bruises, petechiae—small pinpoint hemorrhages just under the skin—painful joints, severe headache, and abdominal pain. Once a day, do dipstick tests for blood in the urine and guaiac tests for blood in the stool.

Check the patient's prothrombin time before giving warfarin and the partial thromboplastin time before giving heparin. Usually the doctor wants to maintain these at one-and-a-half to two-and-a-half times the patient's normal (baseline) level.

Also monitor the patient's hemoglobin, hematocrit, and platelet levels to be sure they don't fall too low. When possible, avoid giving injections and avoid invasive procedures because they increase the risk of bleeding. When injections can't be avoided, firmly compress the injection site a few extra minutes after removing the needle.

If the patient starts to bleed or has a higher than normal clotting time, notify the doctor. He may decide to stop the anticoagulant or decrease the dose. If the patient has been getting IV heparin, the doctor will probably order IV protamine sulfate to counteract the heparin. If the patient has been receiving warfarin, he'll probably prescribe vitamin K to reverse its effects.

Additional nursing care

Your patient will continue to need bedrest until the leg pain or tenderness is gone and the swelling subsides. This usually takes about 10 days. Elevate the patient's legs on pillows to reduce edema and promote good venous circulation. You can also reduce edema by applying continuous moist heat as pre-scribed. This helps dilate the superficial arteries and veins.

Avoid using the knee gatch unless recommended by the doctor to allow the patient to bend his knees slightly to relieve pressure on his popliteal blood vessels. Remind the patient not to cross his legs since doing so can block circulation.

Once the patient's allowed out of bed, warn him not to sit or stand for more than an hour at a time.

If the physician prescribes elastic stockings, the patient should start wearing them only after the swelling has subsided. Some physicians believe the stockings will help compress superficial veins and direct blood flow to the deeper veins. Remove the stockings briefly twice a day to check for inadequate circu-lation and skin irritation. Instruct patients to wash them every three days. If placed in a mesh bag they can go in a washer and dryer at mild temperatures.

Caring for patients with deep vein thrombosis can be a heavy responsibility. But knowing the symptoms, diagnostic tests, treatment, and precautions can arm you with the information you need for giving better care. ■

BIBLIOGRAPHY Bang, N.U. et al. *Thrombosis and Atherosclerosis*. Chicago: Year Book Medical Publishers, Inc., 1982. Bergen, J.J. and Yao, S.T. *Surgery of the Veins*. Orlando, Fla.: Grune and Stratton, Inc., 1985. Faney, V.A. An in-depth look at deep vein thrombosis. *Nursing* 14:35, March, 1984. Kwaan, H.C. and Bowie, A.J. *Thrombosis*. Philadelphia: W.B. Saunders, Co., 1982. Loo, J.V. et al. *The Thromboembolic Diseases*. New York: Verlag Publishing Co., 1983. Wyngaarden, J.B. and Smith, L.H. *Textbook of Medicine*. Philadelphia: W.B. Saunders, Co., 1982.

Gastric surgery:
Your crucial pre- and postop role

Your patient may hardly have had time to realize he's seriously ill before he finds himself facing major surgery. You'll have to sustain him through diagnostic tests, see him through an extended recovery period, and help him adjust to the demands of a new lifestyle.

Donna M. Feickert, MSN, RN, CS

To begin with, the symptoms are so vague—feelings of fullness, abdominal discomfort—that the patient dismisses them. He may not notice that he's becoming malnourished, and he doesn't realize that his health is waning. Then, apparently out of the blue, a terrible episode of pain or gastric bleeding drives him to seek medical help. The next thing he knows he's facing major surgery and an uncertain future.

Such is the recent history of many of the patients you'll nurse through gastric or duodenal surgery. Most have peptic ulcer disease; their abnormally copious gastric secretions digest not only their food but their stomach linings as well. Cancer of the stomach is the second most common diagnosis, followed by trauma and Mallory-Weiss tears in the esophageal wall

resulting from forceful vomiting.

By the time many of these patients get to the operating room, their disease has already weakened them severely, leaving them vulnerable to a variety of postop complications. Clearly, care of such patients is a demanding task. You'll have to sustain them through diagnostic tests, prepare them for surgery, see them through an extended recovery period, and help them adjust to a changed way of life.

Assess and alleviate the patient's pain

Your initial assessment provides baseline data that you'll use in evaluating a patient's postop progress. You need to pay special attention to the patient's pain, nutritional status, and fluid and electrolyte balance.

Pain is your first concern. Patients with a peptic ulcer or advanced cancer usually experience

severe pain. Ask where the pain is located. Would he describe it as dull, stabbing, or aching? What brings it on? What relieves it? Is he taking any medications for it?

The patient with a peptic ulcer may tell you that his pain is sharp and burning. It may increase at night when the stomach empties. Fatty foods, spicy foods, and alcohol make it worse, while carbohydrates seem to help. Warn this patient not to take aspirin for his pain because aspirin will further irritate his already damaged stomach lining. For pain relief, he should take antacids or agents that inhibit the production of peptic acid—for example, cimetidine (Tagamet) and ranitidine (Zantac).

Some cancer patients may feel little pain. Others may need morphine to control intense pain, depending on the location and extent of the malignancy. Cancer pain, often characterized as dull, doesn't

THE AUTHOR is a surgical clinical specialist at the Hospital of the University of Pennsylvania in Philadelphia.

Produced by David Anderson

change with food intake. When a carcinoma metastasizes, the pain spreads beyond the stomach.

The patient's nutritional status

Most patients undergoing gastric surgery have been suffering from nausea, vomiting, and anorexia long enough and severely enough to be malnourished. Take a dietary history and observe the patient for dehydration, weakness, or muscle wasting. If he appears malnourished but says he eats, cancer may be interfering with his body's ability to utilize food.

The patient with a peptic ulcer should eat a bland diet. He may also need iron supplements to offset anemia caused by bleeding. Patients with gastric cancer may eat without restriction; most, however, require parenteral feeding.

To improve your patient's food intake, find out when his appetite peaks and serve his meals then. Try to give him foods he likes. Encourage his family to bring favorite foods from home.

Offer the peptic ulcer patient small, frequent feedings rather than large meals. Smaller meals help reduce gastric secretions. Report the frequency and amount of any vomiting. If your patient vomits a great deal, he may need parenteral feeding before surgery. Vomitus and stool should be guaiaced.

Try to coordinate your patient's preop testing schedule so that he doesn't miss too many meals. For example, make sure tests that call for him to be NPO after midnight are done promptly in the morning so that he doesn't miss breakfast.

How the stomach and duodenum process food

Food passes from the esophagus into the fundus, the antechamber of the stomach. The rhythmic muscle contractions of peristalsis break up the food mechanically as it's propelled from the fundus through the two other chambers of the stomach, the body and antrum.

Meanwhile, the presence of food signals the vagus nerve to stimulate glands in the stomach walls that produce the acids and enzymes that break food down chemically. The fundic glands and glands in the body of the stomach secrete pepsinogen, hydrochloric acid, and intrinsic factor. Glands in the walls of the antrum produce the enzyme gastrin.

After food leaves the stomach, it passes into the duodenum through the pylorus. In the duodenum, it mixes with intestinal secretions.

For a healthy person, a meal of moderate size takes between three and four hours to make this passage.

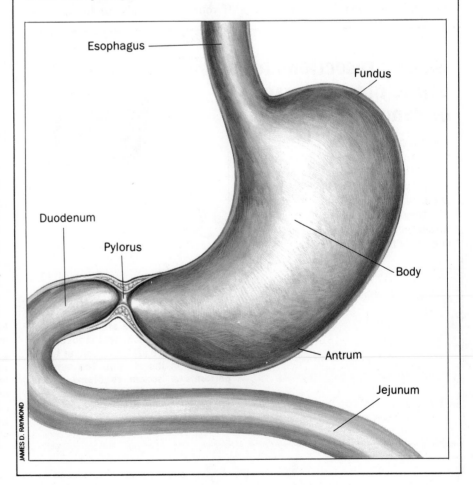

Manage fluids and electrolytes

Fluid and electrolyte balance is your third major concern throughout the patient's hospital stay. Monitor his fluid intake and output including emesis. Excessive fluid loss washes electrolytes out of the body, creating a potential for dangerous imbalances. Fluid and electrolyte imbalance is a particular danger if your patient is bleeding, vomiting, diarrheal, feverish, taking laxatives, or undergoing GI suctioning to remove blood or relieve stomach distention.

If your patient puts out much more fluid than he takes in or if you find signs of dehydration, monitor daily blood samples for electrolyte studies. Watch for signs of hypokalemia—i.e., muscle cramps, confusion, and cardiac arrhythmias.

To test for dehydration, pinch the patient's arm. If the skin feels dry and stays dimpled after you let go, he's dehydrated. Weigh the patient every day at the same time and on the same scale. If he loses two pounds or more in 24 hours or keeps losing day after day, he may need IV fluid replacement.

Tell the patient what to anticipate

If your patient must undergo diagnostic tests before surgery, explain what they entail. Start teaching early so that he'll have time to formulate questions and prepare himself mentally for the procedures. Include his family in all teaching.

The most common gastrointestinal tests:

X-ray studies. An upper GI series outlines the GI tract and shows obstructions, ulcers, and structural defects. Tell the patient he'll have to swallow chalky-tasting barium immediately before this test. Flat plate X-rays will show growths, fluid levels, or gas.

Endoscopic examination. The physician looks directly into the GI

Gastric resections for peptic ulcer disease or cancer

The surgical procedures described at right are used to remove large peptic ulcers that can't be treated in place. The purpose of performing these procedures on cancer patients is to remove the tumor masses, hopefully before cells from the mass metastasize to other parts of the patient's body.

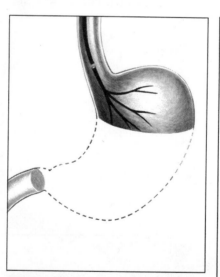

Bilroth I removes the antrum and total body of the stomach. This procedure is used to remove ulcers or cancer that's localized in the antrum. The surgeon performs a truncal vagotomy at the same time to control pain. He attaches the gastric stump to the duodenum.

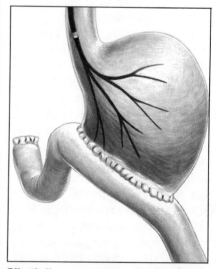

Bilroth II removes the antrum and the lower body of the stomach. The surgeon performs this procedure to remove ulcers or eradicate cancer that's located in the body or fundus. He also performs a truncal vagotomy to control pain. To provide for continuity of the digestive tract, he attaches the gastric stump to the jejunum.

tract through an endoscope—a long, flexible tube with a lighted end. Tell the patient he'll have to swallow one end of the tube and tell him he'll be sedated and given a local anesthetic to suppress his gag reflex.

Biopsy. If X-ray or endoscopy reveals a growth, the physician may remove tissue samples and examine them to see if they're benign or malignant. The endoscope has a special attachment that can be used to take tissue samples. If the size or location of the growth precludes an endoscopic biopsy, the physician may take the patient to the operating room for a surgical biopsy.

Secretory analysis. If the physician suspects a peptic ulcer, he'll expect to find high levels of acid in the patient's gastric secretions. He draws secretions from the stomach through an endoscope—secretory analysis is often combined with endoscopy—or nasogastric tube. The patient must fast for 12 hours before this test. During the test, he may be given crackers, bread, caffeine, or alcohol to stimulate the secretion of gastric acid.

Secretory analysis may be repeated postop to see if surgery has successfully lowered the rate of gastric secretion.

Radionucleic uptake tests. This group of tests measures how well the patient's stomach absorbs nutrients. After fasting, the patient receives vitamin B_{12}, fats, or proteins that have been combined with a radioactive isotope. The absorption of these substances can then be tracked by X-ray.

You should monitor your patient's test schedule to make sure tests are done in proper order. An abdominal X-ray should be taken before any tests requiring a barium swallow or enema. Otherwise, it will have to be put off for two days while residual contrast material washes out of the patient's digestive tract.

The boxes below and on page 27 describe the most common types of gastric operations. Before he goes to surgery, warn your patient that he'll wake up with tubes and drains in place. Tell him he won't be able to eat or drink anything immediately postop. Teach him the turning, coughing, deep breathing, and leg exercises he'll be asked to do. Train him to use an incentive spirometer. Also reassure him that he'll receive pain medication regularly.

Restore mobility, digestion, strength

Most patients remain in the hospital for seven to 10 days after gastric surgery. They—and their nurses— have plenty to do during that time.

As soon as the patient recovers from anesthesia, start coughing and deep breathing exercises to clear his lungs. Listen to his lungs q4h for new sounds that might mean pulmonary congestion.

Turn the patient several times each shift to keep blood clots from

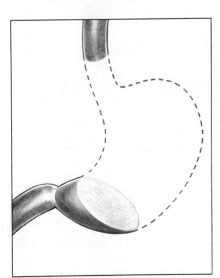

Esophagogastrectomy is used to restore patency to the patient's upper GI tract when it's been blocked by cancer or esophageal stenosis. This operation removes the distal esophagus and most of the stomach, then reconnects the remaining portions of the esophagus and the stomach. Esophageal stenosis occurs when repeated cycles of peptic ulceration and healing cause formation of scar tissue.

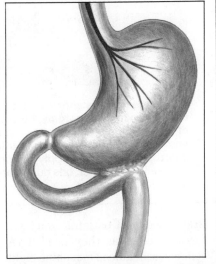

Gastroenterostomy improves gastric drainage when a tumor blocks the way to the pylorus. The surgeon anastomoses a loop of duodenum to the lower border of the stomach. Gastric contents then drain through the anastomosis as well as the pylorus.

Surgery for peptic ulcer disease

Peptic ulcer disease occurs when gastric secretions erode the mucosa lining the wall of the stomach. It warrants surgery when the erosion produces uncontrollable bleeding or perforation of the stomach wall.

This type of surgery reduces gastric secretions by cutting the vagus nerve, which plays an important role in stimulating the production of gastric secretions. The two procedures that are usually used to cut the nerve:

Truncal vagotomy, the more radical of the two procedures, severs the two main branches of the vagus nerve, thereby interrupting all vagal stimulation of the stomach. This procedure is usually coupled with antrectomy—surgical removal of the antrum, or lower portion of the stomach—to arrest bleeding. After removing the antrum, the surgeon restores the continuity of the digestive tract by anastomosing the body of the stomach to the duodenum or jejunum.

Proximal gastric vagotomy disconnects only those vagal branches that stimulate production of peptic acid. Physicians perform this procedure in emergency situations when they close a perforation of the stomach wall.

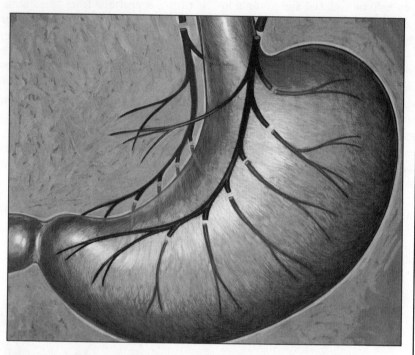

The vagus nerve is shown above in black and grey. If the surgeon does a proximal vagotomy, he severs only the smaller branches of the nerve—as shown above in grey. More commonly, though, he does a truncal vagotomy, cutting the two main trunks. This interrupts the nerve supply not only to the stomach, but also to the liver, gallbladder, bile duct, pancreas, small intestine, and half of the large intestine.

forming and occluding dependent or compressed vessels or migrating to the pulmonary arteries.*

For the same reason, have the patient do leg exercises—bending his knees, lifting each leg from the hip, and flexing the feet. If he's able, have him begin walking the day after surgery.

Give pain medication regularly at

*For a variety of exercises that will help these patients, see "Exercises to ease pain after abdominal surgery" in the July 1986 issue of *RN*.

first, since most patients won't ask for it as often as they need it. A common schedule is morphine eight to 15 mg IM or subcutaneously q3h, switching to prn after 48 hours.

Check your patient's surgical sites frequently for bleeding. Monitor his hemoglobin and hematocrit for signs of anemia that could be due to blood lost in surgery. Also be sure to look for purulent drainage, warmth, tenderness, or erythema that may signal infection.

Expect a temperature of 99° to 100° F (37° to 38° C). If it goes higher, give acetaminophen according to doctor's orders and suspect infection. Palpate your patient's abdomen q4h for undue tenderness and rigidity, an early sign of peritonitis that must be reported to the physician immediately.

Irrigate your patient's nasogastric tube with normal saline according to doctor's orders to keep it patent. If you have trouble irrigating the tube, it may need repositioning. Expect to find small clots and bright red blood in the tube for the first four to six hours postop, but report any fresh blood you find after that.

The trauma and swelling caused by surgery halts peristalsis, the rhythmic muscle contractions that move food through the stomach and intestines. Until it returns, your patient must receive nutrients parenterally. A common physician's order calls for 800 to 1,000 cc of Ringer's lactate or dextrose and saline solution per shift. Monitor the IV carefully to make sure the patient gets the right amount.

Resume monitoring fluid intake and output and serum electrolytes for signs of imbalance. Be sure to figure in the amount of fluid lost through drainage tubes.

Listen q 2 to 4 hours for bowel sounds, which indicate returning peristalsis. This usually happens gradually over the course of a couple of days. Even after peristalsis returns, your patient will still have to build up his oral food intake slowly and carefully because surgery may have decreased his stomach capacity.

Prepare the patient for new habits

Most patients must modify their lifestyles after surgery, and many find it difficult to do so. The ulcer patient, for instance, must learn how to manage stress. The cancer patient must learn to live with pain-control regimens, chemotherapy treatments, and the fact of lethal illness.

Although the physician, dietitian, social worker, and home care nurse may all be involved in helping the patient and his family prepare for discharge, you're the one who's with the patient all day, every day. There's a great deal you can do to help reinforce what the others are teaching.

The diet your patient receives in the hospital is the model for his diet after discharge. The patient with peptic ulcer disease, for example, should continue to eat high-protein, low-carbohydrate foods. Most patients take vitamin and mineral supplements. Arrange to have the dietitian meet with your patient to show him how to obtain maximum satisfaction from his prescribed diet.

Since the patient's stomach may be smaller or may no longer produce normal amounts of enzymes, it may take longer to break down food. Advise him to continue to eat small, frequent meals after he goes home and to avoid taking fluids with meals. Fluids accelerate the passage of solid food out of the stomach into the intestine.

If the patient goes home with a drainage tube in place, teach him how to change the dressing and how to recognize infection.

Management of the patient undergoing gastric surgery demands a great deal of skill and caring. You must not only meet the considerable demands of physical care, but prepare the patient and his family for major changes in lifestyle as well. The establishment of a trusting relationship between you and your patient will help you attain both those objectives. ■

BIBLIOGRAPHY Given, B. and Simmons, S. *Gastroenterology in Clinical Nursing* (3rd ed.). St. Louis: The C.V. Mosby Co., 1979. Greenberger, N. *Gastrointestinal Disorders: A Pathophysiologic Approach* (2nd ed.). Chicago: Yearbook Medical Publishers, 1981. Herrington, L. The surgical management of duodenal ulcer and benign gastric ulcer. *International Surgery*, 68:299, 1983. Holtermuller, K. and Malagelada, J., eds. *Advances in ulcer disease*. Princeton: Excerpta Medica, 1980. Jones D., Dunbar, C., and Jirovec, M. *Medical-Surgical Nursing: A Conceptual Approach*. New York: McGraw Hill, 1982. Schwartz, S. *Principles of Surgery* (4th ed.). New York: McGraw Hill, 1984. Stabile, B. and Passaro, E. Duodenal ulcer: a disease in evolution. *Current Problems in Surgery*, 21(1):1, 1984.

Colorectal cancer: When a polyp is more than a polyp

The publicity generated by President Reagan's surgery plus new technology for diagnosing and removing precancerous polyps could significantly reduce the death rate from colon cancer.
By Sherry Greifzu, RN

Colorectal cancer is one of the five most common types of cancer in both men and women. Despite millions of dollars spent on research, the death rate from this form of cancer remains about the same today as it was 50 years ago.

Yet there are grounds for hope. The American Cancer Society believes that three out of four patients with colorectal cancer could be saved with early detection and treatment. Detection efforts, in fact, are increasing. Perhaps because of the attention focused on President Reagan's colon cancer, patients are coming in for colorectal exams in record numbers.

Colorectal cancer usually begins in polyps that form on the walls of the lower five to six feet of the intestines. Such polyps can remain benign for years. If they're removed during the precancerous stage or even in the early stages of malignancy, the patient's chances of survival are good. That explains why early detection and treatment

THE AUTHOR is head nurse on the medical oncology unit at the Hospital of Saint Raphael in New Haven, Conn.

Produced by Estelle Beaumont, RN, MS

is the goal of today's therapy.

To advance that goal, urge high-risk patients to undergo regular colorectal exams and stool tests. If an initial exam suggests the presence of polyps, you'll have to guide the patient through additional diagnostic tests. If cancer is confirmed, you'll have to provide skillful care during the course of treatment.

Risk factors and symptoms

The people at highest risk of developing colorectal cancer are those over 40 years of age and those with polyps, ulcerative colitis, Crohn's disease, or a personal or family history of cancer.

Of these risk factors, polyps are perhaps the most intriguing. These growths can occur singly or, more often, in groups. They rarely cause pain unless they become large enough to obstruct the colon, but they often cause bleeding. Indeed, bleeding is the single most common early warning sign of precancerous polyps. For a closer look at the different kinds of polyps, see the discussion on page 25.

Other signs and symptoms of colorectal cancer include anemia, abdominal discomfort, intestinal obstruction, unexplained weight loss, and a change in normal bowel habits, such as constipation or diarrhea, lasting for a period of two weeks or more.

Symptoms may vary according to where the cancer is located. Cancer in the sigmoid colon, for instance, usually doesn't cause anemia but can cause "napkin-ring" bowel obstruction and, occasionally, gross bleeding. Cancer of the rectum usually causes pain, gross bleeding, incomplete evacuation, and tenesmus—ineffective straining at stool.

In search of hidden bleeding

Because occult blood in the stool is such a common sign of colon cancer, many physicians recommend annual stool tests for everyone over 45 years of age.

The tests involve placing a stool specimen on a slide impregnated with a reagent called guaiac. To ensure accurate results, the patient should eat no meat and no foods containing vitamin C for at least 48 hours before obtaining the first specimen.

Some tests must be sent to a lab or the physician's office for evaluation. Others are read by the patient at home. Tell the patient to follow the instructions on the test kit.

In addition to guaiac tests, the American Cancer Society recommends an annual digital rectal exam for everyone over 40. The ACS also recommends a sigmoidoscopy every three to five years after two consecutive yearly exams are negative—beginning at age 50.

If these exams suggest that further evaluation is necessary, several other procedures can be done to confirm or rule out a diagnosis of cancer.

A diagnostic workup for colorectal cancer usually includes various X-ray procedures, endoscopy, and blood tests. If a patient is admitted for a such a workup with symptoms of bowel obstruction (e.g., nausea, vomiting, or abdominal pain), you'll probably be asked to insert an IV line for fluids and nourishment. You'll also be asked to withhold food and fluids by mouth in case the patient needs emergency surgery. Often the physician inserts a Cantor tube to decompress the colon through the removal of fluid and flatus.

Exposing cancer with X-rays

X-ray procedures to diagnose colorectal cancer include a barium enema, computerized tomography scanning, and sometimes an intravenous pyelogram. Most physi-

cians also order a routine chest X-ray to check for lung metastasis.

Explain each procedure carefully in advance, and try to coordinate the procedures to decrease the number of enemas needed. Also try to be present to offer the patient support when the physician gives the patient the test results.

Barium enema. The physician will usually order a barium enema to discover if polyps are present or to obtain more information about an abdominal mass.

The success of this method of detecting cancerous lesions depends heavily on good bowel preparation. Explain to the patient that he'll be allowed only clear liquids the day before the test and nothing by mouth for several hours before the X-ray. Tell him that he'll receive laxatives and enemas to clean out his bowel. He will also need laxatives after the test to clear out any residual barium, which can cause constipation.

If the patient is elderly, keep in mind that he can quickly become dehydrated while he's NPO before the test. Watch for poor skin turgor and other signs of dehydration such as dry mouth and fever. Notify the physician if you think the patient needs IV fluids.

CT scan. The physician may order a computerized tomography scan of the abdomen and pelvic area if the barium enema is inconclusive or if he needs information about pelvic lymph nodes. A CT scan combines X-ray technology with a computer's ability to calculate small differences in various tissues to provide clearer images than otherwise possible.

As with the barium enema, the patient's bowel will need a thorough cleaning prior to the CT scan. But if the scan is done on the same day as other tests that call for a bowel prep, the patient probably won't need additional laxatives or enemas.

Sometimes the doctor will do an enhanced CT scan using intravenously injected radiopaque dye. Before this test, ask the patient if he has any allergies. If he's allergic to radiographic dye, the doctor may want to give medications to counteract a possible reaction to the dye.

Intravenous pyelogram. This X-ray of the kidneys, ureters, and bladder can help determine if a colorectal tumor is pushing against the ureters or kidneys.

The patient is given radiopaque dye intravenously so that the urinary system will show up more vividly on the X-ray film. Again, ask him whether he has any allergies that might predispose him to a reaction to the dye.

The physician usually orders laxatives before the examination to clear the patient's colon of feces and gas that might obstruct the view.

The benefits of endoscopy

Endoscopy—examination of the bowel with a sigmoidoscope or colonoscope—can confirm and differentiate tumors when used in combination with biopsy. Many endoscopes can also be equipped to remove or shrink tumors by cautery or laser energy.

Sigmoidoscopy. A sigmoido-

Projecting the patient's prognosis

When the physician discovers a polyp in the patient's bowel, he must determine whether it's neoplastic or non-neoplastic. If it's non-neoplastic, he might not remove it. If it's neoplastic, he'll probably stage it according to Dukes classification system to determine the prognosis.

The Dukes system, named for pathologist Cuthbert Dukes, classifies colorectal tumors into three stages—A, B, and C, as described below. A fourth stage, D, was added later to classify cancers that have metastasized to other organs. When cancer reaches this stage, only about 5% of patients survive for five years without a recurrence of disease.

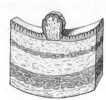

A pseudopolyp is a small, benign growth that resembles inflammation more than a tumor. A growth like this was discovered in President Reagan's colon in May 1984. It resorbed without treatment.

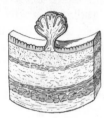

A tubular adenoma is a small, red polyp that's attached to the bowel wall by a stemlike structure called a peduncle. Many physicians consider all such polyps precancerous and recommend that they be removed.

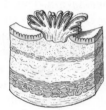

A villous adenoma is a relatively large, soft, spongy polyp with many finger-like projections. It doesn't have a peduncle. Villous adenomas are less common than tubular adenomas but are more likely to become malignant. They may cause diarrhea with resulting protein and electrolyte loss. They also have a strong tendency to recur.

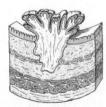

In cancers classified as Dukes stage A, malignant cells have penetrated into the mucosa of the intestinal wall but not into the muscle layer. If such lesions are removed promptly, about 98% of patients survive for five years without recurrence.

In Dukes stage B, malignant cells have penetrated the mucosa and muscle layer of the intestinal wall but haven't metastasized to lymph nodes or other organs. When such lesions are removed, up to 80% of patients survive for five years without recurrence.

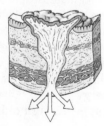

In Dukes stage C, malignant cells have penetrated the entire width of the intestinal wall and have metastasized to the lymph nodes. If the cancer is treated at this stage, up to 40% of patients survive five years without recurrence

JANE HURD

scope enables the physician to find about two-thirds of all tumors in the rectum and lower bowel. Some doctors recommend sigmoidoscopy as part of the annual physical exam for all men and women over 40. Others follow the ACS recommendations mentioned earlier.

When preparing a patient for sigmoidoscopy, explain that the scope is a flexible instrument with a light at the tip that allows the physician to look at the inside of the lower bowel. Tell him he'll receive laxatives or enemas to clean out his bowel. During the exam, which takes about 30 minutes, the physician will pump air into the bowel to straighten the mucosal folds so he can see the lining better. Warn the patient that the instrument and sometimes the air might cause abdominal discomfort.

Tell the patient he'll be asked to breathe deeply from time to time to relieve the discomfort and help relax his bowel.

Colonscopy. Colonoscopy is similar to sigmoidoscopy except that the physician examines both the upper and lower bowel. Modern colonoscopy has revolutionized diagnosis of colon disease because the physician can see polyps through the colonoscope that he can't see via sigmoidoscopy or X-ray.

Colonoscopy requires that the entire length of the bowel be cleaned out. The patient will probably receive liquids or a low-residue diet for 24 to 48 hours. Then he'll receive laxatives and enemas or a colon lavage solution such as Colyte or GoLYTELY. Usually the physician prescribes IV diazepam and meperidine (Demerol) to help relax the patient.

As with sigmoidoscopy, the doctor will pump air into the bowel prior to the examination. If the patient has been having abdominal pain, the doctor may prescribe an analgesic to relieve the added discomfort caused by the air.

Tests to rule out anemia and metastasis

In addition to the foregoing tests, the patient will have blood tests to check for anemia and evaluate liver function. Colon cancer usually spreads to the liver first, so abnormal results from liver-function tests suggest that metastasis has occurred. In that case, the patient would probably undergo further evaluation by liver scan and needle biopsy.

If the IVP indicates that cancer has invaded the bladder, the physician might order a cystoscopy to evaluate the possibility of removing part of the bladder along with the colon.

A positive blood test for carcinoembryonic antigen—CEA—can also suggest metastasis. This test isn't specific enough or sensitive enough to diagnose early cancers, but it can help monitor the course of the metastasis or detect a recurrence.

The prognosis and treatment options

If the diagnostic workup confirms that the patient has cancer, prognosis and treatment are the next issues the physician must consider. Both will depend on the size of the tumor, the degree to which it has invaded the surrounding tissue,

Distribution of colorectal cancers

Three-quarters of all colorectal cancers occur in the descending colon, the sigmoid colon, or the rectum. President Reagan's malignancy belonged to the approximately 16% of cancers that occur in the ascending colon.

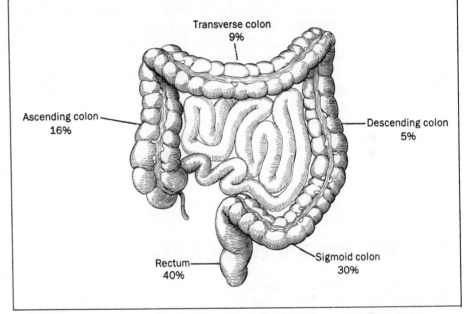

Transverse colon
9%

Ascending colon
16%

Descending colon
5%

Rectum
40%

Sigmoid colon
30%

and the presence or absence of metastasis to lymph nodes or distant organs.

Colorectal tumors are commonly classified according to the Dukes classification system. For a description of the Dukes system, see the preceding page.

Current treatment options for colorectal cancer consist of surgery, radiation therapy, and chemotherapy, used separately or in combination.

When the patient faces bowel surgery

Surgery typically involves the removal of a portion of the patient's colon, with or without the creation of an ostomy. The various surgical procedures are described in the box on page 28.

Prior to surgery, the patient will be given a low-residue diet for three to five days, then clear liquids for one to three days. The physician may order antibiotics to decrease the level of bacteria in the colon. You'll also have to give enemas or lavage solution for four to five days before surgery to thoroughly clean the patient's colon.

Be sure to warn the patient that he'll probably feel nauseated and very tired the day after the operation. Also tell him that he'll probably have a tube inserted through his nose to help remove air and stomach fluids so his colon will heal better.

How to give better stoma care

Patients whose surgery involves creation of a stoma sometimes want to know if they'll have to wear a pouch all the time. Explain that when surgery is in the lower colon, the patient can regulate bowel movements with enemas given once or twice a day. He'll wear a pouch until his bowel regime is established. After that, he need only cover the stoma with a 4x4 gauze pad between enemas, as long as he avoids foods that give him gas or cause diarrhea.

In general, the farther the ostomy is from the stomach the better the chance that the patient will need a pouch only part of the time. That's because intestinal contents become less liquid as they move through the intestines.

Arrange for a member of a local ostomy club to visit patients who are scheduled for ostomy surgery. It's important to the patient's sense of well-being to know that people who have had similar problems are now doing well.

When the patient returns from the recovery room, monitor his vital signs and his intake and output. Teach the patient to cough, deep breathe, and turn every two hours to prevent lung congestion and thrombosis. Help him get out of bed as soon as he's allowed to do so.

Keep the area around an abdominal incision clean and dry. Report any bleeding or abnormal drainage.

If the patient has a perineal incision in addition to an abdominal incision, change dressings as often as necessary to keep the area clean and dry. Drainage can be profuse and very foul smelling the first several days, but it should gradually decrease over a period of weeks. Meanwhile you can order an automatic room deodorizer. Sometimes

Surgery for colorectal cancer

Depending on the nature and extent of the lesions, surgery for colorectal cancer may involve anything from removal of a precancerous polyp with a colonoscope to removal of the entire colon. The surgery may or may not require creation of a stoma.

The illustrations show the major procedures used to treat colorectal cancer. The three procedures on the opposite page require a stoma; the two procedures at right do not.

An ostomy is created for one of two reasons: to rest the bowel prior to surgery, or to provide a means of evacuation when so much of the large intestine has been removed that normal evacuation is impossible. The location of the stoma reflects the extent of the surgery.

In these illustrations, cancerous lesions appear in red. The sections of intestine being removed are shown in yellow.

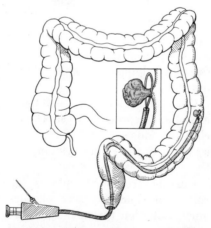

The endoscopist performs a polypectomy, as shown above, by inserting a colonoscope into the bowel through the rectum. He snares the polyp with an attachment on the end of the scope and then severs the growth from the bowel wall. Pedunculated polyps up to 4 cm in diameter and small unpedunculated (sessile) polyps can be removed this way.

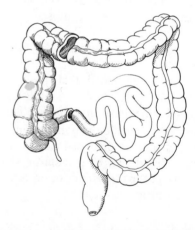

Bowel resection involves removing the section of bowel where a polyp is located as well as a length of bowel on either side. The surgeon then anastomoses the cut ends. Resection is usually done to remove polyps with bases larger than 2 cm in diameter and lesions classified as Dukes stage A.

the physician will prescribe irrigations of half-strength peroxide to keep the area free of infection.

Remember to check the stoma itself. It should be pink or red. If it becomes gray or black, that can mean that necrosis, a serious complication, is taking place.

If the patient has a colostomy, begin bowel irrigations as ordered, keeping the patient's usual elimination pattern in mind. For example, if he's used to having a bowel movement once a day in the evening, irrigate the stoma then. If the patient has a double-barrel colostomy—a temporary colostomy with two openings which will be reanastomosed several weeks later—it's usually the opening on the patient's left that leads to the lower bowel.

If the patient has an ileostomy, it usually means the entire large intestine has been removed. He'll probably have both an abdominal and a perineal incision. At first, he will have only a small amount of drainage from the ileostomy. But when peristalsis returns, drainage can be profuse. At that time, you will need to be especially alert for fluid and electrolyte imbalances.

Report symptoms of electrolyte disturbances, such as headache, fatigue, drowsiness, nausea, and muscle weakness. Be aware that vomiting, diarrhea, or excessive drainage from nasogastric tubes can compound the problem. If the patient's skin turgor is poor, if serum electrolyte levels are abnormal, or if output is greater than intake for more than three shifts, notify the physician. He'll probably prescribe IV infusions to replenish fluids, electrolytes, and nutrients.

Because ileostomy drainage is more liquid and more caustic than colostomy drainage, you need to take special care to prevent skin irritation. Consult an enterostomal

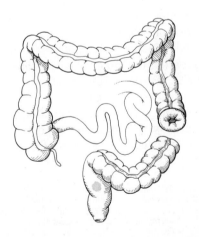

When the surgeon must excise the rectum and part of the descending colon to remove cancer, he creates a colostomy in the descending colon above the excision site.

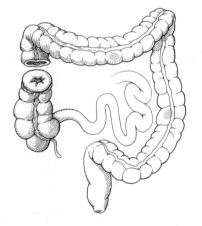

An ostomy in the ascending colon is necessary when the surgeon must remove all of the transverse and descending colon.

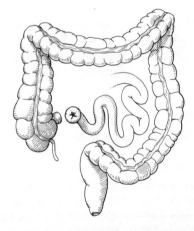

When extensive cancer necessitates removal of the entire large intestine, the surgeon creates an ileostomy in the ileum of the small intestine to drain wastes.

therapist for the appropriate appliance, belt, and skin prep to use.

In fact, with so many different types of ostomy appliances and skin preparations available, it's often best to refer all your ostomy patients to an enterostomal therapist. She'll help each patient find the products that work best for him.

But don't abandon the patient just because an enterostomal therapist is on the scene. He still needs your support and teaching. You can help ease the embarrassment caused by bowel irrigation by emphasizing that bowel function is a normal and necessary way for the body to rid itself of wastes.

Your patient may also worry about sex. Reassure him that most patients are able to resume normal sexual functioning soon after surgery. The exceptions are women who've had their vaginas diverted or removed and men whose parasympathetic nerve has been damaged. But even for these exceptions, counseling or plastic surgery can alleviate the problem.

Radiation therapy and chemotherapy

The patient with colorectal cancer may receive radiation therapy as a preoperative adjunct to surgery or as primary treatment. Some physicans believe that low-dose radiation—500 to 2,000 rads—given before surgery can increase survival.

As primary therapy, many doctors give moderate to full doses—4,000 to 6,000 rads—over a period of five to six weeks. This amount can shrink the tumor. It can also relieve pain, obstruction, or hemorrhage in patients who refuse surgery or who aren't good candidates for surgery.

Chemotherapy is usually given to patients with inoperable cancer or metastasis. The traditional anticancer drug, 5-fluorouracil (5-FU), is sometimes combined with other drugs such as vincristine (Oncovin), BCG, or levamisole. We have found that 5-FU alone is just as effective as any combination.

Besides nausea and vomiting, which can sometimes be relieved with antiemetic drugs, a patient receiving 5-FU may experience mouth soreness and difficulty swallowing after five to eight days of treatment. Rinsing his mouth every three to four hours with a baking soda and salt solution—one teaspoon of each in a glass of warm water—may bring relief.

If discomfort persists, ask the physician to prescribe a mouthwash of diphenhydramine (Benadryl), magnesium and aluminum hydroxide (Maalox), and lidocaine (Xylocaine). This solution relieves inflammation and anesthetizes the mouth and throat. The pharmacist can prepare the mixture for the patient to use every four hours prn or before meals.

Other side effects of 5-FU include rash, diarrhea, itching eyes, hair loss, low WBC and platelet count, hypotension, and pigmented areas on the face and hands.

Ask the physician if it's all right to give the patient diphenoxylate (Lomotil) for diarrhea. Reassure the patient that his hair will probably grow back and that pigmented areas usually return to normal.

Monitor the patient's WBC and platelet count, and check his blood pressure every four hours. If it's low, notify the physician in case he wants to order IV fluids. Don't leave the patient alone. He's at risk of falling because of postural hypotension. Headache, visual disturbances, and a shuffling gait are possible side effects of chemotherapy and should be reported.

One of the sad realities of colorectal cancer is that many patients could probably avoid radiation or chemotherapy—and live longer—if only their disease had been discovered earlier. The five-year survival rate for patients with localized cancer in the colon that's treated promptly is about 76%. If the cancer spreads to other parts of the body before it's diagnosed and treated, the survival rate drops to 28%. Perhaps the greater public awareness of colorectal cancer stemming from President Reagan's surgery will send more people to their doctors' offices before it's too late. ■

BIBLIOGRAPHY Bouchard-Kurtz, R. and Speese-Owens, N. *Nursing Care of the Cancer Patient*. St Louis: C.V. Mosby Co., 1981. Burns, R. *Nursing and Cancer*. Philadelphia: W.B. Saunders Co., 1982. DeVita, V. et al. *Cancer*. Philadelphia: J.B. Lippincott Co., 1985. Griffiths M. et al. *Oncology Nursing*. New York: MacMillan Publishing Co., 1984. Holland, J. et al. *Cancer Medicine*. Philadelphia: Lea and Febiger, 1982. *Neoplastic Disorders*. Springhouse, Pa.: Springhouse Corp., 1985. Rubin, P. *Clinical Oncology*. New York: American Cancer Society, 1983.

Nursing the kidney transplant patient

Replacing a damaged kidney with a healthy one is one of the benchmark achievements of modern medicine —a procedure that makes the utmost demands on nurse, patient, and family.

By Rose Rivers, RN

Now that several thousand kidneys are being transplanted every year, the day may soon come when you'll have an opportunity to nurse a patient through this process. If you do, you'll face a breathtaking array of challenges and satisfactions.

To meet those challenges, you'll need to maintain close personal contact not only with the patient but also with his family. Only by so doing will you be able to give them the support they need to weather preop suspense and psychologically jarring lifestyle adjustments.

Your physical assessment will help establish the patient's readiness for surgery. It will also guide the patient through the postop period. After surgery, maintaining optimum fluid and nutritional status are paramount, and the success of the transplant may hinge on the way you respond to early signs of complications.

Your teaching will help the patient care for himself in the months

THE AUTHOR is nursing supervisor of the renal transplant unit of Shands Hospital in Gainesville, Fla.

Produced by David Anderson

following discharge, when the twin dangers of infection and rejection remain strong.

Helping the patient who's being screened

Not every patient who would benefit from a transplanted kidney receives one. For example, severe cardiac disease, cancer, or other incurable conditions can disqualify a candidate.

To see if a patient is healthy enough for surgery, the doctor will order an exhaustive battery of screening tests—CBC with electrolytes, clotting tests, hepatitis antigen test, liver function tests, and renal function tests including BUN, creatinine, and urinalysis. He'll also want an ECG, chest X-ray, and radiographic studies of bladder function and joint formation. Preop interviews with psychiatrists and social workers will determine whether the patient can be expected to comply with postop treatment.

These tests and any others deemed necessary will enable the

doctor to take preop measures to prevent postop problems. Chief among these is infection, since postop medication will lower the patient's resistance. To eliminate potential infection sites in the mouth, a dentist will fill all cavities, clean abscesses, and perhaps pull loose teeth. Fragile joints may be replaced before the transplant, since postop medications weaken bones.

You'll participate in the screening procedures. You'll also help sustain the patient and his family emotionally.

Make sure they have correct information about the transplant— the procedure itself, its risks and benefits, and the lifestyle changes that will follow. Set aside enough time to listen to their questions, apprehensions, or expressions of doubt.

Once the patient is approved for a transplant, he'll be discharged to continue dialysis as an outpatient. While awaiting a donor kidney he may receive a series of random blood transfusions. For reasons nobody fully understands, such transfusions enhance graft acceptance and survival.

Preop nursing sets postop baselines

When the patient is admitted for the transplant, the doctor repeats many of the screening tests. You assess vital signs and fluid and electrolyte balance. Your findings provide a baseline for measuring postop progress.

Assuming no complications, the transplant procedure, described in the box on page 247, takes about four hours. Afterwards, the patient spends 12 to 24 hours in the post-anesthesia room or ICU. He wakes up with peripheral IV lines to administer and monitor fluid replacement, and a Foley catheter. In some institutions all patients have CVP lines placed during surgery, in others only patients at high risk for fluid imbalance. Some surgeons regularly insert drains in the wound.

When the patient returns to the floor, you should assess the surgical site and change the dressing prn—which will probably be about once a day. In most cases, the wound heals quickly enough to require no dressings after the fifth day postop.

To clear the patient's lungs and prevent atelectasis and pneumonia, have him breathe deeply and cough q2h. You should aim to get him out of bed and walking on the first postop day.

Once you have attended to the care of the wound and prevention of respiratory complications, you can then turn to promoting the three physical requirements for discharge—good fluid and electrolyte balance, acceptance of the graft kidney, and freedom from infection.

Nursing priority: managing fluids

Monitor the patient's vital signs, heart and lung sounds, and fluid intake and output hourly for the first 12 to 24 hours, q4h thereafter. Check renal profile and weight daily. Notify the physician if vital signs or lab values are abnormal, weight gains exceed two pounds in

a day, or intake exceeds output.

To help the patient achieve fluid and electrolyte balance, the doctor may prescribe an anephric diet—one that contains 60 to 80 gm of protein, 2 to 4 gm of sodium, and 40 to 60 mEq of potassium. Until his kidneys are working well, the patient receives phosphate binders such as Amphogel or Basalgel to prevent calcium and phosphorous imbalances. When fluid intake and output balance and renal function tests show that the graft kidney's function is improving, the patient advances to a regular diet with sodium and potassium restrictions. He graduates to a regular diet without restrictions when his creatinine level falls to within normal limits.

By the time the patient returns to the floor, his urine intake and output should be balanced. If so, he doesn't need IV fluid replacement provided he's able to take in enough fluids—around 1,500 cc per day—by mouth. Most kidney transplant patients have their intravenous lines removed on the day after surgery.

If the transplant patient develops oliguria—urine output less than 30 cc/hr—in the immediate postop period, the cause may be an obstructed Foley catheter, hypovolemia, fluid retention, or acute tubular necrosis.

Test the first possibility by irrigating the catheter. Or change it, taking care to first obtain a physician's order if your institution requires one.

If urine still doesn't flow, examine the patient to see if he's dehydrated or retaining fluid. To treat

dehydration, the doctor orders fluids to bring the central venous pressure to 10 mm H_2O or until symptoms resolve. To treat fluid retention, he gives a bolus of the diuretic furosemide (Lasix) to prevent overload by shifting fluid out of the extravascular spaces and stimulating excretion.

If oliguria still persists the patient has probably developed acute tubular necrosis, a temporary failure of the kidney. An ultrasound scan can help confirm this diagnosis by ruling out ureteral compression and other obstructions. Acute tubular necrosis resolves without treatment, usually within a couple of weeks. If it doesn't resolve quickly, however, the physician may have the patient resume dialysis temporarily.

If oliguria develops seven days or so after the transplant procedure, the cause may well be rejection of the graft.

Preventing rejection or reversing it

Graft rejection occurs because the immune system naturally attacks the transplanted tissues just as it does bacteria that are introduced into the body.

One sign of graft rejection is decreased urine output. Other warning signs include increased blood pressure, elevated temperature, tenderness or swelling over the graft, increased serum creatinine, increased BUN, proteinuria, hyperkalemia, and weight gain due to fluid retention.

At the same time you're watching for signs of graft rejection, you will also administer immunosuppressant drugs to prevent it.

Prednisone, which is an anti-inflammatory corticosteroid, will be given 2 mg/kg of body weight per day intravenously or orally in divided doses. To prevent GI irritation, have the patient take his oral doses with food, and maintain him on an antacid. Avoid magnesium-containing antacids such as milk of magnesia or Mylanta, however, if the patient's kidney is not working well. He could develop hypermagnesemia if the kidney doesn't excrete the electrolyte sufficiently.

Prednisone causes decreased resistance to infection, retention of sodium and fluid, slower wound healing, mood changes, and cushingoid appearance. It may cause hypertension, cataracts, and aseptic bone necrosis. It may lead to hyperglycemia by modifying the patient's glucose metabolism, especially if he's diabetic.

Azathioprine (Imuran), a cytotoxic agent, will be given intravenously or orally. The first day's dosage will be 3 mg/kg of body weight. Since this drug disrupts production of white blood cells, the dosage will be changed each day depending on the WBC count. Watch for anemia, anorexia, bleeding, oral lesions, or swelling or other signs of liver toxicity.

Cyclosporine (Sandimmune), a direct inhibitor of immune cell reproduction, will be given intravenously or orally in doses calibrated to achieve ideal serum levels. To give cyclosporine orally, have the patient mix it with milk or orange juice to mask its unpleasant taste. Be sure the liquids are at room temperature since cyclosporine will

The transplant procedure

Kidney transplants are done under general anesthesia and take approximately four hours. The kidney is placed retroperitoneally in the right or left iliac fossa. The renal artery of the donor's kidney is anastomosed to the recipient's internal or external iliac artery, and the renal vein is anastomosed to the recipient's external iliac vein. The donor ureter is implanted into the posterior wall of the recipient's bladder through a submucosal tunnel. The patient's native kidney is left in place unless it contains stones or is a source of infection or uncontrolled high blood pressure.

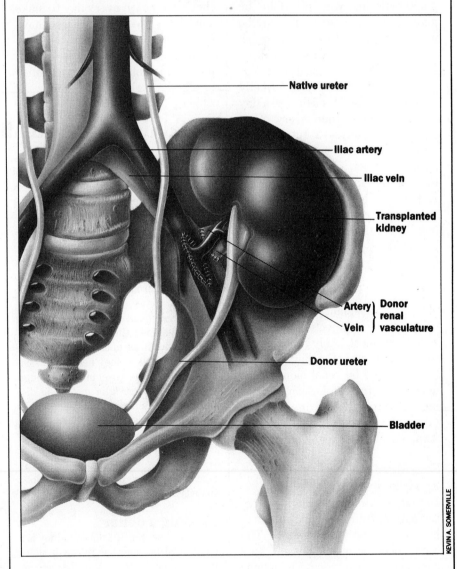

Native ureter

Iliac artery

Iliac vein

Transplanted kidney

Artery
Vein } Donor renal vasculature

Donor ureter

Bladder

KEVIN A. SOMERVILLE

clump in cold liquids. This drug's most serious side effect is nephrotoxicity. Some other potential side effects include GI disturbances, hyperkalemia, tremors, blurred vision, headache, hypertension, gum hyperplasia, hirsutism, and hearing loss.

Methylprednisolone (SoluMedrol), which is an anti-inflammatory glucocorticoid, will probably be given intraoperatively and may be used thereafter to reverse rejection. In the latter case, it will be given in pulses. A typical pulse regimen consists of 20 mg/kg of body weight given by IV push once a day for three days, then every other day for six days—a total of six doses. This drug may well cause hypernatremia, so the patient's intake of sodium should be limited. Euphoria, headaches, insomnia, sweating, hypokalemia, hypocalcemia, hyperglycemia, hypertension, peptic ulcers, and congestive heart failure are other potential side effects.

Despite these drugs, some 50% of kidney transplant patients develop symptoms of rejection. Such episodes will most likely occur seven to 14 days postop; the diagnosis will be confirmed by renal biopsy. The doctor will treat rejection by adding to the patient's immunosuppressant regimen. If caught early, it can usually be reversed.

Standing watch against infection

Immunosuppressant drugs protect the patient from rejection but make him vulnerable to infection. The immunocompromised patient may contract life-threatening infections from pathogens such as *pneumocystis carinii*, *Candida albicans*, *Aspergillis*, and cytomegalovirus that pose little or no threat to people who have normal immune systems.

The patient will be given nystatin (Mycostat, Nilstat) oral suspension after meals to prevent overgrowth of *Candida*. Remember to check his mouth every day to make sure no white fungal lesions have appeared.

To avert *pneumocystis carinii* pneumonia and urinary tract infection, the patient receives trimethoprim-sulfamethoxazole (Septra).

Wash your hands whenever you touch the patient, and use aseptic technique when you touch areas of broken skin. Prepare IV insertion and catheter sites with povidone-iodine (Betadine) rather than alcohol swabs. Wear gloves when you change dressings. Tape catheters and IV needles well to make sure they don't wobble or irritate, which might lead to infection.

You will also have to obtain a clean catch urine specimen for uri-

Obtaining and matching the donor kidney

Mental clouding may be the first sign you'll notice when you're introduced to the kidney transplant candidate. Other signs and symptoms shared by these patients include edema, uremia, anemia, electrolyte disturbances, and serum acid buildup. All of these conditions are caused by the failure of the patient's kidneys to filter blood, excrete waste products, and balance fluid and electrolytes.

The transplant candidate's kidneys have developed the severe degree of failure known as end-stage renal disease. That means they need the assistance of dialysis to eliminate enough toxins to prevent fatal metabolic disturbances. It's not unusual for them to require hemodialysis as often as three times a week or peritoneal dialysis four times a day. Even with such heroic treatment, some patients will still face death from overwhelming blood toxicity.

Finding a donor
The safest source of a donor kidney is a blood relation. Because relatives share many tissue proteins and characteristics, the patient's immune system is more likely to accept such a kidney without mounting an intense rejection reaction.

Only about 40% of patients have blood relatives who can and want to donate kidneys. Others must receive organs from cadavers of recently deceased persons who have signed donor cards or whose relatives agree to the removal. Unfortunately, patients reject cadaver kidneys some 20% of the time, as contrasted to only 10% rejection rates for kidneys from relatives.

Some 50 agencies are involved in soliciting organs from the public. The most prominent of these are UNOS, United Network for Organ Sharing, and NATCO, North American Transplant Coordinators Organization.

Screening the living donor
The relative who offers a kidney becomes the transplant team's second patient. Before plans are made to remove his kidney, the donor undergoes physical and psychological screening. Although the removal of one kidney is unlikely to affect his health over the long

nalysis and culture twice a week.

Keep visitors who have colds or other infections away from the patient. This will be easier to do if you limit visitors to two at a time.

How to prepare for discharge

Most kidney transplant patients are discharged two to three weeks postop, when the period of highest incidence of rejection is past. If the new kidney isn't functioning at full efficiency, the doctor will first perform a fine-needle biopsy to make

sure the problem is due to acute tubular necrosis and not rejection.

The risks of infection and rejection don't disappear when the patient leaves the hospital. That's why you must prepare the patient and family to take over monitoring and managing protective regimens.

This means, first of all, impressing upon them the importance of taking all prescribed drugs and keeping all clinic appointments.

Give the patient a notebook to record each of his medications, their schedules, purposes, and side

effects. He'll use this book for two months or so, while the schedules fluctuate. Eventually he'll shift to maintenance levels of immunosuppressant drugs, which he'll take for the rest of his life.

Patient satisfaction— the nurse's reward

It's thrilling to see the sparkle in the eyes of a transplant patient on the first postop day.

The successful transplant frees the patient from his renal symptoms. It spares him from the need for dialysis, and it also allows him to relax some of his dietary and fluid restrictions.

Most transplant patients will have an easier time controlling the underlying disease—most often diabetes or hypertension—that had caused his kidney deterioration. His energy levels and feeling of well-being will usually increase. The desire to enjoy this improved vitality—and not dull it in any way—may be the reason why few patients ask for any pain medication after the second postop day.

A few patients experience complications that force removal of the graft kidney. Despite the pain, discomfort, and disappointment of their unsuccessful graft, almost all say that they would try a second time, and a third if necessary. ■

term, the patient must be healthy enough to withstand general anesthesia and surgery.

Preop, the nurse makes sure that he understands the removal procedure. She also helps him express his questions and hesitations.

To shield relatives from pressure to donate, they're always interviewed privately. Some hospitals go further, offering to protect dubious donors from recrimination by telling the patient and other family members that they're immunologically incompatible.

Postop, the transplant team follows both the patient and donor to help them with any conflicts or concerns that may develop.

Matching the kidney

When a kidney is found, the doctor orders a series of tests to determine exactly how compatible its blood and tissues are with the patient's. ABO type and crossmatch tests must demonstrate blood and tissue compatibility in order for there to be any chance of success. The doctor also obtains a comparison of the patient's human leukocyte

antigens and those of the available organ. This gives a much more refined indication of how the recipient's immune system will respond to the kidney, since there are hundreds of HLA types as opposed to only four blood types.

If the potential donor is a living relative, the doctor also orders a mixed lymphocyte culture. White cells from the patient and relative are cultured together for several days. The patient's cells may mount a strong antibody reaction to his relative's tissue even if their HLA types are very similar. Such a reaction indicates a likelihood that the patient will reject the offered kidney.

If the available kidney comes from a cadaver, the doctor orders a white cell crossmatch. Again, the purpose is to see if the immune cells attack each other. If they do, the search for a kidney resumes.

Once screening and matching are finished, the living donor may schedule the transplant at a time that's convenient for him and the patient. Transplant from a cadaver must be done within 72 hours of the donor's death or the kidney will deteriorate.

BIBLIOGRAPHY Schoengrund, L. and Balzer, P. *Renal Problems in Critical Care.* New York: John Wiley & Sons, 1985. Jackle, M. and Rosmussen, C. *Renal Problems: A Critical Care Nursing Focus.* London: Prentice-Hall International, Inc., 1980. Glassock, R. *Current Therapy in Nephrology and Hypertension.* St. Louis: C.V. Mosby Company, 1985. DHHS Publication No. HRS-A-OC 85-2, Aug. 1985. *Q & A Organ Transplantation.* Office of Organ Transplantation. Rockville, Md. *Sandimmune (cyclosporine) and Organ Transplants.* East Hanover, N.J.: Sandoz, Inc., 1984.

Nursing the patient in traction

Once you understand the simple principles
behind those ropes, weights, and pulleys,
you can turn to the basic nursing considerations
that will keep your traction patient
safe and comfortable.

By Linda Morris, RN, MSN, CCRN, Shirley Kraft, RN, BS,
Sandra Tessem, RN, BSN, and Susan Reinisch, RN

The patient at the center of that spider's web of steel and rope is benefiting from one of the most common of all orthopedic techniques: traction.

Its pulling force—applied to the skin or to a bone—can immobilize fractures, maintain proper alignment, prevent soft tissue injury, and decrease muscle spasm and pain.

Too much force, however, can cause damage to nerves and tissues, while too little can produce painful muscle spasms and impair healing.

The prolonged bed rest that's required with traction puts the patient at risk for all the complications of immobility as well. Given these facts, you must be as adept at

THE AUTHORS: Ms. Morris is a clinical nurse specialist in critical care at the University of Illinois Hospital in Chicago. Ms. Kraft is the head nurse and Ms. Tessem a staff nurse on the orthopedic unit at Westlake Community Hospital in Melrose Park, Ill. Ms. Reinisch, formerly an orthopedic staff nurse, is now the staffing coordinator at Westlake Community Hospital.

Produced by Mary-Beth Moriarty, RN, CCRN

handling the traction equipment as you are skilled at caring for the patient.

Some basics about skin traction

Skin traction exerts force directly on the surface of the body and indirectly on the underlying muscles and bones. Pulling on a limb with your hands is a simple, temporary method of applying skin traction. A physician, for example, can employ this technique—it is also called manual traction—to realign fractured bones.

To maintain effective skin traction for longer periods of time, a system of ropes, weights, and pulleys is used. Adhesive tape, elastic bandages, or a specially designed covering are first applied to the skin and then attached to the system, creating a constant pull.

Skin traction can be applied to the spine, pelvis, or the long bones

of the extremities. The most common forms and their functions are illustrated on page 28.

What to look for before you apply skin traction

Before you apply traction to an extremity, do a baseline neurovascular assessment. That way you'll be able to detect changes quickly afterward. Palpate the peripheral pulses. Check capillary refill. Note skin color, temperature, and turgor. Compare these findings with those of the unaffected limb.

Check for numbness, tingling, or a decrease in sensation in the extremity. Find out if the patient can move his fingers or toes. Ask him if he has any pain. If so, have him locate and describe the discomfort.

The skin that will bear the brunt of the force of traction also needs special attention. Find out if the patient has any skin allergies. Look for signs of injury or infection. As a rule, skin traction is not used when a patient has hypersensitive skin, an infection, open wound, or soft tissue damage. It is also contraindicated in cases of swelling, neurologic deficits, or vascular insufficiency due to trauma.

How to assemble the equipment

The basic setup for traction includes a standard hospital bed with a firm mattress. If necessary, place a bed board underneath to prevent sagging, which can change the angle and effectiveness of traction.

Fasten the traction frame to the head and the foot of the bed, then secure smaller bars called traction arms to the frame. Screw down all

Assembling traction equipment

For effective traction, you have to assemble the setup of bars, pulleys, ropes, and weights in a precisely prescribed manner. But before you worry about angles, pulling force, and the like, you've got to get the basics in place. You'll start with a traction frame much like the one pictured at the right. The frame includes two horizontal bars, one each at the head and foot of the bed, and two vertical bars, one in the middle of each horizontal bar and at right angles to it. An overhead bar connects the vertical bars and supports a trapeze.

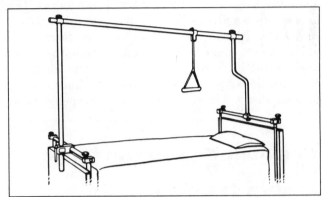

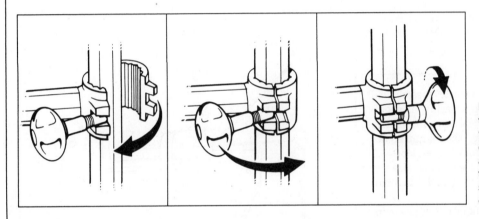

Hinged clamps secure smaller traction arms to the vertical bars of the frame. To attach a traction arm, close the two sides of the clamp around the vertical bar as shown in the picture at the far left. Then swing the screw into the grip. Tighten the clamp by turning the knob.

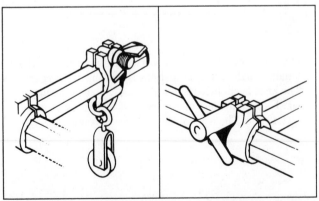

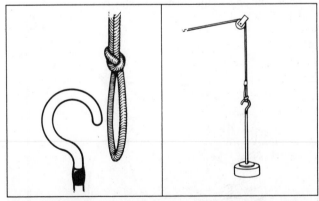

A knob isn't the only kind of fastener used to secure a hinged clamp. You may also use a wing nut, shown at left, or a T bar, at right. The wing nut is used most often to attach a pulley to a traction arm.

The actual pulling force of traction comes from the weights that are suspended from rope threaded through the pulleys. Knot the rope, as shown above, to provide a loop from which to hang the prescribed amount of weight.

the clamps so they fasten tightly.

To maintain proper body alignment, traction must be exerted along the long axis—an imaginary line passing lengthwise through the center of the bone. The placement of the pulleys on the frame and the angle of the involved joints determine the line of pull. The orthopedic specialist will include this information in the orders for traction.

He'll also specify the number of pulleys to use. With a single pulley, the force of traction is equal to the weight applied. With two pulleys, the force of traction doubles. Attach the pulleys to the traction arms. Make sure they roll freely.

Ropes that are threaded through the pulleys convey the force of traction. Look for kinks. Tape ends to prevent fraying. The rope should not touch the traction frame or bed.

Make a loop at the end and knot the rope. Be sure all knots are secure and positioned no closer than 12 inches to the nearest pulley.

Suspend the prescribed amount of weight from the loop. Make sure that the weights hang freely. They

Reviewing common types of skin traction

Skin traction can be applied to the spine, the pelvis, or the long bones of the extremities. The types you'll see most often are shown here.

Cervical traction helps relieve muscle spasms and nerve compression in the neck, upper arms, or shoulders. The front strap of the cervical sling fits underneath the chin with a slight overlap. The rear strap fits at the base of the skull, away from the earlobes. A spreader bar fits into the loops of rope to equalize the pull. The head of the bed is elevated 30 to 40° to maintain the proper angle for traction.

If a patient in cervical traction complains of jaw pain, notify the physician. The weight may be too heavy.

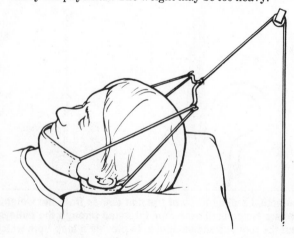

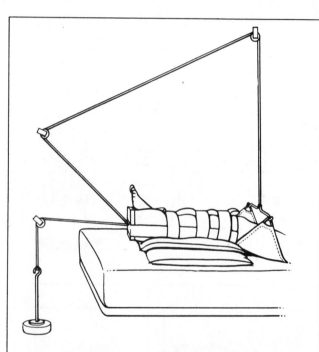

Russell's traction is used to stabilize fractures of the femoral shaft while the patient is waiting for surgery. The knee is slightly flexed. A sling supports the upper leg. Elevate the foot of the bed slightly to provide countertraction. The head of the bed should remain flat.

should not touch the floor, the traction frame, or the bed.

You're now ready to attach the system to the patient.

Attaching traction to the patient

The orthopedist will specify whether he wants to use a sling, bandage, or belt to connect the patient to the traction apparatus. Make sure that the skin under this connector is clean and dry.

In the case of cervical traction, the sling should fit snugly underneath the patient's chin. Make sure that the straps don't press on the earlobes.

If a belt is used for pelvic traction, fasten it securely but not too tightly. Make certain that the buckles are not pressing into the patient's skin.

If you use elastic bandages to apply traction to an extremity, be sure to wrap them smoothly around the limb.

A foam rubber boot is sometimes used to apply skin traction to the lower leg. The boot should fit snug-

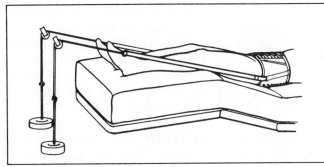

Pelvic traction alleviates low back, hip, and leg pain. It can also reduce muscle spasms and aid in proper skeletal alignment. The patient wears a wide cloth belt that fits snugly around the hips. Long ties on either side of the belt attach to two weight and pulley systems, creating an equal pull on both sides of the body. For countertraction, place the patient in William's position. That is, elevate the head of the bed and the knee gatch to approximately the same angle.

Buck's traction immobilizes fractures of the hip and reduces muscle spasm pending surgical repair. The patient wears a foam rubber boot that's attached to the traction equipment. The force of a single pulley is applied through the boot to hold the leg in a straight line. To create countertraction, elevate the foot of the bed on shock blocks.

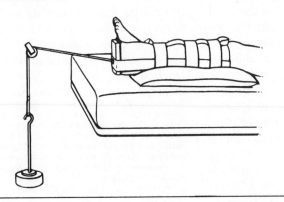

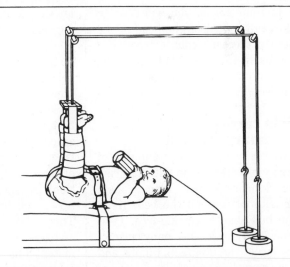

Bryant's traction is used to correct congenital hip dislocations or to stabilize fractured femurs in young children. Flexion at the hips creates a vertical pull to both legs thus maintaining proper alignment of the bones and hip joints. The weight of the child's torso provides countertraction.

SCOTT BODELL

ly but not so tight as to interfere with circulation.

Whatever kind of connector you employ, check to make sure that the body part is aligned properly before you attempt to attach the rope.

Fasten the rope securely to the connector. Then take away your hands slowly. This allows for a gradual pull of traction. A sudden release can cause pain. Remain with the patient after you apply traction.

Assess him for any increased pain or symptoms of neurovascular impairment. These are signs that the traction may require some kind of adjustment.

Check the patient and the equipment at least once a shift—more often if you have to change the patient's position.

In some cases, you will need to elevate the foot or the head of the bed to increase countertraction—the balancing force that keeps the patient from being dragged toward the weights.

Skin care— a primary concern

Bed rest and the constant pull of traction increase the patient's risk for skin breakdown. Place a foam or air mattress on the bed. Keep the bed sheets wrinkle-free. Periodically, check the bony prominences of the unaffected limbs and back as well.

Place a pillow underneath a leg in traction to help relieve pressure on the heel, making sure it extends beyond the popliteal space. A pillow that becomes bunched up underneath the knee keeps the joint flexed and impairs venous flow.

Check with the physician before you remove a traction boot. If he agrees, the boot can be removed once a shift to assess and care for the skin. Remember to maintain traction with your hands. A sudden release can cause painful muscle spasms.

When you inspect the skin, check also for symptoms of circulatory or neurologic impairment. Document and report any changes immediately, especially those that signal possible nerve damage—a loss of mobility, increased pain, or sensory changes.

Promote movement, give moral support

When possible, reposition the patient every two hours. To turn a patient in Buck's traction, place pillows between his legs. Support the leg and maintain the line of traction while the patient turns to the unaffected side. Make sure that the sheets do not interfere with the traction.

Some patients who are unable to turn can use a trapeze bar for repositioning. The bar hangs from the traction frame just below the level of the patient's shoulders. The patient grasps it and pulls himself up—much like doing a chin-up. This relieves pressure on the back and sacrum. Such activity also promotes lung expansion and helps prevent pneumonia—another complication that threatens a bedridden patient.

Use of a trapeze bar is contraindicated with some forms of traction, particularly cervical traction. Be sure to check with the physician before you encourage this kind of activity.

Exercise is also the best way to prevent muscle weakness. A patient can exercise his arms while eating and bathing. To maintain muscle strength in his unaffected leg, show a patient the way to do active range-of-motion exercises. Such activity also improves circulation and thus decreases the risk for thrombophlebitis. Be sure to inform the patient, however, what movements he must avoid. A patient in Russell's traction, for example, should not turn his body below the waist. A patient in Buck's traction must not bend from the waist or sit up.

Patients in traction, especially the elderly, often complain of constipation. If a patient's condition allows, encourage fluids and a high-fiber diet to prevent this problem.

Patients who are confined to bed often feel isolated. When possible make brief visits in addition to providing care. Keep the TV controls, telephone, and bedside table within reach.

Traction is a challenge for both the patient and the nurse. When traction is applied directly to the bone, you'll have some additional concerns. Next month we'll tell you how to care for a patient in skeletal traction. ∎

BIBLIOGRAPHY Brunner, L. and Suddarth, D. *Textbook of Medical-Surgical Nursing* (3rd ed.). Philadelphia: J.B. Lippincott Company, 1975. Brunner, L. and Suddarth, D. *The Lippincott Manual of Nursing Practice* (2nd ed.). Philadelphia: J.B. Lippincott Company, 1978. Carini, G. and Birmingham, J. *Traction Made Manageable: A Self-Learning Module.* New York: McGraw-Hill, Inc., 1980. Hilt, N. and Cogburn, S. *Manual of Orthopedics.* St. Louis: The C.V. Mosby Company, 1980. *Working with Orthopedic Patients, Nurses Reference Library.* Springhouse, Pa.: Intermed Communications, Inc., 1983.

Special care for skeletal traction

Principles described in last month's article on skin traction hold true when the pull is applied directly to a bone. Much of the equipment will be similar, too, but there are added nursing concerns when a patient needs skeletal traction.

By Linda Morris, RN, MSN, CCRN, Shirley Kraft, RN, BS, Sandra Tessem, RN, BSN, and Susan Reinisch, RN

The force of traction—applied to the skin or directly to the bone—corrects deformities, eases muscle spasms, and keeps broken bones in proper alignment.

Adhesive tape, elastic bandages, or special coverings are used to apply skin traction. Skeletal traction, on the other hand, demands metal hardware—pins, wires, or tongs inserted into the bone. In both cases, ropes, weights, and pulleys maintain the constant force needed for effective treatment.

You will ask yourself the same questions when you set up or check the equipment for skin or skeletal traction. Do the angles of the ropes and pulleys create a pull along the long axis of the bone? Is the rope taut and free of kinks and frayed ends? Do the pulleys move easily? Are all clamps and knots secure?

THE AUTHORS: Ms. Morris is a clinical specialist in critical care at the University of Illinois Hospital in Chicago. Ms. Kraft is the head nurse and Ms. Tessem a staff nurse on the orthopedic unit at Westlake Community Hospital in Melrose Park, Ill. Ms. Reinisch, formerly an orthopedic staff nurse, is now the staffing coordinator at Westlake Community Hospital.

Produced by Mary-Beth Moriarty, RN, CCRN

Do the weights hang freely? Is there sufficient countertraction?

You'll also take steps to prevent complications of prolonged bed rest. Repositioning and frequent skin care will help prevent breakdown. Exercises will combat pneumonia, muscle atrophy, bone demineralization, and venous stasis. Adequate fluid intake will ward off constipation and urinary stasis.

But in addition to the care that's common to any traction patient, you'll need to be on the lookout for other problems when you care for a patient in skeletal traction.

Special concerns with skeletal traction

Skeletal traction can be applied to the skull, the proximal end of the ulna, the distal end of the femur, the proximal and distal ends of the tibia, and the calcaneus or heel bone. Since bone can withstand greater stress than skin, heavier weights can be used. As much as 35 pounds can applied to keep fractured bones aligned and to help

prevent damage to the surrounding soft tissues from bone edges or fragments.

Patients may need to remain in skeletal traction for several months. During that time, traction is released only in the event of a life-threatening situation—cardiac arrest, for example. Premature or sudden release can produce strong muscle contractions, which, in turn, can disrupt bone fragments and cause more trauma.

Jarring movements can disrupt traction, too. Approach the patient and equipment with unusual care, and use one smooth coordinated effort whenever you must reposition a patient.

Preventing infection is a major priority

The pins, wires, or tongs used with skeletal traction need special attention. Because the hardware pierces the skin and passes into the bone, an infection at the insertion site can easily spread to the bone itself. Thus, osteomyelitis is a serious complication of skeletal traction.

To prevent infection, you'll give the insertion sites special care. Using Betadine for site care is controversial. Some physicians feel it corrodes the pins. So, the exact steps you'll take will depend on physician preference or hospital policy but are likely to be along these lines:

▶ Remove the dressings. Inspect insertion sites for signs of infection. Notify the doctor if you see bright red blood or purulent drainage.

▶ Put on a mask and sterile gloves. Use sterile applicators dipped in hydrogen peroxide to clean around the pins. Repeat with fresh applicators dipped in sterile water.

▶ Wrap a povodine-iodine gauze around the pin. Leave the gauze in place until the next cleaning.

Document and report at once any signs of infection—fever, redness, swelling, or purulent discharge. Notify the physician, too, if you see any change in the pin's position.

Skeletal traction that prevents spinal injury

When applied to the skull, skeletal traction stabilizes fractured or displaced vertebrae in the neck and upper thorax, preventing injury to the spinal cord. Four types of metal tongs—Blackburn, Gardner-Wells, Crutchfield, and Vinke can be used for cervical traction. The tips of the tongs are inserted into either side of the skull.

The tongs are positioned under local anesthesia. The procedure for inserting each type varies slightly. Placing Crutchfield tongs, for example, requires small scalp incisions and drill holes in the outer layer of the skull, while no drill holes are called for with Gardner-Wells tongs. With any kind of tong traction, meticulous care of the site is absolutely essential to prevent infection.

Trauma is often the cause of fractures of the cervical or thoracic vertebrae. For this reason, when you care for a patient in skeletal tong traction, you'll watch for signs of spinal cord injury.

Assess the patient's neurologic status hourly for the first 24 hours. Look for changes in his level of consciousness, loss of sensation, paralysis, muscle weakness, or pain.

Monitor vital signs, too. A drop in systolic blood pressure can be a symptom of spinal cord damage. Be alert for respiratory distress—a common complication with upper spinal cord injury.

The cervical tongs can loosen or slip out of place. Notify the physician immediately should the patient complain that the tongs feel loose. Caution the patient to remain quiet. Place a small sandbag on either side of his head until the physician replaces the tongs and traction can be resumed.

Check with the physician before you move a patient in cervical tong traction. If repositioning is permitted, never try to turn the patient alone. Logroll or turn the body as a unit. One person should keep the head in a neutral position, while two others move the body. The doctor may order a special bed that allows you to turn a patient while also keeping his body immobilized.

Halo traction can also immobilize a fractured or dislocated cervical vertebrae. With this form of skeletal traction, two anterior and two posterior pins secure a metal ring or halo around the patient's head.

The sterile ends of diagonally opposed pins are first inserted with finger pressure. The physician then tightens the pins simultaneously with a special screwdriver that creates 5 to 6 inch-pounds of pressure. The pins penetrate the skull about one-eighth of an inch. No skin incisions or drill holes are needed, but pin site care is still required.

Halo traction affords more mobility than tong traction. The metal headpiece can be attached to a plastic vest. With the vest secured, traction is maintained and the patient is able to ambulate.

The vest is lined with sheepskin to prevent skin irritation. This does not eliminate the need for good skin care and frequent inspection for signs of breakdown.

The halo apparatus may create a sensation of pressure on the patient's head, but not pain. If he complains of a severe headache, notify the physician. The traction may need to be adjusted.

A form of traction that permits motion

Balanced suspension traction provides a patient with some degree of movement when skeletal traction is applied to the leg. This type of traction may be used in conjunction with skeletal traction for fractures of the hip, femur, tibia, and fibula.

Two pieces of equipment—the Pearson attachment and the Thomas splint—support the leg as shown on page 29. The proximal end of the Thomas splint is a padded ring or half-ring that fits around the upper leg. The distal end is attached to a

Skeletal traction for injured vertebrae

Tongs or a halo ring immobilize fractures of the cervical and upper thoracic vertebrae. When tongs are employed, the center of the curved metal bar is aligned with the spinal column. The tongs are then secured on either side of the skull. The tips are inserted into the bone but do not pierce through to the brain. A weighted rope is then attached to the center of the metal bar, which creates a pull along the long axis of the spine.

For halo ring traction, a metal ring secured by four pins—two anterior and two posterior—encircles the skull. The ring can be attached to a weighted rope or a molded plastic vest. With the vest secured, traction is maintained and the patient may ambulate.

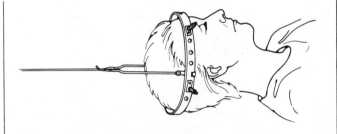

Halo ring traction attached to a weighted rope and pulley system

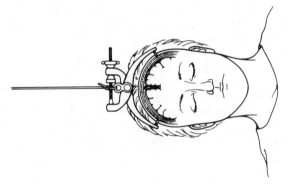

Crutchfield tongs positioned for cervical skeletal traction

KATHY GREY

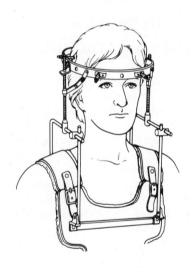

A plastic vest maintains halo ring traction and allows more mobility.

weighted rope for suspension.

The Pearson attachment joins the Thomas splint at knee level and supports the lower leg. The entire setup allows a patient to move his leg within the limits of healing—without altering the position of the broken bones.

Attach a footplate to the apparatus. Show the patient how to flex his foot against the plate to prevent foot drop. Position sheepskin slings on the Pearson attachment so the heel and Achilles tendon do not carry the weight of the lower leg. To prevent skin breakdown, pad the ischial ring of the Thomas splint.

Place the bed in a flat position for 20 minutes once a shift. This extends the hip, reducing the patient's risk for flexion contractures caused by remaining in a semi-Fowler's position for long periods.

When a patient is in balanced suspension traction, make sure the affected leg does not turn outward.

External rotation puts pressure on the head of the fibula, compressing the peroneal nerve. Increased pain, numbness and tingling, or the inability to flex and extend the toes could signal nerve compression.

Too much traction can hurt rather than heal

The same symptoms that signal peroneal nerve compression can also herald the onset of compartment syndrome. This is a serious neurovascular complication that can occur after trauma or fractures of the forearm and the lower leg. It can also result from excessive traction, a constrictive bandage, or a too-tight cast.

Edema in the affected limb increases the pressure in tissue compartments—muscle groups that are surrounded by inelastic connective tissue or fascia. Since the compartment cannot expand to accommodate the swollen tissues, the nerves and blood vessels are compressed and the muscle cells die. The end result is a binding down of tendons and nerve tissues with a permanent paralysis and loss of sensation.

The earliest symptom of compartment syndrome is increasingly severe pain that cannot be relieved by analgesics. As the condition progresses, you may also notice signs that circulation is impaired. The loss of peripheral pulses in the patient's extremity is a late and ominous signal.

Treatment includes measures to decrease edema—elevating the ex-

Balanced suspension and skeletal leg traction

To apply skeletal traction to an extremity, the orthopedist inserts a wire or pin through the bone. The Steinmann pin and the Kirschner or K wire shown below are two examples. This hardware connects to a U-shaped metal traction bow which, in turn, attaches to the weighted rope and pulley system. Both the pin and the wire are available with a threaded surface that prevents slipping.

Because it has a small diameter, the Kirschner wire can cut through the bone when very heavy traction is being appplied. The traction bow that's used with the Kirschner wire exerts a pull on both sides, which keeps the wire from bending.

The Steinmann pin is larger in diameter than the K wire and can withstand greater amounts of traction. It is often used for skeletal leg traction.

When used in conjunction with skeletal leg traction, a balanced suspension system affords the patient greater mobility without the risk of disrupting the traction.

The system includes two large U-shaped metal bars, much like those shown in the third drawing below. The upper bar or Thomas splint has a padded ring or half-ring opening at the

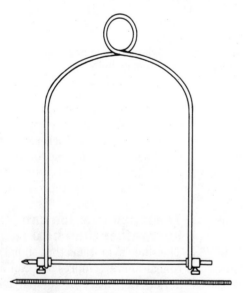

Steinmann pin and traction bow

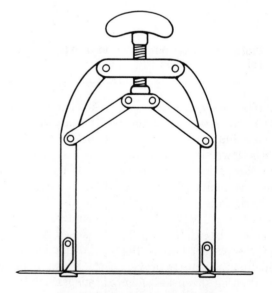

Kirschner wire and traction bow

tremity, decreasing the weight of traction, loosening bandages, or splitting the cast. A fasciotomy is sometimes needed to relieve the compression.

Early detection of compartment syndrome is the key to preventing permanent disability. Do a neurovascular assessment of the affected limb at least once a shift. Most im-portant, never ignore a patient who complains of pain.

When anxiety signals a physical problem

A patient in traction may be quite apprehensive, especially at the beginning of therapy. Give him assurance and emotional support. Keep in mind, though, that there may be a physiological reason for his anxiety—especially if he requires traction for a fractured long bone. His emotional state could stem from hypoxia caused by a fat embolism.

The exact mechanism responsible for the formation of fat emboli remains unclear. In the case of long bone fractures, the source may be fat released from the bone marrow

proximal end. A sling at the top of the splint helps support the thigh. The horizontal bar or Pearson attachment attaches to the Thomas splint at the level of the knee. Sheepskin slings support the lower leg.

To create the balanced suspension, the distal end of the Thomas splint is attached to a weighted rope. That maintains an upward pull, as is shown in the drawing at the far right. The proximal end of the Thomas splint is suspended by ropes that are attached to a spreader bar. The spreader bar, in turn, is attached to a weighted rope that's threaded through the pulleys on the overhead bar of the traction frame.

The angle where the splint and the Pearson attachment join can be adjusted to flex the knee to maintain proper alignment for traction. The Pearson attachment can be suspended by tying ropes to the Thomas splint as shown in the last drawing or by connecting a weighted rope to the distal end of the attachment.

The actual pull of skeletal traction is maintained by a separate weighted rope and pulley system that's connected to the pin in the extremity.

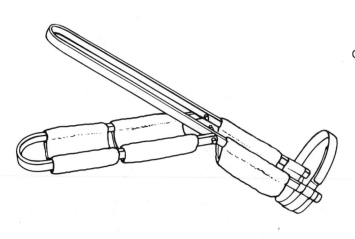

Thomas splint with padded ring and Pearson attachment

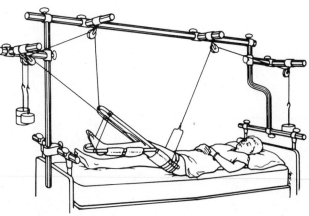

Skeletal leg traction with balanced suspension

at the fracture site. An alteration in fat metabolism in response to trauma may also play a role in emboli formation. In any case, the emboli disrupt normal circulation.

A patient is most likely to develop this complication 12 to 72 hours after his injury but cases have been reported as late as two weeks post injury. The symptoms are similar to those of a pulmonary embolism. The patient becomes anxious, increasingly restless, and dyspneic. His respirations and pulse rate increase. He may complain of chest pain. Arterial blood gas results show a decreased PaO_2.

Emboli that travel to the brain can cause memory loss, confusion, headache, and an elevated temperature. The appearance of petechiae on the neck, axillae, and upper chest is a classic but late sign of fat embolism. Treatment includes oxygen therapy and supportive measures to relieve the symptoms.

Patients who are confined to bed for months in skeletal traction often feel frustrated and helpless. Encourage them to express their feelings and needs. Allow them as much control over their care and their environment as possible. Make brief "social" visits to help decrease isolation and loneliness.

Encourage the family to get involved. Teach both the patient and his family about traction. Explain what traction is, why it's used, and how the family can help. Your encouragement, teaching, and expert nursing care will help a patient get full benefit from skeletal traction. ∎

BIBLIOGRAPHY Brunner, L. and Suddarth, D. *Textbook of Medical-Surgical Nursing* (3rd ed.). Philadelphia: J.B. Lippincott Company, 1975. Brunner, L. and Suddarth, D. *The Lippincott Manual of Nursing Practice* (2nd ed.). Philadelphia: J.B. Lippincott Company, 1978. Carini, G. and Birmingham, J. *Traction Made Manageable: A Self-Learning Module.* New York: McGraw-Hill, Inc., 1980. Farrell, J. *Illustrated Guide to Orthopedic Nursing* (3rd ed.). Philadelphia: J.B. Lippincott Company, 1986. Hilt, N., and Cogburn, S. *Manual of Orthopedics*, St. Louis: The C.V. Mosby Company, 1980. *Working with Orthopedic Patients, Nurses Reference Library.* Springhouse, Pa.: Intermed Communications, Inc., 1983.

THE HIP:
When the joint must be replaced

You and your patient must function as a team. Both training and practice are essential to getting him back on his feet.

By Linda M. Dunajcik, RN,C, BSN

Most nurses enjoy patient education, and few procedures demand more teaching skill than hip replacement. In order to recover fully, patients need to understand and participate actively in their care—just as did Sharon, the patient in the preceding article on hip fractures.

Although total hip arthroplasty is done for some patients who've fractured the femoral neck, surgical advances and improved prosthetic devices are making the procedure an option for an increasing number of patients who have a wide range of complaints. In many cases, osteoarthritis has caused degeneration of the hip joint. In others, the joint has been damaged by rheumatoid or traumatic arthritis, chronic synovitis, congenital hip dysplasia, bone tumor, or aseptic necrosis of the hip. The immediate indication for surgery is usually severe joint degeneration with hip pain that doesn't respond to oral

THE AUTHOR, a former nurse educator for the orthopedic unit at the University of Missouri-Columbia Hospital & Clinics in Columbia, Mo., is now studying for her master's degree at the University of Washington.

Produced by Sigrid Nagle

analgesics, disturbs sleep, and limits the ability to walk or climb stairs.

Giving preop instructions

Show the patient before surgery how to limit movement afterwards. Explain that the femur must be positioned carefully to minimize the chances of dislocating the new hip. Placement differs for anterior and posterior incisions, so find out which approach the surgeon will employ.

After surgery involving an anterior incision, the patient's legs will be spread somewhat and the affected leg turned slightly inward. This minimizes the pressure of the head of the femur against the front of the joint capsule, which has been weakened by the incision. To help the patient maintain the correct position, place an abductor or bed pillow between his legs and a trochanter roll along the outside of the femur.

The legs are also spread when a posterior incision has been used, but the affected leg is turned slightly *outward*. Tell your patient

to be careful not to turn his leg in, cross his legs, or flex his hip more than 90°—or the prosthesis may press on the weakened posterior hip capsule and dislocate. Use pillows between the legs but not a trochanter roll, since you want the leg to turn out.

The patient will have to turn from back to side—supported with a body wedge or pillows—every two hours after surgery. Reassure him that you'll help him, and have him practice a few turns with the abductor pillow in place. Show him how to use the trapeze to pull himself up in bed and to lift himself onto a bedpan, in this case a small fracture pan.

To rehearse the latter, unfasten the abductor strap on the unaffected leg so that he can bend his knee. Have him plant his foot firmly on the bed, lift his upper body on the trapeze, and use his leg muscles to raise the hips high enough to clear the pan.

Demonstrate deep breathing exercises, and emphasize the importance of performing them every two hours. Teach the patient isometric, range-of-motion, and up-

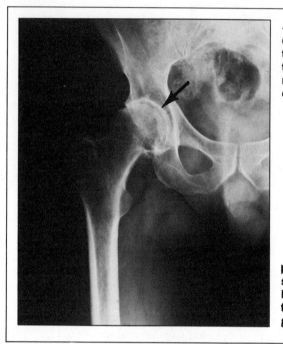

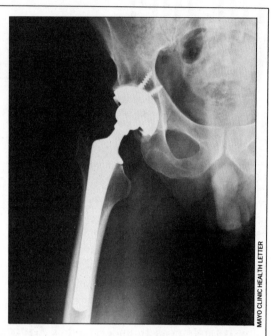

◄ This X-ray shows degeneration of the hip joint where the head of the femur fits into the acetabulum (arrow).

► An X-ray of the same area illustrating a hip prosthesis that has been surgically implanted.

MAYO CLINIC HEALTH LETTER

per-extremity exercises that will help prevent complications from bed rest.

It's best to talk about postop pain *before* the patient experiences it. Explain that you can offer medication to relieve different levels of discomfort; that way he'll know what type to ask for later. Practice with him other methods of pain control, for example, relaxation techniques, imagery, and distraction, and find out which of these he prefers.

Tell your patient that for approximately two days after surgery a suction drain will be in place to prevent pooling of blood, which can cause infection and abscess. There will also be a large pressure dressing over the hip; you'll be checking both drain and dressing every two hours during the first postop day. Let him know that you will be

available then and afterwards to answer his questions and discuss his concerns.

Managing postop complications

When the patient returns from surgery, your vigilance will help ensure a smooth recovery. Here are the main problems to watch for:

Shock. Hypovolemia sometimes occurs if IV or oral fluid replacement is not adequate or if blood loss lowers the hematocrit below 25. Use your patient's I&O records and the lab values from the OR and PAR as a baseline.

As soon as he's able, encourage him to drink plenty of fluids. Tell him to let you know if he has a damp dressing. Record the amount and appearance of the drainage, and, because dressings can absorb a significant amount of drainage,

keep track of the number you use.

Alert the physician that precautions may be in order if blood pressure falls below 90 systolic or 60 diastolic, if more than 200 ml of blood is lost in an eight-hour period, or if the hematocrit is below 30.

Also call if urine output is low—less than 30 ml per hour from an indwelling catheter or less than 240 ml in an eight-hour period from voiding.

Irritability and restlessness are early signs of hypovolemic shock, as are pallor, tachycardia, tachypnea, and decreased blood pressure and temperature. If you suspect this condition, place your patient flat on the bed with the legs elevated 20°. Notify the physician.

Start a large bore IV line if the patient doesn't already have one, and be prepared to administer IV fluids, blood, or blood products as

What happens in hip replacement surgery

The ball-and-socket joint of the hip is formed by the head of the femur and the acetabulum. A fibrous capsule supports this joint, as do ligaments and muscles. If the hip has degenerated, the surgeon is able to replace the head of the femur with a ball-and-stem prosthesis and the acetabulum with a cup prosthesis.

After the area has been prepped, the surgeon makes an anterior or posterior incision through skin, fat, fascia, muscle, and hip capsule. Next, he dislocates the joint by inserting a bone hook under the femoral neck while a surgical assistant applies manual traction and rotates the leg.

To remove the femoral head and expose the acetabulum, the surgeon saws through the neck of the femur. He prepares the acetabulum by reaming it. He then inserts the acetabular cup; when the position is acceptable he press-fits or cements it into place.

The surgeon prepares the femur to accommodate its prosthesis by reaming the spongy bone in the shaft. He inserts a trial ball-and-stem component into the shaft and reduces it into the new cup to determine the fit.

If the fit is good, he again dislocates the hip, removes the trial femoral component, and replaces it with the permanent prosthesis. This he cements or press-fits into place.

He irrigates the wound and, with the help of his assistant, reduces the hip joint. Finally, he inserts a suction drain and closes the wound with sutures and staples.

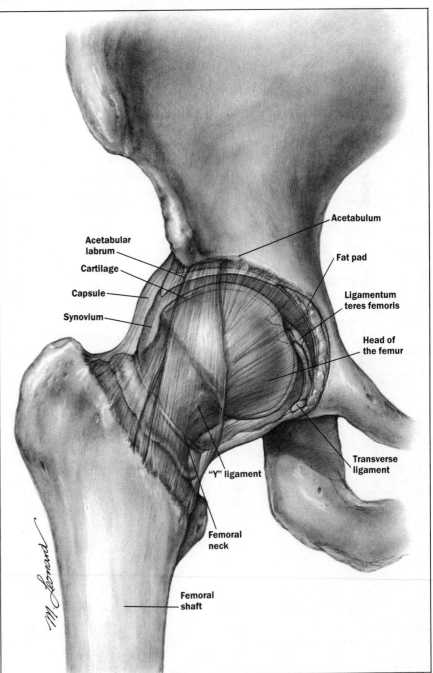

Acetabular labrum

Cartilage

Capsule

Synovium

Acetabulum

Fat pad

Ligamentum teres femoris

Head of the femur

Transverse ligament

"Y" ligament

Femoral neck

Femoral shaft

MICHAEL E. LEONARD

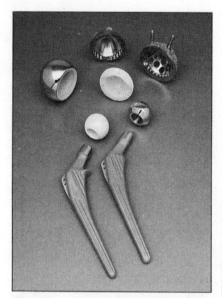

One type of prosthesis is press-fitted into place. Shown here is Richards Medical Co.'s Ti-Fit prosthesis.

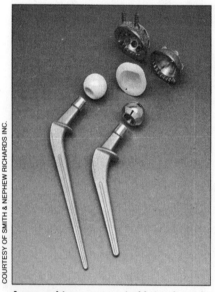

A second type, cemented into place, is exemplified by Richards Spectron EF prosthesis.

instructed. Additionally, oxygen may be ordered via nasal cannula or face mask.

Pain. Some people report pain matter-of-factly; others cry and moan; still others withdraw from their surroundings and hold their bodies stiff. Blood pressure may be elevated and respiration rapid. A simple way to assess the intensity of pain is to have the patient rate it on a scale from 0 to 10.

Give meds as ordered and 30 to 60 minutes before a scheduled therapy session. Help your patient use the relaxation techniques practiced before surgery, and tell him to let you know *before* pain becomes intolerable, so that you can stay on top of it.

If he asks for pain medication at night but goes to sleep before you can administer it, wake him up and give it to him anyway (unless his breathing seems depressed). Even a patient in severe pain can become so fatigued he falls asleep. The sleep will be fitful, however, and the pain may get out of control.

Keep in mind that proper body alignment is essential to comfort.

Dislocation. Have your patient notify you if the new hip hurts despite medication, if he can't straighten his leg, or if his legs don't seem to be the same length. When the head of the femur dislocates anteriorly, the knee flexes and the leg turns outward. It may look longer than the other, and you may be able to feel the head of the femur in the groin area.

When the hip dislocates posteriorly, the leg will turn inward and appear to be shorter than the other. The femoral head will be promi-

nent and the greater trochanter elevated.

Report any signs of dislocation to the physician.

Circulatory problems. To detect vascular complications, assess the affected leg for color, motion, sensation, temperature, pulses, and capillary refill time.

While you're checking, tell the patient what symptoms to report: pale, blue, or cold skin; edema or numbness; or pain or tingling in the groin or calf. Some swelling in the hip region is normal postop, but not in the calf.

To discover thrombophlebitis, check for redness, swelling, and warmth. Caution the patient not to massage or exercise a painful calf muscle, as that might cause the thrombus to break loose. Check the unaffected leg also.

To promote good circulation, keep pressure off the back of the knees. Don't put pillows or blankets under them, and be sure the lower part of the bed remains flat.

Also, be careful that the straps of the abductor pillow are not around the patient's knees, and that they are loose enough so that he can do calf-pumping and ankle rotation exercises. Encourage him to do these exercises every hour while awake.

Apply elastic stockings, ace wraps, or pneumatic compression hose, and explain that these and foot exercises aid venous flow to the heart. Remove these stockings once each shift to check compression points and skin integrity.

Monitor lab work for an elevated hematocrit, an indication that a clot may form. Discourage smoking, which can impede circulation by constricting the blood vessels.

Without alarming him, instruct your patient about the symptoms of pulmonary embolism—chest pain, shortness of breath, and coughing up blood. Other signs the nurse should watch for are pale, cool skin, increased pulse rate, decreased breath sounds, and decreased blood pressure.

To reduce chances of a clot, your patient will probably be on anticoagulant therapy: heparin, aspirin, warfarin, dextran, or a combination of these. Watch his prothrombin·and PTT values, which should be one and a half to two times the control level for effective anticoagulation. Ask him to tell you if he sees bleeding or unusual bruising.

Infection. This is a major concern, since joint infection can lead to systemic infection and even necessitate removal of the new hip.

Your patient may be on IV or oral antibiotics for a few days postop. Watch for and teach him about signs of infection at the incision site—redness, hardness, swelling, increased pain, and excessive or foul-smelling drainage. When you change dressings, use sterile technique and inspect the incision line and surrounding skin. Document your observations.

If you suspect infection, withhold any antipyretic that might mask it by reducing fever, and call the physician. Be prepared to stop the antibiotic and obtain samples for blood and wound cultures and a specimen for urine culture and sensitivity tests; these tests could pick up signs of systemic infection.

Teach your patient that cleanliness, a well-balanced diet high in protein, and adequate rest will prevent infection and promote healing. Tell him not to scratch the incision line, which might introduce bacteria, and not to put lotion or powder on it until it's healed. He shouldn't get the incision line wet until after the sutures are removed.

Skin breakdown. If your patient is allergic to tape, note that on the chart and use paper tape. Elderly, diabetic, thin, or obese patients are at particular risk of pressure sores, therefore you may want to use an eggcrate mattress. Massage bony prominences each time you reposition the patient.

Constipation. Elimination is a problem for many orthopedic patients because of inactivity, drugs, and changes in diet and daily routine. Stress and lack of privacy can also disrupt bowel habits.

Ask the patient if he is constipated, and look for such signs as malaise, dizziness, headache, loss of appetite, indigestion, and abdominal fullness. Stool softeners and prn laxatives will help re-establish a normal daily routine. Explain their use to the patient.

Advise plenty of raw vegetables, fruits, cereals, and fluids. Increased activity will also help solve the problem. If the patient has a posterior incision, be sure the bathroom he will use is equipped with a raised toilet seat.

Small amounts of diarrhea or hard stool may be a sign of fecal impaction. A digital examination is the next step. If you locate hard or firm stool in the lower colon, you can administer an oil-retention or phosphate (Fleet) enema.

Getting the patient back on his feet

Since prolonged bed rest can cause joint contractures, muscle weakness, and bone demineralization, exercise is an important part of the postop routine. Range-of-motion exercises should involve all joints except the new hip. Doing them three times a day will maintain flexibility and muscle tone.

Isometric exercises are also done three times daily. Quadriceps and gluteal sets will strengthen the muscles used for walking. To do the former, the patient tenses the muscles around the knees for five seconds, releases for five seconds, and repeats the exercise nine times. For gluteal sets, he should tighten and release the muscles in the buttocks ten times.

A third exercise is done with the unaffected leg. Have the patient push his foot against the footboard, hold for a count of five, release for a count of five, and repeat. This applies stress to the long bones and helps prevent demineralization.

Your patient may also need to strengthen arms and shoulders to use crutches or a walker. Teach him to push his body up with his arms from a sitting position, leaning back and straightening elbows.

If he needs more help, ask your physical therapist to design exercises he can do with handweights.

When the patient first gets out of bed, teach him how to pivot to a chair on the unaffected leg. To sit, a patient with an anterior incision can flex his hip, but someone with a posterior incision should slowly extend the affected leg and lower himself into the chair without flexing the hip more than 90°.

Explain that this limitation will apply for two months postop. At home, the patient will need a raised toilet seat, an extender arm to retrieve objects out of reach, and assistance bathing the lower body and putting on shoes and socks.

What you tell the patient about weight bearing depends on if the prosthesis has been press-fitted or cemented into place. A press-fitted prosthesis has a porous surface into which new bone grows. Until it solidifies, the patient can touch only the toe of the affected leg to the floor for balance. He'll use crutches for about three months. He can put weight on a cemented prosthesis—usually used for patients over 60—in 24 hours. Crutches, a walker, or cane are utilized for extra support.

Preparing for discharge

Make certain your patient knows how to position his leg as he stands, sits, and lies down and how to use the adaptive equipment he'll be taking home. He must understand the purpose of the prescribed medications, their side effects, and when to take them. He should know how to control pain and prevent constipation.

Review the symptoms of dislocation, circulatory impairment, and infection with him. Tell him to call the physician if he runs a fever over 101.3° F (38.5° C) or gets any kind of infection, even a cold. Before having dental work done, he should ask for prophylactic antibiotics.

With the assistance and instruction you've provided, your patient will soon be back to normal. You can take pride in the contribution your nursing care has made to his recovery. You have made it possible for him to put his "best foot forward." ■

BIBLIOGRAPHY Campbell, C. *Nursing Diagnosis and Intervention in Nursing Practice* (2nd ed.). New York: Wiley Medical Publication, 1984. Carlson, D.C. and Robinson, H.J. Surgical approaches for primary total hip arthroplasty. *Clinical Orthopaedics and Related Research* 222:161, Sept. 1987. Crownshield, R. An overview of prosthetic materials for fixation. *Clinical Orthopaedics and Related Research* 235: 166, Oct. 1988. Doheny, M.O. Porous coated femoral prosthesis: Concepts and care considerations. *Orthopedic Nursing* 1:43, Jan./Feb. 1985. Farrell, J. *Illustrated Guide to Orthopedic Nursing* (3rd ed.). Philadelphia: J.B. Lippincott Co., 1986. Farrell, J. Orthopedic pain: What does it mean? *Am. J. Nurs.* 4:466, April 1984. Lentz, M. Selected aspects of deconditioning secondary to immobilization. *Nurs. Clin. North Am.* 16:729, Dec. 1981. Luckmann, J. and Sorensen, K.C. *Medical-Surgical Nursing: A Pychophysiologic Approach* (3rd ed.). Philadelphia: W.B. Saunders Co., 1987. Meinhart, N.T. and McCaffery, M. *Pain: A Nursing Approach to Assessment and Analysis.* Norwalk, Conn.: Appleton-Century-Crofts, 1983. Morscher, E.W. Cementless total hip arthroplasty. *Clin. Orthop.* 181:76, Dec. 1983. Olson, E.V. The hazards of immobility. *Am. J. Nurs.* 67:780, April 1967. Pellino, T.A., Mooney, N.E., et al., eds. *National Association for Orthopedic Nurses Core Curriculum for Orthopedic Nursing.* Pitman, N.J.: Anthony Jannetti, Inc., 1986. Spotting a dislocated hip. *Emergency Medicine* 16:53, Sept. 30, 1984.

The new challenges of insulin therapy

Although insulin therapy can't perfectly imitate a healthy pancreas,
when properly administered, the hormone can save life and limb.
By Carolyn Robertson, RN, MSN, CDE

Some 20 million people around the world owe a debt of gratitude to Frederick Banting and Charles Best, the scientists who first isolated insulin. While insulin regimens can control diabetes, however, not even the most sophisticated can precisely duplicate the body's ability to secrete the proper amount of hormone at just the right time.

A normal pancreas continuously produces small amounts of insulin to control excess glucose output by the liver. Larger amounts, given off in response to a meal, pull glucose out of the bloodstream, preventing hyperglycemia.

Within five to 15 minutes after a person starts a meal, insulin production increases fortyfold. First-phase insulin secretion moves glucose into the cells, where it's used as fuel or converted to fat tissue. Within 30 minutes, the pancreas enters phase two, releasing a uniform stream of hormone for two hours—about as long as it takes to

digest the average meal. Together, these two "doses" of insulin prevent postprandial blood sugar from varying more than 20 to 40 mg/dl from normal between-meal values.

Injected insulin acts more slowly and reaches the bloodstream in one dose instead of two. For instance, fast-acting, regular insulin, administered subcutaneously, reaches peak blood concentration 20 times more slowly than the natural hormone, and its effects last two to three times as long. Intermediate- and long-acting insulins, because they contain retarding agents that delay absorption, peak even later.

Insulin therapy has come a long way since the crude hormone extracts used decades ago. To help your patient take advantage of recent advances, you'll need to go beyond preparing and injecting the drug and explain the more subtle aspects of insulin therapy.

Know your insulin preparations
The three types of product used in insulin therapy—fast, intermediate, and long-acting—are outlined

in this article. A physician's choice of product, as well as the dose and the timing of injections, depends in part on the patient's ability to manufacture the hormone. A Type I patient makes virtually none, while someone with Type II makes insufficient or nonfunctioning insulin. A patient's age, weight, ability to follow diet and exercise guidelines, and other illnesses help set the regimen.

Insulin preparations are derived from human, pork, or beef sources. Beef and pork insulins, which were developed first, have the same number of amino acids as human insulin but individual acids vary slightly. The more deviation, the more likely the body will create insulin antibodies.

Proinsulin, the hormone's precursor, is a marker for more dangerous impurities. The greater the amount of proinsulin, the greater the risk of an immune reaction. Highly purified insulin has less than 10 parts per million of proinsulin. Some older, conventional insulins containing 50 or more ppm still remain on the market, but those with over 50,000 ppm of proinsulin

THE AUTHOR: Ms. Robertson, a clinical diabetes specialist at New York University Medical Center, is a member of RN's editorial board. She's serving as co-editor of this diabetes series, along with Paul L. Cerrato, BS, MA, director of clinical nutrition and an associate editor of RN.

Types of insulins

Subcutaneous insulin is available in fast-, medium-, and long-acting forms. Examples of the beef and pork versions of all three types are listed below, along with their effects on blood glucose levels. Human insulins are also available in the same three forms but their effects begin, peak, and end sooner than animal products.

A fast-acting IV insulin that begins to work within five minutes is also available for emergencies; it peaks after 15 to 30 minutes and continues to lower bG levels for an hour.

Type	Blood-glucose lowering action		
	Onset	**Peak**	**Duration**
Fast-acting (regular, Semilente) Iletin II Regular (beef) Semilente purified pork	30-60 min.	2-3 hrs.	4-6 hrs.
Intermediate-acting (NPH, Lente) Iletin I Lente (beef/pork) Insulatard NPH (pork)	2-3 hrs.	6-10 hrs.	More than 18 hrs.
Long-acting (Ultralente) Ultralente (beef) Protamine, zinc & Iletin I (beef/pork)	4-6 hrs.	22-26 hrs.	More than 36 hrs.

were discontinued many years ago.

When a patient comes on your unit without specific insulin orders, ask him what type he's been taking and get a doctor's order to continue it during his stay. Changing from animal to human or from conventional to highly purified can disrupt blood sugar levels and require as much as a 20% change in dosage to regain control. If a patient's never been on insulin, ask the attending physician if you can give the least immunogenic product—human or highly purified pork insulin.

When giving the hormone, keep in mind that many factors will influence its effectiveness:

Injection site. Peak insulin concentration is reached most rapidly when the drug is injected in the abdomen, followed by the deltoids, thighs, and buttocks. Choosing a site where subcutaneous fatty tissue has atrophied or thickened from overuse—lipodystrophy—will produce erratic absorption.

Body temperature. Fever or a sauna can increase blood flow, which speeds insulin absorption. Conversely, a hypothermia blanket may impede hormone action by slowing absorption.

Depth of injection. The deeper the shot, the faster the absorption. An injection reaches progressively greater numbers of blood vessels as it moves from intradermal to subcutaneous to intramuscular.

Concentration. A very concentrated solution—500 units/ml, for example—reaches peak blood levels more slowly than a standard 100 units/ml preparation.

Species. Because human insulin is more biologically active than its animal counterparts, its effects begin, peak, and end sooner.

Antibodies. Insulin antibodies blunt the hormone's effect but prolong its duration.

Glucose level. The higher the glucose level at the time of injection, the less potent the hormone.

Be familiar with basic insulin regimens

There are three primary treatment regimens. The first uses a single intermediate insulin such as NPH or Lente. (NPH stands for neutral protamine Hagedorn insulin. It contains protamine, a fish protein that slows down the hormone's absorption, and was developed by a Danish doctor. Lente derives from the Latin word for slow.) When given before breakfast, it provides enough hormone to balance the rise in blood glucose after lunch and meet the patient's basal insulin needs through early evening.

Because this approach doesn't offer round-the-clock coverage or mimic endogenous insulin secretion, it's contraindicated for Type I patients. Most endocrinologists think it's also inappropriate for

Type II patients who require insulin but it's still commonly prescribed in general practice. Patients who take more than 40 units of intermediate insulin in a single dose also risk hypoglycemia before lunch. Many sidestep this danger by eating more at their most vulnerable times, but that encourages weight gain. Reducing or splitting the dose is a better solution.

The second regimen uses a combination of intermediate- and short-acting regular products. It frequently calls for two injections: NPH or Lente plus regular at breakfast and supper. Sometimes, the routine is three injections: intermediate and regular at breakfast, regular at supper, and intermediate at bedtime.

Both protocols more closely mimic normal insulin secretion than a single shot does. The two-shot regimen, however, can cause overnight hypoglycemia because the intermediate-acting insulin given at supper peaks six to 10 hours later. A bedtime snack reduces this risk. Also tell the patient to report morning "hangovers"—headaches and malaise, for instance—or any changes in sleep patterns or dreams; all suggest hypoglycemia. Some experts suggest self-testing of blood glucose between 2:00 a.m. and 3:00 a.m. at least once a week as well.

The third regimen requires intermediate or long-acting insulin one to three times a day to meet the basal needs, plus regular insulin before meals. The subcutaneous insulin infusion pump serves a similar function, delivering a basal dose of regular insulin throughout the day and supplying a bolus on demand

before meals. Both protocols permit the patient to schedule meals whenever he wants.

Don't overlook patient education

All patients using insulin must be taught to use the hormone *safely*. That means knowing how to recognize and correct hypoglycemia. For example, diabetic patients should carry a sugar source at all times— even if they're only leaving the unit to go for an X-ray. Five or six Life Savers or two glucose tablets will usually suffice.

To treat severe hypoglycemia, which can cause loss of consciousness and seizures, the patient's family should be trained to inject glucagon, a hormone that raises blood sugar by stimulating the liver's release of glycogen. The hormone is also sometimes used to maintain normal blood glucose levels when the patient cannot eat.

For insulin to work, it must be synchronized with food intake. With that in mind, tell your patient to eat a full meal within half an hour of taking a short-acting preparation; a snack should follow in two to three hours. Intermediate-acting insulin demands a meal within four to five and a half hours and a snack some two to three hours after that. Long-acting products such as PZI or Ultralente and low doses of intermediate insulin needn't be followed by food as they don't actively lower blood glucose. They only prevent its elevation by inhibiting hepatic glucose output between meals and overnight. For an example of how meals and insulin can be synchronized, see the above box.

Physical activity can lower blood sugar levels by using up calories. Explain to patients that exercise requires adjustments in diet or insulin to prevent hypoglycemia— drink a glass of milk 15 minutes before a vigorous 30-minute walk, for instance. Urge self-monitoring of blood glucose to keep track of exercise-induced fluctuations.

Once patients have learned these safety rules, teach them how to administer the hormone. Do this *before* discussing how to prepare injections or mix products, as detailed instructions will probably fall on deaf ears until the patient gets past the anxiety of giving that first shot.

Instruct lean patients to inject at a 45° angle to prevent the needle from extending below subcutaneous fatty tissue—the proper insulin absorption site. A 90° angle may be all right for obese patients. Teach patients to rotate sites within a specific body area such as the buttocks, thigh, or upper abdomen. Changing from area to area, however, should be done only about once a month because differences in absorption rates among the areas can cause fluctuations in blood glucose.

Explain proper hormone preparation

Once these tasks are mastered, show your patient how to prepare the shot. Insulins can be mixed in the syringe just before injection or mixed in a syringe or vial and stored for future use. When combining products, the patient should draw the short-acting, regular insulin into the syringe first. If an intermediate or long-acting insulin is drawn up first, traces of retarding agent on the needle may contaminate the bottle of regular insulin that's drawn second, converting it into a longer-acting insulin.

Mixing a slow-acting Lente with a regular insulin allows the Lente's excess zinc—its retarding agent—to bind gradually to the regular, decreasing its potency and increasing the potency of the Lente insulin. Such mixtures should either be used immediately or given 24 hours to stabilize.

On the other hand, insulins that contain a phosphate buffer, including NPH, PZI, and all insulins made by Nordisk, Inc., should not be mixed with the Ultralente or Lente. The phosphate would bind to the retarding agent in the Lente products, converting the entire dose into fast-acting insulin. (Even Semilente, although classified as short-acting, may become altered.) However, NPH and regular preparations can be mixed and allowed to stand for an indeterminate period of time without any problems.

Teach patients to store syringes horizontally. Storing with the needle down can clog the tip when the insulin crystals settle out of suspension; storing tip up may cause crystals to adhere to the plunger, lowering the potency upon resuspension. To resuspend a properly stored solution, gently roll or invert the syringe several times.

Stored syringes needn't be refrigerated; a vial of insulin can be kept at room temperature for up to a month without losing potency. When temperatures exceed 86° F (30° C), however, potency declines rapidly. Because this breakdown won't change the appearance of the solution, tell patients to store extra vials in the refrigerator.

Provide extra help for special patients

Visually impaired diabetics and those with sensory or motor neuropathy may need extra assistance to prepare and administer insulin. Several companies make magnifiers for syringe calibrations. Palco Labs and Becton Dickinson also make magnifiers that help the patient guide the syringe into the insulin bottle.

Dos-Aid, the top photo on page 35, lets a visually impaired patient draw up a predetermined volume of insulin. The device is adjustable, so a sighted assistant can reset the volume when a dosage change is needed. It's available through the American Foundation for the Blind, 15 West 16th St., New York, N.Y. 10011, (212) 620-2000.

Squibb-Novo, Inc. markets an insulin delivery device that holds a vial of the hormone and looks like a pen. NovolinPen lets the patient dial his dose and then inject by push button. The device helps ensure accurate dosing for patients who lack the fine motor coordination to measure precise amounts.

If someone finds injections extremely painful, a spring-loaded device (third photo) quickly propels the needle through the skin. Others may prefer a jet injector (bottom photo), which delivers a high-pressure pulse of insulin through a fine nozzle.

The insulin of the future will most likely be administered by newer and more innovative methods. In fact, researchers are already experimenting with nasal sprays, transdermal patches, suppositories, implantable insulin pumps, even transplantation of the pancreas' insulin-secreting beta cells. But until these techniques are perfected, we must teach patients how to use the available insulin to achieve blood sugar levels as close to normal as possible. ∎

BIBLIOGRAPHY Bergman, M., ed. *Principles of Diabetes Management*. New York: Elsevier Science, 1987. Borders, L., Binghamm, P., and Riddle, M. Traditional Insulin-Use Practices and the Incidence of Contamination and Infection. *Diabetes Care* 7:121, March/April 1984. Davidson, J. *Clinical Diabetes Mellitus: A Problem Oriented Approach*. New York: Theime Inc., 1986. Davidson M. *Diabetes Mellitus: Diagnosis and Treatment*. New York: John Wiley and Sons, 1981. Galloway, J., Potvin, J., and Shuman, C., eds. *Diabetes Mellitus*, (9th ed.), Indianapolis: Eli Lilly and Company, 1988. Hare-Joshu D., Flavin, K., and Clutter, W. Controlling the Insulin Balance. *Am. J. Nurs.* 86:1240, Nov. 1986. Oldham, J. and Campbell, R. Treatment of the Hospitalized Hypoglycemic Patient. *Diabetes Educator* 13:310, 1987. Olson, Charles. *Diagnosis and Management of Diabetes Mellitus* (2nd ed.). New York: Raven Press, 1988. Peterson, C. and Jovanovic, L. *The Diabetes Self-Care Method*. New York: Simon & Schuster, 1984. Shade, D., Santiago, J., et al., eds. *Intensive Insulin Therapy*. Amsterdam: Excerpta Medica, 1983.

Nursing implications of today's burn care techniques

Advances in resuscitation techniques have improved survival rates for burn victims. Attention now focuses on early excision and grafting to close the burn wound.
By Lisa Morra Martin, RN, BSN, CCRN

Burn trauma. A devastating event that can happen to anyone at any time. The house fire in the middle of the night, the rush-hour auto accident, the industrial mishap, or the family barbecue that ends in tragedy. All disastrous events producing emotional and physical scars that may last a lifetime.

More than two million people in the United States suffer thermal injuries each year. Approximately 100,000 of them must be admitted to the hospital. If their clinical course remains uncomplicated, victims with major burns can expect to be hospitalized about one day for each percent of body surface injured. Hospital and medical costs are estimated at more than $1 billion a year.

Immediate efforts focus on lifesaving measures and prompt stabilization, followed by a continuous struggle toward progressive rehabilitation and prevention of compli-

THE AUTHOR is an instructor in the critical care and trauma nurse internship program at Parkland Memorial Hospital in Dallas.

Produced by Mary-Beth Moriarty, RN, CCRN

cations. We'll begin with an overview of this complex care, then concentrate on current concepts—and new horizons—in burn wound excision, biologic dressings, and skin substitutes.

Burn injury pathophysiology

During the 48 hours immediately following the injury the patient must be monitored closely for signs of burn shock. Every victim of major burns is at risk for this profound hypovolemia leading to circulatory failure.

The insult begins with destruction of the epidermis, the outermost layer of the skin, eliminating the body's barrier to water evaporation and allowing fluid loss.

The greatest loss of fluid, electrolytes, and protein, however, is caused by volume shifts from the intravascular to the extravascular compartment secondary to an increase in capillary permeability. Heat effects and the release of vasoactive substances from the injured area add to this increase in

permeability also known as capillary leaking. The resulting fluid shifts are directly proportional to the depth and extent of the burn.

The level of tissue involvement determines the burn's depth or degree. First degree burns end at the epidermis. Second degree burns reach into the dermis. Third degree burns destroy the epidermis, dermis, and subcutaneous tissue.

The rule of nines gives a quick, rough estimate of burn size. The Lund and Browder chart permits a more accurate assessment. You'll find details about both methods on the chart titled "Estimating burn size." To double-check your estimate, calculate both the burned and the unburned areas. The sum of the two should equal 100%.

Calculating volume replacement

IV fluids are critical in preventing burn shock. The choice will depend on the physician's preference, but all require that you watch the patient carefully and modify the regimen if his requirements change.

To give you a clearer picture of how this works, we'll apply the Parkland formula to calculate fluid replacement for Mr. Hayes, who weighs 75 kg and has a total body surface area (TBSA) burn of 40%. The accident happened at 9:00 p.m. and Mr. Hayes arrived in the emergency department a half hour later:

According to the formula, Mr. Hayes will receive 12 liters (4 ml × 75 kg × 40% TBSA burn = 12,000 ml) of Lactated Ringer's solution in the first 24 hours after the burn. (The TBSA percentage is used as a whole number rather than a decimal in these calculations.)

Half of the fluid (6,000 ml) will be infused during the first eight hours at 750 ml/hr. One quarter (3,000 ml) will be given over the next eight hours at 375 ml/hr. The remaining quarter (3,000 ml) will be infused at the same rate during the third eight hours. Keep in mind that the periods are calculated from the time of the injury, in this case 9:00 p.m., rather than the time resuscitation began.

After 24 hours the capillary leak begins to seal and fluid requirements decrease. For the next eight hours (24 to 32 hours after the injury) Mr. Hayes will receive 1500 ml of fresh frozen plasma (0.5 ml × 75 kg × 40% TBSA burn = 1500 ml) at 187 ml/hr. That will be followed by D_5W titrated to maintain a urine output of at least 30 ml/hr.

Mr. Hayes needs assessment often during resuscitation. Check vital signs, urine output, and level of consciousness at least every hour. If a patient has deep second or third degree circumferential burns of the extremities, do a neurovascular assessment of these areas every hour to ensure adequate peripheral perfusion. Give morphine intravenously as ordered for pain control.

Look for signs of hypovolemia and inadequate tissue perfusion that signal the need for even greater fluid volume—a heart rate of more than 110 beats a minute, a decrease in urine output below 30 ml/hr, and mental status changes.

Treating the burn wound

Fluid resuscitation techniques have greatly reduced the number of deaths from burn shock. As a result, specialists are focusing on better ways to care for the burn wound.

In the past, topical antimicrobial agents such as silver sulfadiazine (Silvadene) and mafenide acetate (Sulfamylon) have been the mainstays of therapy. Deep second degree burns were treated with these creams and periodic debridement and allowed to heal without grafting, but this technique produced excessive scarring. Research also showed that using antimicrobial agents to treat very large burns did not improve survival rates significantly. These findings stimulated a search for new therapies.

The increased availability of biologic dressings and the development of synthetic skin substitutes have improved our ability to close the burn wound. In addition, the evolution of expansion grafting techniques and the capacity to freeze and bank skin helped pave the way for early excisional therapy—the removal of dead burned tissue by sharp dissection into viable tissue within 72 hours after the injury.

The following findings—some of them proven and others derived from suggestive data and clinical impressions—have led burn specialists to support early excision and grafting as the therapy of choice for deep partial thickness and full thickness burns:

Patients with TBSA of less than 20% heal faster when treated in this manner, shortening their hospital stay. Early excision and grafting reduces the need for painful wound debridements. Covering the wound helps slow the increase in metabolic rate that occurs with burn trauma and decreases pain. Patients who undergo early excision have fewer problems with infection. Early wound closure results in less severe scarring, so that less reconstructive surgery is needed.

Choosing candidates for early excision

Any patient with burns that will take longer than three weeks to heal is considered for early excision. Individual factors such as age, other injuries, and pre-existing medical problems that could complicate surgery or anesthesia are weighed carefully.

The type, extent, and location of the burn are also important. Excision of flat surfaces of the trunk, the arms and legs and, in the case of a thin patient, the abdomen yields the best results. Conservative excision of the face and the

Estimating burn size

To estimate the total area of a burn injury, use either the rule of nines or the Lund and Browder chart. For both methods, you color areas of third degree burns red, areas of second degree burns blue. With the rule of nines you add the percentages listed below for each area of the body burned. Thus, burns on the arm and leg would total 27%. The Lund and Browder chart permits a more accurate assessment of burn size because it divides the body into more sections and takes age-related changes in body proportions into consideration. To use it, mark the appropriate percentages for your patient from the figures listed for each area of the body. Thus an infant who has burns of the head and thigh would be burned on 24½% of its body, an adult with burns in the same areas would have injuries on 16½%.

The Rule of Nines

Head and neck	**9%**
Right arm	**9**
Left arm	**9**
Posterior trunk	**18**
Anterior trunk	**18**
Right leg	**18**
Left leg	**18**
Perineum	**1**
	100%

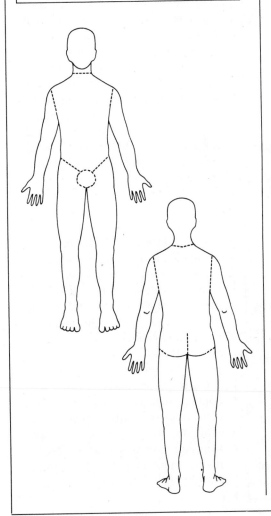

The Lund and Browder Chart

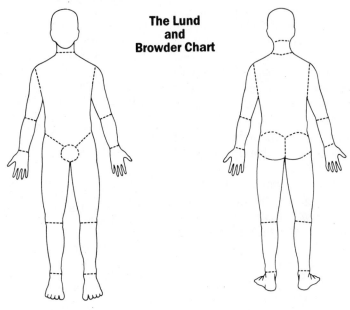

AREA	AGE-YEARS					% 2°	% 3°	% TOTAL
	0-1	**1-4**	**5-9**	**10-15**	**ADULT**			
Head	19	17	13	10	7			
Neck	2	2	2	2	2			
Ant. Trunk	13	17	13	13	13			
Post. Trunk	13	13	13	13	13			
R. Buttock	2½	2½	2½	2½	2½			
L. Buttock	2½	2½	2½	2½	2½			
Genitalia	1	1	1	1	1			
R.U. Arm	4	4	4	4	4			
L.U. Arm	4	4	4	4	4			
R.L. Arm	3	3	3	3	3			
L.L. Arm	3	3	3	3	3			
R. Hand	2½	2½	2½	2½	2½			
L. Hand	2½	2½	2½	2½	2½			
R. Thigh	5½	6½	8½	8½	9½			
L. Thigh	5½	6½	8½	8½	9½			
R. Leg	5	5	5½	6	7			
R. Foot	3½	3½	3½	3½	3½			
L. Foot	3½	3½	3½	3½	3½			
					Total			

Adapted from Lund, C., Browder, N. The estimation of areas of burns. *Surg. Gynecol. Obstet.* 1944.

perineum is performed in many burn centers. Special care is required when excising face and neck burns, as overexcision can limit the success of reconstructive surgery.

When a patient has minor burns, the hands and other joint surfaces are given top priority. Survival is the primary goal with larger burns, and selection of excision sites is based on reducing total burn size and achieving optimal grafting results.

The final decision depends on the depth of the injury, the patient's response to resuscitation, and contraindications to surgery and general anesthesia.

A burn wound can be excised in two ways. For a fascial excision, the surgeon removes the burned tissue and the subcutaneous fat, exposing the fascia. This technique guarantees a bed of viable tissue for grafting, but the healed wound is not cosmetically pleasing.

In sequential excision, the surgeon uses a special knife or a power-driven dermatome to remove layers of burned tissue that are one-hundredth of an inch thick until capillary bleeding indicates that a layer of viable tissue has been reached.

Significant blood loss is a risk with sequential excision. Bleeding is controlled with topical agents such as thrombin solutions, warm laparotomy pads, and compression dressings.

Because subcutaneous fat is left in place, the final results of sequential excision are more attractive than those of fascial excision. But no matter which method is used,

Classifying burns

The American Burn Association defines a burn as minor, moderate, or major, based chiefly on its depth and surface area. Also relevant are the cause of the injury, the involvement of body parts that need special care, and the presence of complications. The chart below lists the criteria for each category.

Minor Burn

Second degree burn of less than 15% TBSA (total body surface area) in adults or less than 10% TBSA in children.

Third degree burn of less than 2% TBSA that does not involve special care areas: face, eyes, ears, hands, feet, or perineum.

Moderate Uncomplicated Burn

Second degree burns of 15 to 25% TBSA in adults; 10 to 20% in children.

Third degree burns of less than 10% TBSA not involving special care areas.

Major Burn

Second degree burns totaling more than 25% TBSA in adults; 20% in children. All third degree burns of 10% TBSA or more.

All burns involving the hands, feet, face, eyes, ears, or perineum. All inhalation injuries, electrical injuries, or burns complicated by fractures or other major trauma. All poor risk patients, i.e. infants, elderly patients, and those patients with other medical problems such as diabetes, heart disease, or renal disorders.

---

the excised wound must be protected until it heals.

Closing the burn wound

The best cover for a wound is, of course, the patient's own skin. Autografting presents few problems when a burn is small and the patient has many areas of intact skin. Patients with major burns, however, may not have enough intact skin to serve as donor sites. Sometimes a small piece of skin can be meshed and expanded to cover the wound. When this isn't possible other coverings must be used.

The ideal substitute would meet many criteria. It would be durable, inexpensive, non-antigenic, non-toxic, tissue compatible, and have a long shelf life. It would be easy to apply and remove but would also adhere well to the wound. It would protect against the loss of protein, electrolytes, and water from the wound while preventing bacteria from entering. Lastly, it should decrease pain.

None of the substitutes currently available meets all of these requirements. Fresh skin from a human cadaver (called homograft or allograft) is considered the best biologic substitute. It provides a bacterial barrier, reduces protein, water, and heat loss, and stimulates the growth of granulation tissue.

Clean burns can be covered with homograft at the bedside or in the operating room after excision. The graft adheres to the wound's surface and becomes vascularized. It may remain in place for approximately three to five weeks, until the host rejects it.

In addition to providing temporary coverage, homograft can test the likelihood of successful autografting. If the homograft adheres and vascularizes in 48 to 72 hours, there's an excellent chance an autograft will do the same.

The drawbacks of homograft include limited supplies, restricted shelf life, and the potential for transmitting infection from donor to host.

Efforts to meet the demand for homograft led to heterografting—transferring tissue between two different species. Pigskin, in fresh or frozen form, is the heterograft used most often in the U.S.

Frozen pigskin is less likely than fresh to be rejected but raises the risk of infection. Therefore, the surgeon or nurse may apply an antimicrobial dressing. For the

Guides to fluid administration

The three formulas listed below are often used to determine volume replacement during the first 48 hours after a burn injury. Note that the post-burn periods are counted from the time the injury occurs, not from the time resuscitation begins.

Evans Formula	Brooke Formula	Parkland Formula

First 24 hours post burn
Colloid-containing fluid equivalent to plasma
1 ml/Kg/% TBSA* burn
    plus
Normal saline (0.9% NACL)
1 ml/Kg/% TBSA burn
    plus
5% dextrose in water (D5W) 200 ml
 	
Give half the fluid in the first eight hours, one quarter in the second eight hours, and one quarter in the third eight hours
	First 24 hours post burn
	Colloid-containing fluid equivalent to plasma
	0.5 ml/Kg/% TBSA* burn
	    plus
	Lactated Ringer's solution
	1.5 ml/Kg/% TBSA burn
	    plus
	D5W 2000 ml
	
	Give half the fluid in the first eight hours, one quarter in the second eight hours, and one quarter in the third eight hours
		First 24 hours post burn
		Lactated Ringer's solution 4 ml/Kg/% TBSA* burn
		
		Give one half of the fluid in the first eight hours, one quarter in the second eight hours, and one quarter in the third eight hours

Second 24 hours post burn
Colloid-containing fluid equivalent to plasma
0.5 ml/Kg/% TBSA burn
    plus
Normal saline (0.9% NACL)
0.5 ml/Kg/% TBSA burn
    plus
5% dextrose in water (D5W) 2000 ml divided evenly over 24 hours
	Second 24 hours post burn
	Colloid-containing fluid equivalent to plasma
	0.25 ml/Kg/% TBSA burn
	    plus
	Lactated Ringer's solution
	0.75 ml/Kg/% TBSA burn
	    plus
	D5W 2000 ml
	divided evenly over 24 hours
		Second 24 hours post burn
		Between 24 and 32 hours post burn administer colloid-containing fluid equivalent to plasma
		0.5 ml/Kg/% TBSA burn for eight hours then D5W at a rate to maintain a urine output of at least 30 ml/hr

*Maximum calculated burn is 50% TBSA

*Maximum calculated burn is 50% TBSA

*Calculation is by absolute percentage of burn. There is *no* maximum.

same reason, the heterograft may be removed every three to four days. At that time the wound is cleansed and evaluated and a new graft applied.

Despite the potential for infection, pigskin heterograft has many advantages. It's readily available, easily stored, and easy to apply and remove. Like homograft, it adheres well to the wound, limits pain, and prevents the loss of fluid, electrolytes, and heat.

Biobrane (Woodroof Laboratories, Inc.), a biosynthetic material, meets many of the requirements of an ideal skin substitute. This combination of collagen and a synthetic membrane is elastic, durable, and relatively inexpensive. It has the crucial quality of adherence and is also non-toxic and non-antigenic.

Biobrane comes in a sterile package and can be stored indefinitely. Unused portions may be resterilized for future application.

The material adheres to a clean wound in two stages. First, fibrin in the wound unites with the nylon and collagen backing of Biobrane. Then cell migration into the nylon mesh aids in binding Biobrane to the wound. Antimicrobial creams can penetrate Biobrane and reduce the risk of infection. Biobrane can be left on for 60 to 80 days, according to some reports, covering the wound until autograft is available.

Nursing care after excision

Keep excised areas immobile and free from pressure to prevent disruption of the graft. Elevate affected extremities to decrease postop edema. Check for bleeding and signs of neurovascular impair-

ment—increasing pain, numbness, or tingling—at least every hour.

The bulky pressure dressings applied in the OR will remain in place for two to three days. The physician may order application of sterile saline or an antibiotic solution every four hours to keep the dressings moist. Because of the risk of infection, use aseptic technique for this or any other procedure involving a burn wound.

After an autograft the donor site also requires special attention. Leave it open to air, keep pressure off it, and apply a heat lamp as ordered. Be alert for any increased bleeding from this area, also. Assess both the donor site and the grafted areas often for signs of infection. Medicate the patient for pain as needed, considering each patient and his pain individually.

What the future holds for burn care

Several important advances have been made in the quest for the perfect skin substitute. Epithelial cells can now be grown in a test tube. That means a piece of a patient's unburned skin approximately one centimeter square can increase many times over in a matter of weeks.

A double-layered artificial skin has also been developed. The temporary epidermis, a thin layer of silastic, blocks bacteria and controls water loss. The dermal layer adheres to the wound. Fibroblasts and capillaries enter this layer and begin to form a new dermal bed, known as the neodermis. When autograft is available, the epidermal layer of silastic is removed and very thin, split-thickness auto-

grafts are then placed over the neodermis.

Both of these techniques are still in the investigational stages, and the preliminary results have been encouraging. These and other developments are starting to change the course of burn wound management. Nurses who care for burn patients can expect new rewards and new challenges as they guide these patients on their long road towards recovery. ■

BIBLIOGRAPHY Arturson, M. The pathophysiology of severe thermal injury. *J. Burn Care and Rehab.* 6:1239, March/April 1985. Baxter, C. Problems and complications of burn shock resuscitation. *Surg. Clin. North Am.* 58(6):1313, 1978. Boswick, J. *The Art and Science of Burn Care.* Rockville, Md.: Aspen Publishers, 1987. Cardona, V., Hurn, P., et al. *Trauma Nursing.* Philadelphia: W.B. Saunders Co., 1988. Demling, R. Fluid and electrolyte management. *Critical Care Clinics* 1:27, March 1985. Fisher, S. and Helm, P. *Comprehensive Rehabilitation of Burns.* Baltimore: Williams and Wilkins Co., 1984. Holloway, N. *Nursing the Critically Ill Adult.* Menlo Park, N.J.: Addison-Wesley Publishing, 1984. Hunt, J., Sato, R., and Baxter, C. Early tangential excision and immediate mesh autografting of deep dermal hand wounds. *Ann. Surg.* 189:141, 1979. Jacoby, F. Care of the massive burn wound. *Crit. Care Q.* 7:44, Dec. 1984. Kenner, C., Guzzetta, C., and Dossey, B. *Critical Care Nursing.* Boston: Little, Brown and Co., 1985. Merrell, S., Saffle, J., et al. Increased survival after major thermal injury. *Am. J. Surg.* 154:623, Dec. 1987. Moore, E., Eisman, B., and Van Way, C. *Critical Decisions in Trauma.* St. Louis: C.V. Mosby Co., 1984. Munster, A. The early management of thermal burns. *Surgery* 87:29, 1980. Morton, J. Fluid replacement in patients with large-area full- and partial-thickness burns. *Arch. Surg.* 114:247, 1979. Nowicki, C. and Sprenger, C. Temporary skin substitutes for burn patients: A nursing perspective. *J. Burn Care and Rehab.* 9:209, Feb. 1988. Pruitt, B. and Levine, N. Characteristics and uses of biologic dressings and skin substitutes. *Arch. Surg.* 119:312, March 1984. Sabiston, D. *Textbook of Surgery.* Philadelphia: W.B. Saunders Co., 1986. Salisbury, R., Newman, N., and Dingeldein, G. *Manual of Burn Therapeutics.* Boston: Little, Brown and Co., 1989. Schwartz, S. *Principles of Surgery.* New York: McGraw-Hill Book Co., 1988. Thompson, P., Herndon, D., et al. Effects of early excision on patients with major thermal injury. *J. Trauma.* 27:205, Feb. 1987. Wagner, M. *Care of the Burn-injured Patient: A Multidisciplinary Approach.* Littleton, Mass.: PSG Publishing Co., 1982.

UNIT 3
PEDIATRIC NURSING

by

Janice Selekman, RN, DNSc
Judy Donlen, RN,C, DNSc
Holly Hillman, RN, MSN
Mary Lou Manning, RN, MSN, PNP

The challenges today's pediatric nurse faces in providing care for children and their families require skills from a wide spectrum of both technologic and psychosocial arenas. To meet the needs of both the child and the family in a variety of settings, the nurse must not only have a thorough understanding of disease processes, but also a knowledge of emotional, social, cultural, and developmental needs.

To provide this essential knowledge base, this unit begins with a review of growth and development, which is basic to understanding the behavior of children and the influences of illness. Disorders related to failure of normal progression through the developmental process are also considered in this section. The next section covers multisystem stressors, such as genetic disorders, fluid and electrolyte and acid-base imbalances, accidents, poisonings, and ingestions.

The unit is then further divided into specific body systems. For each system, there is an initial review of those aspects of anatomy and physiology unique to the child. Each step of the nursing process is then reviewed, followed by discussions of the major health problems of that system.

Throughout the chapter, only information that is specific to children is presented. In many cases, for instance where lab tests or nursing care do not differ from those for the adult, the content is not repeated. Be sure to refer to Unit 2 for background information when needed.

Growth and Development

GENERAL PRINCIPLES

Definition of Terms

A. *Growth:* increase in size of a structure. Human growth is orderly and predictable, but not even; it follows a cyclical pattern.
B. *Development:* maturation of structures. Development includes growth and is a process that continues over time.
C. *Cephalocaudal:* head-to-toe progression of growth and development
D. *Proximodistal:* trunk-to-periphery (fingers and toes) progression of growth and development
E. *Phylogeny:* development or evolution of a species or group; a pattern of development for a species
F. *Ontogeny:* development of an individual within a species
G. *Critical period:* specific time period during which certain environmental events or stimuli have greatest effect on a child's development.

Rates of Development

Growth and development are not synonymous but are closely interrelated processes directed by both genetic and environmental factors. Although changes in growth and development are more obvious in some periods than others, they are important in all periods.
A. Infancy and adolescence: fast growth periods
B. Toddler through school-age: slow growth periods
C. Fetal period and infancy: the head and neurologic tissue grow faster than other tissues.
D. Toddler and preschool periods: the trunk grows more rapidly than other tissue.
E. The limbs grow most during school-age period.
F. The trunk grows faster than other tissue during adolescence.

Child Development Theorists

Also see Unit 5, pages 491–493.

Sigmund Freud (Psychosexual Theory)

A. 0–6 months: oral passive (development of id; biologic pleasure principle)
B. 7–18 months: oral aggressive (teething); oral satisfaction of needs by mother decreases tension
C. 1½–3 years: anal (toilet training); projection of feelings onto others; elimination and retention as ways to control and inhibit
D. 4–5 years: phallic (love of opposite sex, parent-Oedipal complex); ego development: objective conscious reality
E. 6–12 years: latent; sexual drive repressed; socialization occurs; superego and morality development

Erik Erikson (Psychosocial Theory)

Core stages/psychosocial tasks or crises
A. Birth–1 year: trust vs mistrust
B. 1–3 years: autonomy vs shame and doubt
C. 3–6 years: initiative vs sense of guilt
D. 6–12 years: industry vs inferiority
E. 13–18 years: indentity vs confusion (identity diffusion)
F. Young adult: intimacy vs isolation
G. Adult: generativity (intimacy) vs self-absorption
H. Elderly: ego integrity vs despair (disgust)

Jean Piaget (Cognitive Theory)

Development of thought
A. 0–2 years: sensorimotor (reflexes, repetition of acts)
B. 2–4 years: preoperational (preconceptual); no cause and effect reasoning; egocentrism; use of symbols; magical thinking
C. 4–7 years: intuitive/preoperational (beginning of causation)
D. 7–11 years: concrete operations
E. 11–15 years: formal operations (reality, abstract thought)

ASSESSMENT

Developmental Tasks

Developmental tasks are accomplishments normally occurring at one stage and having an effect on the development of subsequent stages; fall into three categories
A. Physical tasks (e.g., learning to sit, crawl, walk; toileting)
B. Psychologic tasks (e.g., learning trust, self-esteem)
C. Cognitive tasks (e.g., acquiring concepts of time and space, abstract thought)

Measurement Tools

There are a number of different assessment tools for measuring the progress of growth and development.

A. Chronologic age: looks at accomplishment of developmental tasks related to birth date

B. Mental age: looks at cognitive development
  1. Measured by variety of standardized intelligence tests (IQ)
  2. Results from at least two separate testing sessions needed before an assessment is made
  3. Uses toys and language based on mental rather than chronologic age

C. *Denver Developmental Screening Test (DDST)*
  1. Generalized assessment tool; measures gross motor, fine motor, language, and personal-social development from 0–6 years
  2. Does not measure intelligence

D. Growth parameters
  1. Bone age: x-ray of tarsals and carpals determines degree of ossification
  2. Growth charts: norms are expressed as percentile of height, weight, head circumference for age; any child who crosses over multiple percentile lines needs further evaluation

Developmental Stages

Infant (Birth through 12 months)

A. Physical tasks
  1. *Neonate (Birth to 1 month)*
    a. Weight: 7–8 lb (3175–3629 gm); gains 5–7 oz (142–198 gm) weekly for first 6 months
    b. Length: 20 inches (50 cm); grows 1 inch (2.5 cm) monthly for first 6 months
    c. Head growth
      1) Head circumference 33–35.5 cm (13–14 inches)
      2) head circumference equal to or slightly larger than chest
      3) increases by ½ inch (1.25 cm) monthly for first 6 months
      4) brain growth related to myelinization of nerve fibers; increase in size of brain reflects this process, reaches 2/3 adult size at 1 year; 90% adult size at 2 years
      5) no control of muscles of the head
    d. Vital signs
      1) pulse: 110–160 and irregular; count for a full minute apically
      2) respirations: 32–60 and irregular; neonates are abdominal breathers, obligate nose breathers
      3) blood pressure: 80/46 mm Hg
      4) poor development of sweating and shivering mechanisms; impaired temperature control
    e. Motor development
      1) behavior is reflex controlled
      2) flexed extremities

      3) can lift head slightly off bed when prone
    f. Sensory development
      1) hearing and touch well developed at birth
      2) sight not fully developed until 6 years
        a) differentiates light and dark at birth
        b) rapidly develops clarity of vision within 1 foot
        c) fixates on moving objects
        d) strabismus due to lack of binocular vision

  2. *1–4 months*
    a. Head growth: posterior fontanel closes
    b. Motor development
      1) primitive reflexes fade (Moro, tonic, neck, Perez, crawling, grasp)
      2) gains head control; balances head in sitting position
      3) rolls from back to side
      4) begins voluntary hand-to-mouth activity
    c. Sensory development
      1) begins to have ability to coordinate stimuli from various sense organs
      2) hearing: locates sounds by turning head and visually searching
      3) vision
        a) binocular vision developing; less strabismus
        b) beginning hand-eye coordination
        c) prefers human face
        d) follows objects 180°
        e) ability to accommodate is equal to adult

  3. *5–6 months*
    a. Weight: birth weight doubled; gains 3–5 oz (84–140 gm) weekly for next 6 months
    b. Length: gains ½ inch (1.25 cm) for next 6 months
    c. Eruption of teeth begins
      1) lower incisors first
      2) causes increased saliva and drooling
      3) enzyme released with teething causes mild diarrhea, facial skin irritation
      4) slight fever may be associated with teething; but not a high fever or seizures
    d. Motor development
      1) intentional rolling over
      2) supports weight on arms
      3) creeping; pushes backwards with hands
      4) can grasp and let go voluntarily
      5) transfers toys from one hand to another
      6) sits with support
    e. Sensory development
      1) hearing: can localize sounds above and below ear
      2) vision: smiles at own mirror image and responds to facial expressions of others
      3) taste: sucking needs have decreased and cup weaning can begin; chewing, biting, and taste preferences begin to develop

  4. *7–9 months*
    a. Teething continues
      1) 7 months: upper central incisors
      2) 9 months: upper lateral incisors

b. Motor development
   1) sits unsupported; goes from prone to sitting upright
   2) crawls; may go backwards initially
   3) pulls self to standing position
   4) develops finger-thumb opposition (pincer grasp)
   5) preference for dominant hand evident
c. Sensory development: vision
   1) can fixate on small objects
   2) beginning to develop depth perception
5. *10–12 months*
   a. Weight: birth weight tripled
   b. Length: 50% increase over birth length
   c. Head and chest circumference equal
   d. Teething
      1) lower lateral incisors erupt
      2) average of eight deciduous teeth
   e. Motor development
      1) creeps with abdomen off floor
      2) walks with help or cruises
      3) may attempt to stand alone
      4) can sit down from upright position
      5) weans from bottle to cup
   f. Sensory development: vision
      1) able to discriminate simple geometric forms
      2) able to follow rapidly moving objects
      3) visual acuity 20/50 or better
      4) binocularity well established; if not, amblyopia may develop
B. Psychosocial tasks
   1. *Neonatal period*
      a. Cries to express displeasure
      b. Smiles indiscriminately
      c. Receives gratification through sucking
      d. Makes throaty sounds
   2. *1–4 months*
      a. Crying becomes differentiated at 1 month
         1) decreases during awake periods
         2) ceases when parent in view
      b. Vocalization distinct from crying at 1 month
         1) squeals to show pleasure at 3 months
         2) coos, babbles, laughs; vocalizes when smiling
      c. Socialization
         1) stares at parents' faces when talking at 1 month
         2) smiles socially at 2 months
         3) shows excitement when happy at 4 months
         4) demands attention, enjoys social interaction with people at 4 months
   3. *5–6 months*
      a. Vocalization: begins to imitate sounds
      b. Socialization: recognizes parents, stranger anxiety begins to develop; comfort habits begin
   4. *7–9 months*
      a. Vocalization: verbalizes all vowels and most consonants
      b. Socialization
         1) shows increased stranger anxiety and anxiety over separation from parent

         2) exhibits aggressiveness by biting at times
         3) understands word "no"
   5. *10–12 months*
      a. Vocalization: imitates animal sounds, can say only 4–5 words but understands many more
      b. Socialization
         1) begins to explore surroundings
         2) plays games such as pat-a-cake, peek-a-boo
         3) shows emotions such as jealousy, affection, anger, fear (especially in new situations)
C. Cognitive tasks
   1. *Neonatal period:* reflexive behavior only
   2. *1–4 months*
      a. Recognizes familiar faces
      b. Is interested in surroundings
      c. Discovers own body parts
   3. *5–6 months*
      a. Begins to imitate
      b. Can find partially hidden objects
   4. *7–9 months*
      a. Begins to understand object permanence; searches for dropped objects
      b. Reacts to adult anger; cries when scolded
      c. Imitates simple acts and noises
      d. Responds to simple commands
   5. *10–12 months*
      a. Recognizes objects by name
      b. Looks at and follows pictures in book
      c. Shows more goal-directed actions
D. Nutrition
   1. Birth to 6 months
      a. Breast milk is a complete and healthful diet; supplementation may include 0.25 mg fluoride, 400 IU vitamin D, and iron after 4 months.
      b. Commercial iron-fortified formula is acceptable alternative; supplementation may include 0.25 mg fluoride if water supply is not fluoridated.
      c. No solid foods before 5 months; too early exposure may lead to food allergies, and protusion reflex will cause food to be pushed out of mouth.
      d. Juices may be introduced at 5–6 months, diluted 1:1 and preferably given by cup.
   2. *6–12 months*
      a. Breast milk or formula continues to be primary source of nutrition.
      b. Introduction of solid foods starts with cereal (usually rice cereal), which is continued until 18 months.
      c. Introduction of other food is arbitrary; most common sequence is fruits, vegetables, meats.
         1) introduce one new food a week.
         2) decrease amount of formula to about 30 oz as foods are added.
      d. Iron supplementation can be stopped.
      e. Finger foods such as cheese, meat, carrots, can be started around 10 months.
      f. Chopped table food or junior food can be introduced by 12 months.

g. Weaning from breast or bottle to cup should be gradual during second 6 months.

E. Safety

    1. *Birth to 4 months*

        a. Use crib and car seat that conform to federal regulations.

        b. Ensure crib mattress fits snugly; do not use a pillow in the crib.

        c. Keep side rails of crib up.

        d. Do not leave infant unattended on bed, couch, table.

        e. Do not tie pacifier on string around infant's neck; remove bib before sleep.

        f. Remove small objects that infant could choke on.

        g. Check temperature of bath water and warmed formula or food.

        h. Use cool mist vaporizer.

        i. Start immunizations (see also Table 3.2, page **288**).

            1) 2 months: first DPT and OPV

            2) 4 months: second DPT and OPV

    2. *5–7 months*

        a. Restrain in high chair or infant seat.

        b. Do not feed hard candy, nuts, food with pits.

        c. Inspect toys for small removable parts.

        d. Be sure paint on furniture does not contain lead.

        e. Keep phone number of poison control center readily available.

        f. Continue immunizations: third DPT at 6 months

    3. *8–12 months*

        a. Keep crib away from other furniture and windows.

        b. Keep gates across stairways.

        c. Keep safety plugs in electrical outlets.

        d. Remove hanging electrical wires and tablecloths.

        e. Use child protective caps and cabinet locks.

        f. Place cleaning solutions and medications out of reach.

        g. Do not let child use fork to self-feed.

        h. Do not leave alone in bathtub.

        i. Tuberculin test at 12 months.

F. Play

    1. *Birth to 4 months*

        a. Provide variety of brightly colored objects, different sizes and textures.

        b. Hang mobiles within 8–10 inches of infant's face.

        c. Expose to various environmental sounds; use rattles, musical toys.

    2. *5–7 months*

        a. Provide brightly colored toys to hold and squeeze.

        b. Allow infant to splash in bath.

        c. Provide crib mirror.

    3. *8–12 months*

        a. Provide toys with movable parts and noisemakers: stack toys, blocks; pots, pans, drums to bang on; walker and push-pull toys.

        b. Plays games: hide and seek, pat-a-cake.

G. Fears

    1. Separation from parents

        a. Searches for parents with eyes.

        b. Shows preference for parents.

        c. Develops stranger anxiety around 6 months.

    2. Pain

        a. Reacts with generalized body movement and loud crying.

        b. Can be distracted with talking, sucking opportunities.

Toddler (12 months to 3 years)

A. Physical tasks: this is a period of slow growth

    1. Weight: gain of approximately ll lb (5 kg) during this time; birth weight quadrupled by $2\frac{1}{2}$ years

    2. Height: grows 20.3 cm (8 inches); adult height about 2 times height at 2 years

    3. Head circumference: $19\frac{1}{2}$–20 inches (49–50 cm) by 2 years; anterior fontanel closes by 18 months

    4. Pulse 110; respirations 26; blood pressure 99/64

    5. Primary dentition (20 teeth) completed by $2\frac{1}{2}$ years

    6. Develops sphincter control necessary for bowel and bladder control

    7. Mobility

        a. Walks alone by 18 months.

        b. Climbs stairs and furniture by 18 months.

        c. Runs fairly well by 2 years.

        d. Jumps from chair or step by $2\frac{1}{2}$ years.

        e. Balances on one foot momentarily by $2\frac{1}{2}$ years.

        f. Rides tricycle by 3 years.

B. Psychosocial tasks

    1. Increases independence; better able to tolerate separation from primary caregiver.

    2. Less likely to fear strangers.

    3. Able to help with dressing/undressing at 18 months; dresses self at 24 months.

    4. Has sustained attention span.

    5. May have temper tantrums during this period; should decrease by $2\frac{1}{2}$ years.

    6. Vocabulary increases from about 10–20 words to over 900 words by 3 years.

    7. Has beginning awareness of ownership (my, mine) at 18 months; shows proper use of pronouns (I, me, you) by 3 years.

    8. Moves from hoarding and possessiveness at 18 months to sharing with peers by 3 years.

    9. Toilet training usually completed by 3 years.

        a. 18 months: bowel control

        b. 2–3 years: daytime bladder control

        c. 3–4 years: nightime bladder control

C. Cognitive tasks

    1. Follows simple directions by 2 years.

    2. Begins to use short sentences at 18 months to 2 years.

    3. Can remember and repeat 3 numbers by 3 years.

    4. Knows own name by 12 months; refers to self, gives first name by 24 months; gives full name by 3 years.

    5. Able to identify geometric forms by 18 months.

    6. Achieves object permanence; is aware that objects exist even if not in view.

7. Uses "magical" thinking; believes own feelings affect events (e.g., anger causes rain).

8. Uses ritualistic behavior; repeats skills to master them and to decrease anxiety.

9. May develop dependency on "transitional object" such as blanket or stuffed animal.

D. Nutrition

    1. Needs 16–24 oz milk/day.

    2. Appetite decreases.

    3. Able to feed self.

    4. Encourage low cariogenic diet.

    5. Negativism may interfere with eating.

E. Safety

    1. Turn pot handles toward back of stove.

    2. Teach swimming and water safety; supervise near water.

    3. Supervise play outdoors.

    4. Avoid large chunks of meat, particularly hotdogs.

    5. Do not allow child to walk around with objects such as lollipops in mouth.

    6. Know when and how to use ipecac.

    7. Immunization

        a. 15 months: measles, mumps, rubella (MMR)

        b. 18 months: DPT, OPV

        c. 24 months: HBPV

F. Play

    1. Predominantly "parallel play" period.

    2. Imitation of adults often part of play.

    3. Begins imaginative and make-believe play.

    4. Provide toys appropriate for increased locomotive skills: push toys, rocking horse; riding toys or tricycles; swings and slide.

    5. Give toys to provide outlet for aggressive feelings: work bench, toy hammer and nails, drums, pots, pans.

    6. Provide toys to help develop fine motor skills, problem-solving abilities: puzzles, blocks; finger paints, crayons.

G. Fears: separation anxiety

    1. Learning to tolerate and master brief periods of separation is important developmental task.

    2. Increasing understanding of object permanence helps toddler overcome this fear.

    3. Potential patterns of response to separation

        a. Protest: screams and cries when mother leaves; attempts to call her back.

        b. Despair: whimpers, clutches transitional object, curls up in bed, decreased activity, rocking.

        c. Denial: resumes normal activity but does not form psychosocial relationships; when mother returns child ignores her.

    4. Bedtime may represent desertion.

Preschooler (3 to 5 years)

A. Physical tasks

    1. Slower growth rate continues

        a. Weight: increases 4–6 lb (1.8–2.7 kg) a year

        b. Height: increases 2–2½ inches (5–6.25 cm) a year

        c. Birth length doubled by 4 years

    2. Vital signs decrease slightly

        a. Pulse 90–100 bpm

        b. Respirations 24–25/minute

        c. Blood pressure: systolic 85–100 mg Hg; diastolic 60–70 mm Hg

    3. Permanent teeth may appear late in preschool period; first permanent teeth are molars, behind last temporary teeth.

    4. Gross motor development

        a. Walks up stairs using alternate feet by 3 years.

        b. Walks down stairs using alternate feet by 4 years.

        c. Rides tricycle by 3 years.

        d. Stands on 1 foot by 3 years.

        e. Hops on 1 foot by 4 years.

        f. Skips and hops on alternate feet by 5 years.

        g. Balances on 1 foot with eyes closed by 5 years.

        h. Throws and catches ball by 5 years.

        i. Jumps off 1 step by 3 years.

        j. Jumps rope by 5 years.

    5. Fine motor development

        a. Hand dominance is established by 5 years.

        b. Builds a tower of blocks by 3 years.

        c. Ties shoes by 5 years.

        d. Ability to draw changes over this time.

            1) copies circles, may add facial features by 3 years.

            2) copies a square, traces a diamond by 4 years.

            3) copies a diamond and triangle, prints letters and numbers by 5 years.

        e. Handles scissors well by 5 years.

B. Psychosocial tasks

    1. Becomes independent.

        a. Feeds self completely.

        b. Dresses self.

        c. Takes increased responsibility for actions.

    2. Aggressiveness and impatience peak at 4 years then abate; by 5 years child is eager to please and manners become more evident.

    3. Gender-specific behavior is evident by 5 years.

    4. Egocentricity changes to awareness of others; rules become important; understands sharing.

C. Cognitive development

    1. Focuses on one idea at a time; cannot look at entire perspective.

    2. Awareness of racial and sexual differences begins.

        a. Prejudice may develop based on values of parents.

        b. Manifests sexual curiosity.

        c. Sexual education begins.

        d. Beginning body awareness.

    3. Has beginning concept of causality.

    4. Understanding of time develops during this period.

        a. Learns sequence of daily events.

        b. Is able to understand meaning of some time-oriented words (day of week, month, etc.) by 5 years.

    5. Has 2000-word vocabulary by 5 years.

    6. Can name 4 or more colors by 5 years.

    7. Is very inquisitive.

D. Nutrition: similar to toddlers

E. Safety
  1. Immunizations: DPT, OPV (4–6 years)
  2. Safety issues similar to toddler
  3. Education of children concerning potential dangers important during this period
F. Play
  1. Predominantly "associative play" period.
  2. Enjoys imitative and dramatic play.
    a. Imitates same sex role functions in play.
    b. Enjoys dressing up, dollhouses, trucks, cars, telephones, doctor and nurse kits.
  3. Provide toys to help develop gross motor skills: tricycles, wagons, outdoor gym; sandbox, wading pool.
  4. Provide toys to encourage fine motor skills, self-expression, and cognitive development: construction sets, blocks, carpentry tools; flash cards, illustrated books, puzzles; paints, crayons, clay, simple sewing sets.
  5. Television, when supervised, can provide a quiet activity; some programs have educational content.
  6. Imaginary playmates common during this period.
    a. More prevalent in bright children
    b. Help child deal with loneliness and fears
    c. Abandoned by school age
G. Fears
  1. Greatest number of imagined and real fears of childhood during this period.
  2. Fears concerning body integrity are common.
    a. Child is able to imagine an event without experiencing it.
    b. Observing injuries or pain in others can precipitate fear.
    c. Magical and animistic thinking allows children to develop many illogical fears (fear of inanimate objects, the dark, ghosts).
  3. Exposing child to feared object in a safe situation may provide a degree of conditioning; child should progress at own rate.

School-age (6 to 12 years)

A. Physical tasks
  1. Slow growth continues.
    a. Height: 2 inches (5 cm) per year
    b. Weight: doubles over this period
    c. At age 9, both sexes same size; age 12, girls bigger than boys
  2. Dentition
    a. Loses first primary teeth at about 6 years.
    b. By 12 years, has all permanent teeth except final molars.
  3. Bone growth faster than muscle and ligament development; very limber but susceptible to bone fractures during this time.
  4. Vision is completely mature; hand-eye coordination develops completely.
  5. Gross motor skills: predominantly involving large muscles; children are very energetic, develop greater strength, coordination, and stamina.
  6. Develops smoothness and speed in fine motor control.

B. Psychosocial tasks
  1. School occupies half waking hours; has cognitive and social impact.
    a. Readiness includes emotional (attention span), physical (hearing and vision), and intellectual components.
    b. Teacher may be parent substitute, causing parents to lose some authority.
  2. Morality develops
    a. Before age 9 moral realism predominates: strict superego, rule dominance; things are black or white, right or wrong.
    b. After age 9 autonomous morality develops: recognizes differing points of view, sees "gray" areas.
  3. Peer relationships
    a. Child makes first real friends during this period.
    b. Is able to understand concepts of cooperation and compromise (assist in acquiring attitudes and values); learns fair play vs competition.
    c. Help child develop self-concept.
    d. Provide feeling of belonging.
  4. Enjoys family activities.
  5. Has some ability to evaluate own strengths and weaknesses.
  6. Has increased self-direction.
  7. Is aware of own body; compares self to others; modesty develops.
C. Cognitive development
  1. Period of industry
    a. Is interested in exploration and adventure.
    b. Likes to accomplish or produce.
    c. Develops confidence.
  2. Concept of time and space develops.
    a. Understands causality.
    b. Masters concept of conservation: permanence of mass and volume; concept of reversibility.
    c. Develops classification skills: understands relational terms; may collect things.
    d. Masters arithmetic and reading.
D. Nutrition
  1. Caloric needs diminish in relation to body size: 85 kcal/kg.
  2. "Junk" food may become a problem; excess sugar, starches, fat.
  3. Obesity is risk in this age group.
  4. Nutrition education should be integrated into school program.
E. Safety
  1. Incidence of accidents is decreased when compared with younger children.
  2. Motor vehicle accidents most common cause of severe injury and death.
  3. Other common activities associated with injuries include sports (skateboarding, rollerskating, etc.).
  4. Education and supervision are key elements in prevention.
    a. Proper use of equipment
    b. Risk-taking behavior

F. Play
   1. Rules and ritual dominate play; individuality not tolerated by peers; knowing rules provides sense of belonging; "cooperative play."
   2. Team play: games or sports
      a. Help learn value of individual skills and team accomplishments.
      b. Help learn nature of competition.
   3. Quiet games and activities: board games, collections, books, television, painting
   4. Athletic activities: swimming, hiking, bicycling, skating
G. Fears: more realistic fears than younger children; include death, disease or bodily injury, punishment; school phobia may develop, resulting in psychosomatic illness.

Adolescent (12 to 18 years)

A. Physical tasks
   1. Fast period of growth
   2. Vital signs approach adult norms
   3. Puberty
      a. Follows same pattern for all races and cultures.
      b. Is related to hormonal changes.
      c. Results in growth spurt, change in body structure, development of secondary sex characteristics, and reproductive maturity.
      d. Girls: height increases approximately 3 inches/year; slows at menarche; stops around age 16.
      e. Boys: growth spurt starts around age 13; height increases 4 inches/year; slows in late teens.
      f. Boys double weight between 12 and 18, related to increased muscle mass.
      g. Body shape changes
         1) boys become leaner with broader chest.
         2) girls have fat deposited in thighs, hips, and breasts; pelvis broadens.
      h. Apocrine glands cause increased body odor.
      i. Increased production of sebum and plugging of sebaceous ducts causes acne (page **355**).
   4. Sexual development: girls
      a. Menarche
         1) onset about 2 years after first of pubescent changes
         2) average age 12½ years
         3) first 1–2 years: menses irregular and infertile
      b. Menstrual cycle: controlled by complex interaction of hormones (see page **382**).
      c. Development of secondary sex characteristics and sexual functioning under hormonal control (see Table 2.4).
      d. Breast development is first sign of puberty.
         1) bud stage: areola around nipple is protuberant.
         2) breast development is complete around the time of first menses.
   5. Sexual development: boys
      a. Development of secondary sex characteristics, sex organs and function under hormonal control (see Table 2.24).
      b. Enlargement of testes is first sign of sexual maturation; occurs at approximately age 13, about 1 year before growth spurt.
      c. Scrotum and penis increase in size until age 18.
      d. Reaches reproductive maturity about age 17, with viable sperm.
      e. Nocturnal emission: a physiologic reflex to ejaculate buildup of semen; natural and normal; occurs during sleep (child should not be made to feel guilty; needs to understand that this is not enuresis).
      f. Masturbation increases (also a normal way to release semen).
      g. Pubic hair continues to grow and spread until mid 20s.
      h. Facial hair; appears first on upper lip.
      i. Voice changes due to growth of laryngeal cartilage.
      j. Gynecomastia: slight hypertrophy of breasts due to estrogen production; will pass within months but causes embarrassment.
B. Psychosocial tasks
   1. Early adolescence (junior-high age group): ages 12–13 years
      a. Starts with puberty.
      b. Physical body changes result in an altered self-concept.
      c. Tends to compare own body to media idols.
      d. Early and late developers have anxiety regarding fear of rejection.
      e. Fantasy life, day dreams, crushes are all normal, help in role play of varying social situations.
      f. Is prone to mood swings.
      g. Needs limits and consistent discipline.
   2. Middle adolescence (high-school age group): ages 14–16 years
      a. Is separate from parents (except financially).
      b. Can identify own values.
      c. Can define self (self-concept, strengths and weaknesses).
      d. Partakes in peer group; conforms to values/fads.
      e. Has increased heterosexual interest; communicates with opposite sex; may form "love" relationship.
      f. Sex education is complete at this point.
   3. Late adolescence: ages 17–19 years
      a. Is physically and financially independent from parents.
      b. Chooses a vocation.
      c. Participates in society.
      d. Finds an identity.
      e. Finds a mate.
      f. Develops own morality.
      g. Completes physical and emotional maturity.
C. Cognitive development
   1. Develops abstract thinking abilities.
   2. Is often unrealistic.
   3. Is capable of scientific reasoning and formal logic.
   4. Enjoys intellectual abilities.
   5. Is able to view problems comprehensively.

D. Nutrition
1. Nutritional requirements peak during years of maximum growth: age 10–12 in girls, 2 years later in boys
2. Appetite increases.
3. Inadequate diet can retard growth and delay sexual maturation.
4. Food intake needs to be balanced with energy expenditure.
5. Increased needs include calcium for skeletal growth; iron for increased muscle mass and blood cell development; zinc for development of skeletal and muscle tissue and sexual maturation.

E. Safety
1. Accidents are leading cause of death: motor vehicle accidents, sports injuries, firearms accidents.
2. Safety measures include education about proper use of equipment and caution concerning risk taking.
3. Drugs and alcohol use may be a serious problem during this period.
4. Adolescent characteristics of poor impulse control and recklessness make prevention complex.

F. Activities: group activities predominate (sports are important); activities involving opposite sex by middle adolescence.

G. Fears
1. Threats to body image: acne, obesity, homosexuality
2. Injury or death
3. The unknown

ANALYSIS

Nursing diagnoses for disorders of growth and development may include
A. Alteration in thought processes
B. Knowledge deficit
C. Disturbance in self-concept
D. Social isolation
E. Potential for violence
F. Alteration in family process
G. Ineffective family coping
H. Alteration in health maintenance
I. Alteration in parenting

PLANNING AND IMPLEMENTATION

Goals

A. Child will achieve appropriate developmental level for age.
B. Family/child will adapt successfully to developmental changes.
C. Family/child will cope successfully with crises of sickness and hospitalization.

Interventions for the Sick or Hospitalized Child

Communicating with Children

A. Speak in quiet, pleasant tones.
B. Bend down, to meet child on own level.
C. Use words appropriate to age/communication ability; do not use clichés.
D. Do not explain more than is necessary.
E. Always explain what you are going to do and give the reason for it.
F. Be honest; do not lie about whether something will hurt.
G. Do not make a promise you known you cannot keep.
H. Observe nonverbal behavior for clues to level of understanding.
I. Do not threaten; and when necessary, punish the act, not the child ("I like you, but not what you did.").
J. Never shame a child by using terms like baby or sissy.
K. Allow child to show feelings (hurt and anger); provide therapeutic play, pounding or throwing toys; allow child to cry; encourage creative writing.
L. Provide time to talk; encourage a trusting environment where the child can talk without embarrassment and confide without fear.
M. Provide support to child and parents/family.
N. Teach parents to anticipate next stage of development.
O. If teaching with a child is interrupted, start over from the beginning.
P. Promote independence; allow the child to perform as many self-care activities as possible.
Q. Do not compare child's progress to that of anyone else.
R. Provide praise at every opportunity.
S. Instead of asking what something is, ask child to give it a name or tell you about it.
T. Allow choices where possible, but do not use yes/no questions unless you can accept a "no" answer ("It is time for your medication now; do you want it with milk or juice?" versus "Do you want your medication now?").
U. Involve parents in child's care.
V. Keep routines as much like home as possible (on admission, ask parents about routines such as toileting, eating, sleeping, and names for bowel movements and urination).
W. Allow parents time and opportunities to ask questions and express themselves.
X. If parents cannot stay with child, encourage them to bring in a favorite toy, pictures of family members, or to make a tape to be played for the child.

Play

A. Play is a way to problem solve, become enculturated, express creativity, decrease stress in the environment, prepare for different situations, sublimate sensations, enhance fine and gross motor development as well as social development.
B. Make play appropriate for mental age and physical/disease state (e.g., appropriate for oxygen tents, isolation, hearing or vision defects).

C. Use multisensory stimulation.
D. Provide toys safe for mental age (no points, sharp edges, small parts, loud noises, propelled objects).
E. Offer play specific to age group.
   1. Toddler: enjoys repetition; solitary play, parallel play.
   2. Preschooler: likes to role play and make believe; associative play.

3. School-age: likes group, organized activities (to enhance sharing); cooperative play, group goals with interaction.

Preparation for Procedures

A. Allow child to play with equipment to be used.

Table 3.1 Communicable Childhood Diseases

Disease	Characteristics	Immunization
Diphtheria	A rare respiratory disease caused by bacteria; life threatening to children under age 5. Bacteria forms a pseudomembrane across the trachea causing respiratory distress; also produces an exotoxin that causes tissue destruction in heart, PNS, and kidney.	Included in DPT* up to 6 years, then in Td*, repeated every 10 years throughout life.
Pertussis (whooping cough)	Common respiratory disease caused by bacteria; life threatening in young children. Severe paroxysmal cough results in severe respiratory distress; sequelae include mental retardation, seizures, cardiac arrest.	Included in DPT*; not given after 6 years because of risk from associated side effects. Do not give pertussis if child has active neurologic disorder.
Tetanus (lockjaw)	Neurologic disorder caused by bacterial exotoxin affects motor neurons, causing rigidity and spastic muscles; first symptom is stiffness of the jaw (trismus). No immunity is conferred after having the disease; associated mortality 25%–50%.	Included in DPT* up to 6 years; included in Td* every 10 years throughout life. May be given with a puncture wound if the wound is dirty and no immunization has been given in 5 years, or if wound is clean but more than 10 years have elapsed since previous immunization.
Measles (rubeola)	Viral infection producing harsh cough, maculopapular rash, photophobia, and Koplik spots; complications may include pneumonia, bacterial superinfections, and encephalitis. Incubation period is 2 weeks. Care includes keeping room darkened and providing antipruritic measures.	Maternal antibodies last for at least a year, then included in MMR* given at 15 months. Do not give measles virus if child has had another viral vaccine within 6 weeks, or will have TB test within 1 month (will convert to negative from measles infection or immunization).
German measles (rubella)	Viral infection causing lymphadenopathy and pink maculopapular rash; very mild disease, no specific care needed; complications may include arthralgia or arthritis, especially if occurring in young adults. Greatest danger is if pregnant woman contracts the disease; causes serious congenital anomalies.	Included in MMR* given at 15 months.
Mumps (parotitis)	Viral infection causing swelling of the parotid glands with painful swallowing, displacement of ear(s), and decreased tolerance of tart or sour foods/fluids. Ice collar may help relieve discomfort. Complications include orchitis (usually unilateral) if disease occurs after puberty, aseptic meningitis, encephalitis.	Included in MMR* given at 15 months.
Poliomyelitis (polio)	Viral infection, passed by fecal-oral route. Virus multiplies in the GI tract and enters the bloodstream to affect the CNS, resulting in paralysis.	OPV* (includes all three types of viruses).
Chickenpox (varicella)	Most common communicable childhood disease, caused by the varicella zoster virus. Causes rash that starts on the trunk and spreads. Rash starts as vesicles, which then erupt and crust over. Highly contagious from 2 days prior to rash to 6 days after rash erupts; incubation period 21 days. Once lesions have crusted or scabbed over they are no longer contagious. Care is directed at relief of itching.	No protection from maternal antibodies. Vaccine available but only recommended for high-risk groups.

*For immunization schedule and additional information about vaccine see Table 3.2

B. Demonstrate procedure first on a doll.

C. Teach child skills that will be needed after the procedure and provide time to practice (crutches, blow bottles).

D. Show the child pictures of staff garb, special treatment room, special machines to be used, etc. before the procedure.

E. Describe sensations the child may experience during or after the procedure.

F. Listen carefully to child to detect misconceptions or fantasies.

G. With younger children, the preparatory information should be simple and as close to the time of the procedure as possible.

H. Parents can often be helpful in preparing child for procedures, but need to be prepared as well.
   1. May need different explanation, away from child.
   2. Should have opportunity to ask questions about what will happen to child.

I. School-age children and adolescents may not wish parents to be present during procedure.
   1. Child's desires should be confirmed.
   2. Parents need to be assured that this is not rejection by child.

J. Inadequate preparation results in heightened anxiety that may result in regressive behavior, uncooperativeness, or acting out.

EVALUATION

A. Child maintains normal developmental level during hospitalization.

B. Parents participate in care of child during hospitalization.

DISORDERS OF GROWTH AND DEVELOPMENT

Communicable Childhood Diseases

A. Table 3.1 Common Childhood Communicable Diseases

B. Types of immunity (see page 14)

C. Immunization schedule (see Table 3.2)

D. Special considerations concerning immunization
   1. If the immunization schedule is interrupted it is not necessary to reinstitute the entire series. Immunization should occur on the next visit as if the usual interval has elapsed
   2. If immunization status is unknown, children should be considered susceptible and appropriate immunizations administered
   3. For children not immunized during the first year of life and who are less than 7 years old the same immunizations are given but following different time schedule
   4. For children 7 years old and older who are not immunized, Td rather than DTP is administered and PRP-D is eliminated
   5. Immunizations should not be given during a febrile illness
   6. Live virus vaccines are contraindicated for children with congenital disorders of the immune system
   7. Live virus vaccines are usually contraindicated for children receiving immunosuppressive therapy

E. Tuberculin testing
   1. Not an immunization, but part of normal screening program for children; included in immunization schedule
   2. Testing recommended at 12 to 15 months of age, before school entry (4 to 6 years of age) and in adolescence (14 to 16 years of age). Skin testing is always indicated for individuals with known contact with a person with tuberculous disease
   3. Positive reaction means that child has been exposed to and has circulating antibodies to tuberculosis but does not necessarily have the disease
   4. Positive reaction indicates need for further testing
   5. Once positive, always positive

Child Abuse

A. General information
   1. Physical, emotional, or sexual abuse of children: may result from intentional and nonaccidental actions; or may be from intentional and nonaccidental acts of omission (neglect)
   2. In sexual abuse, 80% of children know their abuser

Table 3.2   Recommended Schedule for Immunization American Academy of Pediatrics, Committee on Infectious Disease, 1988

Age	Immuni-zation	Comment
2 months	DTP, OPV	DTP = diphtheria and tetanus toxoids with pertusis vaccine OPV = oral poliovirus vaccine containing attenuated poliovirus types 1, 2 and 3 The DTP is given IM. Side effects may include fever or local irritation at the site of injection
4 months	DTP, OPV	6–8 week interval desired for OPV to avoid interference from previous dose
6 months	DTP	A third dose of OPV is not indicated in the United States
15 months	MMR	MMR = measles, mumps, rubella Combined vaccine preferred to individual vaccines. Do not give if child is allergic to eggs
18 months	DTP, OPV PRP-D	PRP-D = haemophilus b diphtheria toxoid conjugate vaccine. The DTP should be given 6 to 12 months after the third dose. The OPV should be given at any time between 12 and 24 months of age. DTP and OPV may be given simultaneously with MMR.
4–6 years	DTP, OPV	Up to 7th birthday but may be required for entrance to school
11–12 years	MMR	Revaccination before entry to junior high or middle school
14–16 years	Td	Td = adult tetanus toxoid and diphtheria toxoid for adult use. Repeat every 10 years

3. Problem usually related to parents' limited capacity to cope with, provide for, or relate to a child and/or to each other

4. Adults who abuse were often themselves victims of child abuse; although abuser may care about child, pattern of response to frustration and discipline is to be abusive.

5. Occurs in all socioeconomic groups.

6. Only 10% of abusers have serious psychologic disturbances, but most have low self-esteem, little confidence, low tolerance for frustration.

7. Abuse is most common among toddlers as they exercise autonomy and parents may sense loss of power.

B. Assessment findings

  1. History may be indicative of child abuse.

    a. No history to explain injury

    b. Delay in seeking medical attention

    c. History changes with repetition

    d. Injury not consistent with history

  2. Skin injuries (bruises, lacerations, burns) are most common; may show outline of instrument used and may be in varying stages of healing.

  3. Musculoskeletal injuries, fractures (especially chip or spiral fractures), sprains, dislocations are also common; x-rays may show multiple old fractures.

  4. Signs of central nervous system (CNS) injuries include subdural hematoma, retinal hemorrhage.

  5. Abdominal injuries may include lacerated liver, ruptured spleen.

  6. Observation of parents and child may reveal interactional problems.

    a. Does parent respond to child's cues?

    b. Does parent comfort child?

    c. Does child respond to parent with fear?

C. Nursing interventions

  1. In emergency room: tend to physical needs of child first; determination of existence of abuse must wait until child's condition is stable.

  2. Report suspected child abuse to appropriate agency.

  3. Provide a role model for parents in terms of communication, stimulation, feeding, and daily care of child.

  4. Encourage parents to be involved in child's care.

  5. Encourage parents to express feelings concerning abuse, hospitalization, and home situation.

    a. Feelings of fear and guilt should be acknowledged.

    b. Provide reassurance.

  6. Provide family education concerning child care, especially safety and nutrition needs, discipline, and age-appropriate stimulation.

  7. Initiate referrals for long-term follow-up (community agencies, pediatric and mental health clinics, self-help groups).

Failure to Thrive (FTT)

A. General information

  1. A condition in which a child fails to gain weight and is persistently less than the 5th percentile on growth charts.

  2. When related to nonorganic cause, it is usually due to a disrupted maternal-child relationship.

  3. Other pathology (especially absorption problems and hormonal dysfunction) must be ruled out before a disorder can be diagnosed as FTT.

  4. Growth and developmental delay usually improve with appropriate stimulation.

B. Assessment findings

  1. Sleep disturbances; rumination (voluntary regurgitation and reswallowing)

  2. History of parental isolation and social crisis, with inadequate support systems

  3. Physical exam reveals delayed growth and development (decreased vocalization, low interest in environment) and characteristic postures (child is stiff or floppy, resists cuddling)

  4. Disturbed maternal-infant interaction may be demonstrated in feeding techniques, amount of stimulation provided by mother, ability of mother to respond to infant's cues.

C. Nursing interventions

  1. Provide consistent care.

  2. Teach parents positive feeding techniques.

    a. Provide quiet environment.

    b. Follow child's rhythm of feeding.

    c. Maintain face-to-face posture with child.

    d. Talk to child encouragingly during feeding.

  3. Involve parents in care.

    a. Provide supportive environment.

    b. Give positive feedback.

    c. Demonstrate and reinforce responding to child's cues.

  4. Refer to appropriate community agencies.

Learning Disabilities

A. General information

  1. A heterogeneous group of disorders manifested by significant difficulties in acquisition and use of listening, speaking, writing, reasoning, or math skills

  2. Presumed to be due to CNS dysfunction

  3. Children of average or above-average IQ

  4. Affects all aspects of learning, not just academics

  5. Boys affected 6 times more often than girls

  6. Categories include

    a. Receptive/sensory: perceptual problem (dyslexia, visual misperception)

    b. Integrative: difficulty processing information (analysis, organization, sequencing, abstract thought)

    c. Expressive: motor dysfunction (aphasia, writing or drawing difficulties, difficulty in sports or games)

    d. Diffuse: combination of above

B. Assessment findings

  1. Poor attention span

  2. Poor grades, normal IQ

  3. Low general information scores on standardized IQ tests

  4. Decreased participation in extracurricular activities or hobbies

  5. Low self-esteem due to multiple failures

  6. Diagnostic tests: specific testing to confirm diagnosis and determine type of defect

C. Medical management: psychostimulants may be prescribed to reduce hyperactivity and frustration and to increase attention span and self-control; side effects include anorexia.
D. Nursing interventions
   1. Environmental manipulation for behavior management
      a. Limit external stimuli.
      b. Maintain predictable routines.
      c. Enforce limits on behavior.
   2. Teaching strategies tailored for child's specific defects
      a. Repeat directions often.
      b. Elicit feedback from child.
      c. Give time to ask questions.
      d. Keep teaching sessions short.
      e. Do not give nonessential information.

Sudden Infant Death Syndrome (SIDS)

A. General information
   1. Sudden death of any young child that is unexpected by history and in which thorough post mortem examination fails to demonstrate adequate cause of death
   2. Cannot be predicted; cannot be prevented (unexpected and unexplained)
   3. Peak age: 3 months; 90% by 6 months
   4. Usually occurs during sleep; there is no struggle and death is silent
   5. Diagnosis made at autopsy
   6. Although cause of death is not known, chronic hypoxemia related to periodic apnea has been suggested; suffocation and DPT reactions are *not* causes of SIDS.
B. Assessment findings
   1. Incidence higher in preterm infants, twins or triplets, low-birth-weight infants
   2. Infant with abnormalities in respiration, feeding or other neurologic symptoms at higher risk
C. Nursing interventions
   1. Nursing care is directed at supporting parents/family; parents usually arrive at emergency department.
   2. Provide a room for the family to be alone if possible, stay with them; prepare them for how infant will look and feel (baby will be bruised and blanched due to pooling of blood until death was discovered; also will be cold).
   3. Let parents say good-bye to baby (hold, rock).
   4. Reinforce that death was not their fault.
   5. Provide appropriate support referrals: clergy, notification of significant others, local SIDS program.
   6. Explain how parents can receive autopsy results.
   7. Notify family physician or pediatrician.

Multisystem Stressors

GENETIC DISORDERS

A. Genes are functional units of heredity, capable of replication, mutation, and expression.

B. Teratology is the branch of embryology that deals with the study of abnormal development and congenital malformations.

    1. *Congenital disorders:* present at birth, although may not be noticeable until later; may be caused by genetic factors, nongenetic factors, or a combination.

    2. *Genetic disorders:* caused by a single aberrant gene or a deviation in chromosome structure or number.

C. In humans there are normally 46 chromosomes (23 pairs) that contain the genes.

    1. *Genotype:* the gene constitution of an individual

    2. *Phenotype:* the outward visable physical appearance/expression of a person's genes (color, size, allergies)

    3. *Karyotype:* the number and pattern of chromosomes in a cell

    4. *Allele:* one of two or more forms of a gene that controls expression of specific characteristic (e.g., genes for eye color)

        a. *Mendel's law:* for each hereditary property we receive 2 genes, l from each parent; l is dominant and expressed; l is recessive and not expressed.

        b. *Homozygous:* alleles for characteristic are identical; both dominant (DD) or both recessive (dd).

        c. *Heterozygous:* alleles are different (Dd).

D. Normal cell division

    1. *Meiosis:* cell division that produces gametes, each with a haploid set of chromosomes (one-half the number of the parent cell); this is reductional division, occurs in the ova and sperm.

    2. *Mitosis:* cell division that produces two cells (daughter cells) each with a full complement of chromosomes, identical to the composition of the parent cell.

Principles of Inheritance

Traits that are controlled by genes located on autosomes are inherited according to dominant or recessive patterns. Most cases of autosomal inheritance in humans involve traits controlled by one gene.

Autosomal Dominant

A. General information

    1. Allele responsible for the trait (or disease) is dominant.

    2. Only one parent needs to pass on the gene (child may be heterozygous for trait).

    3. Examples of inherited diseases: Huntington's chorea, myotonic muscular dystrophy, night blindness, osteogenesis imperfecta, neurofibromatosis.

B. Genetic counseling: advise parents that if one of them has a disease inherited through autosomal dominant pattern, there is a 50% chance with each pregnancy that the child will have the disease/disorder.

Autosomal Recessive

A. General information

    1. Allele responsible for trait (or disease) will not result in expression if the other allele in the pair is dominant.

    2. Both parents must pass on the gene(s) (child is homozygous for trait).

    3. Examples of inherited diseases: cystic fibrosis, PKU, sickle cell anemia, albinism, Tay-Sachs, microcephaly, cretinism.

B. Genetic counseling: advise parents that if one of them has a disease inherited by autosomal recessive pattern

    1. There is a 25% chance with each pregnancy of having a child with the disease/disorder.

    2. There is a 50% chance with each pregnancy of having a child who is a carrier of the disease but who will not have the symptoms.

    3. There is a 25% chance with each pregnancy of having a child who will neither have the disease nor be a carrier.

Sex-linked (X-linked) Inheritance

A. General information

    1. Inheritance of characteristics located on X and Y chromosomes

    2. Only known genetic locus on the Y chromosome is associated with determination of male sex.

3. X chromosome carries other traits in addition to determination of female sex.
4. Sex-linked inheritance in males: even a recessive defective gene on X chromosome can manifest itself in males because there is no opposing normal gene on Y chromosome.
5. Sex-linked inheritance in females: recessive defective gene can be masked by a normal dominant gene.
6. Examples of sex-linked inherited disorders: color blindness, baldness, hemophilia A and B, Duchenne's muscular dystrophy, G_6PD deficiency.

B. Genetic counseling
1. If a woman is a carrier for a sex-linked disorder and her partner does not have the disorder
   a. There is a 50% chance with each pregnancy that her son will have the disorder.
   b. There is a 50% chance her daughter will become a carrier.
2. If a man has a sex-linked disorder all his daughters will be carriers, but none will manifest the disease.

Chromosome Alterations

A. General information: deviations from normal chromosome complement may be numeric or structural.
1. *Mutation:* spontaneous alteration in genetic material not present in previous generation
2. *Nondisjunction:* failure of a pair of chromosomes to separate during meiosis; results in a numeric change called trisomy (47 chromosomes); can be passed on by either parent (one parent would pass 24 chromosomes).
3. *Translocation:* the transfer of all or part of a chromosome to another location on the same chromosome or to a different chromosome after chromosome breakage
4. *Mosaicism:* the presence in the same individual of two or more genotypically different cell lines

B. Genetic counseling: varies depending on the origin of the alteration
1. Random risk: chromosome alterations caused by environmental agents are not likely to occur in subsequent pregnancies. Therefore, the risk of the same defect recurring is no more than for any person in the general population.
2. High risk: at least one parent carries a chromosomal aberration or mutant gene and passes it on to the offspring (e.g., if a parent is a balanced translocation carrier, the risk of a child being affected is 1 in 4)
3. Moderate risk: largest group; includes multifactorial disorders. Risk recurrence in these disorders is empiric, based not on genetic theory but on prior experience and observation.

Assessment

History

A. Careful, detailed history is the basis of genetic counseling; can help confirm diagnosis and establish recurrence risk in multifactorial disorders.

B. Family history (pattern of affected family members) is recorded in form of pedigree chart or family tree.
1. Information about affected child and immediate family: history of this pregnancy and all previous pregnancies, including stillbirths and abortions; information about siblings
2. Information about maternal relatives
   a. Mother's siblings
   b. Outcome of maternal grandmother's pregnancies
   c. Health status of maternal relatives
3. Information about paternal relatives: same as maternal

Laboratory/Diagnostic Tests

A. Amniocentesis
1. Examination of amniotic fluid to screen for
   a. Some inborn errors of metabolism
   b. Chromosomal abnormalities
   c. Some CNS disorders
   d. Sex of infant in sex-related disorders
2. Indications
   a. One parent is chromosome mosaic or has balanced translocation.
   b. Mother is age 35 or older.
   c. Both parents are heterozygous for an autosomal recessive disorder.
   d. Mother is carrier of an X-linked disorder.
   e. Couple already has an affected child.

B. Karyotyping (chromosomal analysis)
1. Confirms or refutes probable diagnosis of chromosomal abnormality.
2. Identifies whether individual is a carrier of chromosomal abnormality.
3. Determines infant's sex if necessary.

Analysis

Nursing diagnoses for the family/individual with a genetic disorder may include
A. Alteration in thought processes
B. Knowledge deficit
C. Self-care deficit
D. Potential alteration in parenting

Planning and Implementation

Goals

A. Child will achieve maximum potential for cognitive and motor development.
B. Family will develop effective coping strategies.

Interventions

A. Provide community health agency referral.
B. Support family in identification of appropriate stimulation programs for child.
C. Communicate with and provide support for parents.
D. Offer genetic counseling (see Principles of Inheritance).

Evaluation

A. Optimum level of motor and cognitive developments is attained.

B. Self-care is performed at satisfactory level.

C. Family is able to function appropriately.

D. Parents demonstrate ability to meet child's physical and developmental needs.

E. Parents derive comfort/satisfaction from parenting affected child.

Chromosome Disorder

Down's Syndrome

A. General information
1. One of the most common causes of mental retardation; incidence: about 1 in 600 live births
2. Caused by an extra chromosome 21 (total 47)
   a. Most cases associated with nondisjunction; incidence increased with maternal, and to some degree paternal, age; incidence in women over age 35 markedly increased
   b. Also associated with translocation; hereditary type, incidence not increased with parental age

B. Assessment findings
1. Head and face
   a. Small head, flat facial profile, broad flat nose
   b. Small mouth, normal-size protruding tongue
   c. Upward slanting palpebral fissure
   d. Brushfield's spots
   e. Low-set ears
2. Extremities
   a. Short, thick fingers and hands
   b. Simian creases (single crease across palms)
3. Associated anomalies and disorders
   a. Congenital heart defects (40% incidence)
   b. GI structural defects
   c. Increased incidence of leukemia
   d. Increased incidence of respiratory infection
   e. Visual defects: strabismus, myopia, nystagmus, cataracts
4. Retardation usually moderate, IQ 50–70

C. Nursing interventions: see also Mental Retardation, page 502
1. Provide parent education concerning
   a. Increased susceptibility to respiratory infection
   b. Nutritional needs, feeding techniques
   c. Medication administration if necessary.
2. Provide genetic counseling.

FLUID AND ELECTROLYTE, ACID-BASE BALANCES

General Principles and Variations from Adult

A. Percent body water compared to total body weight
1. Premature infant: 90% water
2. Infant: 75%–80% water
3. Child: 64% water

B. Infant also has a higher percentage of water in extracellular fluid compared to adults (therefore infant has less fluid reserve).

C. Renal function
1. Concentrating ability of kidney does not reach adult levels until approximately age 2; specific gravity of infant's urine is 1.003.
2. Glomerular filtration rate does not reach adult levels until approximately age 2.
3. Average urine output
   a. Infant: 5–10 cc/hour
   b. 1–10 years: 10–25 cc/hour
   c. 35 cc/hour thereafter

D. Metabolic rate in children is 2–3 times that of adults; children therefore have an increased need for nutrients and fluids, and an increased amount of waste to excrete.

E. Fluid is not conserved; there is less reserve, and children more prone to fluid volume deficit than adults; $\frac{1}{2}$ of infant's extracellular fluid is exchanged each day compared with only $\frac{1}{5}$ of adult's.

F. Children have faster respiratory rate than adults, causing more water loss through breathing.

G. Infants have a greater body surface area per kg body weight than adults, therefore fluid loss through skin (evaporation) is greater in children.

Assessment

Health History

A. Ascertain age, recent weight, usual feeding habits/patterns, amount and type of daily intake.

B. Determine usual voiding/stooling habits and volume of urine/stool output.

C. Identify any recent illnesses or medications taken.

D. Ascertain usual activity level.

Physical Examination

A. Measure present weight and vital signs.

B. Observe general appearance.
1. Muscle tone
2. Reflex responses
3. Activity level

C. Inspect skin and mucous membranes for turgor, color, temperature.

D. Head and face
1. Inspect fontanels, eye orbits.
2. Ascertain presence of tears, saliva.

E. Abdomen/genitalia
1. Auscultate for bowel sounds, peristaltic waves.
2. Inspect for diaper rash, urine stream.

Laboratory/Diagnostic Tests

A. Hematologic studies
1. Hbg and Hct
2. Sodium, potassium, chloride, calcium, magnesium
3. pCO_2 and CO_2
4. pH

B. Urine studies: specific gravity, glucose, ketones, osmolarity, pH

C. Stool studies: culture, reducing substances, blood, sodium, potassium, pH

Analysis

Nursing diagnoses for children with fluid/electrolyte and acid-base imbalances may include

A. Alteration in bowel elimination: diarrhea

B. Alteration in comfort: pain

C. Fluid volume deficit

D. Alteration in nutrition

E. Alteration in oral mucous membrane

F. Impairment of skin integrity

G. Alteration in tissue perfusion

H. Alteration in pattern of urinary elimination

Planning and Implementation

Goals

A. Child will have normal hydration status.

B. Parents will demonstrate knowledge of child's disorder, prescribed treatment, and prevention of complications.

Interventions

A. Maintain strict I&O.
   1. Weigh diapers.
   2. Monitor urine specific gravity.
   3. Hematest stools.

B. Take daily weights.

C. Keep NPO for bowel rest.

D. Administer IV fluids.
   1. Maintenance plus replacement
   2. Generally use hypotonic solutions (0.25 NSS, 0.33 NSS, or 0.45 NSS)

E. Provide pacifier for infant.

F. Reintroduce oral fluids slowly.
   1. In children under 2 years use Pedialyte, a balanced electrolyte solution.
   2. In children over 2 use weak tea, flat soda.
   3. Do not use
      a. Broth (high sodium)
      b. Milk/formula (high solute)
      c. Water, glucose water, Jell-O (no electrolytes).

Evaluation

A. Child has adequate hydration status.
   1. Adequate I&O
   2. Normal stooling pattern
   3. Good skin turgor
   4. Normal vital signs
   5. Normal serum laboratory values

B. Parents participate in care, demonstrate understanding of signs and symptoms of disorder and treatment.

Disorders

Dehydration

A. The most common fluid and electrolyte disturbance in infants and children

B. Osmotic factors, particularly sodium, control the movement of fluid between extracellular and intracellular compartments and influence the types of dehydration
   1. *Isotonic dehydration*
      a. Plasma sodium level is normal (130–150 mEq/liter).
      b. Water and electrolyte lost in proportionate amounts; net loss is isotonic.
      c. Major loss is from extracellular fluid; loss of circulating blood volume.
      d. Shock may develop if losses are severe.
   2. *Hypotonic dehydration*
      a. Plasma sodium level is less than 130 mEq/liter.
      b. Electrolyte deficit exceeds water deficit.
      c. May occur when fluid and electrolyte losses are replaced with plain or glucose water.
      d. Fluid lost from extracellular compartment; also moves from extracellular to intracellular compartment.
      e. Signs of decreased fluid appear sooner with smaller fluid losses than in isotonic dehydration.
      f. Shock is a frequent finding.
   3. *Hypertonic dehydration*
      a. Plasma sodium exceeds 150 mEq/liter.
      b. Water loss exceeds electrolyte loss; may occur when fluid and electrolyte losses are replaced with large amount of solute (hypertonic formula).
      c. Fluid shifts from the intracellular to the extracellular compartments.
      d. Physical signs of dehydration may be less apparent.
      e. Neurologic symptoms (e.g., seizures) often occur.

Diarrhea

A. General information
   1. A change in consistency and frequency of stool
   2. Very common in young children
   3. Caused by bacteria and viruses, parasites, poisons, inflammation, malabsorption, allergies, abnormal bowel motility, and anatomic alterations
   4. Infants can easily lose 5% of their body weight in 1 day
   5. Intestines are alkaline; large loss causes metabolic acidosis
   6. Also causes bicarbonate and potassium loss
   7. Body may use its own fat for energy leading to ketosis

B. Assessment findings
   1. History of frequent stools; child may complain of or indicate abdominal cramping by guarding, weight loss; child may be lethargic and irritable
   2. Decreased urine output, decreased tears and saliva, dry mucous membranes, dry skin with poor tissue turgor
   3. In children less than 18 months, may find depressed anterior fontanel
   4. Soft eyeballs with sunken appearance
   5. Ashen skin color; cold extremities

6. High-pitched cry
7. Increased pulse rate and decreased blood pressure
8. Diagnostic tests
    a. Hct elevated if dehydrated
    b. Serum sodium and potassium decreased
    c. BUN elevated if renal circulation is decreased
    d. CBC will show increased bands if caused by bacterial infection
    e. Low pH and positive sugar with disaccharide intolerance
    f. Stool culture will identify specific microorganism
    g. Leuokcytes in stool if caused by enteroinvasive organisms
C. Nursing interventions
    1. Keep NPO to rest bowel, if ordered.
    2. Administer IV fluid therapy as ordered.
    3. Resume oral feedings slowly; provide foods such as bread, rice, tea.
    4. Provide skin care to prevent/treat excoriation of diaper area.
    5. Test all stool and chart results.
    6. Isolation may be ordered with infectious cause.

Vomiting

A. General information
    1. Common symptom during childhood; usually not a cause for concern
    2. Differs from spitting up (dribbling of undigested formula, often with burping)
    3. If prolonged may result in metabolic alkalosis or aspiration
B. Assessment findings: in addition to vomiting, child may have fever, abdominal pain and distension.
C. Nursing interventions
    1. Assist with identification and treatment of underlying cause.
        a. Assess for accompanying diarrhea that may indicate gastroenteritis.
        b. Determine if others in family/school/etc. are also sick; may indicate food poisoning.
        c. Assess for history of anxiety-producing life events.
        d. Assess amount and force of vomitus; forceful, projectile vomiting may indicate pyloric stenosis (page 314).
        e. Determine frequency and character of vomitus (color, whether formula or food, presence of bile or blood, relationship to feeding (new foods, overeating).
    2. Prevent complications: monitor fluid/electrolyte and acid-base status
    3. Administer antiemetics if ordered; trimethobenzamide HCl (Tigan) and promethazine HCl (Phenergan) recommended for children.

ACCIDENTS, POISONINGS, AND INGESTION

A. Accidents are the main cause of death in children over the age of 1 year.

B. 90% of accidents are preventable.
C. Interaction among host (the child), agent (the principle cause), and environment ($\frac{2}{3}$ of accidents occur in the home); safeguard the host while the agent and environment are made safer.
D. Methods of prevention
    1. Childproofing the environment
    2. Educating parents and child
    3. Legislation (e.g., seat belts, safe toys)
    4. Anticipatory guidance
    5. Understanding and applying growth and development principles
        a. Infant: totally dependent on adults for maintenance of safe environment
        b. Toddler: more mobile, impatient; urge to investigate and imitate; climbing, running, jumping
        c. Preschooler: very curious, exploring neighborhood, running, climbing, riding bikes; can accept and respond to teaching but still needs protection
        d. School-age and adolescent: taking dares, sports injuries, peer pressure, learning to drive
E. Precipitating factors
    1. Arguments or tension in the home
    2. Change in routines
    3. Tired child/tired parents
    4. Inadequate babysitting
    5. Hungry child
    6. Illness in immediate family member
F. Potential outcomes include temporary incapacitation, permanent disfigurement, and death

Specific Disorders

Pediatric Poisonings

A. General information
    1. Toddlers and suicidal adolescents most often involved
    2. Deaths have declined due to continued efforts in prevention and the establishment of poison control centers
    3. Modes of exposure: ocular, skin, ingestion (vast majority)
    4. Types of substances ingested: drugs, household products (cleaning agents), garden supplies, plants and berries
    5. Most ingestions are acute in nature and accompanied by a history of invasion of the medicine chest or cabinet where household cleansers are kept.
    6. Chronic ingestions result in accumulation of toxic substance, such as lead.
B. General assessment findings
    1. Signs vary depending on substance ingested
    2. May evidence bradycardia; tachycardia; tachypnea; slow, depressed respiration; hypotension or hypertension; hypothermia or hyperpyrexia
    3. Confusion, disorientation, coma, ataxia, seizures
    4. Miosis, mydriasis, nystagmus
    5. Jaundice, cyanosis
    6. Child may have a distinctive odor: hydrocarbons, alcohol, garlic, sweat.

C. General interventions
  1. Resuscitate child and stabilize condition: establish patent airway and provide measures to restore circulation as indicated.
  2. Prevent absorption.
    a. Determine what, when, and how much was ingested; will frequently not be able to identify substance.
    b. Induce emesis.
      1) indicated in all cases *except* caustic material ingestion, or in a child who is comatose, experiencing seizures, or lacks gag reflex
      2) drug of choice is syrup of ipecac.
        a) administer 30 cc for adolescents, 15 cc for children, 10 cc for children under 1 year.
        b) follow with 100–300 cc water.
        c) if no response in 20–30 minutes, repeat dose.
        d) produces vomiting almost 100% of time.
    c. Gastric lavage: may also be used to prevent absorption
      1) use largest nasogastric (NG) or orogastric tube possible.
      2) aspirate gastric contents.
      3) use water or $\frac{1}{2}$ normal saline.
      4) continue until return is clear.
    d. Activated charcoal: minimizes absorption of toxins by binding them on its surface
      1) administer after vomiting with ipecac treatment
      2) administer 5–10 gm for each gram of drug or chemical ingested.
      3) mix charcoal with water to make a syrup that can be given by mouth or NG tube.
    e. Catharsis: may be used after emesis or lavage to speed elimination of ingested substance; recommended agents are sodium or magnesium sulfate.
  3. Provide treatment and prevention information to parents.
    a. Parents should always be instructed to save container, vomitus, spills on clothing for analysis.
    b. Teach parents about safety practices that will decrease chances of accidental poisonings; educate as to use of drugs, labeling, storage, and handling of household products, importance of child-resistant safety packaging.
    c. Stress importance of having syrup of ipecac in the home (30 cc can be purchased over the counter) and instruct parents on proper administration.
    d. Advise parents to keep poison control center phone number readily available.
    e. Incorporate anticipatory guidance related to developmental stage of child.
    f. Discuss general first aid measures with parents.

Aspirin Ingestion

A. General information
  1. Toxicity begins at doses of 150–200 mg/kg.
  2. Products include not only aspirin but oil of wintergreen and analgesic cold medicines.
  3. Peak effect of aspirin is 2–4 hours and effects may last 8 hours.
  4. Ingestion may be accidental or due to therapeutic overdosing.
  5. Aspirin causes CNS stimulation, fluid and electrolyte loss, respiratory alkalosis, metabolic acidosis and impaired glucose metabolism.
B. Assessment findings
  1. Hyperventilation, hyperpyrexia, hyperglycemia, tinnitus, headache, bleeding
  2. Vomiting, sweating, dehydration
  3. Decreased level of consciousness (LOC), confusion, seizures, coma
C. Nursing interventions: in addition to general measures outlined above
  1. Provide emotional support to child and family.
  2. Monitor for latent effects (especially if time-release capsules ingested).
  3. Seriously ill children may require hemodialysis to promote salicylate elimination.
  4. Administer IV therapy as ordered, to correct fluid and electrolyte imbalances.
  5. Provide information to parents concerning products containing aspirin with proper dosages.

Acetaminophen Ingestion

A. General information
  1. Has become a commonly used analgesic-antipyretic
  2. Little associated morbidity or mortality in accidental ingestion
  3. Major risk is severe hepatic damage.
B. Assessment findings
  1. Vague and nonspecific initially; nausea, vomiting, anorexia, sweating
  2. Jaundice, liver tenderness, increase in liver enzymes, abdominal pain
  3. Progression to hepatic failure
C. Nursing interventions
  1. Emesis or lavage; do *not* use activated charcoal (will bind antidote).
  2. Administer antidote (acetylcysteine [Mucomyst]): lessens hepatic damage if given within 16 hours of ingestion. *Note:* antidote is still under investigation, use requires permission from Rocky Mountain Poison Control Center.

Lead Poisoning

A. General information
  1. Increased blood lead levels resulting from ingestion and absorption of lead-containing substances
  2. Most common source is lead-based paint (used in houses prior to 1950)
  3. Toddlers and preschoolers most often affected; many have pica (tendency to eat nonfood substances)
  4. Lead range of 5–30 mg/dl not dangerous
  5. Symptoms usually appear once level is 70 mg/dl

6. Lead is absorbed through the GI tract and pulmonary system; it is then deposited in bone, soft tissue, and blood; excretion occurs via urine, feces, and sweat; toxic effects are due to enzyme inhibition.
7. Low dietary iron and calcium may enhance toxic effects.
8. Widespread screening programs have diminished severe effects.

B. Assessment findings
  1. Abdominal complaints including colicky pain, constipation, anorexia, vomiting, weight loss
  2. Pallor, listlessness, fatigue
  3. Clumsiness, irritability, loss of coordination, ataxia, seizures
  4. Encephalopathy
  5. Identification of lead in the blood
  6. Erythrocyte protoporphyrin (EP) levels increased

C. Nursing interventions
  1. Administer chelating agents as ordered: dimercaprol (BAL in Oil); edatate calcium disodium (calcium EDTA).
    a. Prepare child for multiple injections; involve parents.
    b. Relieve pain at injection sites by applying warm soaks, rotating sites.
    c. Maintain hydration, measure I&O, encourage fluids (chelation is toxic to kidney).
  2. Provide nutritional counseling.
  3. Aid in eliminating environmental conditions that led to lead ingestion.

Aspiration of a Foreign Object

A. General information
  1. Relatively common airway problem
  2. Severity depends on object (e.g., pins, coins, nuts, buttons, parts of toys) aspirated and the degree of obstruction.
  3. Depending on object aspirated, symptoms will increase over hours or weeks.
  4. The curious toddler is most frequently affected.
  5. If object does not pass trachea immediately, respiratory distress will be evident.
  6. If object moves beyond tracheal region, it will pass into one of the main stem bronchi; symptoms will be vague, insidious.
  7. Causes 400 deaths per year in children under age 4.

B. Medical management
  1. Objects in upper airway require immediate removal.
  2. Lower airway obstruction is less urgent (bronchoscopy or laryngoscopy).

C. Assessment findings
  1. Sudden onset of coughing, dyspnea, wheezing, stridor, apnea (upper airway)
  2. Persistent or recurrent pneumonia, persistent croupy cough or wheeze
  3. Object not always visible on x-ray
  4. Secondary infection

D. Nursing interventions
  1. Perform Heimlich maneuver if indicated.
  2. Reassure the scared toddler.

3. After removal, place child in high-humidity environment and treat secondary infection if applicable.
4. Counsel parents regarding age-appropriate behavior and safety precautions.

SAMPLE QUESTIONS

1. You have assessed four children of varying ages, which one would require further evaluation?
   o 1. A 7-month-old who is afraid of strangers
   o 2. A 4-year-old who talks to an imaginary playmate
   o 3. A 9-year-old with enuresis
   o 4. A 16-year-old male who has nocturnal emissions

Jeffrey, age 17, has Down's syndrome. He is 57 inches tall and weighs 155 pounds.

2. In planning his care, it is most important for the nurse to take into consideration
   o 1. his mental age.
   o 2. his chronologic age.
   o 3. his bone age.
   o 4. growth chart percentiles.

3. Down's syndrome is caused by
   o 1. an autosomal recessive defect.
   o 2. an extra chromosome.
   o 3. a sex-linked defect.
   o 4. a dominant gene.

The Nervous System

VARIATIONS FROM THE ADULT

Brain and Spinal Cord

Size and Structure

A. Rapid head growth in early childhood: brain is 25% of adult weight at birth, 75% at 2½ years, and 90% at 6 years

B. Head growth results from development of nerve tracts within the brain and an increase in nerve fibers, not an increase in the number of neurons.

C. Infant's skull is not a rigid structure.
   1. Bones of skull are not fused until 18 months.
   2. Head circumference will increase with increase in intracranial volume in infants.
   3. Sutures may separate if there is significant gradual increase in intracranial volume up to age 12.

D. Fontanels ("soft spots"): areas of head not covered by skull
   1. Anterior fontanel
      a. Diamond-shaped opening at junction of parietal and frontal bones
      b. Closes between 9 and 18 months
   2. Posterior fontanel
      a. Triangular-shaped opening at junction of occipital and parietal bones
      b. Closes by 2 months
   3. Should feel flat and firm
   4. May be sunken with severe dehydration
   5. Will bulge with increased intracranial pressure (ICP)

Function

A. Cortical functions (e.g., fine motor coordination) are incompletely developed at birth.

B. The autonomic nervous system (ANS) is intact but immature.
   1. Infant has limited ability to control body temperature
   2. Infant's heart rate very sensitive to parasympathetic stimulation

C. Infant's behavior primarily reflexive
   1. Neurologic exam consists of evaluating reflexes
   2. Babinski's reflex normal in infant; disappears after child begins to walk

D. Peripheral neurons not myelinated at birth

   1. Myelinization occurs in later infancy
   2. Motor skill development depends on myelinization

E. Infant usually demonstrates a dominance of flexor muscles; extremities will be flexed even when infant is sleeping.

F. Small tremors are normal findings during first few months of life: not considered seizure activity if occurring in response to environmental stimuli, if they are not accompanied by abnormal eye movements, and if movements cease with passive flexion.

Eye and Vision

A. Vision changes as the eye and eye muscles undergo physiologic change.

B. Visual function becomes more organized.
   1. Binocular vision developed by 4 months
   2. Maturation of eye muscles by 1 year
      a. Nystagmus common in infant
      b. Strabismus (eyes out of alignment when fixating on an object): due to imbalance in extraocular muscles, common up to 6 months
   3. Visual acuity changes
      a. 16 weeks: 20/50 to 20/100
      b. 1 year: 20/50+
      c. 2 years: 20/40
      d. 3 years: 20/30
      e. 4 years: nearly 20/20

Ear and Hearing

A. Hearing is fully developed at birth.

B. Abnormal physical structure of ears may indicate genetic problems (low-set ears often associated with renal problems or mental retardation).

ASSESSMENT

History

A. Most important part of neurologic evaluation

B. Family history: seizure disorders, degenerative neurologic diseases, mental retardation, sensory defects

C. History of pregnancy: maternal illness, placental dysfunction, fetal movements, nuchal cord, intrapartal fetal distress, prematurity, meconium staining, Apgar scores
D. Child's health history: delayed motor or speech development, hypotonia, seizures, childhood illnesses
E. Parental concerns: development, vision, hearing

Physical Examination

A. Inspect size and shape of head: note fontanels in infants, chart head circumference on growth chart.
B. Observe posture and activity: note flexed posture versus hypotonia or opisthotonos, symmetry of movement of extremities, excessive tremors or twitching, abnormal eye movements, ineffective suck or swallow, high-pitched cry.
C. Observe respiratory pattern: note apnea, ataxic breathing, asymmetric or paradoxic chest movement.
D. Determine developmental level with DDST.
E. Vision tests
  1. Binocularity
    a. Corneal light reflex test: performed by shining a light at the bridge of the nose as the child looks straight ahead; light reflex should fall at the same point in both pupils; deviation indicates strabismus
    b. Cover test: performed by getting the child to fixate on an object and then covering one eye and uncovering that eye quickly to determine if child remains fixated on that object; normally both eyes will remain fixated without drifting.
  2. Visual acuity
    a. Snellen E chart for preschoolers
    b. Snellen alphabet chart for older children
  3. Peripheral vision
  4. Color vision
F. Auditory tests
  1. Audiometry: perception of sound
  2. Tympanometry: conduction of sound in middle ear
  3. Crib-o-gram: neonatal motor response to sound
  4. Conduction tests

Laboratory/Diagnostic Tests

A. Same tests that are used in adults are used in children
B. Child should be carefully prepared and informed of what to expect during the test
C. Sedation may be required for tests requiring child to be immobile for extended period.
D. Positioning and immobilization is crucial to the success of lumbar puncture.

ANALYSIS

Nursing diagnoses for the child with a disorder of the nervous system may include
A. Impaired physical mobility
B. Alteration in thought processes
C. Self-care deficit
D. Sensory-perceptual alteration
E. Knowledge deficit
F. Alteration in health maintenance
G. Alteration in comfort: pain
H. Ineffective family coping: compromised or disabling
I. Potential for injury
J. Impaired verbal communication
K. Potential for impairment of skin integrity

PLANNING AND IMPLEMENTATION

Goals

A. Child will be protected from injury.
B. Child will be free from signs and symptoms of increased ICP.
C. Normal respiratory function will be maintained.
D. Optimum developmental level will be achieved.
E. Family will be able to care for child at home.

Interventions

Care of the Child with Increased Intracranial Pressure

A. General information
  1. Intracranial volume and pressure can increase as a result of
    a. Increased brain volume (cerebral edema)
    b. Increased cerebral blood volume (hematoma or hemorrhage)
    c. Increased cerebrospinal fluid (CSF) volume (hydrocephalus)
    d. Mass lesions (tumors)
  2. Herniation of brain tissue: most serious complication of increased ICP; may result in life-threatening deterioration of vital functions
B. Medical management
  1. Directed towards reducing intracranial volume and controlling underlying disorder
  2. Drug therapy
    a. Osmotic diuretics (mannitol, glycerol) to reduce acute brain edema; for short-term use only
    b. Corticosteroids (dexamethasone) to reduce brain swelling
      1) may be used for longer periods than osmotic diuretics
      2) antacids may be given concomitantly to prevent gastric irritation
  3. Fluid restriction, hyperventilation, temperature regulation may all be used to control increased ICP
  4. Surgery: if increased ICP caused by obstruction to CSF, shunt procedures may be performed
C. Assessment findings
  1. Infants
    a. Lethargy, poor feeding, anorexia or vomiting
    b. High-pitched cry
    c. Tense, bulging fontanel; increased head circumference; separation of cranial sutures

2. Children
   a. Anorexia, nausea, vomiting, irritability or lethargy
   b. Headache, blurred vision, papilledema
   c. Separation of cranial sutures
3. Late signs
   a. Altered LOC
   b. Pupil dilation and sluggish response to light
   c. Tachycardia then bradycardia
   d. Altered respiratory rate then apnea
D. Nursing interventions
   1. Administer medications as ordered.
      a. With osmotic diuretics, monitor fluid and electrolyte balance carefully.
      b. With corticosteroids, monitor for signs of gastric bleeding.
   2. Monitor hydration status carefully.
      a. Administer IV fluids as ordered, assess carefully for fluid overload.
      b. Assess for fluid and electrolyte imbalances.
      c. Monitor for hypovolemic shock if on strict fluid restriction.
   3. Assist with hyperventilation if ordered; monitor arterial blood gases (ABGs).
   4. Assist with reduction of body temperature as needed.
      a. Administer antipyretics as ordered.
      b. Use sponge baths, hypothermia pads as necessary.
   5. Monitor LOC and behavioral/mental changes carefully.
   6. Elevate head of bed 30°–45° unless contraindicated (e.g., possible spinal injury); keep neck in neutral alignment and avoid flexion.
   7. Arrange nursing care activities to minimize stimulation and keep environment as quiet as possible.
   8. Prepare for shunt surgery (page 303) if needed.

EVALUATION

A. Head growth progresses normally, fontanels are flat, and seizure activity is controlled.
B. Child maintains an appropriate activity level.
C. Child is placed in an appropriate special program or school, if needed.
D. Parents demonstrate ability to perform treatments and administer appropriate medications.

DISORDERS OF THE NERVOUS SYSTEM

Disorders of the Brain and Spinal Cord

Hydrocephalus

A. General information
   1. Increased amount of CSF within the ventricles of the brain
   2. May be caused by obstruction of CSF flow or by overproduction or inadequate reabsorption of CSF

3. May result from congenital malformation or be secondary to injury, infection, or tumor
4. Classification
   a. Noncommunicating: flow of CSF from ventricles to subarachnoid space is obstructed.
   b. Communicating: flow is not obstructed, but CSF is inadequately reabsorbed in subarachnoid space.
B. Assessment findings: depend on age at onset, amount of CSF in brain
   1. Infant to 2 years: enlarging head size; bulging, nonpulsating fontanels; downward rotation of eyes; separation of cranial sutures; poor feeding, vomiting, lethargy, irritability; high-pitched cry and abnormal muscle tone
   2. Older children: changes in head size less common; signs of increased ICP (vomiting, ataxia, headache) common; alteration in consciousness and papilledema late signs
   3. Diagnostic tests
      a. Serial transilluminations detect increases in light areas
      b. CT scan shows dilated ventricles as well as presence of tumor; with dye injection shows course of CSF flow
C. Nursing interventions: provide care for the child with increased ICP and for the child undergoing shunt procedures.

Shunts

A. General information
   1. Insertion of a flexible tube into the lateral ventricle of the brain
   2. Catheter is then threaded under the skin and the distal end positioned in the peritoneum (most common type) or the right atrium; a subcutaneous pump may be attached to ensure patency.
   3. Shunt drains excess CSF from the lateral ventricles of the brain in communicating or noncommunicating hydrocephalus; fluid is then absorbed by the peritoneum or enters the general circulation via the right atrium
B. Nursing interventions
   1. Provide routine pre-op care with special attention to monitoring neurologic status.
   2. Provide post-op care.
      a. Maintain patency of the shunt.
         1) position child off the operative site.
         2) pump the shunt as ordered.
         3) observe for signs of infection of the incision.
         4) observe for signs of increased ICP.
         5) position the child flat or with head slightly elevated, as ordered.
   3. Instruct parents regarding
      a. Wound care, positioning of infant, and how to pump the shunt
      b. Signs of infection
      c. Signs of increased ICP
      d. Need for repeated shunt revisions as child grows or if shunt becomes blocked or infected
      e. Expected level of developmental functioning
      f. Availability of support groups and community agencies.

Spina Bifida

A. General information
   1. Failure of posterior vertebral arches to fuse during embryologic development
   2. Incidence: 2 in 1,000 infants in the U.S.
   3. Although actual cause is unknown, frequency of the defect is increased if a sibling has had a neural tube defect; radiation, viral, and environmental factors have been suggested as causative.
   4. Site of the lesion and the contents of the spinal column that may protrude through the defect vary
      a. Lumbosacral vertebrae are the most common sites.
      b. Cervical and thoracic lesions are less common.

B. Types
   1. *Spina bifida occulta*
      a. Spinal cord and meninges remain in the normal anatomic position.
      b. Defect may not be visible, or may be identified by a dimple or a tuft of hair on the spine.
      c. Child is asymptomatic or may have slight neuromuscular deficit.
      d. No treatment needed if asymptomatic; otherwise treatment aimed at specific symptoms.
   2. *Spina bifida cystica*
      a. *Meningocele*
         1) sac (meninges) filled with spinal fluid protrudes through opening in spinal canal; sac is covered with thin skin.
         2) no nerves in sac
         3) no motor or sensory loss
         4) good prognosis after surgery
      b. *Myelomeningocele/meningomyelocele*
         1) same as meningocele except there are spinal nerves in the sac (herniation of dura and meninges).
         2) child will have sensory/motor deficit below site of the lesion.
         3) 80% of these children have multiple handicaps.

C. Medical management
   1. Surgery
      a. Closure of the sac within 48 hours of birth to prevent infection and leakage of fluid and for cosmetic reasons
      b. Shunt procedure if accompanying hydrocephalus
      c. Urinary diversion/colostomy for incontinence
      d. Orthopedic procedures to correct defects of hips, knees, or feet
   2. Drug therapy
      a. Antibiotics for prevention of meningitis, urinary tract infections (UTI), pneumonitis
      b. Bethanechol (Urecholine), propantheline (Pro-Banthine), phenoxybenzamine (Dibenzyline), ephedrine for prevention of urinary complications
   3. Immobilization (casts, braces, traction) for defects of hips, knees, or feet

D. Assessment findings
   1. Depend on site and extent of defect

2. Sac covering: skin may be intact, or may be open and leaking fluid
3. Motor/sensory involvement may include
   a. Voluntary movement of lower extremities
   b. Withdrawal of lower extremities or crying after pin prick
   c. Paralysis of lower extremities
   d. Joint deformities
   e. Hydrocephalus
   f. Bladder/bowel incontinence
4. Diagnostic tests
   a. Prenatal
      1) ultrasound image of the pregnant uterus shows fetal spinal defect and sac
      2) amniocentesis: increased alpha-fetoprotein (AFP) level prior to 18th week of gestation
   b. Postpartal
      1) x-ray of spine shows vertebral defect; x-ray of skull may show hydrocephalus
      2) myelogram shows extent of neural defect
      3) encephalogram may show hydrocephalus
      4) urinalysis, culture and sensitivity (C&S) may identify organism and indicate appropriate antibacterial therapy
      5) BUN may be increased
      6) creatinine clearance rate may be decreased

E. Nursing interventions
   1. Prevent trauma to the sac.
      a. Cover with sterile dressing moistened with normal saline.
      b. Position infant on abdomen with legs abducted.
      c. Keep the area free from contamination by urine or feces.
      d. Inspect the sac for intactness or signs of infection.
      e. Administer antibiotics as ordered.
   2. Prevent complications.
      a. Observe for signs of hydrocephalus, meningitis, joint deformities.
      b. In infants bladder may be emptied by Credé method.
      c. Administer medications to prevent urinary complications as ordered.
      d. Perform passive ROM exercises to lower extremities.
   3. Provide adequate nutrition: adapt diet and feeding techniques according to the child's position.
   4. Provide sensory stimulation.
      a. Adjust objects for visual stimulation according to child's position.
      b. Provide stimulation for other senses.
   5. Provide emotional support to parents/family.
   6. Provide patient teaching and discharge planning to parents concerning
      a. Wound care
      b. Application and care of immobilization devices
      c. Signs of complications
      d. Medication regimen: schedule, dosage, effects and side effects
      e. Availability of appropriate support groups/community agencies/genetic counseling.

Brain Tumors

A. General information
   1. A space-occupying mass in the brain tissue; may be benign or malignant
   2. Males affected more often; peak age 3–7 years
   3. Second most prevalent type of cancer in children
   4. Cause unknown; genetic and environmental factors may play a role; familial tendency for brain tumors, which are found with preexisting neurocutaneous disorders.
   5. Two-thirds of all pediatric brain tumors are beneath the tentorium cerebelli (in the posterior fossa), often involving the cerebellum or brain stem.
   6. Three-fourths of brain tumors in children are gliomas (medulloblastoma and astrocytoma).
B. Types
   1. *Medulloblastoma:* higly malignant tumor usually found in cerebellum; runs a rapid course
      a. Findings include increased ICP plus unsteady walk, ataxia, anorexia, early morning vomiting
      b. Treated with radiation since complete removal is impossible
   2. *Astrocytoma:* a benign, cystic, slow-growing tumor usually found in cerebellum
      a. Onset of symptoms is insidious.
      b. Findings include focal disturbances, papilledema, optic nerve atrophy, blindness.
   3. *Ependymoma:* a usually benign tumor that arises in the ventricles of the brain causing noncommunicating hydrocephalus and damage (by pressure) to other vital tissues of the brain
   4. *Craniopharyngioma:* tumor that arises from remnants of embryonic tissue near the pituitary gland in the sella turcica, causes pressure on the third ventricle
      a. Decreased secretion of ADH causes diabetes insipidus (these children may need Pitressin).
      b. Additional symptoms include altered growth pattern, visual difficulties, difficulty regulating body temperature.
   5. *Brain stem glioma:* slow growing tumor, indicated by cranial nerve palsies, ataxia
C. Medical management: see also Pediatric Oncology (page 356)
   1. Surgery: some tumors entirely or partially resected; others are not amenable to surgery because of proximity to vital brain parts
   2. Radiation therapy: often used to shrink tumors
   3. Chemotherapy: vincristine, lomustine (CCNU), procarbazine, intrathecal methotrexate; not as effective with brain tumors as with other childhood cancers
D. Assessment findings
   1. Symptoms dependent on location and type of tumor
   2. A definite diagnosis is difficult in children because of the elasticity of child's skull and generally poor coordination of the young child.
   3. A decrease in school performance may be the first sign.
   4. Increased ICP
      a. Morning headache
      b. Morning vomiting without nausea; vomiting without relation to feeding schedule; projectile vomiting
      c. Personality changes
      d. Diploplia
         1) difficult to assess in young children
         2) observe child for tilting of head, closing or covering one eye, rubbing the eyes, or impaired eye-hand coordination
      e. Papilledema: a late sign
      f. Increased blood pressure with decreased pulse: also a late sign
      g. Cranial enlargement
         1) more readily noticeable prior to 18 months when suture lines are still open
         2) bulging, tense, pulsating fontanels
         3) widened suture lines
         4) 90% or more on head circumference chart
   5. Focal signs and symptoms
      a. Ataxia
         1) in cerebellar tumors
         2) may not be readily identified because of uncoordinated movements of young children
      b. Muscle strength
         1) weakness with cerebellar tumors
         2) weakness, spasticity, and paralysis of lower extremities with cerebrum or brainstem tumors
         3) change in handedness, posture, or manual coordination: may be early signs
      c. Head tilt
         1) in posterior fossa tumors
         2) early sign of visual impairment
         3) associated with nuchal rigidity
         4) due to traction on the dura
      d. Ocular signs
         1) nystagmus: corresponds to the same side as the infratentorial lesion
         2) diploplia/strabismus: from palsy of cranial nerve VI with brain stem glioma or increased ICP
         3) visual field deficit (child does not react to activity on periphery of vision): with craniopharingiomas
      e. Seizures: with cerebral tumors
   6. Diagnostic tests
      a. Skull x-ray reveals presence and location of tumor
      b. CT scan (with or without contrast dye) reveals position, consistency, size of tumor, and effect on surrounding tissue
      c. EEG may show seizure activity
E. Nursing interventions
   1. Obtain baseline vital signs and perform thorough neurologic assessment; monitor vital signs and neurologic status frequently.
   2. Prevent injury/complications.
      a. Institute seizure precautions.
      b. Monitor for fluid and electrolyte imbalance from vomiting.
      c. Observe for increased ICP.

d. Provide safety measures (bed rails up).
3. Promote comfort/relief of headache.
    a. Decrease environmental stimuli.
    b. Administer analgesics as ordered.
4. Prevent constipation (straining increases ICP).
    a. Provide appropriate foods and fluids as ordered.
    b. Provide stool softeners as ordered.
    c. Avoid enemas, which increase ICP.
5. Provide care for the child undergoing brain surgery (below).
6. Provide care for the child undergoing radiation or chemotherapy.
7. Provide patient teaching and discharge planning concerning
    a. Diagnostic tests (instruction needs to be appropriate to the child's developmental level)
        1) machines will make clicking sounds
        2) wires attached to the head for an EEG will not electrocute child
        3) head is immobilized for a CT scan
        4) the use of contrast dye and expected sensations if used
        5) need to lie still with the technician out of the room for most tests (younger children will be sedated for fuller cooperation)
    b. Importance of family discussion of fears/anxiety about surgery and prognosis
    c. Need to assist in implementing child's interaction with peers
    d. Available support groups and community agencies.

Brain Surgery

A. General information
    1. Indications
        a. Removal of a tumor
        b. Evacuation of a hematoma
        c. Removal of a foreign body or skull fragments resulting from trauma
        d. Aspiration of an abscess
        e. Insertion of a shunt
B. Nursing interventions: preoperative
    1. Assess the child's understanding of the procedure; have the child draw a picture, tell a story; observe doll play.
    2. Explain the procedure in terms according to the child's developmental level.
    3. Allow the child to visit the operating room/intensive care unit, if permitted, depending on the child's emotional and developmental levels.
    4. Explain that pre-op symptoms such as headache and ataxia may be temporarily aggravated.
    5. Advise child/parents that blindness may result, depending on the location of the tumor.
    6. Inform the child/parents that the head will be shaved; long hair may be saved; hats or scarves may be used to cover the head once the dressings are removed.

7. Support the child/family if a tumor cannot be totally removed.
8. Provide instruction about radiation and chemotherapy (may need to be delayed since detail may be overwhelming).
9. Explain to the child/parents about the post-op dressing, monitoring devices, and possibility of facial edema.
C. Nursing interventions: postoperative
    1. Prevent injury/complications.
        a. Monitor vital signs and neuro status frequently until stable.
        b. Apply hypothermia blanket as ordered.
        c. Assess respiratory status/signs of infection.
        d. Observe the dressing for discharge/hemorrhage.
        e. Close or cover eyes, apply ice, instill saline drops or artificial tears.
        f. Position as ordered according to the location of the tumor and type of surgery.
        g. Assess for increased ICP.
        h. Institute seizure precautions.
    2. Promote comfort.
        a. Decrease environmental stimuli.
        b. Administer analgesics as ordered, first assessing LOC.
    3. Promote adequate nutrition.
        a. Administer fluids as ordered.
        b. Monitor I&O.
        c. Provide diet as ordered.
    4. Provide emotional support and encourage child/family to discuss prognosis.
    5. Provide patient teaching and discharge planning concerning
        a. Wound care
        b. Signs of increased ICP
        c. Activity level
        d. Sensation and time period of hair growth
        e. Peer acceptance
        f. Radiation/chemotherapy, if indicated
        g. Availability of support groups/community agencies.

Neuroblastoma

A. General inforamtion
    1. A highly malignant tumor that develops from embryonic neural crest tissue; arises anywhere along the craniospinal axis, usually from the adrenal gland
    2. Incidence
        a. One in 10,000
        b. Males slightly more affected
        c. From infancy to age 4
    3. Staging
        a. Stage I: tumor confined to the organ of origin
        b. Stage II: tumor extends beyond primary site but not across midline
        c. Stage III: tumor extends beyond midline
        d. Stage IV: tumor metastasizes to skeleton (bone marrow), soft tissue (liver), and lymph nodes
B. Medical management: depends on the staging of tumor and

age of child; includes surgery, radiation therapy, chemotherapy

C. Assessment findings vary, depending on the tumor site and stage
1. If in the abdomen, may initially resemble Wilm's tumor
2. Local signs and symptoms caused by pressure of the tumor on surrounding tissue
3. Metastatic manifestations
    a. Ocular: supraorbital ecchymosis, periorbital edema, exophthalmos
    b. Cervical or supraclavicular lymphadenopathy
    c. Bone pain: may or may not occur with bone metastasis
    d. Nonspecific complaints: pallor, anorexia, weight loss, irritability, weakness
4. Diagnosis usually made after metastasis has occurred
5. Diagnostic tests
    a. X-rays of the head, chest, or abdomen reveal presence of primary tumor or metastases
    b. IVP: if tumor is adrenal, shows a downward displacement of the kidney on the affected side
    c. Bone marrow aspiration: to rule out metastasis, neuroblasts have a clumping pattern
    d. CBC: RBCs and platelets decreased
    e. Coagulation studies: abnormal due to thrombocytopenia
    f. Catecholamine excretion: VMA levels in urine increased
        1) child must not ingest vanilla, chocolate, bananas, or nuts for 3 days prior to the test
        2) 24-hour urine specimen needed

D. Nursing interventions: same as for leukemia (page **321**) and brain tumors.

Meningitis

See page 50.

Encephalitis

See page 50.

Reye's Syndrome

A. General information
1. An acute encephalopathy with fatty degeneration of the liver
2. Reye's syndrome is a true pediatric emergency: cerebral complications may reach an irreversible state.
3. Major cause of death in children ages 2–10 years
4. Increased ICP secondary to cerebral edema is major factor contributing to morbidity and mortality.
5. Etiology unknown

B. Medical management
1. Proper initial staging essential
2. Treatment is supportive, based on stage of coma and level of blood ammonia.
3. Treatment should take place in a pediatric intensive care unit.

C. Assessment findings
1. Child appears to be recovering from a viral illness, such as influenza or chickenpox, during which salicylates have been administered; symptoms then appear that follow a definite pattern, which has led to clinical staging.
    a. Stage I: sudden onset of persistent vomiting, fatigue, listlessness
    b. Stage II: personality and behavior changes, disorientation, confusion, hyperreflexia
    c. Stage III: coma, decorticate posturing
    d. Stage IV: deeper coma, decerebrate rigidity
    e. Stage V: seizures, absent deep tendon reflexes, respiratory reflexes, flaccid paralysis
2. Pathophysiologic changes include
    a. Increased free fatty acid level
    b. Hyperammonemia due to reduction of enzyme that converts ammonia to urea
    c. Impaired liver function
    d. Structural changes of mitochondria in muscle and brain tissue
    e. Significant swelling of the brain

D. Nursing interventions (depend on stage)
1. Stage I: assess hydration status: monitor skin turgor, mucous membranes, I&O, urine specific gravity; maintain IV therapy.
2. Stages I-V: assess neurologic status: monitor LOC, pupils, motor coordination, extremity movement, orientation, posturing, seizure activity.
3. Stages II-V
    a. Assess respiratory status: note changing rate and pattern, presence of circumoral cyanosis, restlessness, agitation.
    b. Assess circulatory status: frequent vital signs, note neck vein distension, skin color and temperature, abnormal heart sounds.
    c. Support child/family.
        1) explain all treatments and procedures.
        2) incorporate family members in treatment as applicable.
        3) organize regular family and patient care conferences.
        4) use support services as needed.
    d. Provide additional parental and community education to assure early recognition and treatment.

Seizure Disorders

A. General information
1. *Seizures*: recurrent sudden changes in consciousness, behavior, sensations, and/or muscular activities beyond voluntary control that are produced by excess neuronal discharge
2. *Epilepsy*: chronic recurrent seizures
3. Incidence higher in those with family history of idopathic seizures
4. Cause unknown in 75% of epilepsy cases

5. Seizures may be symptomatic or acquired, caused by
   a. Structural or space-occupying lesion (tumors, subdural hematomas)
   b. Metabolic abnormalities (hypoglycemia, hypocalcemia, hyponatremia)
   c. Infection (meningitis, encephalitis)
   d. Encephalopathy (lead poisoning, pertussis, Reye's syndrome)
   e. Degenerative diseases (Tay-Sachs)
   f. Congenital CNS defects (hydrocephalus)
   g. Vascular problems (intracranial hemorrhage)
6. Pathophysiology
   a. Normally neurons send out messages in electrical impulses periodically, and the firing of individual neurons is regulated by an inhibitory feedback loop mechanism
   b. With seizures, many more neurons than normal fire in a synchronous fashion in a particular area of the brain; the energy generated overcomes the inhibitory feedback mechanism
7. Classification (Table 3.3)
   a. Generalized: initial onset in both hemispheres, usually involves loss of consciousness and bilateral motor activity
   b. Partial: begins in focal area of brain and symptoms are appropriate to a dysfunction of that area; may progress into a generalized seizure, further subdivided into simple partial or complex partial

B. Medical management
   1. Drug therapy
      a. Phenytoin (Dilantin)
         1) often used with phenobarbital for its potentiating effect
         2) inhibits spread of electrical discharge
         3) side effects include gum hyperplasia, hirsutism, ataxia, gastric distress, nystagmus, anemia, sedation
      b. Phenobarbital: elevates the seizure threshhold and inhibits the spread of electrical discharge
   2. Nutrition: ketogenic diet (fasting causes decrease in seizure activity)
   3. Surgery: to remove the tumor, hematoma, or epileptic focus
C. Assessment findings
   1. Clinical picture varies with type of seizure (see Table 3.3)
   2. Diagnostic tests
      a. Blood studies to rule out lead poisoning, hypoglycemia, infection, or electrolyte imbalances
      b. Lumbar puncture to rule out infection or trauma
      c. Skull x-rays, CT scan, or ultrasound of the head, brain scan, arteriogram, or pneumoencephalogram to detect any pathologic defects
      d. EEG may detect abnormal wave patterns characteristic of different types of seizures
         1) child may be awake or asleep; sedation is ordered

Table 3.3   Types of Seizures

Type of Seizure	Clinical Findings
Generalized seizures	
Major motor seizure (grand mal)	May be preceded by aura; tonic and clonic phases. *Tonic phase:* limbs contract or stiffen; pupils dilate and eyes roll up and to one side; glottis closes causing noise on exhalation; may be incontinent; occurs at same time as loss of consciousness; lasts 20–40 seconds *Clonic phase:* repetitive movements, increased mucus production; slowly tapers Seizure ends with postictal period of confusion, drowsiness
Absence seizure (petit mal)	Usually nonorganic brain damage present; must be differentiated from day dreaming. Sudden onset, with twitching or rolling of eyes; lasts a few seconds.
Myoclonic seizure	Associated with brain damage, may be precipitated by tactile or visual sensations. May be generalized or local. Brief flexor muscle spasm; may have arm extension, trunk flexion. Single group of muscles affected; involuntary muscle contractions; myoclonic jerks.
Akinetic seizure (tonic)	Related to organic brain damage. Sudden brief loss of postural tone, and temporary loss of consciousness.
Febrile seizure	Common in 5% of population under 5, familial, nonprogressive; does not generally result in brain damage. Seizure occurs only when fever is rising. EEG is normal 2 weeks after seizure.
Partial seizures	
Psychomotor seizure	May follow trauma, hypoxia, drug use. Purposeful but inappropriate, repetitive motor acts. Aura present; dreamlike state.
Simple partial seizure	Seizure confined to one hemisphere of brain. No loss of consciousness. May be motor, sensory, or autonomic symptoms.
Complex partial seizure	Begins in focal area but spreads to both hemispheres. Impairs consciousness. May be preceded by an aura.
Status epilepticus	Usually refers to generalized grand mal seizures. Seizure is prolonged (or there are repeated seizures without regaining consciousness) and unresponsive to treatment. Can result in decreased oxygen supply and possible cardiac arrest.

and child may be sleep deprived the night before the test

    2) evocative stimulation: flashing strobe light, clicking sounds, hyperventilation

D. Nursing interventions

  1. During seizure activity

    a. Protect from injury.

      1) prevent falling, gently support head.

      2) decrease external stimuli; do not restrain.

      3) do not use tongue blades (they add additional stimuli).

      4) loosen tight clothing.

    b. Keep airway open.

      1) place in side-lying position.

      2) suction excess mucous.

    c. Observe and record seizure.

      1) note any preictal aura.

        a) affective signs: fear, anxiety

        b) psychosensory signs: hallucinations

        c) cognitive signs: "déjà-vu" symptoms

      2) note nature of the ictal phase.

        a) symmetry of movement

        b) response to stimuli; LOC

        c) respiratory pattern

      3) note postictal response: amount of time it takes child to orient to time and place; sleepiness.

  2. Provide patient teaching and discharge planning concerning

    a. Care during a seizure

    b. Need to continue drug therapy

    c. Safety precautions/activity limitations

    d. Need to wear Medic-Alert identification bracelet or carry identification card

    e. Potential behavioral changes and school problems

    f. Availability of support groups/community agencies

    g. How to assist the child in explaining disorder to peers.

Cerebral Palsy (CP)

A. General information

  1. Neuromuscular disorder resulting from damage to or altered structure of the part of the brain responsible for controlling motor function

  2. Incidence: 1.5–5 in 1,000 live births

  3. May be caused by a variety of factors resulting in damage to the CNS; possible causes include

    a. Prenatally: genetic, altered neurologic development, or trauma or anoxia to mother (toxemia, rubella, accidents)

    b. Perinatally: during the birth process (drugs at delivery, precipitate delivery, fetal distress, breech deliveries with delay)

    c. Postnatally: kernicterus or head trauma (child falls out of crib or is hit by a car)

B. Medical management

  1. Drug therapy

    a. Antianxiety agents

    b. Skeletal muscle relaxants

    c. Local nerve blocks

  2. Physical/occupational therapy

  3. Speech/audiology therapy

  4. Surgery: muscle- and tendon-releasing procedures

C. Assessment findings: disease itself does not progress once established; progressive complications, however, cause changes in signs and symptoms

  1. Spasticity: exaggerated hyperactive reflexes (increased muscle tone, increase in stretch reflex, scissoring of legs, poorly coordinated body movements for voluntary activities)

    a. Occurs with pyramidal tract lesion

    b. Found in 40% of all CP

    c. Results in contractures

    d. Also affects ability to speak: altered quality and articulation

    e. Loud noise or sudden movement causes reaction with increased spasm

    f. No parachute reflex to protect self when falling

  2. Athetosis: constant involuntary, purposeless, slow, writhing motions

    a. Occurs with extrapyramidal tract (basal ganglia) lesion

    b. Found in 40% of all CP

    c. Athetosis disappears during sleep, therefore contractures do not develop

    d. Movements increase with increase in physical or emotional stress

    e. Also affects facial muscles

  3. Ataxia: disturbance in equilibrium; diminished righting reflex (lack of balance, poor coordination, dizziness, hypotonia)

    a. Occurs with extrapyramidal tract (cerebellar) lesion

    b. Found in 10% of all CP

    c. Muscles and reflexes are normal

  4. Tremor: repetitive rhythmic involuntary contractions of flexor and extensor muscles

    a. Occurs with extrapyramidal tract (basal ganglia) lesion

    b. Found in 5% of all CP

    c. Interferes with performance of precise movements

    d. Often a mild disability

  5. Rigidity: resistance to flexion and extension resulting from simultaneous contraction of both agonist and antagonist muscle groups

    a. Occurs with extrapyramidal tract (basal ganglia) lesion

    b. Found in 5% of all CP

    c. Diminished or absent reflexes

    d. Potential for severe contractures

  6. Associated problems

    a. Mental retardation: the majority of CP patients are of normal or higher than average intelligence, but are unable to demonstrate it on standardized tests; 18%–50% have some form of mental retardation

b. Hearing loss in 13% of CP patients
c. Defective speech in 75% of CP patients
d. Dental anomalies (from muscle contractures)
e. Orthopedic problems from contractures or inability to mobilize
f. Visual disabilities in 28% due to poor muscle control
g. Disturbances of body image, touch, perception
h. Feelings of worthlessness
D. Nursing interventions
   1. Obtain a careful pregnancy, birth, and childhood history.
   2. Observe the child's behavior in various situations.
   3. Assist with activities of daily living (ADL), help child to learn as many self-care activities as possible; CP patients cannot do any task unless they are consciously aware of each step in the task; careful teaching and demonstration is essential.
   4. Provide a safe environment (safety helmet, padded crib).
   5. Provide physical therapy to prevent contractures and assist in mobility (braces if necessary).
   6. Provide patient teaching and discharge planning concerning
      a. Nature of disease: CP is a nonfatal, noncurable disorder
      b. Need for continued physical, occupational, and speech therapy
      c. Care of orthopedic devices
      d. Provision for child's return to school
      e. Availability of support groups/community agencies.

Tay-Sachs Disease

A. General information
   1. Degenerative brain disease, caused by absence of hexosaminidase A from all body tissues
   2. Autosomal recessive inheritance
   3. Occurs predominantly in children of Eastern European Jewish ancestry
   4. A fatal disease; death usually occurs before age 4
B. Assessment findings
   1. Progressive lethargy in a previously healthy 2- to 6-month-old infant
   2. Loss of developmental accomplishments
   3. Loss of visual acuity
   4. Hyperreflexia, decerebrate posturing, dysphagia, malnutrition, seizures
   5. Diagnosis confirmed by classic cherry red spot on the macula and by enzyme measurements in serum, amniotic fluid, or white cells
C. Nursing interventions
   1. Support parents at time of diagnosis; help them cope with feelings of anger and guilt.
   2. Assist parents in planning long-term care for the child.
   3. Provide genetic counseling and psychologic follow-up as needed

Disorders of the Eye

Blindness

A. Causes
   1. Genetic disorders: Tay-Sachs disease, inborn errors of metabolism
   2. Maternal infections during pregnancy: TORCH syndrome
   3. Perinatal: prematurity, retrolental fibroplasia
   4. Postnatal: trauma, childhood infections
B. Medical management: treatment of causative disorders
C. Assessment findings
   1. Vacant stare; obvious failure to look at objects
   2. Rubbing eyes, tilting head, examining objects very close to the eyes
   3. Does not reach for objects (over 4 months)
   4. Does not smile when mother smiles (over 3 months), but does smile in response to mother's voice
   5. Crawls or walks into furniture (over 12 months)
   6. Does not respond to the motions of others
   7. No concept of the look of an object, no concept of color or reflection of self
   8. Other senses become more keenly developed to compensate
   9. Unable to copy the actions of others; delayed motor milestones in accomplishing tasks but are not mentally handicapped
   10. Various degrees (20/200 O.U. and worse)
D. Nursing interventions
   1. For hospitalized child, find out parents' usual method of care.
   2. Encourage infant to be active; use multisensory stimulation (rocking, water play, musical toys, touch).
   3. From ages 2–5 arrange environment for maximum autonomy and safety (e.g., avoid foods with seeds and bones).
   4. Speak before you touch the child, announce what you plan to do.
   5. Do not rearrange furniture without first telling child.
   6. For a partially sighted child
      a. Encourage child to sit in front of classroom.
      b. Speak directly to child's face; do not look down or turn back.
      c. Use large print and provide adequate nonglare lighting.
      d. Use contrasting colors to help locate areas.
   7. Provide patient teaching and discharge planning concerning
      a. General child care, with adaptations for safety and developmental/functional level
      b. Availability of support groups/community agencies
      c. Special education programs
      d. Interaction with peers; assist child as necessary.

Conjunctivitis

A. General information: infection of membrane covering anterior surface of eye globe and inner surface of eyelid due to multiple causes (bacterial, viral, allergic)

B. Medical management: ophthalmic antibiotics, steroids, anesthetics

C. Assessment findings: weeping eye, reddened conjunctiva, sensitivity to light, eyelid stuck shut with exudate

D. Nursing interventions
1. Administer medications as ordered: apply ophthalmic antiobiotic ointments from inner to outer canthus (do not let container touch eye).
2. Provide patient teaching and discharge planning concerning measures to prevent spread of infection
    a. Very contagious if bacterial or viral; no school until antibiotics have been taken for 24–48 hours
    b. Should not share pillows, tissues, toys
    c. Good handwashing technique
    d. Medication regimen: schedule, dosage, desired and side effects.

Disorders of the Ear

Deafness

A. Causes
1. Conductive: interference in transmission from outer to middle ear from chronic otitis media, foreign bodies
2. Sensorineural: dysfunction of the inner ear (noise, including the noise of ICUs and ventilators); damage to cranial nerve VIII (from rubella, meningitis, drugs)

B. Medical management
1. Treatment of causative disorders
2. Speech/auditory therapy
3. Hearing aids
4. Surgery, depending on the cause

C. Assessment findings
1. Infant
    a. Fails to react to loud noises (does have a Moro reflex, but not to noise)
    b. Makes no attempt to locate sound
    c. Remains in babbling stage or ceases to babble
    d. Fails to develop speech
    e. Startled by sudden appearances
2. All children
    a. Responds only when speaker's lips are visible
    b. Cannot concentrate for long on visual images; constantly scans the surroundings for change
    c. May have slow motor development
    d. Appears puzzled, withdrawn, or strains to hear
    e. Uses high volume on TV/radio
3. Audiologic testing
    a. Slight hearing deficit: difficulty hearing faint sounds, very little interference in school, no speech defect, benefits from favorable seating
    b. Mild hearing deficit: can understand conversational speech at 3–5 feet when facing the other person,

decreased vocabulary, may miss half of class discussions
    c. Marked hearing deficit: misses most of conversation, hears loud noises, needs special education for language skills

D. Nursing interventions
1. Speak slowly, not more loudly.
2. Face child.
3. Get child's attention before talking; let child see you before performing any care.
4. Get feedback from child to make sure child has understood.
5. Decrease outside noises that could interfere with child's ability to discern what you are saying.
6. Be careful not to cover your mouth with hands.
7. Teach language through visual cues, touch, and kinesthetics.
8. Use body demonstrations or use doll play.
9. Provide appropriate stimulation (puppets and musical toys are inappropriate).
10. Provide patient teaching and discharge planning concerning
    a. General child care, with adaptation for safety and developmental/functional levels
    b. Availability of support groups/community agencies
    c. Special education programs
    d. Care and use of hearing aids
    e. Interaction with peers: assist child as needed.

Otitis Media

A. General information
1. Bacterial or viral infection of the middle ear
2. More common in infants and preschoolers as the ear canal is shorter and more horizontal than in older children; also found in children with cleft lip/palate
3. Blockage of eustachian tube causes lymphedema and accumulation of fluid in the middle ear

B. Medical management
1. Drug therapy
    a. Systemic and otic antibiotics
    b. Analgesics/antipyretics
2. Surgery: myringotomy, with or without insertion of tubes (incision into the tympanic membrane to relieve the pressure and drain the fluid)

C. Assessment findings
1. Dysfunction of eustachian tube
2. Ear infection usually related to respiratory infection
3. Increased middle ear pressure; bulging tympanic membrane
4. Pain; infant pulls or touches ear frequently
5. Irritability; cough; nasal congestion
6. Diagnostic tests: C&S of fluid reveals causative organism

D. Nursing interventions
1. Administer antibiotics as ordered, for a full 10-day course. When administering ear drops pull ear lobe up and back for older children and down and back for infants.

2. Administer acetaminophen for fever and discomfort.

3. Administer decongestants to relieve eustachian tube obstruction as ordered.

4. Provide care for child with a myringotomy tube insertion (day surgery)

   a. Use ear plugs if showering or washing child's hair; do not permit diving.

   b. Be aware that tubes may fall out for no reason.

5. Provide patient teaching and discharge planning concerning

   a. Medication administration

   b. Post-op care, depending on the type of surgery.

SAMPLE QUESTIONS

Louise was born with a myelomeningocele with accompanying hydrocephalus. She has had a shunt procedure to alleviate the hydrocephalus.

4. Louise should be placed in which of the following positions?
   o 1. Trendelenburg's
   o 2. On her back
   o 3. With her legs adducted
   o 4. On her abdomen

5. Which of the following signs indicate that Louise's shunt is functioning properly?
   o 1. The sunset sign
   o 2. A bulging anterior fontanel
   o 3. Decreasing daily head circumference
   o 4. Widened suture lines

Henry is a 13-year-old who has been diagnosed as having epilepsy.

6. A positive sign that Henry is taking his Dilantin properly is
   o 1. hair growth on his upper lip.
   o 2. absence of seizures.
   o 3. lowered hemoglobin and hematocrit.
   o 4. drowsiness.

The Cardiovascular System

VARIATIONS FROM THE ADULT

Fetal Circulation

A. Fetal circulation differs from adult circulation in several ways, and is designed to assure a high-oxygen blood supply to the brain and myocardium.

B. Characteristics
1. Placenta is the source of oxygen for the fetus.
2. Fetal lungs receive less than 10% of the blood volume; lungs do not exchange gas.
3. Right atrium of fetal heart is the chamber with the highest oxygen concentration.

C. Pattern of altered blood flow and facilitating structures
1. Blood is carried from the placenta through umbilical vein and enters the inferior vena cava through the *ductus venosus*.
2. This permits most of the highly oxygenated blood to go directly to the right atrium, bypassing the liver.
3. This right atrial blood flows directly into the left atrium through the *foramen ovale*, an opening between the right and left atria.
4. From the left atrium, blood flows into the left ventricle and aorta, through the subclavian arteries, to the cerebral and coronary arteries, resulting in the brain and heart receiving the most highly oxygenated blood.
5. Deoxygenated blood returns from the head and arms through the superior vena cava, enters the right atrium, and passes into the right ventricle.
6. Blood from the right ventricle flows into the pulmonary artery, but because fetal lungs are collapsed, the pressure in the pulmonary artery is very high.
7. Because pulmonary resistance is high, most of the blood passes into the distal aorta through the *ductus arteriosus*, which connects the pulmonary artery and the aorta distal to the origin of the subclavian arteries.
8. From the aorta, blood flows to the rest of the body.

Normal Circulatory Changes at Birth

A. When the umbilical cord is clamped or severed, the blood supply from the placenta is cut off, and oxygenation must then take place in the newborn's lungs.

B. As the lungs expand with air, the pulmonary artery pressure decreases and circulation to lungs increases.

C. Structural changes
1. Ductus venosus: after the umbilical cord is severed, flow through the ductus venosus decreases and eventually ceases; it constricts within 3–7 days after birth and eventually becomes ligamentum venosum.
2. Foramen ovale
   a. Functional closure of this valvelike opening occurs when pressure in the left atrium exceeds pressure in the right.
   b. Expansion of the pulmonary artery causes a drop in pulmonary artery pressure and in right atrial and ventricular pressure.
   c. At the same time there is increased pulmonary blood flow to the left atrium and increased aortic pressure (from clamping of the umbilical cord), which in turn raises left ventricular and left atrial pressure.
   d. Anatomic closure of the foramen ovale occurs within the first few weeks after birth with the deposit of fibrin.
3. Ductus arteriosus
   a. Increase in aortic blood flow increases aortic pressure and decreases right-to-left shunt through the ductus arteriosus; shunt becomes bidirectional.
   b. Increased pulmonary blood flow increases arterial oxygen, causing vasoconstriction of ductus arteriosus within hours of birth.
   c. Functional closure occurs when this constriction causes cessation of blood flow, usually by about 1 week after birth.
   d. Anatomic closure occurs when there is growth of fibrous tissue in the lumen of the ductus arteriosus, by 4–6 weeks.

Abnormal Circulatory Patterns after Birth

A. Normal blood flow in the child may be disrupted as a result of abnormal openings between the pulmonary and systemic circulations.

B. Any time there is a defect connecting systemic and pulmonary circulation, blood will go from high to low pressure (the path of least resistance).

1. Normally pressure is higher in the systemic circulation, so blood will be shunted from systemic to pulmonary (left to right).
2. An obstruction to pulmonary blood flow, however, may cause increased pressure proximal to the site of the obstruction.
3. With an obstruction to pulmonary blood flow, as well as an opening between ventricles, the blood flow may be right to left (if right-sided pressure exceeds left-sided pressure).

ASSESSMENT

History

A. Family history: congenital defects in siblings, history of genetic problems in family
B. History of pregnancy: maternal rubella or other problems of pregnancy
C. Child's health history
   1. Presenting problem: symptoms may include
      a. Frequent respiratory infections
      b. Intolerance to physical activity
      c. Fatigue with eating, poor feeding habits
      d. Poor weight gain
   2. Past medical history: rheumatic fever; associated chromosomal abnormalities (e.g., Down's syndrome)
   3. Ask about child's tendency to squat (helps to decrease the right-to-left cardiac shunt and increase oxygen delivery to tissues).

Physical Examination

A. Plot height and weight on growth chart; measure respiratory rate and rhythm; inspect for chest enlargement or asymmetry.
B. Inspect for presence of cyanosis: lips, mucous membranes, extremities.
C. Inspect for clubbing of fingers (thought to be caused by increased capillary formation and soft tissue fibrosis).
D. Observe for distended veins.
E. Palpate/percuss quality and symmetry of pulses, size of liver and spleen, presence of thrill over heart during expiration.
F. Auscultate for heart rate and rhythm.
G. Auscultate for abnormal heart sounds and murmurs; murmurs are caused by abnormal flow of blood between chambers or vessels; classified as
   1. Innocent: no anatomic or physiologic abnormality
   2. Functional: no anatomic defect, but may be caused by a physiologic abnormality
   3. Organic: caused by a structural abnormality
H. Measure blood pressure in both arm and thigh.
   1. In infants under 1 year, arm and thigh blood pressure should be the same.
   2. In children over 1 year, systolic pressure in leg is usually higher by 10–40 mm Hg.

3. A wide pulse pressure (greater than 50 mm Hg) or a narrow pulse pressure (less than 10 mm Hg) may be associated with a heart defect.

Laboratory/Diagnostic Tests

A. Hgb and Hct: polycythemia is often associated with cyanotic heart defects
B. Cardiac catheterization
   1. Femoral vein often used for access
   2. Catheter often threaded into the right side of the heart, since septal defects permit entry into the left side
   3. Nursing care: pretest
      a. Child's preparation should be based on developmental level, level of understanding, and past experiences.
      b. Use doll play and pictures as appropriate.
      c. Describe sensations child will feel in simple terms.
   4. Nursing care: post-test
      a. Check extremity color, temperature, and pulse.
      b. Check catheter site for bleeding and swelling.

ANALYSIS

Nursing diagnoses for the child with a disorder of the cardiovascular system may include
A. Activity intolerance
B. Alteration in cardiac output: decreased
C. Alteration in fluid volume
D. Impaired gas exchange
E. Altered tissue perfusion

PLANNING AND IMPLEMENTATION

Goals

A. Tissue will be adequately oxygenated.
B. Child will achieve normal growth and development milestones.
C. Child will be free from symptoms of complications of heart disease.
D. Parents will understand child's condition.
E. Parents will be able to care for child at home.

Interventions

Surgery

A. General information
   1. A group of closed-heart procedures to improve hemodynamics
   2. Surgery is palliative; symptoms can be decreased even though defect is not corrected
   3. Generally present less risk than corrective surgery
B. Types
   1. Systemic to pulmonary shunts: used to increase pulmonary blood flow

a. Blalock-Taussig: anastomosis of right or left subclavian artery to the pulmonary artery

b. Potts: anastomosis of descending aorta to the main pulmonary artery

c. Waterston: anastomosis of ascending aorta to the right pulmonary artery

2. Interatrial communication: used to increase mixing of arterial and venous blood in atria

a. Rashkind balloon septostomy: a balloon-tipped catheter is used to create hole in atrial septum

b. Blalock-Hanlon septectomy: surgical creation of a large septal defect

C. Nursing care: same as for cardiac surgery (see page 314).

EVALUATION

A. Child reaches optimum cardiac status.
1. Normal color
2. Easy respirations
3. Increased exercise tolerance
4. Satisfactory growth

B. No evidence of complications such as signs and symptoms of congestive heart failure (CHF), infection, or electrolyte imbalance.

C. Parents demonstrate ability to care for child, perform necessary treatments, and administer prescribed medications.

DISORDERS OF THE CARDIOVASCULAR SYSTEM

Congenital Heart Defects

See Figure 3.1.

Classification

A. Acyanotic heart defects
1. Oxygenated blood is shunted from the systemic to pulmonary circulation (left-to-right shunt) and blood leaving the aorta is completely oxygenated.
2. Increased blood volume on right side of heart results in hypertrophy of right ventricle.
3. Eventually, most acyanotic heart defects will result in CHF.

B. Cyanotic heart defects
1. Unoxygenated blood is shunted from the right to the left side of the heart where it mixes with oxygenated blood.
2. The blood pumped to the peripheral tissues has a much lower oxygen content than normal, causing the bluish color called cyanosis.

Acyanotic Heart Defects

A. General information and medical management
1. *Atrial septal defect (ASD):* abnormal hole in the septum between left and right atria causing a left-to-right shunt
a. May be patent foramen ovale
b. May be asymptomatic

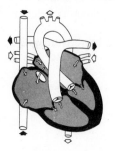

a. Atrial septal defect.

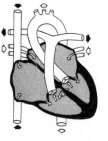

b. Ventricular septal defect.

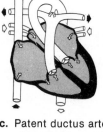

c. Patent ductus arteriosus.

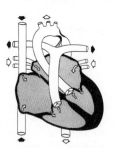

d. Coarctation of the aorta.

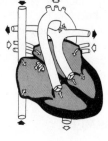

e. Transposition of the great arteries.

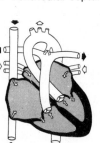

f. Truncus arteriosus.

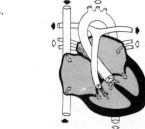

g. Tetralogy of Fallot.

Figure 3.1 Congenital heart defects.
(Courtesy of Ross Laboratories, Columbus, OH, from Clinical Aid, #7.)

c. Open-heart surgery to close the hole is performed in all females and in males with defects of significant size; usually performed at 4–6 years.

2. *Ventricular septal defect (VSD):* hole in the septum between ventricles causing a left-to-right shunt
   a. Most common congenital cardiac abnormality
   b. Small VSDs may be asymptomatic; larger holes may cause hypertrophy and potential failure of right ventricle and CHF.
   c. Surgical repair by sewing a graft over the hole is performed as early as possible.
   d. If an infant is a poor surgical risk, pulmonary artery banding (a constricting band around pulmonary artery to reduce blood flow and prevent heart failure) may be performed; complete repair is undertaken when the child is older.

3. *Patent ductus arteriosus (PDA):* failure to close at birth
   a. Allows oxygenated blood pumped into the aorta from the left ventricle to return to the lungs
   b. A small PDA may be asymptomatic; larger PDAs cause excess blood in lungs and volume overload, leading to CHF.
   c. In premature infants treatment with indomethacin (prostaglandin inhibitor) sometimes causes closure.
   d. Definitive surgery is ligation of PDA (closed-heart procedure), relatively safe at all ages.

4. *Pulmonary stenosis (pulmonic valve stenosis)*
   a. Abnormally narrowed valvular orifice
   b. If stenosis is mild to moderate children may be asymptomatic and require no treatment.
   c. More severe pulmonic valve stenosis can result in right ventricular hypertrophy and even hepatomegaly.
   d. Severe stenosis requires valvotomy.

5. *Aortic stenosis*
   a. Abnormally small valve orifice, valve may be bicuspid rather than tricuspid
   b. Mild to moderate stenosis may not produce symptoms, more severe stenosis produces left ventricular hypertrophy, left heart failure, decreased cardiac output.
   c. Valvotomy is preferred treatment for children, but valve replacement may be necessary later.

6. *Coarctation of aorta*
   a. Narrowing of the aorta usually just beyond the left subclavian artery
   b. Causes a significant decrease in blood flow to abdomen and legs, with majority of blood shunted to head and arms
   c. Clinical manifestations depend on degree of narrowing, may include
      1) blood and pulse pressure higher in arms than legs; high pulse pressure in carotid and radial pulses; low pulse pressure in femoral pulses
      2) warm upper body and cool lower body, nosebleeds and headaches (from increased blood pressure in top half of body)
      3) predisposition to strokes
   d. Surgical treatment dependent on location of coarctation

7. *Endocardial cushion defects*
   a. Altered development of the core of the heart from which septum and valves originate
   b. Causes mixing of oxygenated and unoxygenated blood in the heart chambers
   c. Most common cardiac defects in Down's Syndrome

B. Assessment findings
   1. Signs of CHF: respiratory distress, diaphoresis, congested cough (see also Congestive Heart Failure, page 73)
   2. Increased blood flow to lungs leads to right-sided heart failure
   3. Enlargement of liver (hepatomegaly) due to backup of blood
   4. Increase in pulse and respiratory rate

C. Nursing interventions
   1. Administer medications as ordered.
      a. Digoxin (see Table 2.17, Antiarrhythmic Drugs)
         1) take apical pulse for 1 full minute; do not give if pulse is less than 100.
         2) monitor carefully for digitalis toxicity.
      b. Lasix (see Table 2.18, Antihypertensive Drugs)
         1) monitor I&O carefully, weigh diapers.
         2) restrict fluids as ordered.
         3) weigh daily on same scale.
   2. Monitor vital signs.
   3. Prevent cold stress; maintain body temperature.
   4. Provide adequate rest.
      a. Provide passive age-appropriate play.
      b. Organize care to decrease child's energy expenditure.
      c. Try to anticipate child's needs; prevent crying.
      d. In infants, use soft nipple to decrease work during feeding; gavage feedings may be necessary.
   5. Position child properly.
      a. Use orthopneic position; elevate head and trunk.
      b. Allow child to squat if desired.
   6. Give high-calorie foods that are easy to ingest and digest.
   7. Prevent infection (excess secretions make child susceptible to respiratory infections).

Cyanotic Heart Defects

See Figure 3.1.

A. General information and medical management
   1. *Transposition of the great vessels*
      a. Aorta arises from right ventricle; pulmonary artery arises from left ventricle
      b. Oxygenated blood therefore circulates through left side of heart to lungs and back to left side; unoxygenated blood enters right atrium from body, goes to right ventricle, and back out to the body without being oxygenated.
      c. Child cannot live without a communication between atria or ventricles.
      d. Foramen ovale remains open for short while as pressure in heart is not sufficient to close it.
      e. Poor oxygenation makes these children cyanotic.
      f. Treatment includes surgical incision or balloon septostomy to create an ASD.

g. When child is old enough, defect will be corrected surgically (Mustard procedure) to redirect blood flow.

2. *Truncus arteriosus*

   a. Only one vessel exits heart from both ventricles; always associated with a large VSD.

   b. As there is no septum to divide aorta and pulmonary trunk, oxygenated and unoxygenated blood mix, causing cyanosis.

   c. Medical treatment includes digitalis and diuretics; if growth failure occurs despite treatment surgical intervention is necessary.

   d. Until recently, pulmonary banding was the only surgical option; some centers now perform complete intracardiac repair.

3. *Tetralogy of Fallot*

   a. Concomitant presence of four defects: pulmonary stenosis, VSD, hypertrophy of right ventricle, malposition of the aorta

   b. Aorta sits near core of heart over the VSD and therefore receives blood from both ventricles.

   c. Decreased blood flow to lungs; mixture of unoxygenated blood going to aorta causes cyanosis and dyspnea.

   d. Children may tend to squat, especially after exertion; may show failure to thrive.

   e. Treatment is open-heart surgical correction (Blalock-Taussig).

4. *Hypoplastic left heart syndrome*

   a. Concomitant presence of aortic valve atresia, mitral atresia or stenosis, diminutive or absent left ventricle, severe hypoplasia of ascending aorta, and aortic arch

   b. Usually fatal, few infants survive past 6 weeks

   c. No satisfactory treatment; surgical corrections have had limited success, heart transplant presently the only option

B. Assessment findings

   1. Cyanosis

   2. Polycythemia (low oxygen output triggers increase in RBC production to attempt to increase body's oxygen-carrying capacity

   3. Clubbing of digits (poor circulation to extremities)

   4. Poor growth and little tolerance for activity

   5. Increased pulse and respiratory rate

   6. Poor feeding; weak cry

   7. Squatting (especially in tetralogy) helps to decrease blood flow to extremities and to keep oxygenated blood for brain and trunk

   8. These children at risk for left-sided heart failure, brain infarctions, and blood clots

   9. Development of collateral circulation

   10. Laboratory tests: Hct increased (increased sludging/concentration of blood from increased RBC)

C. Nursing interventions

   1. Do not interfere when child is squatting; as long as child appears comfortable, no intervention other than observation required.

   2. Organize care to decrease child's expenditure of energy.

3. Administer oxygen as ordered.

4. Meet needs quickly; prevent crying.

5. Provide passive stimulation.

6. Use soft "preemie" nipple to decrease energy in sucking.

7. Provide careful skin care; decreased blood flow to periphery predisposes these children to circulatory problems.

Cardiac Surgery

A. General information

   1. Surgical correction of congenital defects within the heart, or surgery of the great vessels in the immediate area surrounding of the heart

   2. *Open-heart surgery* (uses cardiopulmonary bypass): provides a relatively blood-free operative site; heart-lung machine maintains gas exchange during surgery

   3. *Closed-heart surgery* does not use cardiopulmonary bypass machine; indicated for ligation of a patent ductus arteriosus or coarctation of the aorta

B. Nursing interventions: preoperative

   1. Determine the child's level of understanding; have child draw a picture, tell you a story, or use doll play.

   2. Correct misunderstandings/teach the child about the surgery using diagrams and play therapy; use terms appropriate to developmental level.

   3. Accompany the child to the operating and recovery rooms and the intensive care unit, explaining the various equipment; allow child to handle/experience it, if possible, and introduce staff and patients, depending on child's developmental/emotional levels.

   4. Have child practice post-op procedures (turning, coughing, deep breathing, etc.).

   5. Include parents in teaching sessions, but have separate sessions for the parents only.

   6. Establish pre-op baseline data for vital signs, activity/sleep patterns, I&O.

C. Nursing interventions: postoperative

   1. Prevent injury/complications.

     a. Monitor vital signs and circulatory pressure readings frequently until stable.

     b. Assess neurologic status frequently.

     c. Observe dressing for intactness/drainage.

   2. Promote gas exchange (patient may be on mechanical ventilation).

     a. Position as ordered.

     b. Administer oxygen at prescribed rate.

     c. Provide humidification.

     d. Suction as necessary.

     e. Perform postural drainage and chest percussion as ordered.

     f. Turn, cough, and deep breathe hourly.

     g. Perform routine care of chest tubes and drainage system, depending on the type of surgery.

   3. Monitor I&O.

   4. Provide nutrition as ordered.

   5. Provide psychologic support of the child/family.

6. Allow activity as tolerated.
7. Provide patient teaching and discharge planning concerning
   a. Need for child/family to express feelings/fears
   b. Resumption of ADL
   c. Assisting child in dealing with peers/returning to school
   d. Referral for parents to support groups/community agencies.

Acquired Heart Disease

Rheumatic Fever (RF)

A. General information
   1. An inflammatory disorder that may involve the heart, joints, connective tissue, and the CNS
   2. Peaks in school-age children; linked to environmental factors and family history of disorder
   3. Thought to be an autoimmune disorder
      a. Preceded by an infection of group A beta-hemolytic streptococcus (usually a strep throat); the heart itself is not infected, however.
      b. Antigenic markers for strep toxin closely resemble markers for heart valves; this resemblance causes antibodies made against the strep to also attack heart valves
   4. Prognosis depends on degree of heart damage
B. Medical management
   1. Drug therapy
      a. Penicillin
         1) used in the acute phase
         2) used prophylactically for several years after the attack
         3) erythromycin substituted if child is sensitive to penicillin
      b. Salicylates: for analgesic, anti-inflammatory, antipyretic effects
      c. Steroids: for anti-inflammatory effect
   2. Decrease cardiac workload: bedrest until lab studies return to normal
C. Assessment findings
   1. Major symptoms (Jones' criteria)
      a. Carditis
         1) seen in 50% of patients
         2) Aschoff nodules (areas of inflammation and degeneration around heart valves, pericardium, and myocardium)
         3) valvular insufficiency of mitral and aortic valves possible
         4) cardiomegaly
         5) shortness of breath, hepatomegaly, edema
      b. Polyarthritis
         1) migratory, therefore no contractures develop
         2) most common in large joints, which become red, swollen, painful
         3) synovial fluid is sterile
         4) no arthralgia

c. Chorea (Sydenham's chorea, St. Vitus' dance): CNS disorder characterized by abrupt, purposeless, involuntary muscular movements
   1) gradual, insidious onset: starts with personality change or clumsiness
   2) mostly seen in prepubertal girls
   3) may appear months after strep infection
   4) movements increase with excitement
   5) lasts 1–3 months
d. Subcutaneous nodules
   1) usually a sign of severe disease
   2) occur with active carditis
   3) firm, nontender nodes on bony prominences of joints
   4) last for weeks
e. Erythema marginatum: transient, nonpruritic rash starting with central red patches that expand; results in series of irregular patches with red, raised margins and pale centers (resemble giraffe spots)
   2. Minor symptoms
      a. Reliable history of RF, fever
      b. Recent history of strep infection
      c. Diagnostic tests: erythrocyte sedimentation rate (ESR) and anti-streptolysin O (ASO) titer increased; changes on ECG
D. Nursing interventions
   1. Carditis
      a. Administer penicillin as ordered.
         1) used prophylactically to prevent future attacks of strep and further damage to the heart
         2) to be taken until age 20 or for 5 years after attack, whichever is longer
      b. Promote bedrest until ESR returns to normal.
   2. Arthritis: administer aspirin as ordered, change child's position in bed frequently.
   3. Chorea
      a. Decrease stimulation.
      b. Provide a safe environment: no forks with meals, assistance with mobility.
      c. Provide small, frequent meals; increased muscle activity causes increased kcal requirements.
   4. Nodules and rash: none.
   5. Alleviate child's anxiety about the ability of heart to continue to function.
   6. Prevent recurrent infection.
   7. Minimize boredom with age-appropriate sedentary play.
   8. Provide patient teaching and discharge planning concerning
      a. Adaptation of home environment to promote bedrest (commode, call bell, diversional activities)
      b. Importance of prophylactic medication regimen
      c. Diet modification in relation to decreased activity/cardiac demands
      d. Avoidance of reinfections
      e. Home-bound education
      f. Availability of community agencies.

SAMPLE QUESTIONS

Two-week-old Jonathon has a patent ductus arteriosus.

7. Prior to administering digoxin the nurse should
   - o 1. take the apical pulse for 30 seconds and multiply by 2.
   - o 2. give the medication if his pulse is 92, but notify the physician.
   - o 3. take the radial pulse for 1 full minute.
   - o 4. give the medication after finding that the pulse is 135 beats/minute.

8. In planning Jonathon's care, which of the following interventions is NOT appropriate?
   - o 1. Using a soft "preemie" nipple for feedings
   - o 2. Providing passive stimulation
   - o 3. Allowing him to cry to promote increased oxygenation
   - o 4. Placing him in orthopneic position

The Hematologic System

VARIATIONS FROM THE ADULT

A. In the young child all the bone marrow is involved in blood cell formation.

B. By puberty, only the sternum, ribs, pelvis, vertebrae, skull, and proximal epiphyses of femur and humerus are involved.

C. During the first 6 months of life, fetal hemoglobin is gradually replaced by adult hemoglobin, and it is only after this that hemoglobin disorders can be diagnosed.

ASSESSMENT

History

A. Family history: genetic hematologic disorders, anemia or jaundice

B. History of pregnancy: parents' blood types, anemia, infection or drug ingestion, course of labor and delivery

C. Child's health history

1. Neonatal course: occurrence, duration, and treatment of jaundice; bleeding episodes; blood transfusions

2. Accidents, operations, hospitalizations (any blood transfusions or unusual bleeding)

3. Nutrition: dietary intake of iron and vitamin B_{12}; history of pica

4. Ingestions: lead-based paint; drugs

5. Ability to participate in age-appropriate activities

Physical Examination

A. General appearance

1. Skin: note whether cyanotic, pale, ruddy, jaundiced; note bruises or petechiae, other evidence of hemorrhage; pain, swelling around joints.

2. Neurologic status: note listlessness or fatigue, irritability, dizziness or lightheadedness.

B. Measure vital signs; note tachycardia or tachypnea.

C. Plot height and weight on growth chart.

D. Inspect and palpate abdomen; note enlargement of liver and spleen, pain or tenderness on palpation.

ANALYSIS

Nursing diagnoses for the child with a disorder of the hematologic system may include

A. Activity intolerance

B. Alteration in comfort: pain

C. Impaired gas exchange

D. Alteration in tissue perfusion: cardiopulmonary

E. Alteration in nutrition

PLANNING AND IMPLEMENTATION

Goals

A. Child will have adequate tissue oxygenation.

B. Child will be free from complications associated with hematologic diseases.

C. Child will be free from pain, or have pain controlled.

D. Optimal growth and developmental level will be achieved.

E. Parents will participate in care of child.

Interventions

Bone Marrow Transplant

A. General information

1. Relatively new treatment alternative for a variety of childhood diseases including

a. Definite: acute lymphoblastic leukemia, acute nonlymphocytic leukemia, severe aplastic anemia, immunodeficiencies, and malignant infantile osteopetrosis

b. Possible: chronic myelogenous leukemia, solid tumors, some hematologic disorders, and some inherited metabolic disorders

2. Types

a. Autologous: patient transplanted with own harvested marrow

b. Syngeneic: transplant between identical twins

c. Allogeneic: transplant from a genetically nonidentical donor

      1) most common transplant type
      2) sibling most common donor
   3. Procedure
      a. Donor suitability determined through tissue antigen typing; includes histocompatibility antigens (HLA) and mixed leukocyte culture (MLC) typing.
      b. Donor bone marrow is aspirated from multiple sites along the iliac crests under general anesthesia.
      c. Donor marrow is infused IV into the recipient.
   4. Early evidence of engraftment seen during the second week post-transplant; hematologic reconstitution takes 4–6 weeks; immunologic reconstitution takes months.
   5. Hospitalization of 2 or 3 months required.
   6. Prognosis is highly variable depending on indication for use.
 B. Complications
   1. Failure of engraftment
   2. Infection: highest risk in first 3–4 weeks
   3. Pneumonia: nonbacterial or interstitial pneumonias are principle cause of death during first 3 months post-transplant
   4. *Graft vs host disease (GVHD):* principle complication; caused by an immunologic reaction of engrafted lymphoid cells against the tissues of the recipient
      a. Acute GVHD: develops within first 100 days post-transplant and affects skin, gut, liver, marrow, and lymphoid tissue
      b. Chronic GVHD: develops 100–400 days post-transplant; manifested by multi-organ involvement
   5. Recurrent malignancy
   6. Late complications such as cataracts, endocrine abnormalities
 C. Nursing care: pretransplant
   1. Extensive time must be spent with child/parents in preparing for this procedure.
   2. Recipient immunosuppression attained with total body irradiation (TBI) and chemotherapy to eradicate existing disease and create space in host marrow to allow transplanted cells to grow.
   3. Provide protected environment.
      a. Child should be in a laminar air flow room or on strict reverse isolation; surveillance cultures done twice a week.
      b. Encourage use of toys and familiar objects; they must be sterilized before being brought into the room.
      c. Encourage frequent contact with school teacher/play therapist.
      d. Introduce new people where they can be seen, but outside child's room so child can see what they look like without isolation garb.
   4. Monitor central lines frequently; check patency and observe for signs of infection (fever, redness around site).
   5. Provide care for the child receiving chemotherapy and radiation therapy to induce immunosuppression (see also Pediatric Oncology, page **356**).
      a. Administer chemotherapy as ordered, assist with radiation therapy if required.

      b. Monitor side effects and keep child as comfortable as possible.
      c. Monitor carefully for potential infection.
      d. Child will become very ill; prepare parents.
 D. Nursing care: post-transplant
   1. Prevent infection.
      a. Maintain protective environment.
      b. Administer antibiotics as ordered.
      c. Assess all mucous membranes, wounds, catheter sites for swelling, redness, tenderness, pain.
      d. Monitor vital signs frequently (every 1–4 hours as needed).
      e. Collect specimens for cultures as needed and twice a week.
      f. Change IV set-ups every 24 hours.
   2. Provide mouth care for stomatitis and mucositis (severe mucositis develops about 5 days after irradiation).
      a. Note tissue sloughing, bleeding, changes in color.
      b. Provide mouth rinses, viscous lidocaine, and antibiotic rinses.
      c. Do not use lemon and glycerin swabs.
      d. Administer parenteral narcotics as ordered if necessary to control pain.
      e. Provide care every 2 hours or as needed.
   3. Provide skin care: skin breakdown may result from profuse diarrhea from the TBI.
   4. Monitor carefully for bleeding.
      a. Check for occult blood in emesis and stools.
      b. Observe for easy bruising, petechiae on skin, mucous membranes.
      c. Monitor changes in vital signs.
      d. Check platelet count daily.
      e. Replace blood products as ordered (all blood products should be irradiated).
   5. Maintain fluid and electrolyte balance and promote nutrition.
      a. Measure I&O carefully.
      b. Provide adequate fluid, protein, and caloric intake.
      c. Weigh daily.
      d. Administer fluid replacement as ordered.
      e. Monitor hydration status: check skin turgor, moisture of mucous membranes, urine output.
      f. Check electrolytes daily.
      g. Check urine for glucose, ketones, protein.
      h. Administer antidiarrheal agents as needed.
   6. Provide patient teaching and discharge planning concerning
      a. Home environment (e.g., cleaning, pets, visitors)
      b. Diet modifications
      c. Medication regimen: schedule, dosages, effects and side effects
      d. Communicable diseases and immunizations
      e. Daily hygiene and skin care
      f. Fever
      g. Activity.

EVALUATION

A. Serum values of hematologic components are normal.
B. Child is free from signs or symptoms of infection.
C. Child has no abnormal bleeding episodes.
D. Normal activity level is maintained without pain or fatigue.
E. Parents are able to describe symptoms of disease and complications.
F. Parents are able to administer medications and participate in child's care.

DISORDERS OF THE HEMATOLOGIC SYSTEM

Anemias

Iron Deficiency Anemia

A. General information: iron deficiency is most common cause of anemia in children; children whose diet consists mainly of cow's milk, which is low in absorbable iron, are especially vulnerable.
B. Assessment findings
　1. Pallor, fatigue, irritability
　2. History of iron-deficient diet
　3. Diagnostic tests
　　a. RBC normal or slightly reduced
　　b. Hgb below normal range for child
　　c. Hct below normal
C. Nursing interventions
　1. Add iron to formula, food, or by vitamins by age 4–6 months.
　　a. Oral iron
　　　1) give iron with citrus juice and on empty stomach (iron is best absorbed in an acidic environment).
　　　2) have child use straw if possible, since iron stains teeth and skin.
　　b. Administer IM iron if ordered.
　2. Provide iron-rich foods: liver (muscle meats), nuts, dried beans/legumes, dried fruit, dark green leafy vegetables (spinach), whole grains (farina), egg yolk, potatoes, shellfish.

Sickle Cell Anemia

A. General information
　1. Most common inherited disorder in U.S. black population; sickle cell trait found in 10% of black Americans
　2. Autosomal recessive inheritance pattern
　3. Individuals who are homozygous for the sickle cell gene have the disease (more than 80% of their hemoglobin is abnormal [HgbS]).
　4. Those who are heterozygous for the gene have sickle cell trait (normal hemoglobin predominates, may have 25%–50% HgbS). Although sickle cell trait is not a disease, carriers may exhibit symptoms under periods of severe anoxia or dehydration.
　5. In this disease, the structure of hemoglobin is changed; the sixth rung of the beta chain changes glutamine for valine.
　6. HgbS (abnormal Hgb), which has reduced oxygen-carrying capacity, replaces all or part of the hemoglobin in the RBCs.
　7. When oxygen is released, the shape of the RBCs changes from round and pliable to crescent shaped, rigid, and inflexible.
　8. Local hypoxia and continued sickling lead to plugging of vessels.
　9. RBCs live for 6–20 days instead of 120, causing hemolytic anemia.
　10. Usually no symptoms prior to age 6 months; presence of increased level of fetal hemoglobin tends to inhibit sickling.
　11. Death often occurs in early adulthood due to occlusion or infection.
　12. *Sickle cell crisis*
　　a. Vaso-occlusive (thrombocytic) crisis: most common type
　　　1) crescent-shaped RBCs clump together; agglutination causes blockage of small blood vessels.
　　　2) blockage causes the blood viscosity to increase, producing sludging and resulting in further hypoxia and increased sickling.
　　b. *Splenic sequestration*: often seen in toddler/preschooler
　　　1) sickled cells block outflow tract resulting in sudden and massive collection of sickled cells in spleen.
　　　2) blockage leads to hypovolemia and severe decrease in hemoglobin and blood pressure, leading to shock.
B. Medical management: sickle cell crisis
　1. Drug therapy
　　a. Urea: interferes with hydrophobic bonds of the HgbS molecules
　　b. Analgesics/narcotics to control pain
　　c. Antibiotics to control infection
　2. Exchange transfusions
　3. Hydration: oral and IV
　4. Bedrest
　5. Surgery: splenectomy
C. Assessment findings
　1. First sign in infancy may be "colic" due to abdominal pain (abdominal infarct)
　2. Infants may have dactylitis (hand-foot syndrome): symmetrical painful soft tissue swelling of hands and feet in absence of trauma (aseptic, self-limiting)
　3. Splenomegaly: initially due to hemolysis and phagocytosis; later due to fibrosis from repeated infarct to spleen
　4. Weak bones or spinal defects due to hyperplasia of marrow and osteoporosis
　5. Frequent infections, especially with *H. influenzae* and *D. pneumoniae*.
　6. Leg ulcers, especially in adolescents, due to blockage of blood supply to skin of legs

7. Delayed growth and development, especially delay in sexual development
8. CVA/infarct in the CNS
9. Renal failure: difficulty concentrating urine due to infarcts; enuresis
10. Heart failure due to hemosiderosis
11. Priapism: may result in impotence
12. Pain wherever vaso-occlusive crisis occurs
13. Development of collateral circulation
14. Diagnostic tests
    a. Hgb indicates anemia, usually 6–9 gm/dl
    b. Sickling tests
       1) sickle cell test: deoxygenation of a drop of blood on a slide with a cover slip; takes several hours for results to be read; false negatives for the trait possible.
       2) Sickledex: a drop of blood from a fingerstick is mixed with a solution; mixture turns cloudy in presence of HgbS; results available within a few minutes; false negatives in anemic patients or young infants possible.
    c. Hgb electrophoresis: diagnostic for the disease and the trait; provides accurate, fast results.
D. Nursing interventions: sickle cell crisis
1. Keep child well hydrated and oxygenated.
2. Avoid tight clothing that could impair circulation.
3. Keep wounds clean and dry.
4. Provide bedrest to decrease energy expenditure and oxygen use.
5. Correct metabolic acidosis.
6. Administer medications as ordered.
   a. Analgesics: acetaminophen, meperidine, morphine (avoid aspirin as it enhances acidosis, which promotes sickling)
   b. Avoid anticoagulants (sludging is not due to clotting)
   c. Antibiotics
7. Administer blood transfusions as ordered.
8. Keep arms and legs from becoming cold.
9. Decrease emotional stress.
10. Provide good skin care, especially to legs.
11. Test siblings for presence of sickle cell trait/disease.
12. Provide patient teaching and discharge planning concerning
    a. Pre-op teaching for splenectomy if needed
    b. Genetic counseling
    c. Need to avoid activities that interfere with oxygenation, such as mountain climbing, flying in unpressurized planes.

Disorders of Platelets or Clotting Mechanism

Idiopathic Thrombocytopenic Purpura (ITP)

A. General information
1. Increased destruction of platelets with resultant platelet count of less than 100,000 μ/liter; characterized by petechiae and ecchymoses of the skin

2. Exact cause unknown; may be an autoimmune mechanism; onset sudden, often preceded by a viral illness
3. The spleen is the site for destruction of platelets; spleen is not enlarged.
B. Medical management
1. Drug therapy: steroids and immunosuppressive agents
2. Platelet transfusion
3. Surgery: splenectomy
C. Assessment findings
1. Petechiae: spider-web appearance of bleeding under skin due to small size of platelets
2. Ecchymosis
3. Blood in any body secretions, bleeding from mucous membranes, nosebleeds
4. Diagnostic tests: platelet count decreased, anemia
D. Nursing interventions
1. Control bleeding.
   a. Administer platelet transfusions as ordered.
   b. Apply pressure to bleeding sites as needed.
   c. Position bleeding part above heart level if possible.
2. Prevent bruising.
3. Provide support to patient and be sensitive to change in body image.
4. Protect from infection.
5. Measure normal circumference of extremities for baseline.
6. Administer medications orally, rectally or IV, rather than IM; if administering immunizations, give subcutaneously (SC) and hold pressure on site for 5 minutes.
7. Administer analgesics (acetaminophen) as ordered; avoid aspirin.
8. Provide care for the patient with a splenectomy (see page 93).
9. Provide patient teaching and discharge planning concerning prevention of trauma
   a. Pad crib and playpen, use rugs wherever possible.
   b. Provide soft toys.
   c. Sew pads in knees and elbows of clothing.
   d. Provide protective headgear during toddlerhood.
   e. Use soft Toothettes instead of bristle toothbrushes.
   f. Keep weight to low normal to decrease extra stress on joints.
   g. Use stool softeners to prevent straining.
   h. Avoid contact sports; suggest swimming, biking, golf, pool.

Hemophilia

A. General information
1. A group of bleeding disorders where there is a deficit of one of several factors in clotting mechanism
2. Sex-linked, inherited disorder; classic form affects males only
3. Types
   a. *Hemophilia A:* factor VIII deficiency (75% of all hemophilia)

b. *Hemophilia B (Christmas disease):* factor IX deficiency (10%–12% of all hemophilia)

c. *Hemophilia C:* factor XI deficiency (autosomal recessive, affects both sexes)

4. Only the intrinsic system is involved; platelets are not affected, but fibrin clot does not always form; bleeding from minor cuts may be stopped by platelets.

5. If individual has less than 20%–30% of factor VIII or IX, there is an impairment of clotting and clot is jelly-like.

6. Bleeding in neck, mouth, and thorax requires immediate professional care.

B. Assessment findings

1. Prolonged bleeding after minor injury

a. At birth after cutting of cord

b. Following circumcision

c. Following IM immunizations

d. Following loss of baby teeth

e. Increased bruising as child learns to crawl and walk

2. Bruising and hematomas but no petechiae

3. Peripheral neuropathies (due to bleeding near peripheral nerves): pain, paresthesias, muscle atrophy

4. Hemarthrosis

a. Repeated bleeding into a joint results in a swollen and painful joint with limited mobility

b. May result in contractures and possible degeneration of joint

c. Knees, ankles, elbows, wrists most often affected

5. Diagnostic tests

a. Platelet count normal

b. Prolonged coagulation time: PTT increased

c. Anemia

C. Nursing interventions

1. Control acute bleeding episode.

a. Apply ice compress for vasoconstriction.

b. Immobilize area to prevent clots from being dislodged.

c. Elevate affected extremity above heart level.

d. Provide manual pressure or pressure dressing for 15 minutes; do not keep lifting dressing to check for bleeding status.

e. Maintain calm environment to decrease pulse.

f. Avoid sutures, cauterization, aspirin: all exacerbate bleeding.

g. Administer hemostatic agents as ordered.

1) fibrin foam

2) topical application of adrenalin/epinephrine to promote vasoconstriction

2. Provide care for hemarthrosis.

a. Immobilize joint and control acute bleeding.

b. Elevate joint in a slightly flexed position.

c. Avoid excessive handling of joint.

d. Administer analgesics as ordered, pain relief will minimize increases in pulse rate and blood loss.

e. Instruct to avoid weight bearing for 48 hours after bleeding episode if bleeding is in lower extremities.

f. Provide active or passive ROM exercises after bleeding has been controlled (48 hours), as long as exercises do not cause pain or irritate trauma site.

3. Administer cryoprecipitate (frozen factor VIII) as ordered.

a. Thaw slowly.

b. Gently rotate bottle; shaking deteriorates antihemophilic factor.

c. Infuse immediately when thawed; factor VIII deteriorates at room temperature.

4. Provide patient teaching and discharge planning concerning

a. Prevention of trauma (see Idiopathic Thrombocytopenic Purpura)

b. Genetic counseling

1) when mother is carrier: 50% chance with each pregnancy for sons to have hemophilia, 50% chance with each pregnancy for daughters to be carriers

2) when father has hemophilia, mother is normal: no chance for children to have disease, but all daughters will be carriers

c. Availability of support/counseling agencies

Disorder of White Blood Cells

Infectious Mononucleosis

A. General information

1. Viral infection that causes hyperplasia of lymphoid tissue and a characteristic change in mononuclear cells of the blood

2. Affects adolescents and young adults most commonly

3. Caused by the Epstein Barr virus, which is not highly contagious, but is transmitted by saliva (the "kissing" disease)

4. Incubation period 2–6 weeks

5. Pathophysiology: mononuclear infiltration of lymph nodes and other body tissue

B. Assessment findings

1. Lethargy

2. Sore throat/tonsilitis

3. Lymphadenopathy; enlarged spleen, liver involvement

4. Diagnostic tests

a. Atypical WBCs increased

b. Heterophil antibody and Monospot tests positive

Malignancies

Leukemia

A. General information

1. Most common form of childhood cancer

2. Uncontrolled proliferation of WBC precursors that fail to mature

3. Normal cells are crowded out by leukemia cells; bone marrow becomes packed with abnormal cells (blasts).

4. Symptoms reflect marrow failure and associated involvement of other organ tissues.

5. Liver, spleen, and lymph nodes are the most commonly infiltrated organs.

6. Types: distinguished by type of cell proliferating

a. *Myelocytic (acute myelogenous) leukemia (AML)*

1) average age 11 years
2) 50%–70% get a first remission
3) median survival: 25 years
b. *Acute lymphocytic leukemia (ALL)*
  1) average age 4 years
  2) 90% get first remission
  3) 50% live 5 years
  4) abrupt sudden onset
  5) accounts for 80% of childhood leukemia
7. Affects boys more than girls; incidence higher in children with Down's syndrome
8. Prognosis depends on initial WBC, child's age at diagnosis, and histologic type of disease

B. Assessment findings
  1. Anemia (due to decreased production of RBCs), weakness, pallor, dyspnea
  2. Bleeding (due to decreased platelet production), petechiae, spontaneous bleeding, ecchymoses
  3. Infection (due to decreased WBCs production), fever, malaise
  4. Enlarged lymph nodes
  5. Enlarged spleen and liver
  6. Abdominal pain with weight loss and anorexia
  7. Bone pain due to expansion of marrow

C. Nursing interventions
  1. Provide care for the child receiving chemotherapy and radiation therapy (see Pediatric Oncology).
  2. Provide support for child/family; needs will change as treatment progresses.
  3. Support child during painful procedures (frequent bone marrow aspirations, lumbar punctures, venipunctures needed).
    a. Use distraction, guided imagery.
    b. Allow child to retain as much control as possible.
    c. Administer sedation prior to procedure as ordered.

Hodgkin's Lymphoma

A. General information
  1. Malignant neoplasm of lymphoid tissue, usually originating in localized group of lymph nodes; a proliferation of lymphocytes
  2. Metastasizes first to adjacent lymph nodes
  3. Cause unknown
  4. Most prevalent in adolescents; accounts for 5% of all malignancies
  5. Prognosis now greatly improved for these children; influenced by stage of disease and histologic type
  6. Long-term treatment effects include increased incidence of second malignancies, especially leukemia and infertility

B. Medical management
  1. Diagnosis: extensive testing to determine stage, which dictates treatment modality
    a. Lymphangiogram determines involvement of all lymph nodes (reliable in 90% of patients); is helpful in determining radiation fields
    b. Staging via laparotomy and biopsy

    1) stage I: single lymph node involved; usually in neck; 90%–98% survival
    2) stage II: involvement of 2 or more lymph nodes on same side of diaphragm; 70%–80% survival
    3) stage III: involvement of nodes on both sides of diaphragm; 50% survival
    4) stage IV: metastasis to other organs
  c. Laparotomy and splenectomy
  d. Lymph node biopsy to identify presence of Reed-Sternberg cells and for histologic classification
  2. Radiation: used alone for localized disease
  3. Chemotherapy: used in conjunction with radiation therapy for advanced disease; MOPP (nitrogen mustard [mechlorethamine], vincristine [Oncovin], procarbazine and prednisone) is drug combination of choice

C. Assessment findings
  1. Major presenting symptom is enlarged nodes in lower cervical region; nodes are nontender, firm, and moveable
  2. Recurrent, intermittent fever
  3. Night sweats
  4. Weight loss, malaise, lethargy
  5. Pruritus
  6. Diagnostic test: presence of Reed-Sternberg cells

D. Nursing interventions
  1. Provide care for child receiving radiation therapy.
  2. Administer chemotherapy as ordered and monitor/alleviate side effects.
  3. Protect patient from infection, especially if splenectomy performed.
  4. Provide support for child/parents; specific needs of adolescent patient must be considered.

Non-Hodgkin's Lymphoma

A. General information
  1. Tumor originating in lymphatic tissue
  2. Significantly different from Hodgkin's lymphoma
    a. Control of primary tumor is difficult
    b. Disease is diffuse, cell type undifferentiated
    c. Tumor disseminates early
    d. Includes wide range of disease entities: lymphosarcoma, reticulum cell sarcoma, Burkitt's lymphoma
  3. Primary sites include GI tract, ovaries, testes, bone, CNS, liver, breast, subcutaneous tissues
  4. Affects all age groups.

B. Medical management
  1. Chemotherapy: multiagent regimens including cyclophosphamide (Cytoxan), vincristine, prednisone, procarbazine, doxorubicin, bleomycin
  2. Radiation therapy: primary treatment in localized disease
  3. Surgery for diagnosis and clinical staging

C. Assessment findings
  1. Depend on anatomic site and extent of involvement
  2. Rapid onset and progression
  3. Many have advanced disease at diagnosis

D. Nursing interventions: see Pediatric Oncology, page **356.**

SAMPLE QUESTIONS

John is 4 years old and has been diagnosed as having iron deficiency anemia.

9. A liquid iron preparation has been prescribed. When administering John's medication the nurse should
   - o 1. ask him if he wants to take his medicine.
   - o 2. mix the medication in his milk bottle and give it to him at nap time.
   - o 3. allow him to sip the medication through a straw.
   - o 4. give the medication after lunch with a sweet dessert to disguise the taste.

Todd, age 10, has hemophilia A and is admitted to the hospital for hemarthrosis of the right knee. He is in a great deal of pain.

10. Which of the following interventions would aggravate his condition?
    - o 1. Applying an ice bag to the affected knee
    - o 2. Administering children's aspirin for pain relief
    - o 3. Elevating the right leg above the level of his heart
    - o 4. Keeping the right leg immobilized

The Respiratory System

VARIATIONS FROM THE ADULT

A. Infants are obligatory nose breathers and diaphragmatic breathers

B. Number and size of alveoli continue to increase until age 8 years.

C. Until age 5, structures of the respiratory tract have a narrower lumen and children are more susceptible to obstruction/distress from inflammation.

D. Normal respiratory rate in children is faster than in adults
  1. Infants: 40–60/minute
  2. 1 year: 20–40/minute
  3. 2–4 years: 20–30/minute
  4. 5–10 years: 20–25/minute
  5. 10–15 years: 17–22/minute
  6. 15 and older: 15–20/minute

E. Most episodes of acute illness in young children involve the respiratory system due to frequent exposure to infection and a general lack of immunity

ASSESSMENT

History

A. Presenting problem: symptoms may include cough, wheezing, dyspnea

B. Medical history: incidence of infections, respiratory allergies or asthma, prescribed and OTC medications, recent immunizations

C. Exposure to other children with respiratory infections or other communicable diseases

Physical Examimation

A. Inspect shape of chest; note
  1. Barrel chest: occurs with chronic respiratory disease.
  2. Pectus carinatum (pigeon breast): sternum protrudes outward producing increased A-P diameter; usually not significant.
  3. Pectus excavatum (funnel chest): lower part of sternum is depressed; usually does not produce symptoms; may impair cardiac function.

B. Note pattern of respirations.
  1. Rate
  2. Regularity
     a. Periodic respirations (periods of rapid respirations, separated by periods of slow breathing or short periods of no respirations) normal in young infants
     b. Apnea episodes (cessation of breathing for 20 seconds or more accompanied by color change or bradycardia) an abnormal finding
  3. Respiratory effort
     a. Nasal flaring: attempt to widen airway and decrease resistance
     b. Open-mouth breathing: chin drops with each inhalation
     c. Retractions: from use of accessory muscles

C. Observe skin color and temperature, particularly mucous membranes and peripheral extremities.

D. Note behavior: position of comfort, signs of irritability or lethargy, facial expression (anxiety).

E. Note speech abnormalities: hoarseness or muffled speech.

F. Observe presence and quality of cough: productive; paroxysmal, with inspiratory "whoop" characteristic of pertussis.

G. Auscultate for abnormal breath sounds (auscultation may be more difficult in infants and young children because of shallowness of respirations).
  1. Grunting on expiration
  2. Stridor: harsh inspiratory sound associated with obstruction or edema
  3. Wheezing: whistling noise during inspiration or expiration due to narrowed airways, common in asthma
  4. "Snoring": noisy breathing associated with nasal obstruction

Laboratory/Diagnostic Tests

A. Pulmonary function testing should not be done under age 6 years since children have difficulty following directions.

B. Chest x-rays: avoid unnecessary exposure; protect gonads and thyroid.

ANALYSIS

Nursing diagnoses for the child with a disorder of the respiratory system may include
A. Activity intolerance
B. Alteration in respiratory functions: ineffective airway clearance, ineffective breathing pattern, impaired gas exchange, mechanical ventilation
C. Anxiety
D. Alteration in comfort
E. Alteration in oral mucous membrane
F. Alteration in nutrition
G. Sleep pattern disturbance

PLANNING AND IMPLEMENTATION

Goals

A. Child will have patent airway and satisfactory oxygenation.
B. Child will be free from symptoms of respiratory distress.
C. Child will have improved ability to tolerate exercise, conserve energy.
D. Parents will participate in caring for child.

Interventions

Oxygen Tent (Croup Tent, Mist Tent, Oxygen Canopy)

A. General information
1. Used when desired oxygen concentration is 40% or less as oxygen concentration can be difficult to control
2. Primarily used for croup, when mist is to be delivered
B. Nursing care
1. Keep sides of plastic down and tucked in.
2. If tent has been opened for a while, increase oxygen flow to raise concentration quickly.
3. If child has been out of the tent, return oxygen concentration to ordered percent before returning child to tent.
4. If tent enclosure gets too warm, add ice to cooling chamber as needed.
5. Mist is usually prescribed in addition to oxygen
   a. Keep reservoir for humidification filled.
   b. Do not allow condensation on tent walls to obstruct view of child.
   c. Keep clothes and bedding dry to avoid chilling.
6. Provide safety measures.
   a. Keep plastic away from child's face.
   b. Avoid toys that produce spark or friction, such as mechanical toys.
   c. Avoid stuffed toys because of tendency to absorb moisture.
   d. Encourage use of one or two favorite toys or transitional object in tent; other toys may be kept outside of tent in child's view.

Vaporizers

A. General information
1. Same principle as oxygen tent.
2. Used at home; placed at bedside; mist directed into room around child
3. Usually cool mist
B. Nursing responsibilities: teach parents to clean frequently because bacteria that grow in vaporizer can be dispersed into air.

Chest Physical Therapy

A. Postural drainage: infants and young children do not have enough rib cage for a lower front position
1. Combine side and lower front positions
2. 5 positions: upper front, upper back, lower back, right side and front, and left side and front
3. 2–5 minutes per position
B. Percussion
1. Do not use with patients with an acute attack of asthma or croup (dislodged mucus may cause plugging because of bronchial edema).
2. Use percussion 30 minutes before meals to clear mucus before eating, thus enhancing intake.
3. If aerosol medications are being used, administer immediately before percussion.
4. Percussion is done with cupped hand, never on bare skin, over the rib cage only
   a. Use an undershirt, gown, or diaper over skin.
   b. If infant's chest is too small for nurse's hand, a small face mask can be substituted.
   c. Be careful to avoid spine and neck during percussion.
   d. Infants can be percussed while being held on nurse's lap.
   e. If child is unable to cough during and after percussion, suction as needed.

Suctioning

A. Bulb syringes can be used to clear nasal stuffiness.
B. For nasotracheal suction, use low pressure.

Deep Breathing Exercises

A. Encourage use by making exercises into games (e.g., touch toes, sit-ups, jumping jacks, blowing out "flashlight," ping pong ball games using blowing).
B. Encourage use of toys that require blowing (harmonicas, bubbles).
C. Laughing and crying also stimulate coughing and deep breathing.

Apnea Monitor

A. General information: monitors often use same three chest leads for simultaneous cardiac and respiratory rate monitoring
1. Lead placement will differ from that usually prescribed for cardiac monitoring if apnea monitoring is also required.

2. To monitor respiratory rate, chest leads will need to be where chest moves during inspiration.
3. As chest wall movement rather than air entry is monitored, obstruction and dyspnea may not be recognized early.
4. Most useful for early recognition of cessation of breathing.

B. Nursing care: when alarm sounds
  1. Note whether cardiac or respiratory rate has triggered alarm.
  2. Assess child's color, activity, and presence of respiratory effort.
  3. Auscultate cardiac and respiratory sounds.
  4. If no physical distress, check lead placement.

EVALUATION

A. Child is satisfactorily oxygenated.
  1. Absence of respiratory distress
  2. Normal color and activity
  3. Decreased need for supplementary oxygen therapy
B. Parents are able to care for child at home.
  1. Identify symptoms of increased oxygen need
  2. Perform prescribed treatments
  3. Have obtained and demonstrated use of necessary equipment

DISORDERS OF THE RESPIRATORY SYSTEM

Tonsillitis

A. General information
  1. Inflammation of tonsils often as a result of a viral or bacterial pharyngitis
  2. 10%–15% caused by group A beta-hemolytic streptococci
B. Medical management
  1. Comfort measures and symptomatic relief
  2. Antibiotics for bacterial infection, usually penicillin or erythromycin
  3. Surgery: removal of tonsils/adenoids if necessary
C. Assessment findings
  1. Enlarged, red tonsils; fever
  2. Sore throat, difficulty swallowing, mouth breathing, snoring
  3. White patches of exudate on tonsillar pillars, enlarged cervical lymph nodes
D. Nursing interventions
  1. Provide soft or liquid diet.
  2. Use cool-mist vaporizer.
  3. Administer salt water gargles, throat lozenges.
  4. Administer analgesics (acetaminophen) as ordered.
  5. Administer antibiotics as ordered; stress to parents importance of completing entire course of medication.

Tonsillectomy

A. General information
  1. One of the most common operations performed on children

2. Indications for tonsillectomy include recurrent tonsillitis, peritonsillar abscess, airway or esophageal obstruction
3. Indications for adenoidectomy include nasal obstruction due to hypertrophy

B. Nursing interventions: preoperative
  1. Make pre-op preparation age-appropriate; child enters the hospital feeling well and will leave with a very sore throat.
  2. Obtain baseline bleeding and clotting times.
  3. Check for any loose teeth.
C. Nursing interventions: postoperative
  1. Position on side or abdomen to facilitate drainage of secretions.
  2. Avoid suctioning if possible; if not, be especially careful to avoid trauma to surgical site.
  3. Provide ice collar/analgesia for pain.
  4. Observe for hemorrhage; signs may include frequent swallowing, increased pulse, vomiting bright red blood (vomiting old dried blood or pink-tinged blood is normal).
  5. Offer clear, cool, noncitrus, nonred fluids when awake and alert.
  6. Provide patient teaching and discharge planning concerning
     a. Need to maintain adequate fluid and food intake and to avoid spicy and irritating foods
     b. Quiet activity for a few days
     c. Need to avoid coughing, mouth gargles
     d. Chewing gum (but not Aspergum): can help relieve pain and difficulty swallowing and aids in diminishing bad breath
     e. Mild analgesics for pain
     f. Signs and symptoms of bleeding and need to report to physician.

Epiglottitis

A. General information
  1. Life-threatening bacterial infection of epiglottis and surrounding structures
  2. Primary organism: *H. influenzae*, type B
  3. Often preceded by upper respiratory infection
  4. Rapid progression of swelling causes reduction in airway diameter; may lead to sudden respiratory arrest
  5. Affects children ages 3–7 years
B. Assessment findings
  1. Fever, tachycardia, inspiratory stridor, labored respirations with retractions, sore throat, dysphagia, drooling
  2. Irritability, restlessness, anxious looking
  3. Position: sitting upright, head forward and jaw thrust out
  4. Diagnostic tests
     a. WBC increased
     b. Lateral neck X-ray reveals characteristic findings
C. Nursing interventions
  1. Provide mist tent with oxygen.
  2. Administer IV antibiotics as ordered.
  3. Provide tracheostomy or endotracheal tube care (page 105); note the following
     a. Restlessness, fatigue, dyspnea, cyanosis, pallor,

tachycardia, tachypnea, diminished breath sounds, adventitious lung sounds.

    b. Need for suctioning to remove secretions; note amount, color, consistency.

4. Reassure child through touch, sound, and physically being present.

5. Involve parents in all aspects of care.

6. Avoid direct examination of the epiglottis as it may precipitate spasm and obstruction.

7. Remember this is extremely frightening experience for child and parents; explain procedures and findings; reinforce explanations of physician.

Acute Spasmodic Laryngitis (Croup)

A. General information

    1. Respiratory distress characterized by paroxysmal attacks of laryngeal obstruction

    2. Etiology unclear but familial predisposition, allergy, viruses, psychologic factors, and anxious temperament have been implicated

    3. Common in children ages 1–3 years

    4. Attacks occur mostly at night; onset sudden and usually preceded by a mild upper respiratory infection

    5. Respiratory symptoms last several hours; may occur in a milder form on a few subsequent nights

B. Assessment findings

    1. Inspiratory stridor, hoarseness, barking cough, anxiety, retractions

    2. Afebrile, skin cool

C. Nursing interventions

    1. Instruct parents to take the child into the bathroom, close the door, turn on the hot water, and sit on floor of the steamy bathroom with child.

    2. If the laryngeal spasm does not subside the child should be taken to the emergency department.

    3. After the spasm subsides, provide cool mist with a vaporizor.

    4. Provide clear fluids.

    5. Try to keep child calm and quiet.

    6. Assure parents this is self-limiting.

Laryngotracheobronchitis

A. General information

    1. Viral infection of the larynx that may extend into trachea and bronchi

    2. Most common cause for stridor in febrile child

    3. Parainfluenza viruses most common cause

    4. Infection causes endothelial insult, increased mucus production, edema

    5. Affects children ages 6 months to 3 years

    6. Onset more gradual than with croup, takes longer to resolve; usually develops over several days with upper respiratory infection.

    7. Usually treated on outpatient basis; indications for admission include dehydration and respiratory compromise.

B. Medical management

    1. Drug therapy

        a. Racemic epinephrine via positive pressure nebulizer, in hospitalized child only

        b. Antibiotics only if secondary bacterial infection present

        c. Steroids: still controversial

    2. Oxygen therapy: low concentrations to relieve mild hypoxia (concentrations greater than 30% may mask signs of obstruction and should not be used)

    3. Oral or nasotracheal intubation for moderate hypoxia

    4. IV fluids to maintain hydration

C. Assessment findings

    1. Fever, coryza, inspiratory stridor, barking cough, tachycardia, tachypnea, retractions

    2. May have difficulty taking fluids

    3. WBC normal

D. Nursing interventions

    1. Instruct parents to take child into steamy bathroom for acute distress.

    2. Keep child calm.

    3. After distress subsides, use cool mist vaporizer in bedroom.

    4. Child may vomit large amounts of mucus after the episode; reassure parents that this is normal.

    5. For hospitalized child

        a. Monitor vital signs, I&O, skin color, and respiratory effort.

        b. Provide care for the intubated child.

        c. Plan care to disturb the child as little as possible.

        d. Avoid direct examination of the epiglottis as it may precipitate spasm and obstruction.

Bronchiolitis

A. General information

    1. Pulmonary viral infection characterized by wheezing

    2. Usually caused by respiratory syncytial virus

    3. Virus invades epithelial cells of nasopharynx and spreads to lower respiratory tract causing increased mucus production, decreased diameter of bronchi, hyperinflation, and possible atelectasis.

    4. Affects infants ages 2–8 months

    5. Increased incidence of asthma as child grows older

B. Medical management: IV epinephrine (if provides relief, follow with epinephrine suspension (Sus-Phrine), which is longer acting, then theophylline); if no response to epinephrine, all treatment is supportive

C. Assessment findings

    1. Difficulty feeding, fever

    2. Cough, coryza

    3. Wheezing, prolonged expiratory phase, tachypnea, nasal flaring, retractions (intercostal more pronounced than supraclavicular retractions)

    4. Diagnostic tests

        a. WBC normal

        b. X-ray reveals hyperaeration

D. Nursing interventions
1. Provide high-humidity environment, with oxygen in some cases (instruct parents to take child into steamy bathroom if at home).
2. Offer small, frequent feedings; clear fluids if trouble with secretions.
3. Provide adequate rest.
4. Administer antipyretics as ordered to control fever.

Cystic Fibrosis (CF)

A. General information
1. Disorder characterized by dysfunction of the exocrine glands (mucus-producing glands of the respiratory tract, GI tract, pancreas, sweat glands, salivary glands)
2. Transmitted as an autosomal recessive trait
3. Incidence: 1 in 1500–2000 live births
4. Most common lethal genetic disease among Caucasians in U.S. and Europe
5. No test to detect carriers
6. Prenatal diagnosis of CF is not reliable
7. Secretions from mucus glands are thick, causing obstruction and fibrosis of tissue
8. Sweat and saliva have characteristic high levels of sodium chloride
9. Affected organs
   a. Pancreas: 85% of CF patients have pancreatic involvement
      1) obstruction of pancreatic ducts and eventual fibrosis and atrophy of the pancreas leads to little or no release of enzymes (lipase [fats], amylase [starch], and trypsin [protein])
      2) absence of enzymes causes malabsorption of fats and proteins
      3) unabsorbed food fractions excreted in the stool produce steatorrhea
      4) loss of nutrients and inability to absorb fat-soluble vitamins causes failure to thrive
   b. Respiratory tract: 99.9% of CF patients have respiratory involvement
      1) increased production of secretions causes increased obstruction of airway, air trapping, and atelectasis
      2) pulmonary congestion leads to cor pulmonale
      3) eventually death occurs by drowning in own secretions
   c. Reproductive system
      1) males are sterile
      2) females can conceive, but increased mucus in vaginal tract makes conception more difficult
      3) pregnancy causes increased stress on respiratory system of mother
   d. Liver: one-third of patients have cirrhosis/portal hypertension
10. The disease is ultimately fatal; average age of death is 20 years; 95% of deaths are from abnormal mucus secretion and fibrosis in the lungs.

B. Medical management
1. Pancreatic involvement: aimed at promoting absorption of nutrients
   a. Diet modification
      1) infant: predigested formula
      2) older children: may require high-calorie, high-protein, or low/limited-fat diet, but many CF patients tolerate normal diet
   b. Pancreatic enzyme supplementation: enzyme capsules, tablets or powders (Pancrease, Cotazym, Viokase) given with meals and snacks
2. Respiratory involvement: goals are to maintain airway patency and to control lung infection
   a. Chest physiotherapy
   b. Antibiotics for infection

C. Assessment findings: symptoms vary greatly in severity and extent
1. Pancreatic involvement
   a. Growth failure; failure to thrive
   b. Stools are foul smelling, large, frequent, foamy, fatty (steatorrhea), contain undigested food
   c. Meconium ileus (meconium gets stuck in bowel due to lack of enzymes) in newborns
   d. Rectal prolapse is possible due to greasy stools
   e. Voracious appetite
   f. Characteristic protruding abdomen with atrophy of extremities and buttocks
   g. Symptoms associated with deficiencies in the fat soluble vitamins
   h. Anemia
   i. Diagnostic tests
      1) trypsin decreased to absent in aspiration of duodenal contents
      2) fecal fat in stool specimen increased
2. Respiratory involvement
   a. Signs of respiratory distress
   b. Barrel chest due to air trapping
   c. Clubbing of digits
   d. Decreased exercise tolerance due to distress
   e. Frequent productive cough
   f. Frequent pseudomonas infections
   g. Diagnostic tests
      1) chest x-ray reveals atelectasis, infiltrations, emphysemic changes
      2) pulmonary function studies abnormal
      3) ABGs show respiratory acidosis
3. Electrolyte involvement
   a. Hyponatremia/heat exhaustion in hot weather
   b. Salty taste to sweat
   c. Diagnostic tests
      1) pilocarpine iontophoresis sweat test: indicates 2–5 times normal amount of sodium and chloride in the sweat
      2) fecal fat elevated
      3) fecal trypsin absent or decreased

D. Nursing interventions

1. Pancreatic involvement
   a. Administer pancreatic enzymes with meals as ordered: do not mix enzymes until ready to use them; best to mix in applesauce.
   b. Provide a high-calorie, high-carbohydrate (no empty-calorie foods), high-protein, normal-fat diet.
   c. Provide a double dose of multivitamins per day, especially fat-soluble vitamins (A, D, E, K), in water-soluble form.
   d. If low-fat diet required, MCT (medium-chain triglycerides) oil may be used.
2. Respiratory involvement
   a. Administer antibiotics as ordered (all antibiotics for pseudomonas are given IV).
      1) doses may be above recommended levels (for virulent organisms)
      2) multiple drugs used to prevent resistance to any one medication
   b. Administer expectorants, mucolytics (rarely used) as ordered.
   c. Avoid cough suppressants and antihistamines.
   d. Encourage breathing exercises.
   e. Provide percussion and postural drainage 4 times a day.
   f. Provide aerosol treatments as needed: hand-held nebulizers, mask, intermittent positive pressure breathing (IPPB), mist tent.
3. Electrolyte involvement
   a. Add salt to all meals, especially in summer.
   b. Give salty snacks (pretzels).
4. Provide appropriate long-term support to child and family.
5. Provide patient teaching and discharge planning concerning
   a. Genetic counseling
   b. Promotion of child's independence
   c. Avoidance of cigarette smoking in the house
   d. Availability of support groups/community agencies
   e. Alternative school education during extended hospitalization/home recovery.

Asthma

A. General information
   1. Obstructive disease of the lower respiratory tract
   2. Most common chronic respiratory disease in children, in younger children affects twice as many boys as girls; incidence equal by adolescence
   3. Often caused by an allergic reaction to an environmental allergen, may be seasonal or year round
   4. Immunologic/allergic reaction results in histamine release, which produces three main airway responses
      a. Edema of mucous membranes
      b. Spasm of the smooth muscle of bronchi and bronchioles
      c. Accumulation of tenacious secretions
   5. *Status asthmaticus* occurs when there is little response to treatment and symptoms persist.

B. Medical management
   1. Drug therapy
      a. Bronchodilators to relieve bronchospasm
         1) theophylline: check pulse and blood pressure
         2) epinephrine: in emergency department
         3) metaproterenol (Alupent), isoetharine (Bronkosol)
      b. Corticosteroids to relieve inflammation and edema
      c. Expectorants (acetylcysteine [Mucomyst]) to decrease congestion
      d. Antibiotics
      e. Sedatives
      f. Cromolyn sodium: not used during acute attack; inhaled; inhibits histamine release in lungs and prevents attack
   2. Physical therapy
   3. Allergy testing/sensitization
C. Assessment findings
   1. Family history of allergies
   2. Patient history of eczema
   3. Respiratory distress: shortness of breath, expiratory wheeze, prolonged expiratory phase, air trapping (barrel chest if chronic), use of accessory muscles, irritability (from hypoxia), diaphoresis, change in sensorium if severe attack
   4. Diagnostic tests: ABGs indicate respiratory acidosis
D. Nursing interventions
   1. Place patient in high-Fowler's position.
   2. Administer oxygen as ordered.
   3. Administer medications as ordered.
   4. Provide humidification/hydration to loosen secretions.
   5. Provide chest percussion and postural drainage when bronchodilation improves.
   6. Monitor for respiratory distress.
   7. Provide patient teaching and discharge planning concerning
      a. Modification of environment
         1) ensure room is well ventilated.
         2) stay indoors during grass cutting or when pollen count is high.
         3) use damp dusting.
         4) avoid rugs, draperies or curtains, stuffed animals.
         5) avoid natural fibers (wool and feathers).
      b. Importance of moderate exercise (swimming is excellent)
      c. Purpose of breathing exercises (to increase the end expiratory pressure of each respiration)

SAMPLE QUESTIONS

Kevin is 7 years old and has been diagnosed as having cystic fibrosis. Chest physiotherapy has been ordered.

11. Kevin's chest percussion should be performed
    - o 1. before postural drainage.
    - o 2. ½ hour before meals.
    - o 3. before an aerosol treatment.
    - o 4. after suctioning.

12. Kevin's left lower lobe is particularly congested and needs to be drained. The nurse should position Kevin on his
    - o 1. left side in semi-Fowler's position.
    - o 2. right side in semi-Fowler's position.
    - o 3. left side in Trendelenburg's position.
    - o 4. right side in Trendelenburg's position.

13. Kevin's sweat test will show an elevation of which electrolyte?
    - o 1. Chloride
    - o 2. Fluoride
    - o 3. Potassium
    - o 4. Calcium

The Gastrointestinal System

VARIATIONS FROM THE ADULT

A. Mechanical functions of digestion are immature at birth.
  1. No voluntary control over swallowing until 6 weeks
  2. Stomach capacity decreased
  3. Peristalsis increased, faster emptying time, more prone to diarrhea
  4. Relaxed cardiac sphincter contributes to tendency to regurgitate food
B. Liver functions (glyconeogenesis and storage of vitamins) are immature throughout infancy.
C. Production of mucosal lining antibodies is decreased.
D. Gastric acidity is low in infants, slowly rises until age 10, and then increases again during adolescence to reach adult levels.
E. Secretory cells are functional at birth, but efficiency of enzymes impaired by lower gastric pH.
F. Infant has decreased saliva, which causes decreased ability to digest starches.
G. Digestive processes are mature by toddlerhood.
H. Completion of myelinization of spinal cord allows voluntary control of elimination.

ASSESSMENT

History

A. Presenting problem: symptoms may include
  1. Vomiting: type, color, amount, relationship to eating or other events
  2. Abnormal bowel habits: diarrhea, constipation, bleeding
  3. Weight loss or growth failure
  4. Pain: location; relationship to meals or other events; effect on sleep, play, appetite
  5. Any other parental concerns
B. Diet/nutrition history: appetite, daily caloric intake, food intolerances, feeding schedule, nutritional deficits

Physical Examination

A. General appearance
  1. Plot height and weight on growth chart.
  2. Measure midarm circumference and tricep skinfold thickness.
  3. Observe color; jaundiced or pale.
B. Mouth
  1. Note level of dentition, presence of dental caries.
  2. Observe mucosal integrity.
C. Abdomen
  1. Observe skin integrity.
  2. Note abdominal distention or visible peristaltic waves (seen in pyloric stenosis).
  3. Inspect for hernias (umbilical, inguinal).
  4. Auscultate for bowel sounds (a sound every 10–30 seconds is normal).
  5. Palpate for tenderness.
  6. Palpate for liver (inferior edge normally palpated 1–2 cm below right costal margin).
  7. Palpate for spleen (may be felt on inspiration 1–2 cm below left costal margin).
D. Vital signs: note presence of fever.

ANALYSIS

Nursing diagnoses for the child with a disorder of the gastrointestinal system may include
A. Alteration in bowel elimination: constipation, diarrhea
B. Alteration in comfort: pain
C. Potential fluid volume deficit
D. Alteration in nutrition: less than body requirements
E. Alteration in oral mucous membrane
F. Potential impairment of skin integrity
G. Alteration in tissue perfusion: gastrointestinal
H. Alteration in family process

PLANNING AND IMPLEMENTATION

Goals

A. Child will maintain adequate nutritional intake.
B. Child will be free from complications of inadequate nutritional intake.
C. Pain will be relieved/controlled.
D. Child will reach optimal developmental level.
E. Parents will be able to care for child at home.

Interventions

Nasogastric Tube Feeding

A. Provide continuous NG tube feedings when child needs high-calorie intake.

B. Use infusion pump to ensure sustained intake.

C. Check tube placement every 4 hours.

D. Check residuals and refeed every 4 hours.

Gastrostomy

A. Used for patients at high risk for aspiration.

B. Regulate height of tube so feeding flows in over 20–30 minutes.

Parenteral Nutrition

A. Use central venous line for high dextrose solutions (greater than 10%).

B. Check infusion rate and amount every 30 minutes.

C. Monitor urine sugar and acetone every 4 hours for 24 hours after a solution change, then every 8 hours.

D. Monitor for signs of hyperglycemia (nausea, vomiting, dehydration).

E. Provide sterile care for insertion site.

  1. Change solution and tubing every 24 hours.

  2. Change dressing every 1–3 days.

  3. Apply restraints (if needed) to prevent dislodgment of central line.

F. Provide infants who are not receiving oral feedings with a pacifier to satisfy sucking needs.

EVALUATION

A. Child is receiving adequate nourishment as evidenced by normal growth and development.

B. Skin is intact, free from signs of redness or inflammation.

C. Child is free from infection, diarrhea, or vomiting.

D. Child is free from pain.

  1. Relaxed facial expression

  2. Level of activity

  3. No guarding of abdomen

E. Parents participate in care of child.

F. Child participates in normal daily activities with family and peers.

DISORDERS OF THE GASTROINTESTINAL TRACT

Congenital Disorders

Cleft Lip and Palate

A. General information

  1. Nonunion of the tissue and bone of the upper lip and hard/soft palate during embryologic development

  2. Familial disorder, often associated with other congenital abnormalities; incidence higher in Caucasians

    a. Cleft lip/palate: 1 in 1000 births

    b. Cleft palate: 1 in 2500 births

    c. Cleft lip with or without cleft palate affects more boys; cleft palate affects more girls

  3. With cleft palate, the failure of the bone and tissues to fuse results in a communication between the mouth and nose

B. Medical management: team approach for therapy

  1. Speech therapist

  2. Dentist and orthodontist

  3. Audiologist, otolaryngologist, pediatrician (these children are prone to otitis media and possible hearing loss)

  4. Surgical correction

    a. Timing varies with severity of defect; early correction helps to avoid speech defects.

    b. Cheiloplasty: correction of cleft lip

      1) goal is to unite edges to allow lips to be both functional and cosmetically attractive.

      2) usually performed approximately age 2 months (to prepare gums for eruption of teeth) when child is free from respiratory infection.

      3) Steri-Strips or Logan bar usually used to take tension off suture line.

    c. Cleft palate repair is usually not done until age 18 months in anticipation of speech development.

      1) between lip and palate repair child is maintained on normal nutritional and respiratory status; also maintains normal immunization schedule.

      2) child should be weaned and able to take liquids from a cup before palate repair.

C. Assessment findings

  1. Facial abnormality visible at birth: cleft lip or palate or both, unilateral or bilateral, partial or complete

  2. Difficulty sucking, inability to form airtight seal around nipple (size of defect may preclude breast-feeding)

  3. Formula/milk escapes through nose in infants with cleft palate

  4. Predisposition to infection because of free communication between mouth and nose

  5. Possible difficulty swallowing

  6. Abdominal distension due to swallowed air

D. Nursing interventions: pre-op cleft lip repair

  1. Feed in upright position to decrease chance of aspiration and decrease amount of air swallowed.

  2. Burp frequently; increased swallowed air causes abdominal distension and discomfort.

  3. Use a large-holed nipple; press cleft lip together with fingers to encourage sucking and to strengthen muscles needed later for speech.

  4. If infant unable to suck, use a rubber-tipped syringe and drip formula into side of mouth.

  5. Administer gavage feeding as ordered if necessary.

  6. Finish feeding with water to wash away formula in palate area.

  7. Provide small, frequent feedings.

  8. Provide emotional support for parents/family.

    a. Demonstrate benefits of surgery by showing before and after pictures.

    b. Reinforce that disorder is not their fault and that it will not affect child's life span or mental ability.

E. Nursing care: post-op cleft lip repair

  1. Maintain patent airway (child may appear to have respiratory distress because of closure of previously open space; adaptation occurs quickly).

  2. Assess color; monitor amount of swallowing to detect hemorrhage.

  3. Do not place in prone position or with pressure on cheeks; avoid any pressure or tension on suture line.

  4. Avoid straining on suture line by anticipating child's needs.

    a. Prevent crying.

    b. Keep child comfortable and content.

  5. Use elbow restraints or pin sleeves of shirt to diaper to keep child's hands away from suture line.

  6. Resume feedings as ordered.

  7. Keep suture line clean; clean after each feeding with saline, peroxide, or water to remove crusts and prevent scarring.

  8. Provide pain control/relief.

F. Nursing interventions: pre-op cleft palate repair

  1. Prepare parents to care for child after surgery

  2. Instruct concerning feeding methods and positioning.

G. Nursing interventions: post-op cleft palate repair

  1. Position on side for drainage of blood/mucus.

  2. Have suction available but use only in emergency.

  3. Prevent injury or trauma to suture line.

    a. Use cups only for liquids; no bottles.

    b. Avoid straws, utensils, Popsicle sticks, chewing gum.

    c. Provide soft toys.

    d. Use elbow restraints.

    e. Provide liquid diet initially, then progress to soft before returning to normal.

    f. Give water after each feeding to clean suture line.

    g. Hold and cuddle these babies to help distract them.

Altered Connections between Trachea, Esophagus, and Stomach

A. General information

  1. Types (Figure 3.2)

    a. *Esophageal atresia:* esophagus ends in a blind pouch; no entry route to stomach

    b. *Tracheoesophageal fistula (TEF):* open connection between trachea and esophagus

    c. *Esophageal atresia with TEF:* esophagus ends in a blind pouch; stomach end of esophagus connects with trachea

  2. These deformities are found more often in low-birth-weight or premature infants, and are associated with polyhydramnios in the mother and multiple congenital anomalies.

B. Medical management

  1. Drug therapy: antibiotics for respiratory infections

  2. Surgery

    a. Palliative

      1) gastrostomy for placement of a feeding tube

      2) esophagostomy to drain secretions

    b. Corrective

      1) end-to-end anastomosis to correct the defect and restore normal anatomy

      2) colon transplant for defects where there is insufficient tissue for an end-to-end anastomosis

C. Assessment findings

  1. Esophageal atresia

    a. History of polyhydramnios in mother (from infant's inability to swallow and excrete amniotic fluid)

    b. Inability to pass an NG tube

    c. Increased drooling and salivation

    d. Immediate regurgitation of undigested formula/milk when fed

    e. Intermittent cyanosis from choking on aspirated secretions

  2. TEF

    a. Normal swallowing but some food/mucus crosses fistula, causing choking and intermittent cyanosis

    b. Distended abdomen from inhaled air crossing fistula into stomach

    c. Aspiration pneumonia from reflux of gastric secretions into the trachea

  3. Esophageal atresia with TEF

    a. All findings for esophageal atresia

    b. Abdominal distension and aspiration pneumonia from gas and reflux of gastric acids into trachea

  4. Diagnostic tests: fluoroscopy with contrast material reveals type of defect

D. Nursing interventions: preoperative

  1. Maintain patent airway.

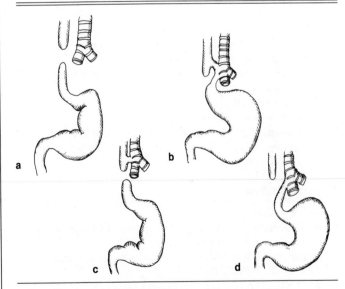

Figure 3.2 Esophageal defects.
a. Esophageal atresia. **b, c, d.** Esophageal atresia with tracheoesophageal fistula.

    a. Position according to type of defect (usually 30° head elevation).

    b. Provide continuous or PRN nasal suctioning.

  2. Keep NPO.

  3. Administer IV fluids as ordered.

E. Nursing interventions: postoperative

  1. Provide nutrition.

    a. Provide gastrostomy tube feedings until the anastomosis site has healed.

    b. Start oral feedings when infant can swallow well.

    c. Progress from glucose water to small, frequent formula feedings.

  2. Promote respiratory function.

    a. Position properly.

    b. Suction as needed.

    c. Provide chest tube care (page 101).

  3. Provide patient teaching and discharge planning concerning

    a. Alternative feeding methods

    b. Signs of respiratory distress and suctioning technique.

Gastroesophageal Reflux (Chalasia)

A. General information

  1. Reversal of flow of stomach contents into lower portion of esophagus

  2. More common in premature infants due to hypotonia

  3. Caused by relaxed cardiac sphincter or overdistension of stomach by gas or overfeeding

  4. Results in local irritation of the lining of the esophagus from backflow of acidic gastric contents; sometimes causes aspiration pneumonia

B. Assessment findings

  1. Irritability

  2. "Spitting up" (versus vomiting or projectile vomiting); note relationship to feedings

  3. Diagnostic tests

    a. Muscle tone of cardiac sphincter reduced

    b. Esophageal pH: contents acidic

    c. Fluoroscopy: presence of refluxed contrast material not quickly cleared or repeated reflux

C. Nursing interventions

  1. Position with head elevated 30°–45°.

  2. Give small, frequent feedings with adequate burping.

  3. Provide patient teaching and discharge planning: teach parents how to position and feed infant.

Pyloric Stenosis

A. General information

  1. Hypertrophy (thickening) of the pyloric sphincter causing stenosis and obstruction

  2. Incidence: 5 in 1000 births; more common in Caucasian, firstborn, fullterm boys

  3. Cause unknown; possibly familial

B. Medical management

  1. Noninvasive: thickened feedings

  2. Surgery: pyloromyotomy (Fredet-Ramstedt procedure)

C. Assessment findings

  1. Olive-size bulge under right rib cage

  2. Vomiting

    a. As obstruction increases, vomiting becomes more forceful and projectile.

    b. Vomitus does not contain bile (bile duct is distal to the pylorus).

  3. Peristaltic waves during and after feeding (look like rolling balls under abdominal wall)

  4. Failure to thrive, even though infant appears hungry after vomiting

  5. Dehydration: sunken fontanels, poor skin turgor, decreased urinary output

  6. Diagnostic tests

    a. Upper GI series reveals narrowing of the diameter of the pylorus

    b. Sodium, potassium, chloride decreased

    c. Hct increased

    d. Metabolic alkalosis

D. Nursing interventions: preoperative

  1. Administer replacement fluids and electrolytes as ordered.

  2. Prevent vomiting.

    a. Give thickened feedings.

    b. Keep in high-Fowler's position.

    c. Place on right side after feedings.

    d. Minimize handling.

    e. Record strict I&O, daily weights, and urine specific gravity.

  3. Observe for symptoms of aspiration of vomitus.

E. Nursing interventions: postoperative

  1. Advance diet as tolerated.

  2. Monitor strict I&O, daily weights.

  3. Observe incision for signs of infection.

  4. Provide patient teaching and discharge planning concerning feeding and positioning of infant.

Intussusception

A. General information

  1. Telescoping of bowel into itself (usually at the ileocecal valve) causing edema, obstruction, and possible necrosis of the bowel

  2. Most common at about age 6 months; occurs more often in boys than in girls; associated with cystic fibrosis and celiac disease

  3. Cause unknown

B. Medical management

  1. Barium enema to reduce telescoping by hydrostatic pressure

  2. Surgery if barium enema unsuccessful or if signs of peritonitis

C. Assessment findings

  1. Piercing cry

  2. Severe abdominal pain (pulls legs up)

  3. Vomiting of bile-stained fluid

  4. Bloody mucus in stool

  5. "Currant-jelly" stool

D. Nursing interventions
  1. Provide routine pre- and post-op care for abdominal surgery.
  2. Monitor for fluid and electrolyte imbalance and intervene as needed.
  3. Monitor for peritonitis and intervene as needed.

Hirschsprung's Disease (Aganglionic Megacolon)

A. General information
  1. Absence of autonomic parasympathetic ganglion cells in a portion of the large colon (usually occurs 4–25 cm proximally from anus) resulting in decreased motility in that portion of the colon and signs of functional obstruction
  2. Usually diagnosed in infancy
  3. Familial disease; more common in boys than girls; associated with Down's syndrome
  4. When stool enters the affected part of the colon, lack of peristalsis causes it to remain there until additional stool pushes it through; colon dilates as stool is impacted.
B. Medical management
  1. Drug therapy: stool softeners
  2. Isotonic enemas
  3. Diet therapy: low residue
  4. Surgery
    a. Palliative: loop or double-barrel colostomy
    b. Corrective: abdominal-perineal pull through; bowel containing ganglia is pulled down and anastomosed to the rectum.
C. Assessment findings
  1. Failure or delay in passing meconium
  2. Abdominal distension; failure to pass stool
  3. Temporary relief following digital rectal exam
  4. Loose stools; only liquid can get around impaction (may also be a ribbonlike stool).
  5. Nausea, anorexia, lethargy
  6. Possibly bile-stained or fecal vomiting
  7. Loss of weight, failure to grow
  8. Volvulus (bowel twists upon itself causing obstruction and necrosis) and enterocolitis due to fecal stagnation
  9. Diagnostic tests: rectal biopsy confirms presence of aganglionic cells
D. Nursing intereventions
  1. Administer enemas as ordered.
    a. Use mineral oil or isotonic saline.
    b. Do not use tap water or soap suds enemas in infants because of danger of water intoxication.
    c. Use volume commensurate with size of child.
      1) infants: 150–200 cc
      2) children: 250–500 cc
  2. Do not treat the loose stools; the child is really constipated.
  3. Administer TPN as ordered.
  4. Provide a low-residue diet.
  5. Provide patient teaching and discharge planning concerning colostomy care and low-residue diet.

Imperforate Anus

A. General information
  1. Congenital malformation caused by abnormal fetal development
  2. Many variations; anal agenesis most frequent
  3. Often associated with fistula formation to rectum or vagina and other congenital anomalies
  4. Surgical correction performed in stages with completion at about age 1 year
  5. May need temporary colostomy
B. Medical management
  1. Manual dilatation
  2. Surgery: anoplasty (reconstruction of anus)
  3. Prophylactic antibiotics
C. Assessment findings
  1. No stool passage within 24 hours of birth
  2. Meconium stool from inappropriate orifice
  3. Inability to insert thermometer
D. Nursing interventions
  1. If suspected, do not take rectal temperature because of risk of perforating wall and causing peritonitis.
  2. Perform manual dilatation as ordered; instruct parents in proper technique.
  3. After surgery prevent infection; keep anal incisional area as clean as possible.
  4. After surgery use side-lying position, or have child lie prone with hips elevated.

Acquired Gastrointestinal Disorders

Celiac Disease

A. General information
  1. Malabsorption syndrome characterized by intolerance of gluten, found in rye, oats, wheat, and barley
  2. Familial disease, found more commonly in Caucasians
  3. Cause unknown; thought to be an inborn error of metabolism or an immunologic disorder
  4. Characterized by flat mucosal surface and atrophy of villi of the intestine; reduced absorptive surface causes marked malabsorption of fats.
B. Medical management: diet therapy main intervention; gluten-free diet, TPN in children who are severely malnourished
C. Assessment findings
  1. Steatorrhea: frothy, pale, bulky, foul-smelling, greasy stools
  2. Chronic diarrhea during late infancy and throughout toddlerhood
  3. Failure to thrive
  4. Grossly distended abdomen; muscle wasting of limbs and buttocks
  5. Abdominal pain, irritability, listlessness, vomiting
  6. Symptoms of vitamin A, D, E, and K deficiency
  7. Diagnostic tests
    a. Pancreatic enzymes and sweat chloride test normal (performed to rule out the possibility of cystic fibrosis)
    b. Jejunal and duodenal biopsies show characteristic atrophy of the mucosa

D. Nursing interventions
1. Monitor gluten-free diet (no wheat, barley, oats, and rye products).
2. Provide supplemental fat-soluble vitamins in water-soluble form.
3. Provide patient teaching and discharge planning concerning
   a. Gluten-free diet; stress allowed foods and importance of reading labels carefully
   b. Avoidance of infection
   c. Assisting child to feel like a "normal" peer
   d. Importance of adhering to diet even though symptoms are controlled
   e. Importance of long-term follow-up management.

Appendicitis

A. General information
1. Inflammation of the appendix that prevents mucus from passing into the cecum; if untreated, ischemia, gangrene, rupture, and peritonitis occur
2. Most common in school-age children
3. May be caused by mechanical obstruction (fecaliths, intestinal parasites) or anatomic defect; may be related to decreased fiber in the diet

B. Assessment findings
1. Diffuse pain, localizes in lower right quadrant
2. Nausea/vomiting
3. Guarding of abdomen, rebound tenderness, walks stooped over
4. Decreased bowel sounds
5. Fever
6. Diagnostic tests
   a. WBC increased
   b. Elevated acetone in urine

C. Nursing interventions
1. Administer antibiotics/antipyretics as ordered
2. Prevent perforation of the appendix; do not give enemas or cathartics or use heating pad
3. In addition to routine pre-op care for appendectomy
   a. Give support to parents if seeking treatment was delayed.
   b. Explain necessity of obtaining lab work prior to surgery.
4. In addition to routine post-op care
   a. Monitor NG tube (usually with low suction).
   b. Monitor Penrose drains.
   c. Position in semi-Fowler's or lying on right side to facilitate drainage.
   d. Administer antibiotics as ordered.

Parasitic Worms

A. General information
1. A parasite is an organism that lives in, on, or at the expense of the host.
2. Common human GI parasites are pinworms and roundworms.
3. Medication varies depending on type of parasite.

B. Assessment findings
1. Pinworms: anal irritation, itching, disturbed sleep
2. Roundworm: colic, abdominal pain, lack of appetite, weight loss

C. Nursing interventions
1. Obtain stool culture.
2. Observe for worms in all excreta (Scotch-tape test for stool).
3. Instruct parents to change clothing, bed linens, towels and launder in hot water.
4. Clean toilets with disinfectant.
5. Instruct all family members to scrub hands and fingernails prior to eating and after using toilet.
6. Follow specific medication and hygiene orders given by physician.

Constipation

A. General information
1. Decrease in number of bowel movements with large, hard stools
2. May be caused by high fat and protein and low fluid in diet
3. May cause bowel obstruction if severe

B. Medical management
1. Drug therapy: stool softeners, suppositories, enemas
2. Diet therapy: increased fluids and fiber

C. Assessment findings
1. Less frequent stools, difficulty eliminating stool, hard consistency compared to normal pattern (children do not have to stool every day)
2. Bleeding with stooling
3. Abdominal pain

D. Nursing interventions
1. Assess for other pathologic causes of constipation.
2. Apply lubricant around anus.
3. Remove stool digitally if possible.
4. Provide prune juice (1 oz); add fruits to diet.
5. Add small amount of Karo syrup to formula.
6. Teach parents methods to prevent further episodes.

SAMPLE QUESTIONS

Janie, age 9, has celiac disease which has been in good control since it was diagnosed six years ago. She has now been admitted to the hospital for an emergency appendectomy.

14. Which preoperative procedure should the nurse withhold?
    - o 1. A cleansing enema
    - o 2. Starting an IV
    - o 3. Keeping her NPO
    - o 4. Obtaining a blood sample for a CBC

15. Janie's recovery is progressing well and she is having her first meal. Which food should the nurse remove from her tray?
    - o 1. Chicken rice soup
    - o 2. Crackers
    - o 3. Hamburger patty
    - o 4. Fresh fruit cup

The Genitourinary System

VARIATIONS FROM THE ADULT

A. Nephrons continue to develop after birth.
B. Glomerular filtration rate is 30% below adult levels at birth; reaches normal level by age 2 years.
C. Tubular functions immature at birth; tubular absorption and secretion reach adult levels by age 1 year.
D. Urethra is shorter in children and more prone to ascending infection (particularly true in girls); the urethra is also closer to anus as source of contamination.
E. Many GU conditions in children become chronic.

ASSESSMENT

History

A. Presenting problem: symptoms may include
   1. Change in appearance, color, or smell of urine
   2. Change in amount, frequency, or pattern of urination
   3. Abdominal or back pain
   4. Anorexia, nausea, vomiting, weight loss
   5. Headaches, seizures
   6. Fatigue, lethargy
   7. Excessive thirst
   8. Drug use or accidental ingestions
B. Family history: kidney disease, hypertension

Physical Examination

A. General appearance: note presence of edema.
B. Abdomen and genitalia: note abdominal distension, presence of undescended testicle, tenderness to palpation, placement of urinary meatus, urinary stream during voiding.
C. Vital signs: note presence of fever; increased blood pressure (common in renal disease)

ANALYSIS

Nursing diagnoses for the child with a disorder of the genitourinary tract may include
A. Alteration in fluid volume: excess
B. Alteration in pattern of urinary elimination
C. Alteration in comfort: pain
D. Activity intolerance
E. Alteration in family process

PLANNING AND IMPLEMENTATION

Goals

A. Child will have normal urinary function.
B. Child's fluid and electrolyte and acid-base balances will be normal.
C. Child will be free from signs of infection.
D. Child's blood pressure will be within normal limits.
E. Parents will be able to care for child at home.

Intervention

Pediatric Urine Collector (PUC)

A. Used when child is not toilet trained
B. Nursing care
   1. Wash genitalia as for clean catch specimens.
   2. Apply bag directly to dry skin; do not use powder or creams.
   3. If child has not voided within 45 minutes, remove bag and repeat process.

EVALUATION

A. Child is adequately hydrated as evidenced by normal serum electrolyte and blood gas values, and normal urine output.
B. Child is free from complications such as infection, skin breakdown, or hypertension.
C. Parents demonstrate ability to administer appropriate medications and treatments.

DISORDERS OF THE GENITOURINARY TRACT

Urinary Tract Infection (UTI)

A. General information
   1. Bacterial invasion of the kidneys or bladder

2. More common in girls, preschool and school-age children

3. Usually caused by *E. coli*; predisposing factors include poor hygiene, irritation from bubble baths, urinary reflux

4. The invading organism ascends the urinary tract, irritating the mucosa and causing characteristic symptoms.

B. Assessment findings

  1. Low-grade fever

  2. Abdominal pain

  3. Enuresis, pain/burning on urination, frequency, hematuria

C. Nursing interventions

  1. Administer antibiotics as ordered; prevention of kidney infection/glomerulonephritis important. (*Note:* obtain cultures before starting antibiotics.)

  2. Provide warm baths and allow child to void in water to alleviate painful voiding.

  3. Force fluids.

  4. Encourage measures to acidify urine (cranberry juice, acid-ash diet).

  5. Provide patient teaching and discharge planning concerning

    a. Avoidance of tub baths (contamination from dirty water may allow microorganisms to travel up urethra)

    b. Avoidance of bubble baths that might irritate urethra

    c. Importance for girls to wipe perineum from front to back

    d. Increase in foods/fluids that acidify urine.

Vesicoureteral Reflux

A. General information

  1. Regurgitation of urine from the bladder into the ureters due to faulty valve mechanism at the vesicoureteral junction

  2. Predisposes child to

    a. UTIs from urine stasis

    b. Pyelonephritis from chronic UTIs

    c. Hydronephrosis from increased pressure on renal pelvis

B. Assessment findings: same as for Urinary Tract Infections

C. Nursing interventions for surgical reimplantation of ureters

  1. Assist with preoperative studies as needed (IVP, voiding cystourethrogram, cystoscopy).

  2. Provide postoperative care.

    a. Monitor drains; may have one from bladder and one from each ureter (ureteral stents).

    b. Check output from all drains (expect bloody drainage initially) and record carefully.

    c. Observe drainage from abdominal dressing; note color, amount, frequency.

    d. Administer medication for bladder spasms as ordered.

Exstrophy of the Bladder

A. General information

  1. Congenital malformation in which nonfusion of abdominal and anterior walls of the bladder during embrylogic development causes anterior surface of bladder to lie open on abdominal wall

  2. Varying degrees of defect

B. Assessment findings

  1. Associated structural changes

    a. Prolapsed rectum

    b. Inguinal hernia

    c. Widely split symphysis

    d. Rotated hips

  2. Associated anomalies

    a. Epispadias

    b. Cleft scrotum or clitoris

    c. Undescended testicles

    d. Chordee (downward deflection of the penis)

C. Medical management: two-stage reconstructive surgery, possibly with urinary diversion; usually delayed until age 3–6 months

D. Nursing interventions: preoperative

  1. Provide bladder care; prevent infection.

    a. Keep area as clean as possible; urine on skin will cause irritation and ulceration.

    b. Change diaper frequently; keep diaper loose-fitting.

    c. Wash with mild soap and water.

    d. Cover exposed bladder with Vaseline gauze.

E. Nursing interventions: postoperative

  1. Design play activities to foster toddler's need for autonomy (e.g., Play-Doh, talking toys, books); child will be immobilized for extended period of time.

  2. Prevent trauma; as child gets older and more mobile, trauma more likely; teach parents to avoid areas such as sandboxes.

Undescended Testicles (Cryptorchidism)

A. General information

  1. Unilateral or bilateral absence of testes in scrotal sac

  2. Testes normally descend at 8 months of gestation, will therefore be absent in premature infants

  3. Incidence increased in children having genetically transmitted diseases

  4. Unilateral cryptorchidism most common

  5. 75% will descend spontaneously by age 1 year

B. Medical management

  1. Whether or not to treat is still controversial; if testes remain in abdomen, damage to the testes (sterility) is possible because of increased body temperature.

  2. If not descended by age 8 or 9, chorionic gonadatropin can be given.

  3. Orchipexy: surgical procedure to retrieve and secure testes placement; performed between ages 1–3 years.

C. Assessment findings: unable to palpate testes in scrotal sac (when palpating testes be careful not to elicit cremasteric reflex, which pulls testes higher in pelvic cavity)

D. Nursing interventions

  1. Advise parents of absence of testes and provide information about treatment options.

  2. Support parents if surgery is to be performed.

  3. Post-op, avoid disturbing the tension mechanism (will be in place for about 1 week).

  4. Avoid contamination of incision.

Hypospadias

A. General information
  1. Urethral opening located anywhere along the ventral surface of penis
  2. Chordee (ventral curvature of the penis) often associated, causing constriction
  3. In extreme cases, child's sex may be uncertain
B. Medical management
  1. Minimal defects need no intervention
  2. Neonatal circumcision delayed, tissue may be needed for corrective repair
  3. Surgery performed at about age 6–18 months
C. Assessment findings
  1. Urinary meatus misplaced
  2. Inability to make straight stream of urine
D. Nursing interventions
  1. Diaper normally without extra care (voiding presents no problem).
  2. Provide support for parents who will be distraught over defect and sexual overtones; refer for counseling as needed.
  3. Provide support for child at time of surgery; fears of mutilation are prominent.
  4. After surgery check orders for dressing changes; monitor catheter drainage.

Enuresis

A. General information
  1. Involuntary passage of urine after the age of control is expected (about 4 years)
  2. Types
     a. Primary: in children who have never achieved control
     b. Secondary: in children who have developed complete control and lose it
  3. May occur at any time of day but is most frequent at night
  4. More common in boys
  5. No organic cause can be identified; familial tendency
  6. Etiologic possibilities
     a. Sleep disturbances
     b. Delayed neurologic development
     c. Immature development of bladder leading to decreased capacity
     d. Psychologic problems
B. Medical management
  1. Bladder-stretching exercises
  2. Bed alarm devices
  3. Drug therapy: results are temporary; side effects may be unpleasant or even dangerous
     a. Tricyclic antidepressants: imipramine HCl (Tofranil)
     b. Amphetamines
     c. Axiolytic agents
C. Assessment findings
  1. Physical exam normal
  2. History of repeated involuntary urination
D. Nursing interventions
  1. Provide information/counseling to family as needed.

a. Confirm that this is not conscious behavior and that child is not purposefully misbehaving.
     b. Assure parents that they are not responsible and that this is a relatively common problem.
  2. Involve child in care; give praise and support with small accomplishments.
     a. Age 5–6 years: can strip bed of wet sheets.
     b. Age 10–12 years: can do laundry and change bed.
  3. Avoid scolding and belittling child

Nephrosis (Nephrotic Syndrome)

A. General information
  1. Autoimmune process leading to structural alteration of glomerular membrane that results in increased permeability to plasma proteins, particularly albumin
  2. Course of the disease consists of exacerbations and remissions over a period of months to years
  3. Commonly affects preschoolers, boys more often than girls
  4. Pathophysiology
     a. Plasma proteins enter the renal tubule and are excreted in the urine causing proteinuria.
     b. Protein shift causes altered oncotic pressure and lowered plasma volume.
     c. Hypovolemia triggers release of renin and angiotensin, which stimulates increased secretion of aldosterone; aldosterone increases reabsorption of water and sodium in distal tubule.
     d. Lowered blood pressure also stimulates release of ADH, further increasing reabsorption of water; together with a general shift of plasma into interstitial spaces, results in edema.
  5. Prognosis is good unless edema does not respond to steroids.
B. Medical management
  1. Drug therapy
     a. Corticosteroids to resolve edema
     b. Antibiotics for bacterial infections
     c. Thiazide diuretics in edematous stage
  2. Bedrest
  3. Diet modification: high protein, low sodium
C. Assessment findings
  1. Proteinuria, hypoproteinemia, hyperlipidemia
  2. Dependent body edema
     a. Puffiness around eyes in morning
     b. Ascites
     c. Scrotal edema
     d. Ankle edema
  3. Anorexia, vomiting, and diarrhea, malnutrition
  4. Pallor, lethargy
  5. Hepatomegaly
D. Nursing interventions
  1. Provide bedrest.
     a. Conserve energy.
     b. Find activities for quiet play.
  2. Provide high-protein, low-sodium diet during edema phase only.

3. Maintain skin integrity.
   a. Do not use Band-Aids.
   b. Avoid IM injections (medication is not absorbed into edematous tissue).
   c. Turn frequently.
4. Obtain morning urine for protein studies.
5. Provide scrotal support.
6. Monitor I&O, vital signs and weigh daily.
7. Administer steroids to suppress autoimmune response as ordered.

Acute Glomerulonephritis (AGN)

A. General information
   1. Immune complex disease resulting from an antigen-antibody reaction
   2. Secondary to a beta-hemolytic streptococcal infection occurring elsewhere in the body
   3. Occurs more frequently in boys, usually between ages 6–7 years
   4. Usually resolves in about 14 days, self-limiting
B. Medical management
   1. Antibiotics for streptococcal infection
   2. Antihypertensives if blood pressure severely elevated
   3. Digitalis if circulatory overload
   4. Fluid restriction if renal insufficiency
   5. Peritoneal dialysis if severe renal or cardiopulmonary problems develop
C. Assessment findings
   1. History of a precipitating streptococcal infection, usually upper respiratory infection or impetigo
   2. Edema, anorexia, lethargy
   3. Hematuria or dark-colored urine, fever
   4. Hypertension
   5. Diagnostic tests
      a. Urinalysis reveals RBCs, WBCs, protein, cellular casts
      b. Urine specific gravity increased
      c. BUN and serum creatinine increased
      d. ESR elevated
      e. Hgb and Hct decreased
D. Nursing interventions
   1. Monitor I&O, blood pressure, urine; weigh daily.
   2. Provide diversional therapy.
   3. Provide patient teaching and discharge planning concerning
      a. Medication administration
      b. Prevention of infection
      c. Signs of renal complications
      d. Importance of long-term follow-up.

Hydronephrosis

A. General information
   1. Collection of urine in the renal pelvis due to obstruction to outflow
   2. Obstruction most common at ureteral-pelvic junction (see Vesicoureteral Reflux, page **339**) but may also be caused by adhesions, ureterocele, calculi, or congenital malformation
   3. Obstruction causes increased intrarenal pressure, decreased circulation, and atrophy of the kidney leading to renal insufficiency
   4. May be unilateral or bilateral, occurs more often in left kidney
   5. Prognosis good when treated early
B. Medical management: surgery to correct or remove obstruction
C. Assessment findings
   1. Repeated UTIs
   2. Failure to thrive
   3. Abdominal pain, fever
   4. Fluctuating mass in region of kidney
D. Nursing interventions: prepare child for multiple urologic studies (see also Vesicoureteral Reflux).

Wilm's Tumor (Nephroblastoma)

A. General information
   1. Large, encapsulated tumor that develops in the renal parenchyma, more frequently in left kidney (usually unilateral)
   2. Originates during fetal life from undifferentiated embryonic tissues
   3. Peak age of occurrence: 1–3 years
   4. Prognosis good if there are no metastases.
B. Medical management
   1. Nephrectomy, with total removal of tumor
   2. Postsurgical radiation in treatment of stages II, III, and IV; stage I disease does not usually require radiation, but it may be used if the tumor histology is unfavorable.
   3. Postsurgical chemotherapy: vincristine and daunorubicin, doxorubicin
C. Assessment findings
   1. Staging
      a. Stage I: limited to kidney
      b. Stage II: tumor extends beyond kidney, but is completely encapsulated
      c. Stage III: tumor confined to abdomen
      d. Stage IV: tumor has metastasized to lung, liver, bone, or brain
      e. Stage V: bilateral renal involvement at diagnosis
   2. Usually mother notices mass while bathing or dressing child; nontender, usually midline near liver
   3. Hypertension and possible hematuria, anemia, and signs of metastasis
   4. Diagnostic test: IVP reveals mass
D. Nursing interventions
   1. Do not palpate abdomen to avoid possible dissemination of cancer cells.
   2. Handle child carefully when bathing and giving care.
   3. Provide care for the patient with a nephrectomy (page 147); usually performed within 24–48 hours of diagnosis.
   4. Provide care for the child receiving chemotherapy and radiation therapy.

SAMPLE QUESTIONS

Lisa is 2 years old and has been admitted to the pediatric unit with a diagnosis of Wilm's tumor.

16. Which would be the MOST important nursing intervention for Lisa?
    - o 1. Empty the bladder using Credé maneuver for a urine specimen.
    - o 2. Record daily abdominal girths.
    - o 2. Auscultate the abdomen for bowel sounds.
    - o 4. Post a sign over the crib advising that her abdomen should not be palpated.

Walter is 20 months old and admitted to the hospital with a diagnosis of cryptorchidism.

17. Surgical correction is performed at this time to prevent
    - o 1. difficulty in urinating.
    - o 2. sterility.
    - o 3. herniation.
    - o 4. peritonitis.

The Musculoskeletal System

VARIATIONS FROM THE ADULT

Bones

A. Linear growth results from skeletal development
  1. Centers of ossification
    a. Primary centers in diaphyses
    b. Secondary centers in epiphyses
    c. Used in assessment of bone age; number of ossification centers in wrist equals age in years plus 1
    d. Centers appear earlier in girls than in boys
  2. Metaphysis
    a. Cartilaginous plate between diaphysis and epiphysis
    b. The site of active growth in long bones
    c. Disappears over time with bony fusion of diaphysis and epiphysis
    d. Linear growth ends with epiphyseal fusion
    e. Assessment of bone age includes the advancing bone edges
B. Bone circumference growth occurs as new bone tissue is formed beneath the periosteum.
C. Skeletal maturity is reached by age 17 in boys and 2 years after menarche in girls.
D. Certain characteristics of bone in children affect injury and healing, bones are more prone to injury, and injury results from relatively minor accidents.
  1. Metaphysis
    a. Absorbs shock, protects joints from injury.
    b. Traumatic injury or infection to this growth plate can cause deformity.
    c. If not injured, this growth plate participates in healing and straightening of limbs by process of remodeling.
  2. Porous bone
    a. Increases flexibility; absorbs force on impact.
    b. Allows bones to bend, buckle, and break in "greenstick" or incomplete fracture.
  3. Thicker periosteum
    a. More active osteogenic potential
    b. Healing more rapid
      1) neonatal period: may take 2–3 weeks
      2) early childhood: may take 4 weeks
      3) later childhood: may take 6 weeks
      4) adolescence: 8–10 weeks
    c. Stiffness after immobilization is rare unless joint has been injured.
E. Bone growth is affected by Wolff's law: bone will grow in the direction in which stress is placed on it.

Muscles

A. Muscle growth is responsible for a large part of increase in body weight.
B. The number of muscle fibers is constant throughout life; growth results from an increase in the size of the muscle fibers and by an increased number of nuclei per fiber.
C. Muscle growth most apparent in adolescence, influenced by growth hormone, adrenal androgens, and in boys by testosterone.

ASSESSMENT

History

A. Presenting problem: symptoms may include
  1. Delayed motor development
  2. Injury
  3. Pain, loss of sensation, tingling
  4. Muscle weakness, loss of function of an extremity
  5. Interference with normal activity or play
  6. Other parental concerns
B. Family history: genetic disorders, skeletal deformities

Physical Examination

A. General appearance: note any asymmetry, visible deformities, swelling (of joints or over bones), quality of movement (ROM, gait, guarding).
B. Measure muscle strength.
C. Identify warmth or tenderness over bones and joints.
D. Assess pain: note type, location, onset, relationship to activity.

ANALYSIS

Nursing diagnoses for the child with a disorder of the musculoskeletal system may include

A. Potential for activity intolerance
B. Alteration in comfort: pain
C. Diversional activity deficit
D. Potential for injury
E. Impaired physical mobility
F. Self-care deficit
G. Disturbance in self-concept: body image
H. Potential impairment of skin integrity
I. Alteration in tissue perfusion: peripheral

PLANNING AND IMPLEMENTATION

Goals

A. Injury or deformity will be identified and treated early.
B. Child will achieve maximum level of mobility.
C. Pain will be relieved/controlled.
D. Child will be free from injury.
E. Parents will be able to care for child at home.

Interventions

Care of the Child with a Cast

Also see page 154.
A. General information
   1. Initial chemical hardening reaction may cause a change in an infant's body temperature; monitor and intervene as needed.
   2. Choose toys too big to fit down cast.
   3. Do not use baby powder near cast since it clumps and provides a medium for bacterial growth.
   4. Prepare for anticipated casting by having child help apply a cast to a doll the day before.
   5. Demonstrate the use of a cast cutter on a doll before using on child to show it does not cut skin.
B. Care of child in hip spica cast (cast encases child from nipples to knees; legs are abducted with a bar between the thighs) (Figure 3.3)
   1. Use firm mattress to allow for increased weight of plaster cast.
   2. Do not lift cast by crossbar.
   3. Protect cast from water and urine.
      a. Put waterproof material over petaling (Chux, plastic diapers).
      b. Elevate head of bed slightly to prevent urine and stool from seeping under cast; confirm that entire body is on a slant, not just the head.
      c. Use Bradford frame (canvas board with opening near genitalia) and place a bedpan under opening.
   4. Use pillows to support all parts of the cast.
   5. Keep towel or Chux across top of chest part of cast during feedings to prevent crumbs from entering cast.
   6. Monitor for pain/pressure points due to growth if cast is on for a long time.

Care of the Child in Traction

Also see page 154.

A. General information
   1. Infants and young toddlers do not have enough body weight to use traditional tractions effectively.
   2. Children do not understand the necessity of maintaining proper body alignment and will need frequent repositioning.
B. Bryant's traction: used primarily in children
   1. Child is own counterweight.
   2. Both legs are at 90° angle to bed.
   3. Buttocks must be slightly off mattress in order to ensure sufficient traction on legs.
   4. Used with children under age 2 years whose weight is too low (under 30 lb [14 kg]) to counterbalance without additional gravitational force.
   5. Used for fractured femur and dislocated hip.
   6. Monitor for vascular injury to feet with frequent neurovascular checks.

Care of the Child with a Brace

A. General information
   1. Orthopedic device made of metal or leather applied to the body, particularly the trunk and lower extremities, to support the weight of the body, to corrrect or prevent deformities, and to prevent involuntary movements in spastic conditions
   2. Types
      a. Milwaukee brace
         1) steel and leather brace fitted and adapted to child individually
         2) extends from chin cup and neck pad to pelvis
         3) used in scoliosis to correct curvature
         4) worn 23 hours/day, removed once daily for bathing
         5) causes little interference with activity

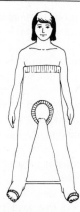

Figure 3.3 Hip spica cast.

    b. Rotowalker
      1) used to provide upright mobility in children with lower limb paralysis
      2) child shifts weight to achieve mobility
    c. Leg brace
      1) designed to stabilize extremity and offer support during ambulation
      2) special hinges permit hip, knee and ankle to flex during sitting
B. Nursing care: provide patient teaching and discharge planning concerning
  1. Importance of meticulous skin care
  2. Need to wear protective clothing under brace
  3. Potential problems of ill-fitting braces
    a. Difficulty in balancing
    b. Muscle stress and skin breakdown
  4. Need for frequent checking and adjustment of braces with growth.

EVALUATION

A. Child's musculoskeletal development is normal as evidenced by normal growth and activity.
B. Child experiences minimal discomfort.
C. Injuries are prevented.
D. Parents demonstrate ability to identify complications and administer treatments correctly.

DISORDERS OF THE MUSCULOSKELETAL SYSTEM

Congenital Dislocation of the Hip

A. General information
  1. Displacement of the head of the femur from the acetabulum; present at birth, although not always diagnosed immediately
  2. One of the most common congenital malformations; incidence is 1 in 500–1000 live births
  3. Familial disorder, more common in girls; may be associated with spina bifida
  4. Cause unknown; may be fetal position in utero (breech delivery), genetic predisposition, or laxity of ligaments
  5. The acetabulum is shallow and the head of the femur cartilaginous at birth, contributing to the dislodgment.
B. Medical management
  1. Goal is to enlarge and deepen socket by pressure.
  2. The earlier treatment is initiated, the shorter and less traumatic it will be.
  3. Early treatment consists of positioning the hip in abduction with the head of the femur in the acetabulum and maintaining it in position for several months.
  4. If these measures are unsuccessful, traction and casting (hip spica) or surgery may be successful.

C. Assessment findings
  1. May be unilateral or bilateral, partial or complete
  2. Limitation of abduction (cannot spread legs to change diaper)
  3. Ortolani's click (should only be performed by an experienced practitioner)
    a. With infant in supine position (on the back), bend knees and place thumbs on bent knees, fingers at hip joint.
    b. Bring femurs 90° to hip, then abduct.
    c. With dislocation there is a palpable click where the head of the femur snaps over edge of acetabulum.
  4. Barlow's test
    a. With infant on back, bend knees.
    b. Affected knee will be lower because the head of the femur dislocates towards bed by gravity (referred to as telescoping of limb).
  5. Additional skin folds with knees bent, from telescoping
  6. When lying on abdomen, buttocks of affected side will be flatter because head of femur falls toward bed from gravity
  7. Trendelenburg test (used if child is old enough to walk)
    a. Have child stand on affected leg only.
    b. Pelvis will dip on normal side as child attempts to stay erect.
D. Nursing interventions
  1. Maintain proper positioning: keep legs abducted.
    a. Use triple diapering.
    b. Use Frejka pillow splint (jumperlike suit to keep legs abducted).
    c. Place infant on abdomen with legs in "frog" position.
    d. Use immobilization devices (splints, casts, braces).
  2. Provide adequate nutrition; adapt feeding position as needed for immobilization device.
  3. Provide sensory stimulation; adapt to immobilization device and positioning.
  4. Provide patient teaching and discharge planning concerning
    a. Application and care of immobilization devices
    b. Modification of child care using immobilization devices.

Clubfoot (Talipes)

A. General information
  1. Abnormal rotation of foot at ankle
    a. Varus (inward rotation): would walk on ankles, bottoms of feet face each other
    b. Valgus (outward rotation): would walk on inner ankles
    c. Calcaneous (upward rotation): would walk on heels
    d. Equinas (downward rotation): would walk on toes
  2. Most common deformity (95%) is talipes equinovarus.
  3. Deformity almost always congenital; usually unilateral
  4. Occurs more frequently in boys than in girls; may be associated with other congenital disorders but cause unknown
  5. General incidence: 1 in 700–1000

B. Medical management
  1. Exercises
  2. Casting (cast is changed periodically to change angle of foot)
  3. Denis Browne splint (bar shoe): metal bar with shoes attached to the bar at specific angle
  4. Surgery and casting for several months
C. Assessment findings: foot cannot be manipulated by passive exercises into correct position (differentiate from normal clubbing of newborn's feet)
D. Nursing interventions
  1. Perform exercises as ordered.
  2. Provide cast care or care for child in a brace.
  3. Child who is learning to walk must be prevented from trying to stand; apply restraints if necessary.
  4. Provide diversional activities.
  5. Adapt care routines as needed for cast or brace.
  6. Assess toes to be sure cast is not too tight.
  7. Provide skin care.
  8. Provide patient teaching and discharge planning concerning
    a. Application/care of immobilization device
    b. Preparation for surgery if indicated
    c. Need to monitor special shoes for continued fit throughout treatment.

Tibial Torsion

A. General information
  1. Rotational deformity of tibia (greater than that normally found in newborn)
  2. Types
    a. Internal: knee forward and foot inward
    b. External: knee forward and foot outward (rare, associated with muscle paralysis)
  3. Majority of cases resolve without treatment
B. Medical management
  1. Splinting: use of Denis Browne splint at night
  2. Surgical correction if still evident by age 3 years
C. Assessment findings: with child lying supine, assess for straight line between tibial tuberosity and 2nd toe; in tibial torsion, the line intersects the 4th or 5th toe.
D. Nursing interventions
  1. If no treatment needed, encourage parents to be patient and emphasize that condition usually resolves by itself
  2. If stretching exercises are recommended, teach parents normal ROM exercises and how to carry them out.
  3. Instruct parents on use of Denis Browne splint if needed.

Legg-Calvé-Perthes Disease

A. General information
  1. Aseptic necrosis of femoral head due to disturbance of circulation to the area
  2. Primarily affects boys ages 4–10 years
  3. Stages: lasting from 18 months to a few years
    a. Initial stage: may not be distinguishable from transient synovitis

b. Avascular stage: often the first stage noticed
    c. Revascularization stage: regeneration of vascular and connective tissue
    d. Regeneration stage: formation of new bone
B. Medical management: goal is to minimize deformity until healing process is completed
  1. Initial bedrest with traction and then an abduction brace
  2. Possible surgery
C. Assessment findings
  1. Limp, limitation of movement
  2. Pain in groin, hip, and referred to knee; often difficult for child to localize pain
  3. Diagnostic test: x-ray reveals opaque ossification center of head of the femur (softened in avascular stage)
D. Nursing interventions
  1. Provide care for a child with a cast or brace.
  2. Provide diversional activities.

Slipped Femoral Capital Epiphysis

A. General information
  1. Spontaneous displacement of proximal femoral epiphysis in a posterior and inferior direction
  2. Onset insidious; usually occurs during fast growth period of adolescence (growth hormones weaken epiphyseal plate)
  3. Occurs most often in very tall and very obese adolescents; boys affected more frequently
B. Medical management
  1. Skeletal traction
  2. Surgical stabilization with pinning
C. Assessment findings
  1. Limp and referred pain to groin, hip, or knee
  2. Limited internal rotation and abduction of hip
D. Nursing interventions
  1. Suggest weight reduction program for obese children to decrease stress on bones.
  2. Provide care for the child with a cast or traction.

Osteogenesis Imperfecta

A. General information
  1. An inherited disorder affecting collagen formation and resulting in pathologic fractures
  2. Types
    a. Osteogenesis imperfecta congenita: autosomal recessive, prognosis poor
    b. Osteogenesis imperfecta tarda: autosomal dominant, less severe form, involvement of varying degrees
  3. Classic picture includes soft, fragile bones; blue sclera; otosclerosis
  4. Severity of symptoms decreases at puberty due to hormone production and child's ability to prevent injury.
B. Medical management
  1. Magnesium oxide supplements
  2. Reduction and immobilization of fractures
C. Assessment findings

1. Osteogenesis imperfecta congenita
   a. Multiple fractures at birth
   b. Possible skeletal deformity due to intrauterine fracture
   c. Bones of skull are soft
   d. Occasional intracranial hemorrhage
2. Osteogenesis imperfecta tarda
   a. Delayed walking, fractures, structural scoliosis as child grows
   b. Lower limbs more frequently affected
   c. Hypermobility of joints
   d. Prone to dental caries
D. Nursing interventions
   1. Support limbs, do not stretch.
   2. Position with care; use blankets to aid in mobility and provide support.
   3. Instruct parents in bathing, dressing, diapering.
   4. Support parents; encourage expression of feelings of anger or guilt (parents may have been unjustly suspected of child abuse).

Scoliosis

A. General information
   1. Lateral curvature of the spine
   2. Most commonly occurs in adolescent girls
   3. Disorder has a familial pattern; associated with other neuromuscular disorders
   4. Majority of the time (75% of cases) disorder is idiopathic; other causes include congenital abnormality of vertebrae, neuromuscular disorders, and trauma
   5. May be functional or structural
      a. Nonstructural/functional: "C" curve of spine
         1) due to posture, can be corrected voluntarily and disappears when child lies down
         2) not progressive
         3) treated with posture exercises
      b. Structural/progressive: "S" curve of spine
         1) usually idiopathic
         2) structural change in spine, does not disappear with position changes
         3) more aggressive intervention needed
B. Medical management
   1. Stretching exercises of the spine for nonstructural changes
   2. Milwaukee brace worn for 23 hours/day for 3 years
   3. Plaster jacket cast
   4. Halo-pelvic or halo-femoral traction
   5. Spinal fusion with insertion of Harrington rod
C. Assessment findings (structural scoliosis)
   1. Failure of curve to straighten when child bends forward with knees straight and arms hanging down to feet (curve disappears with functional scoliosis)
   2. Uneven bra strap marks
   3. Uneven hips
   4. Uneven shoulders
   5. Asymmetry of rib cage
   6. Diagnostic test: x-ray reveals curvature
D. Nursing interventions

1. Teach/encourage exercises as ordered.
2. Provide care for child with Milwaukee brace.
   a. Child wears brace 23 hours/day; is removed once a day for bathing.
   b. Monitor pressure points, adjustments may be needed to accommodate increase in height or weight.
   c. Promote positive body image with brace.
3. Provide cast/traction care.
4. Assist with modifying clothing for immobilization devices.
5. Adjust diet for decreased activity.
6. Provide diversional activities.
7. Provide care for child with Harrington rod insertion (below).
8. Provide patient teaching and discharge planning concerning
   a. Exercises
   b. Brace/traction/cast care
   c. Correct body mechanics
   d. Alternative education for long-term hospitalization/home care
   e. Availability of community agencies.

Harrington Rod Insertion

A. General information
   1. Spinal fusion and installation of a permanent steel rod along spine
   2. Used for moderate to severe curvatures
   3. Usually results in increase in height; positive body image changes
B. Nursing interventions (see also Laminectomy, page 160)
   1. Provide general pre-op teaching and care.
   2. In addition to routine post-op care.
      a. Log roll.
      b. Do not raise head of bed.
      c. Discuss adapting home environment to allow for privacy yet interaction with family during long-term recovery.
      d. Discuss alternative methods of education during recovery period.

Muscular Dystrophy

A. General information
   1. A group of muscular diseases in children characterized by progressive muscle weakness and deformity
   2. Genetic in origin; biochemical defect is suspected
   3. Types
      a. *Pseudohypertrophic (Duchenne type):* most frequent type
         1) x-linked recessive
         2) affects only boys
         3) usually manifests in first 4 years
      b. *Facioscapulohumeral*
         1) autosomal dominant
         2) mild form, with weakness of facial and shoulder girdle muscles
         3) onset usually in adolescence

    c. *Limb girdle*
      1) autosomal recessive
      2) affects boys and girls
      3) onset usually in adolescence
    d. *Congenital*
      1) autosomal recessive
      2) onset in utero
    e. *Myotonic*
      1) autosomal dominant
      2) more common in boys
      3) onset in infancy or childhood, or adult onset
      4) prognosis in childhood form is guarded

4. Disease causes progressive disability throughout childhood; most children with Duchenne's muscular dystrophy are confined to a wheelchair by age 8–10 years

5. Death occurs by age 20 in 75% of patients with Duchenne's muscular dystrophy.

B. Assessment findings (Duchenne type)

1. Pelvic girdle weakness is early sign (child waddles and falls)

2. Gower's sign (child uses hands to push up from the floor)

3. Scoliosis (from weakness of shoulder girdle)

4. Contractures and hypertrophy of muscles

5. Diagnostic tests

    a. Muscle biopsy reveals histologic changes: degeneration of muscle fibers and replacement of fibers with fat.

    b. EMG shows decrease in amplitude and duration of potentials.

6. Serum enzymes increased, especially CPK

C. Nursing interventions

1. Prepare child for EMG and muscle biopsy.

2. Maintain function at optimal level; keep child as active and independent as possible.

3. Plan diet to prevent obesity.

4. Continually evaluate capabilities.

5. Support child and parents and provide information about availability of community agencies and support groups.

Juvenile Rheumatoid Arthritis (JRA)

A. General information

1. Systemic, chronic disorder of connective tissue, resulting from an autoimmune reaction

2. Results in eventual joint destruction

3. Affected by stress, climate, and genetics

4. More common in girls; peak ages 2–5 and 9–12 years

5. Types

    a. *Mono/pauciarticular JRA*
      1) fewer than 4 joints involved (usually in legs)
      2) asymmetric; rarely systemic
      3) generally mild signs of arthritis
      4) symptoms may decrease as child enters adulthood
      5) prognosis good

    b. *Polyarticular JRA*
      1) multiple joints affected
      2) symmetrical symptoms of arthritis, disability may be mild to severe

      3) involvement of temporomandibular joint may cause earaches
      4) characterized by periods of remissions and exacerbations
      5) prognosis poorer
      6) treatment symptomatic for arthritis: physical therapy, ROM exercises, aspirin

    c. *Systemic disease with polyarthritis (Still's disease)*
      1) explosive course with remissions and exacerbations lasting for months
      2) begins with fever, rash, lymphadenopathy, anorexia and weight loss

B. Medical management, assessment findings, and nursing interventions: see Rheumatoid Arthritis, page 155.

Bone Tumors

Osteogenic Sarcoma

A. General information

1. Primary bone tumor arising from the mesenchymal cells and characterized by formation of osteoid (immature bone)

2. Invades ends of long bones, most frequently distal end of femur or proximal end of tibia

3. Occurs more often in boys, usually between ages 10–20 years

4. Lungs most frequent site of metastasis

5. 5-year survival rate is 10%–20%

B. Medical management

1. Surgery: treatment of choice

    a. Amputation: temporary prothesis used immediately after surgery; permanent one usually fitted a few weeks later

    b. Limb salvage procedures

    c. Lung surgery if there are metastases

2. Radiation: only in areas where tumor is not accessible to surgery

3. Chemotherapy: adjuvant therapy being studied

C. Assessment findings

1. Insidious pain, increasing with activity, gradually becoming more severe

2. Tender mass, warm to touch; limitation of movement

3. Pathologic fractures

D. Nursing interventions: see also Pediatric Oncology, page **356**.

1. Prepare child for amputation: discuss fears, concerns and facts of procedure; answer questions regarding prosthetic devices, limited activity.

2. Assure child that phantom limb pain will subside.

Ewing's Sarcoma

A. General information

1. Primary tumor arising from cells in bone marrow

2. Invades bone longitudinally, destroying bone tissue; no new bone formation

3. Femur most frequently affected site

4. More common in males, between ages 5–15 years

5. Lungs most frequent site of metastasis

B. Medical management
  1. High-dose radiation is primary treatment
  2. Chemotherapy
  3. Value of surgery presently being reassessed
C. Assessment findings
  1. Pain and swelling
  2. Palpable mass, may be tender, warm to touch
  3. 15%–35% of patients have metastatic disease at time of diagnosis
D. Nursing interventions: see also Pediatric Oncology.
  1. Promote exercise of affected limb to maintain function.
  2. Avoid activities that may cause added stress to affected limb.

SAMPLE QUESTIONS

Doug, age 3, has a fractured femur and is in Bryant's traction.

18. To evaluate correct application of the traction the nurse should note that
  ○ 1. Doug is being continuously and gradually pulled towards bottom of bed.
  ○ 2. Doug's buttocks are raised slightly.
  ○ 3. Doug's leg is at a 45° angle to the bed.
  ○ 4. Doug can move the unaffected leg freely.

Ethel, age 14, is in a hip spica cast.

19. To turn her correctly, the nurse should
  ○ 1. use the cross bar.
  ○ 2. turn her upper body first, then turn the lower body.
  ○ 3. log roll her.
  ○ 4. tell her to pull on the trapeze and sit up to help in turning.

The Endocrine System

VARIATIONS FROM THE ADULT

A. Adenohypophysis (anterior lobe of pituitary gland)
1. Growth hormone
   a. Does not affect prenatal growth.
   b. Main effect on linear growth is through increase of cells in skeletal bones.
   c. Maintains rate of synthesis of body protein.
2. Thyroid stimulating hormone (TSH)
   a. Important for normal development of bones, teeth and brain.
   b. Secretion decreases throughout childhood, then increases at puberty.
3. Adrenocorticotropic hormone (ACTH)
   a. Little is produced throughout childhood.
   b. Becomes active in adolescence.
   c. Stimulates adrenals to secrete sex hormones
   d. Influences production of gonadotropic hormone by hypothalmus.
      1) gonadotropic hormones activate gonads.
      2) gonads secrete estrogen or testosterone, which stimulate development of secondary sex characteristics.
4. Estrogen has an inhibitory effect on epiphyseal growth.

ANALYSIS

Nursing diagnoses for the child with a disorder of the endocrine system may include
A. Alteration in health maintenance
B. Impaired home maintenance management
C. Noncompliance
D. Disturbance in self-concept: body image, self-esteem

PLANNING AND IMPLEMENTATION

Goals

A. Any endocrine imbalance in childhood will be identifed and treated.
B. Child will achieve a normal metabolic state.
C. Child will develop successful coping mechanisms for manifestations of disease.
D. Child will have no signs of complications of the disease.

EVALUATION

A. Child receives appropriate medication, and nutritional requirements are met; symptoms of endocrine disease are controlled.
B. Child is free from complications of disease.
C. Child is achieving growth and developmental tasks on as normal a timetable as possible.
D. Child discusses feelings about body image and uses coping mechanisms that promote a positive self-image.

DISORDERS OF THE ENDOCRINE SYSTEM

Juvenile Diabetes Mellitus

Also see Diabetes Mellitus, page 173.
A. General information
1. Most common endocrine disorder of children, onset may be at any age
2. All juvenile diabetics are Type I (insulin dependent)
3. Possible genetic predisposition to disease
4. Treatments vary based on rapid growth rate in children, increased incidence of infections, and dietary fads of peers; all include insulin administration.
5. Life expectancy shortened by one-third
6. Risk of complications is high; most commonly retinopathy, neuropathy, nephropathy, skin changes, predisposition to infection
7. Children sometimes have one honeymoon period that occurs shortly after a child is regulated on insulin for the first time
   a. Lasts from 1 month to 1 year.
   b. Represents final effort of pancreas to provide insulin until beta cells are completely destroyed.
   c. During this time child does not need insulin; may be maintained on oral hypoglycemics.

d. Parents may distrust the diagnosis of diabetes and need to be reminded that symptoms will reappear and child will need insulin for life.

B. Medical management
  1. Insulin
  2. Diet therapy
  3. Exercise
  4. Prevention of complications
C. Assessment findings
  1. Rapid onset
  2. Polyuria, polydipsia, polyphagia
  3. Ketosis
  4. Normal weight or weight loss
  5. Dry, flushed skin with hyperglycemia
D. Nursing interventions
  1. Administer insulin (regular and NPH) as ordered.
  2. Force fluids without sugar.
  3. Monitor blood glucose levels daily.
  4. Observe for hypoglycemia (insulin shock): behavior changes, sweating.
  5. Provide patient teaching and discharge planning concerning
    a. Daily regimen for home care
    b. Need to wear an identification or Medic-Alert band
    c. The importance of regular meals, especially with adolescents
    d. Methods to instruct/inform relatives, neighbors, baby sitters, and teachers about care requirements
    e. Ways for child to interact normally with peers.

Congenital Hypothyroidism (Cretinism)

A. General information
  1. Disorder related to absent or nonfunctioning thyroid
  2. Newborns are supplied with maternal thyroid hormones that last up to 3 months
B. Medical management
  1. Prevention: neonatal screening blood test (mandatory in many states)
  2. Drug therapy: thyroid hormone replacement
  3. Without treatment mental retardation and developmental delay will occur after age 3 months
C. Assessment findings
  1. Alteration in body proportions; short stature with legs shorter than they should be in proportion to trunk.
  2. Tongue is enlarged and protrudes from mouth; may result in breathing and feeding difficulties.
  3. Hypothermia with cool extremities
  4. Short, thick neck; delayed dentition
  5. Hypotonia
  6. Low levels of T_3 and T_4
D. Nursing interventions
  1. Administer oral thyroxine and vitamin D as ordered to prevent mental retardation.
  2. Provide patient teaching and discharge planning concerning
    a. Medication administration and side effects
    b. Importance of continued therapy.

Hypopituitarism (Pituitary Dwarfism)

A. General information
  1. Hyposecretion of growth hormone by the anterior lobe of the pituitary gland
  2. Cause may be unknown or it may be due to craniopharyngioma
B. Medical management: administration of growth hormone (limited in supply since it is rendered from human cadavers)
C. Assessment findings
  1. Newborn is of normal size, but child falls below the third percentile by age 1.
  2. Child is well proportioned, but may be overweight for height.
  3. Underdeveloped jaw, abnormal position of teeth, high voice, delayed puberty
  4. Diagnostic tests
    a. X-rays reveal delayed closing of epiphyseal plates of long bones
    b. Normal IQ
D. Nursing interventions
  1. Interact with child according to chronologic age/developmental level, and not according to physical appearance.
  2. Administer growth hormone as ordered (because of delay in bone development, these children can still grow even when their peers have stopped).
  3. Monitor for signs and symptoms of additional neurologic disorders.
  4. Keep careful records of height and weight.
  5. Encourage child/parents to express feelings.
  6. Assist child in learning to interact normally with peers.

Hyperpituitarism (Gigantism)

A. General information
  1. Hypersecretion of growth hormone (usually related to a tumor of the anterior pituitary) resulting in enlargement of bones of head, hands, and feet, and overgrowth of long bones
  2. Especially noticeable at puberty
B. Medical management
  1. Surgery to remove tumor
  2. Radiation therapy if there is no tumor
C. Assessment findings
  1. Height beyond maximum upper percentile
  2. Proportional weight and muscle growth
  3. Coarse facial features
  4. Signs of increased ICP if caused by a tumor
D. Nursing interventions
  1. Record height and head circumference.
  2. Provide nursing care for a patient receiving radiation therapy.
  3. Provide care for the child with a brain tumor.
  4. Assist child in interacting normally with peers.

SAMPLE QUESTIONS

Jenny, age 8, is newly diagnosed with diabetes mellitus.

20. Which of the following symptoms is different from what you would expect to find in maturity-onset diabetes?
    - ○ 1. Increased appetite
    - ○ 2. Increased thirst
    - ○ 3. Increased urination
    - ○ 4. Weight loss

21. Jenny had an injection of regular and NPH insulin at 7:30 A.M. At 3:10 P.M. she complains that she does not feel well. She is pale, perspiring, and trembling. The nurse should
    - ○ 1. tell her to lie down and wait for the dinner trays to arrive.
    - ○ 2. ask her to give a urine specimen and test it for sugar and acetone.
    - ○ 3. give her a carbohydrate snack.
    - ○ 4. administer the afternoon dose of regular insulin.

22. As Jenny learns to administer her insulin she wants to know why she cannot take pills, like her grandmother, for her diabetes. The nurse's response should be
    - ○ 1. How long has your grandmother been taking oral medication?
    - ○ 2. You'll be able to stop taking insulin once you stop growing.
    - ○ 3. You have a different kind of diabetes and you will need to take insulin throughout your life.
    - ○ 4. You'll be able to switch to pills when you reach your grandmother's age.

The Integumentary System

VARIATIONS FROM THE ADULT

A. Skin is only 1 mm thick at birth; approximately twice as thick at maturity.

B. Evaporative water loss is greater in infants and small children.

C. Skin is more susceptible to bacterial infection in children.

D. Children are more prone to toxic erythema as a result of drug reactions and skin eruptions.

E. Children's skin is more susceptible to sweat retention and maceration.

ASSESSMENT

History

A. Medical history: previous skin disease, allergic conditions

B. History of present condition: onset, relationship to eating or other activities, medication usage

Physical Examination

A. Lesion type: note petechiae, erythema, ecchymosis; note secondary symptoms from rubbing, scratching, or healing.

B. Observe distribution pattern.

C. Note presence of pain or altered sensation.

D. Check scalp for signs of lice or nits.

ANALYSIS

Nursing diagnoses for the child with a disorder of the integumentary system may include

A. Alteration in comfort: pain

B. Disturbance in self-concept: body image, self-esteem

C. Sensory-perceptual alteration: kinesthetic

D. Actual and potential impairment of skin integrity

PLANNING AND IMPLEMENTATION

Goals

A. Child will be free from discomfort.

B. Skin integrity will be restored.

C. Spread of infection and secondary infection will be prevented.

EVALUATION

A. Child is free from discomfort.
  1. Minimal scratching or rubbing
  2. Relaxed facial expression
  3. Minimal restlessness

B. Child's skin is clean, dry, and free from redness or signs of irritation.

C. Child is free from complications such as spread of infection.

D. Parents demonstrate satisfactory hygiene measures when caring for child with disorder of skin or scalp.

DISORDERS OF THE SKIN

Burns

Also see page 180.

A. For children, the rule of nines is modified; the head of a small child is 18%–19%, the trunk 32%, each leg 15%, each arm 9½%.

B. Burns in infants and toddlers are frequently due to spills (pulling hot fluids on them or falling into hot baths); for older children, flame burns are more frequent.

Impetigo

A. General information
  1. Superficial bacterial infection of the outer layers of skin (usually staphylococcus or streptococcus)
  2. Common in toddlers and preschoolers
  3. Related to poor sanitation
  4. Very contagious

B. Medical management: topical and systemic antibiotics

C. Assessment findings
  1. Well-demarcated lesions
  2. Macules, papules, vesicles that rupture, causing a superficial moist erosion
  3. Moist area dries, leaving a honey-colored crust

4. Spreads peripherally
5. Most commonly found on face, axillae, and extremities
6. Pruritus
D. Nursing interventions
  1. Implement skin isolation techniques.
  2. Soften the skin and crusts with Burrow's solution compresses.
  3. Remove crusts gently.
  4. Cover draining lesions to prevent spread of infection.
  5. Administer antibiotics as ordered, both orally and as bacteriocidal ointments.
  6. Prevent secondary infection.
  7. Provide patient teaching and discharge planning concerning
    a. Medication administration
    b. Proper hygiene techniques.

Ringworm

A. General information
  1. Dermatomycosis due to various species of fungus
  2. Infected sites include
    a. Scalp (tinea capitis)
    b. Body (tinea corporis)
    c. Feet (tinea pedis or athletes foot)
  3. May be transmitted from person to person or acquired from animals or soil
B. Assessment findings
  1. Scalp
    a. Scaly circumscribed patches on the scalp
    b. Base of hair shafts are invaded by spores of the fungus; causes hair to break off resulting in alopecia
    c. Spreads in a circular pattern
    d. Detected by Wood's lamp (fluoresces green at base of the affected hair shafts)
  2. Skin: red ringed patches of vesicles; pain, scaling, itching
C. Nursing interventions
  1. Prevention: isolate from known infected persons.
  2. Apply antifungal ointment as ordered.
  3. Administer oral griseofulvin as ordered.

Pediculosis (Head Lice)

A. General information
  1. Parasitic infestation
  2. Adult lice are spread by close physical contact (sharing combs, hats, etc.)
  3. Occurs in school-age children, particularly those with long hair
B. Medical management: special shampoos followed by use of fine-tooth comb to remove nits
C. Assessment findings
  1. White eggs (nits) firmly attached to base of hair shafts
  2. Pruritus of scalp
D. Nursing interventions
  1. Institute skin isolation precautions (especially head

coverings and gloves to prevent spread to self, other staff and patients).
  2. Use special shampoo and comb the hair.
  3. Provide patient teaching and discharge planning concerning
    a. How to check self and other family members and how to treat them
    b. Washing of clothes, bed linens, etc; discourage sharing of brushes and combs.

Allergies

Diaper Rash

A. General information
  1. Contact dermatitis
  2. Plastic/rubber pants and linings of disposable diapers exacerbate the condition by prolonging contact with moist, warm environment; skin is further irritated by acidic urine.
  3. May also be caused by sensitivity to laundry soaps used
B. Medical management: exposure of skin to air/heat lamp
C. Assessment findings
  1. Erythema/excoriation in the perineal area
  2. Irritability
D. Nursing interventions
  1. Keep area clean and dry; clean with mild soap and water after each stool and as soon as child urinates.
  2. Take off diaper and expose area to air during the day.
  3. Use heat lamp as ordered.
  4. Provide patient teaching and discharge planning concerning
    a. Proper hygiene/infant care
    b. Diaper laundering methods
    c. Need to avoid use of plastic pants or disposable diapers with a plastic lining
    d. Need to avoid use of cornstarch (a good medium for bacteria once it becomes wet)
    e. Need to avoid use of commercially prepared diaper wipes since they contain chemicals and alcohol, which may be irritating.

Poison Ivy

A. General information
  1. Contact dermatitis; mediated by T-cell response so rash is not seen for 24–48 hours after contact.
  2. Poison ivy is not spread by the fluid in the vesicles; can be spread by clothes and animals that retain the plant resin.
B. Assessment findings: very pruritic impetigo-like lesions
C. Nursing interventions
  1. Administer antihistamines and cortisone as ordered.
  2. Provide patient teaching and discharge planning concerning
    a. Plant identification
    b. Need to wash with soap and water after contact with plant
    c. Importance of washing clothes to get the resin out.

Eczema

A. General information
  1. Atopic dermatitis, often the first sign of an allergic predisposition in a child; many later develop respiratory allergies
  2. Usually manifests during infancy
B. Medical management
  1. Drug therapy
    a. Topical steroids
    b. Antihistamines
    c. Coal tar preparations
    d. Cautious administration of immunizations
    e. Medicated or colloid baths
  2. Diet therapy: elimination diet to detect offending foods
C. Assessment findings
  1. Erythema, weeping vesicles that rupture and crust over
  2. Usually evident on cheeks, scalp, behind ears, and on flexor surfaces of extremities (rarely on diaper area)
  3. Severe pruritus; scratching causes thickening and darkening of skin
  4. Dry skin, sometimes urticaria
D. Nursing interventions
  1. Avoid heat and prevent sweating; keep skin dry (moisture aggravates condition).
  2. Monitor elimination diet to detect food cause.
    a. Remove all solid foods from diet (formula only).
    b. If symptoms disappear after 3 days, start 1 new food group every 3 days to see if symptoms reappear.
    c. The food that is suspected of causing the rash is withdrawn again to make sure symptoms go away in 3 days and is then introduced a second time (challenge test).
  3. Check materials in contact with child's skin (sheets, lotions, soaps).
  4. Avoid frequent baths.
    a. Add Alpha Keri to bath.
    b. Provide lubricant immediately after bath.
    c. Pat dry gently with soft towel (do not rub) and pat in lubricant.
    d. Avoid the use of soap (dries skin).
  5. Administer topical steroids as ordered (penetrate better if applied within 3 minutes after bath).
  6. Use cotton instead of wool clothing.
  7. Keep child's nails short to prevent scratching and secondary infection; use gloves or elbow restraints if needed.
  8. Apply wet saline or Burrow's solution compresses.

Acne

A. General information
  1. Skin condition associated with increased production of sebum from sebaceous glands at puberty
  2. Lesions include pustules, papules, and comedones
  3. Majority of adolescents experience some degree of acne, mild to severe.
  4. Lesions occur most frequently on face, neck, shoulders and back.
  5. Caused by a variety of interrelated factors including increased activity of sebaceous glands, emotional stress, certain medications, menstrual cycle.
  6. Secondary infection can complicate healing of lesions.
  7. There is no evidence to support the value of eliminating any foods from the diet; if cause and effect can be established, however, a particular food should be eliminated.
B. Assessment findings
  1. Appearance of lesions is variable and fluctuating
  2. Systemic symptoms absent
  3. Psychologic problems such as social withdrawal, low self-esteem, feelings of being "ugly"
C. Nursing interventions
  1. Discuss OTC products and their effects.
  2. Instruct child in proper hygiene (handwashing, care of face, not to pick or squeeze any lesions).
  3. Demonstrate proper administration of topical ointments and antibiotics if indicated.

Care of the Terminally Ill Child

PEDIATRIC ONCOLOGY

Overview

A. Cancer is the leading cause of death from disease in children from 1–14 years.
B. Incidence
  1. 6000 children develop cancer per year.
  2. 2500 children die from cancer annually.
  3. Boys are affected more frequently.
C. Leukemia is the most frequent type of childhood cancer, followed by tumors of the CNS.
D. Etiologic factors include environmental agents, viruses, familial/genetic factors and host factors.

Major Stressful Events

Five events have been identified as major stressors:
A. *Diagnosis:* child is initially hospitalized to determine extent of disease, plan course of treatment, and to educate child and family.
B. *Treatment:* multimodal
  1. May include surgery, radiation, chemotherapy
  2. Side effects are serious and unpleasant; child/family may complain that the "treatment is worse than the disease."
C. *Remission:* child is without evidence of disease, treatment continues; goals for this period include
  1. Maintenance of normal family patterns: discipline and usual household chores
  2. Maintenance of relationships among family and friends
    a. Parents' marriage may be strained
    b. Siblings may feel neglected or jealous
  3. Attendance at school
    a. Child may fear rejection by peers due to change in appearance or not being able to keep up
    b. Teacher may be unsure as to what to say or how to treat the child
    c. Classmates need to be prepared for child's return; may have fears/concerns about whether the disease is catching and whether their friend will die
D. *Recurrence*
  1. An event of enormous magnitude and a cause of severe disappointment
  2. May occur while still on treatment or after treatment has been completed
E. *Death*

Modes of Cancer Treatment

Surgery

A. May be performed for tumor removal, to obtain a biopsy, to determine extent of disease, or for palliation
B. Often used in conjunction with radiation or chemotherapy

Radiation Therapy

A. Primarily used in children to improve prognosis
B. Goal is to achieve maximum effect on tumor while sparing normal tissue
  1. May be used for palliative relief from pain, disfigurement
  2. May be curative, destroys cancer cells/reduces size of tumor
  3. Frequently used as an adjunct to chemotherapy and surgery
  4. Must weigh gain versus risks of permanent damage to normal tissue
  5. Infants particularly susceptible to developing skeletal deformities in later years as a result of radiation
  6. Complications to growing child include scoliosis, arrested skeletal development, and pulmonary fibrosis (depends on site radiated)
  7. Dosage range varies; may be as low as 1000 rads to relieve bone pain in a specific area, to as high as 7000 rads to achieve a cure in Ewing's sarcoma
  8. Usually performed 5 days a week for 2–6 weeks

Chemotherapy

Almost all pediatric cancer patients receive some form of drug therapy.
A. Childhood cancers are more sensitive and responsive to drugs than are adult cancers.
B. Childhood cancers tend to metastasize early and systemic treatment is needed in addition to localized treatment.

Stages of Cancer Treatment

A. Induction
1. Goal: to remove bulk of tumor
2. Methods: surgery, radiation/chemotherapy
3. Effects: often the most intensive phase; side effects of treatment are potentially life threatening

B. Consolidation
1. Goal: to eliminate any remaining malignant cells
2. Methods: often chemotherapy/radiation therapy
3. Effects: side effects will still be evident

C. Maintenance
1. Goal: to keep child disease free
2. Method: chemotherapy (this phase may last for several years)

D. Observation
1. Goal: to monitor the child at intervals for evidence of recurrent disease and complications of treatment
2. Method: treatment is complete; child may continue in this stage indefinitely

E. Late effects of treatment
1. Impaired growth and development, usually related to radiation of growth centers
2. CNS damage resulting in intellectual, psychologic, or neurologic sequelae
3. Impaired pubertal development including hormonal or reproductive problems
4. Development of secondary malignancy
5. Psychologic problems (poor self-esteem, depression, anxiety) related to living with a life-threatening disease and complex treatment regimen

Side Effects

A. From combined effects of treatment: nausea, vomiting, diarrhea, alopecia, anemia (low RBCs), increased susceptibility to infection (low WBCs), bleeding (low platelets), stomatitis, mucositis, pain, learning problems

B. From radiation (findings differ according to site radiated): sleepiness, reddened skin

C. From chemotherapy: drug toxicity specific to agents used

D. Developmental: behavior problems, avoidance of school and friends, low self-esteem or self-image

Nursing Interventions

A. Help child cope with intrusive procedures.
1. Provide information geared to developmental level and emotional readiness.
2. Explain what is going to happen, why it is necessary, and how it will feel.
3. Allow child to handle and manipulate equipment.
4. Use needle play as indicated.
5. Allow child some control in situations (e.g., positioning, selecting injection site).

B. Support child and parents.
1. Maintain frequent clinical conferences to keep all informed.
2. Always tell the truth.
3. Acknowledge feelings and encourage child/family to express them, assure them that feelings are normal.
4. Provide contact with another parent or an organized support group such as Candlelighters.
5. Try to keep daily life as normal as possible.

C. Minimize side effects of treatment.
1. Skin breakdown
   a. Keep clean and dry; wash with warm water, no soaps or creams.
   b. Do not wash off radiation markings.
   c. Avoid exposure to sunlight.
   d. Avoid all topical agents with alcohol (perfumes and powders).
   e. Do not use electric heating pads or hot water bottles.
2. Bone marrow suppression
   a. Decreased RBCs
      1) allow child to determine activities.
      2) provide frequent rest periods.
   b. Decreased WBCs
      1) avoid crowds, isolate from children with known communicable disease.
      2) evaluate any potential site of infection.
      3) monitor temperature elevations.
   c. Decreased platelets
      1) make environment safe.
      2) select activities that are physically safe.
      3) avoid use of salicylates.
   d. Administer transfusions as ordered.
   e. Interpret peripheral blood counts to guide specific interventions and precautions.
3. Nausea and vomiting
   a. Administer antiemetic at least half an hour before chemotherapy; repeat as necessary.
   b. Encourage relaxation techniques.
   c. Eat light meal prior to administration of therapy.
   d. Ensure adequate oral intake or administer IV fluids as necessary.
4. Alopecia
   a. Reduce trauma of hair loss (especially in children over age 5 years).
   b. Buy wig before hair falls out.
   c. Discuss various head coverings with boys and girls.
   d. Avoid exposing head to sunlight.
   e. Discuss feelings.
5. Stomatitis, mucositis (see Bone Marrow Transplant, page 317).
6. Nutrition deficits
   a. Establish baseline prior to start of treatment.
   b. Measure height and weight regularly.
   c. Provide small, frequent meals.
   d. Consult dietician as needed.
   e. Provide high-calorie, high-protein supplements.
7. Developmental delays
   a. Discuss limit setting, discipline.
   b. Some behavior problems might be side effects of drug therapy.
   c. Facilitate return to school as soon as able.
   d. Realize changing needs of child.

DEATH AND DYING

Overview

Parental Reponse to Death

A. Major life stress event
B. Initially parents experience grief in response to potential loss of child
  1. Acknowledgement of terminal disease is a struggle between hope and despair with resultant awareness of inevitable death.
  2. Parents will be at different stages of grief at different times and constantly changing.
C. Parental response is related to age of child, cause of death, available social support and degree of uncertainty; response might include denial, shock, disbelief, guilt.
D. Parents often confronted with major decisions such as home care versus hospital care, use of investigational drugs, and continuation of life supports.
E. May have long-term disruptive effects on family system
  1. Stress may result in divorce.
  2. May contribute to behavioral problems or psychosomatic symptoms in siblings.
F. Bereaved parents experience intense grief of long duration.

Child's Response to Death

A. Child's concept of death depends on mental age.
  1. Infants and toddlers
    a. Live only in present.
    b. Are concerned only with separation from mother and being alone and abandoned.
    c. Can sense sadness in others and may feel guilty (due to magical thinking).
    d. Do not understand life without themselves.
    e. Can sense they are getting weaker.
    f. Healthy toddlers may insist on seeing a significant other long after that person's death.
  2. Preschoolers
    a. See death as temporary; a type of sleep or separation.
    b. See life as concrete; they know the word "dead" but do not understand the finality.
    c. Fear separation from parents; want to know who will take care of them when they are dead.
    d. Dying children may regress in their behavior.
  3. School-age
    a. Have a concept of time, causality, and irreversibility (but still question it).
    b. Fear pain, mutilation, and abandonment.
    c. Will ask directly if they are dying.
    d. See death as a period of immobility.
    e. Interested in the death ceremony; may make requests for own ceremony.
    f. Feel death is punishment.
    g. May personify death (bogey man, angel of death).
    h. May know they are going to die but feel comforted by having parents and loved ones with them.
  4. Adolescents
    a. Are thinking about the future and knowing they will not participate.
    b. May express anger at impending death.
    c. May find it difficult to talk about death.
    d. Have an accurate understanding of death.
    e. May wish to write something for friends and family, make things to leave, or make a tape.
    f. May wish to plan own funeral.

Nursing Implications

Communicating with Dying Child

A. Use the child's own language.
B. Do not use euphemisms.
C. Do not expect an immediate response.
D. Never give up hope.

Care Guidelines at Impending Death

A. Do not leave child alone.
B. Do not whisper in the room (increases fears).
C. Know that touching child is important.
D. Let the child and family talk and cry.
E. Continue to read favorite stories to child or play favorite music.
F. Let parents participate in care as far as they are emotionally capable.
G. Be aware of the needs of siblings who are in the room with the family.

SAMPLE QUESTIONS

14-year-old Louise has had an exacerbation of acute lymphocytic leukemia. She is terminal and has been hospitalized.

22. An appropriate nursing action would be to
    ○ 1. leave her alone as much as possible and whisper when in her room in order not to disturb her.
    ○ 2. assist her in giving away her possessions to friends and family.
    ○ 3. encourage Louise's parents to explain to her 5-year-old sister that Louise will be asleep for a long time.
    ○ 4. reduce emotional stress by not having Louise's parents/family participate in her care.

Jack is 10 years old and is receiving cranial irradiation for a brain tumor. He has developed alopecia.

23. Which of the following is an appropriate nursing intervention?
    ○ 1. Have Jack identify famous movie stars and sports heroes who are bald.
    ○ 2. Assure Jack that his hair will grow in before he leaves the hospital.
    ○ 3. Wrap a bandage around his head.
    ○ 4. Help him select a variety of hats.

REFERENCES AND RECOMMENDED READINGS

Athreya, B., & Silberman, B. (1985). *Pediatric/physical diagnosis*. Norwalk, CT: Appleton-Century-Croft.

Broadribb, V. (1983). *Introductory pediatric nursing* (4th ed.) Philadelphia: Lippincott.

Hayman, L. & Sporing, E. (1985). *Handbook of pediatric nursing*, New York: Wiley.

Petrillo, M., & Sanger, S. (1981). *Emotional care of hospitalized children* (2nd ed.). Philadelphia: Lippincott.

Steele, S. (1984). *Nursing care of the child with a long term illness* (3rd ed.). Norwalk, CT: Appleton-Century-Croft.

Whaley, L. & Wong, D. (1983). *Nursing care of infants and children* (2nd ed.). St. Louis: Mosby.

UNIT 3: Reprints

Are you sure it's only croup?

What looks at first like croup may be a far more dangerous condition.
Learning to make an accurate diagnosis and provide
the proper treatment can save your pediatric patient's life.

By Donna Ojanen Thomas, RN, MS, CEN

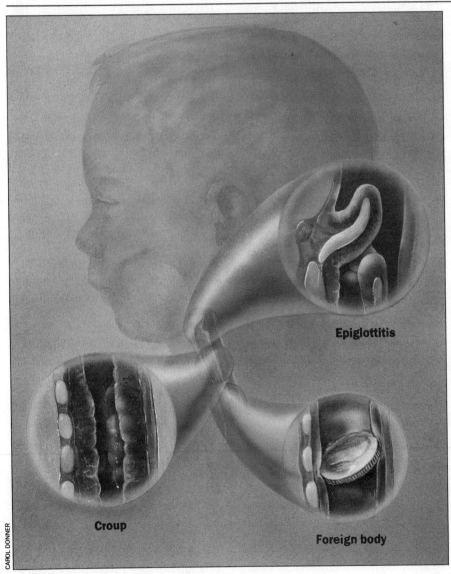

Croup

Epiglottitis

Foreign body

CAROL DONNER

Billy Peterson's parents rush him to the ED because his breathing is so labored they fear he may suffocate. "He's had a cold and slight fever for two days," Billy's mother tells you. "Tonight he got up with this awful cough, and his chest caves in whenever he breathes."

When you examine Billy you find nasal flaring and inspiratory stridor, accompanied by a hoarse cry and a cough that sounds a lot like the bark of a seal. You suspect moderately severe croup.

But are you sure it's croup? This child's life may depend on the accuracy of your assessment. And the symptoms of croup all too closely mimic those of two other conditions: epiglottitis—a medical emergency—and an object obstructing the airway. You must be alert to these two possibilities if you hope to avoid respiratory arrest.

How to tell croup from epiglottitis

The term croup usually encompasses two illnesses, spasmotic croup and acute laryngotracheobronchitis. Both are common in

THE AUTHOR is director of the emergency department at Primary Children's Medical Center in Salt Lake City.

Produced by Paul L. Cerrato

children under three years of age. Spasmotic croup, the milder form of the disease, shows up as the classic "croupy cough" with inspiratory stridor. These symptoms usually spring up suddenly, waking the child in the middle of the night. The patient doesn't have nasal congestion or other signs of upper respiratory infection, and he rarely has a fever. The cause is probably laryngeal edema and vocal cord spasm of unknown origin. Most cases of spasmotic croup are mild and respond to home treatment.

Laryngotracheobronchitis, usually more prevalent in late autumn, is an acute viral infection that begins with upper respiratory symptoms and a low-grade, variable fever. The first sign that the disease has spread to the larynx is the gradual development of a "barky" cough and hoarse voice. As mucous secretions thicken and build up below the epiglottis, the patient's airway narrows and he develops inspiratory stridor. This airway narrowing produces the classic "steeple sign" on a chest X-ray.

The violent coughing characteristic of the disease brings on inflammation and edema of the surrounding mucous membranes, narrowing the airway still further. Severe airway obstruction causes the areas above and below the sternum to recede during inspiration as the patient uses accessory muscles to help him breathe.

If not properly treated, a severe case of croup can lead to hypoxemia, cyanosis, and respiratory arrest. Fortunately, most children with croup don't follow this pattern and can be treated on an outpatient basis. The disease usually runs its course in less than a week.

The dangers of croup pale next to those of epiglottitis, which develops much more rapidly. Epiglottitis, a bacterial infection that's most prevalent between ages two and seven, can turn into a life-threatening emergency only hours after the first symptoms appear. The child has a high fever and difficulty swallowing, may be cyanotic, and adopts a characteristic position—sitting up and leaning forward with his chin thrust forward, drooling saliva. Total airway obstruction may occur without warning.

In earlier stages of epiglottitis, the child will exhibit a softer, lower-pitched stridor and a less severe cough than the patient with croup. His cry will be muffled, not hoarse. These differences in respiratory symptoms probably result from the fact that epiglottitis attacks the area above the vocal cords while the swelling and inflammation of croup affect only the area below the epiglottis and vocal cords. A lateral neck X-ray will distinguish epiglottitis from croup because the swollen epiglottis appears prominently, resembling an adult thumbprint.

One of the most dramatic signs of epiglottitis, a cherry red epiglottis, is one that you'll rarely see—and shouldn't look for. It's *extremely dangerous* to peer down a child's throat when you suspect epiglottitis because the maneuver could cause complete airway obstruction.

Because of the danger of sudden airway obstruction, never place a child with suspected epiglottis in a supine position or leave him unattended, even for a moment or two.

All children with this virulent disease require an artificial airway. Once the patient is intubated, make sure you restrain him. A child who extubates himself may be impossible to reintubate because of the severe swelling of the epiglottis and surrounding tissue.

After inserting the artifical airway, we admit the patient to our ICU and give IV antibiotics. He can usually be extubated in 24 to 48 hours.

Another cause of airway obstruction

Don't forget one other possibility to consider when evaluating the child with croup-like symptoms. A foreign object lodged in the airway closely mimics both croup and epiglottitis and is a common cause of upper airway blockage.

A six-year-old girl was brought to our ED one night with crowing respirations and extreme cyanosis. We tried to intubate her but she vomited during the attempt. After vomiting, her color improved dramatically. An X-ray revealed an earring in her stomach. As it turned out, the earring had been stuck in her larnyx and she swallowed it after our intubation attempt dislodged it from her airway.

Since foreign objects lodged in the airway pose one of the greatest dangers to young children, it's essential to know when to suspect such a problem. Always suspect a foreign object when the patient has a history of swallowing objects. If possible, find out from the parents when the symptoms began. With this kind of obstruction, symptoms

Keeping a scorecard on croup

To measure the severity of croup, we assign each of the most important physical signs a point rating. For example, if the patient has stridor while inhaling (one point), a barking cough (two points), and nasal flaring with suprasternal, subcostal, and intercostal retractions (two points), his score is five.

Signs	Point rating	
	One point	**Two points**
Stridor	inspiratory	inspiratory and expiratory
Cough	hoarse cry	bark
Retractions and nasal flaring	flaring with suprasternal retractions	flaring with suprasternal, subcostal, and intercostal retractions
Cyanosis	in room air	in 40% O_2
Inspiratory breath sounds	harsh sounds with wheezing or rhonchi	delayed breath sounds

Source: Downes, J. *Acute Upper-Airway Obstruction in the Child.* American Society of Anesthesiology, 1980.

often start shortly after eating or while the child is playing with small toys.

How to assess the severity of croup

Once you've determined that your patient's symptoms are indeed caused by croup, the next step is to assess the severity of the condition. We use the scoring system described above to assess all patients suspected of having upper airway obstruction. When a child scores four or more, he's examined by the ED physician and given a vasoconstricting drug such as racemic epinephrine (MicroNEPHRINE). A score of seven or more requires *immediate* attention by a physician and possibly an anesthesiologist.

This scoring system not only standardizes ED assessment but also provides guidelines for admitting the more serious cases. We usually admit patients who score above four if they haven't responded to two treatments in the ED. Children under a year old are usually admitted regardless of how they respond to treatment.

Should you give meds by IPPB or aerosol?

Unlike epiglottitis patients, our more seriously ill croup patients usually respond well to racemic epinephrine, administered by intermittent positive pressure breathing. Two of our former staff anesthesiologists have had a perfect track record for 10 years using this approach in our hospital—not one patient needed a tracheostomy.

We use the IPPB route for patients scoring four or more. The respiratory therapist gives 2.25% racemic epinephrine for 15 to 20 minutes through a Bird Mark 7 respirator. Milder cases and children under four years old usually do well with the aerosol mist. For either route the dosage is the same: 0.25 to 0.5 cc in 3 cc of D5W. Observe and record the patient's croup score before and after each treatment. Also watch for such side effects of the drug as tachycardia, dizziness, nausea, and headache. Racemic epinephrine is contraindicated in children with tetralogy of Fallot, a congenital heart defect, because the drug may precipitate a sudden drop in cardiac output.

When we treat children with croup in the ED, we use racemic epinephrine very cautiously because of its rebound effect: Symptoms initially improve, then return, usually within two hours. To avoid adverse effects, we keep these patients in the ED at least four hours and only release them with physician approval, provided their croup scores are four or less.

In the worst cases—patients with scores of seven or more—we give racemic epinephrine only after the ED physician and the anesthesiologist evaluate the child. Until epiglottitis is ruled out we don't lie the child supine, peer down his throat, or leave him unattended.

If a patient with a score of seven

or more doesn't improve after two or three treatments with medication at less than one-hour intervals, we insert an artificial airway.

Severe croup can be a terrifying experience for both the child and his parents so be sure to give them lots of emotional support. They'll also need information. At Primary Children's Medical Center we give parents a discharge instruction sheet like the one above. It tells them how to treat the disease at home and when to seek medical attention. With a measure of control over their child's condition, most parents feel more secure.

The symptoms of croup can be unsettling even for nurses who are no strangers to respiratory problems. However, if you use the croup scoring system and keep in mind the subtle distinctions between croup and epiglottitis, you'll be able to assess and care for your young patients rapidly and confidently—before the situation gets out of hand. ■

BIBLIOGRAPHY Adair, J. and Ring, W. Management of epiglottitis in children. *Anesthesia and Analgesia* 54: 622, 1975. Barker, G.A. Current management of croup and epiglottitis. *Pediatr. Clin. North. Am.* 26:656, 1979. Fogel, J., Berg, I., et al. Racemic epinephrine in the treatment of croup: nebulization alone versus nebulization with intermittent positive pressure breathing. *J. Pediatr.* 101: 1028, 1982. Newth, C. and Levison, H. Diagnosing and managing croup and epiglottitis. *Journal of Respiratory Diseases* 2:22, Feb. 1981.

Fever in children

By Donna Ojanen Thomas, RN, MS, CEN

Children tend to run higher temperatures than adults would for relatively minor ailments. For this reason, fever is the complaint that most often leads parents to seek health care for their children. The most common cause of fever in children is a viral infection, such as a cold. However, a bacterial infection or some of the same noninfectious conditions that produce fevers in adults can also cause fevers in children.

As with adults, fever itself usually isn't harmful to the child unless it remains above 106° F—a very rare occurrence. Temperature elevations can, however, cause some problems of which you should be aware.

One such problem is dehydration. A child's rate of metabolism is normally twice that of an adult. A fever will raise the child's metabolic rate higher still, which can lead to tachypnea and tachycardia. Tachypnea contributes to fluid loss in children whose fluid intake may already be below normal and further increases the likelihood of dehydration.

Fever can also cause convulsions in children between the ages of six months and six years, possibly because their central nervous systems are immature. These febrile seizures usually do no harm provided they're not prolonged. Any child who has a history of febrile seizures should, of course, receive prompt treatment at the slightest sign of fever.

Fever also requires special attention in infants who are younger than three months. These very young babies are especially susceptible to infections for which they haven't yet developed immunity. Because these infections often don't localize the way they do in older people, the infant may not look sick. The fever may be the only clue that something is wrong. Any child under three months of age with a fever should therefore have a complete physical exam and diagnostic workup.

Children younger than two years who are running unexplained high fevers also require careful evaluation to rule out serious infections such as meningitis and septicemia.

Because of the special problems fever can cause in children, it's best to treat all children with temperatures above 101° F—as well as any child who is very uncomfortable. The usual treatment is 10 to 15 mg/kg of acetaminophen.

You should avoid giving aspirin because of its association with Reye's syndrome in children with viral illnesses.

Before recommending antipyretics, however, ask the parents whether the child is taking any other medications. Many over-the-counter cough preparations and decongestants contain acetaminophen. If the child receives too much you run the risk of overdose.

One of your biggest tasks may be to reassure the parents that the fever itself won't harm the child. Remind them that how the child acts and looks is more important than how high his fever is. If the child's temperature is above 104°F, you can suggest that the parents give him a lukewarm sponge bath. Tell them not to listen to grandma who wants to sponge the child with alcohol. With alcohol sponge baths you run the risk of poisoning the child by inhalation.

A temperature of 104 or above should always be reported to the child's physician. Tell the parents they should also notify their doctor if the fever will not go down, if the child is very listless, or if he has other symptoms, such as a sore throat, vomiting, diarrhea, or a cold.

Remind parents of children three months of age or younger always to report all fevers, no matter how slight, to the doctor. ■

THE AUTHOR is director of the emergency department at Primary Children's Medical Center in Salt Lake City.

Produced by Estelle Beaumont, RN, MS

BIBLIOGRAPHY Long, S.S. Approach to the febrile patient with no obvious focus of infection. *Pediatrics in Review* 5:10, April 1984. Schmitt, B.D. Fever phobia. *American Journal of Diseases of Children* 134, February 1980.

Epilepsy: Putting the patient back in control

Epilepsy is a susceptibility to disturbances in the electrical activity of the brain. You'll need technical knowledge to help the patient control the seizures, and compassionate understanding to help him cope with his condition.

By Mimi Callanan, RN, MSN

A tonic-clonic seizure can be a frightening sight, especially when it is witnessed for the first time. Some people are so terrified by the experience, in fact, that they're convinced the cause must be demonic possession.

The fleeting incapacitation of an absence seizure, on the other hand, can easily be dismissed as a mere lapse of attention. That's the reason why so many children with epilepsy are wrongly thought to be inattentive or uncooperative in the classroom.

While awe, terror, and dismissal are frequent reactions to epileptic seizures, they can often lead to prejudice against people who have epilepsy. A more subtle—but still harmful—misunderstanding is the

THE AUTHOR is a clinical specialist at the Mid-Atlantic Regional Epilepsy Center of the Medical College of Pennsylvania in Philadelphia.

Produced by David Anderson

commonly held belief that epilepsy is a disease. In fact, it's a susceptibility to recurrent seizures that can occur as a symptom of various disturbances of the central nervous system.

When you know the facts about seizures and epilepsy, you can give your patient the protection and support he needs. You can also teach the general public to accept him as he is.

How to protect the seizing patient

The event that precipitates a seizure is a sudden, rapid, disorderly discharge of neurons in the cerebral cortex.

Observation, common sense, and prudence dictate what measures to take to protect your patient during a seizure.

If the patient is standing, help him to the ground. Be sure the air-

way remains open. Turn him on his side to prevent aspiration and allow for drainage of secretions. Pillow his head on something soft and loosen his collar. Clear away furniture and other objects so he won't hurt himself if he thrashes about.

Tempting as it is, do not restrain the patient. He may react with instinctive self-protective violence.

Don't put anything in his mouth. It's better for him to bite his tongue than to break a tooth.

Talk reassuringly. Most seizures resolve within a very few minutes.

How to resolve status epilepticus

Intensive nursing and medical interventions are called for when one tonic-clonic seizure follows another in rapid succession. The patient is then in status epilepticus, a life-threatening emergency. He may stop breathing. Muscle spasms can create an excessive oxygen demand that may induce severe hypoxia, kill nerve cells, and cause cardiac arrhythmias.

Call for help, and have someone contact a physician. Assess the patient's airway. If necessary use an Ambu bag to aid ventilation, or take advantage of the brief relaxation period between seizures to place an oral airway. In some cases a breathing tube may be needed.

Insert an intravenous line. Draw blood for antiepilepsy drug levels and drug screening tests. Status epilepticus often occurs when a patient's medication concentrations fall below the effective minimum, or when alcohol or some other drug alters his metabolism. The physician will also order serum electrolytes, glucose, BUN, creatinine, and SGOT to look for metabolic imbalances. He'll also obtain baseline

arterial blood gases.

Standard orders call for glucose 50 grams and thiamine 100 mg by IV bolus. If the patient is hypoglycemic or alcoholic, his seizure may abate as this infusion moves his metabolism back toward normal.

To stop the seizures, you may—with a doctor's orders—infuse diazepam (Valium) 5 to 20 mg no faster than 1 to 2 mg/min.

To ensure that seizure activity

The classes and types of seizures

A seizure may be as mild as butterflies in the stomach, as subtle as a fleeting fugue state, or as dramatic as a tonic-clonic episode. Almost every seizure, however, fits into one of three major classes defined by the International League for Epilepsy. Each class is further subdivided into types:

Partial seizures (also called focal seizures) begin in a localized area of the brain.

▶ Simple partial seizures are those where the patient remains conscious throughout. If the area—or focus—of the abnormal discharge controls motor function in a part of the body, you'll observe spasms there. One side of the face may begin to shake, for instance, followed by other muscles on the same side of the body as the cerebral discharge spreads out.

If the epileptic discharge affects a different area of the brain, the patient may experience somatosensory effects such as tingling, a metallic taste, or seeing flashing lights. Psychic symptoms such as déjà vu, dreamy states, anger, or hallucinations are usual for some patients. For others, autonomic symptoms such as nausea, pallor, or sweating are typical.

Simple partial seizures may develop into complex partial seizures or generalized seizures.

▶ Complex partial seizures are those where the patient loses consciousness. The blackout may be obvious or so brief that only the patient is aware of it. You should suspect that your patient's seizure is complex partial if he displays repetitive gestures such as lip-smacking or picking at his clothes. These seizures are followed by a period of confusion, agitation, and possibly bizarre behavior.

Complex partial seizures may develop into secondarily generalized seizures.

Generalized seizures result from an abrupt, unruly firing of neurons over a widespread area on both sides of the brain. All generalized seizures will also include certain periods of unconsciousness.

▶ Generalized absence—or petit mal—seizures, most frequently afflict children. They consist of seconds-long periods of unconsciousness, which usually occur without warning and leave no aftereffects. Sometimes the episode also produces atonia, or clonus—alternating spasm and relaxation of muscles. Lip-smacking or other automatisms occasionally occur. Because of their subtlety, absence seizures often persist for a long time before they're recognized and diagnosed. This is regrettable, since they can be a major handicap to learning and social adjustment. Some children may experience as many as a hundred a day.

▶ Generalized tonic-clonic seizures begin with a tonic phase in which you may see the patient throw his arms up and then extend them down rigidly. He loses consciousness immediately and falls to the ground. A clonic phase of rhythmic jerking of all extremities ensues. He may issue a cry or moan as he expels air at the beginning of the seizure, and he may develop apnea or cyanosis. When the sphincter relaxes at the end of this phase, he may be incontinent. In the aftermath, the patient may display confusion, irritability, and memory loss. He'll probably also be sore and tired.

▶ Other generalized seizures include tonic (the only symptom is stiffening), clonic (only rhythmic contraction), myoclonic (single or multiple jerks), and atonic (the patient loses all tone and falls to the ground).

Unclassified seizures are those—such as neonatal seizures—that can't be assigned to one of the preceding classes because of insufficient data.

stays suppressed, you'll follow diazepam with phenytoin (Dilantin) 18 mg/kg of body weight in normal saline. Give it by IV push no faster than 50 mg/min. A second dose may be necessary if seizures resume or continue. Continue to assess respiration; obtain ABGs every half hour if it's compromised. Monitor frequently for cardiac arrhythmias.

If phenytoin fails, some doctors set up a diazepam drip—100 mg in 500 ml of solution. Use only glass bottles if you infuse diazepam. It will precipitate in plastic bags.

If diazepam and phenytoin fail to control tonic-clonic status epilepticus, the doctor may turn to phenobarbital, paraldehyde, or general anesthesia.

Find the source and underlying cause

When the seizure subsides, the process of diagnosis begins.

The first step is to locate the site of the discharge that set off the seizure. Your observation and the history you collect from witnesses will help determine whether your patient had a partial or generalized seizure. The hallmarks of these seizure classes and their subtypes are described on the preceding page.

A very precise description of the seizure's progression, starting with the very first symptom, is critical to the diagnosis. Record everything that happens to the patient—including, for example, changes in motor activity, loss of consciousness, tongue-biting, incontinence, or any kind of injury he may sustain—and note the duration of the episode. Report whether he's sore, confused, lethargic, or exhausted

afterwards, and also, for how long.

A complete nursing history should indicate whether your patient's seizure was an isolated occurrence or whether he has epilepsy. Find out if he has experienced seizures in the past. If so, find out when and obtain full descriptions.

In taking the history, remember that any problem that affects the brain can cause seizures and epilepsy. Inquire about episodes of perinatal trauma or anoxia, genetic defects, lead and mercury poisoning, or degenerative diseases. Question whether he has suffered head trauma or cerebral infections such as meningitis or encephalitis. Has the patient ever abused alcohol or other drugs? Is there a family history of epilepsy or febrile convulsions?

To pinpoint the location of the seizure-provoking discharge more precisely, the doctor orders electroencephalographic studies. The brain waves of most patients with epilepsy continue to show abnormal activity interictally—that is, between seizures. Hyperventilation and photic stimulation with strobe lights are part of a routine EEG.

To seek out the underlying cause

Antiepilepsy drugs and their side effects

Drug	Side effects
Carbamazepine (Tegretol)	Dizziness, drowsiness, unsteadiness, vomiting, double vision, leukopenia
Phenytoin (Dilantin)	Nystagmus, ataxia, slurred speech, mental confusion, dizziness, insomnia
Primidone (Mysoline)	Vertigo and drowsiness
Phenobarbital	Drowsiness
Clorazepate (Tranxene)	Drowsiness
Ethosuximide (Zarontin)	Vague gastric upset
Valproic acid (Depakene)	Anorexia with some weight loss, increased appetite with weight gain
Acetazolamide (Diamox)	Polyuria
Clonazepam (Klonopin)	Drowsiness

of the seizure, the doctor obtains a medical history and also conducts a thorough neurological exam. He orders lab studies such as electrolytes, BUN, ABGs, cerebrospinal fluid, and drug screens to help identify possible metabolic, toxic, or infectious causes. He may order CT scans, MRI, or angiography to rule out infarcts, hemorrhages, tumors, or other brain lesions.

Controlling epilepsy: drugs and surgery

The first line of treatment for epilepsy is medication. The doctor prescribes the appropriate drug for the specific type of seizure.

The patient with epilepsy who has motor seizures receives carbamazepine (Tegretol), phenobarbital, phenytoin (Dilantin), or primidone (Mysoline). The drugs most commonly used to control absence seizures are ethosuximide (Zarontin) and valproic acid (Depakene).

Patients often respond differently to equal doses of these drugs, and some patients tolerate them better than others. For this reason, the patient who is starting an antiepilepsy medication needs to have blood levels monitored according to his physician's guidelines. Teach him the adverse reactions he may experience—and tell him to notify the doctor of any changes in the way he feels. Stress that he'll need to take all doses without fail. The patient should be reminded of what his physician wants him to do if he misses a dose. Advise him to plan to refill prescriptions a week before his supply runs out.

About one patient in five does

Controlling epilepsy with surgery

By Diane Friedman, RN, MSN, CS

Some 60% of patients completely control their seizures with antiepilepsy medications, while another 20% experience nearly complete control. Unfortunately 20% of patients continue to experience seizures despite optimum use of anticonvulsants. For a few of these patients, neurosurgery may help. These procedures are currently being performed at Cleveland Clinic Foundation and some other centers:

Lobectomy and hemispherectomy are methods for shutting down partial seizure activity by removing the brain tissue where the seizure originates.

In order to plan either procedure, the neurosurgeon must first locate the region of the brain—called the focus—where seizures originate. To do so, he admits the patient to the hospital for round-the-clock monitoring to record abnormal brain activity, identify its source, and correlate it with the clinical signs of a seizure. The monitoring is done by EEG, observation by nurses, and sometimes videotape.

Once the seizure focus is located, its extent must be precisely defined. Before the surgeon can operate, moreover, he needs to determine that the focus doesn't overlap into brain areas that control important functions such as speech, movement, or vision. To achieve these dual ends, the neurosurgeon takes the patient to surgery, where he removes the skull over the focal area and places electrodes directly onto the surface of the brain or into the brain tissue.

With these electrodes in place, several more weeks of monitoring ensue, during which each new seizure provides an opportunity for closer mapping of the focal outline. The electrodes don't hinder the patient's movements, but someone must be with him whenever he's up and about. This precaution, taken to prevent the patient from dislodging the electrodes during a seizure, must be observed tactfully to allow the patient to maintain a sense of independence. Nurses also watch closely for signs of increased intracranial pressure and infection.

Finally the patient returns to surgery. The surgeon removes the electrodes and excises the piece of brain tissue from which the seizures originate. When the surgeon removes the entire focal area, the patient will have a 60% to 70% chance of being seizure free. Even when the surgeon can't remove the entire seizure focus—perhaps because it overlaps into areas governing important brain functions—most patients have at least a reduction in seizure activity.

Corpus callosotomy is performed when severe tonic-clonic and atonic (drop attack) seizures are so frequent that the patient is disabled and at high risk for serious injury. The neurosurgeon severs the corpus callosum, a bridge of neurons connecting the two hemispheres of the brain. By preventing neuronal discharges from passing between hemispheres, this procedure reduces the severity and often the frequency of seizures. The patient can present a challenge to nurses during the first postop weeks because he's likely to be apathetic and will need to relearn right-left coordination. Soon, however, all faculties return to normal.

THE AUTHOR is a clinical specialist in epilepsy at the Cleveland Clinic Foundation, Cleveland.

not obtain satisfactory seizure control with antiepilepsy medications. Some of these patients may be helped by temporal lobe resection, or corpus callosotomy. Others may benefit from experimental drugs such as GABA agonists. These treatments are available primarily in specialized epilepsy centers.

Controlling epilepsy through education

Whether or not medications fully control the patient's epilepsy, there are several methods that you can use to help him manage his condition better.

Discuss his seizures with him. Try to ascertain if there are any precipitating factors. For instance, some patients may need to exercise caution with alcohol intake, while others shouldn't consume it at all. Some patients must take special care to avoid fatigue. Others may have to keep away from too much excitement.

Teach the patient to recognize his seizure warning signs. When he starts to feel an episode coming on, he may be able to take precautions to protect himself from possible injury. Be sure to make the patient aware that there are medic-alert identification bracelets and necklaces available for epilepsy—even though it appears that the majority of patients prefer not to wear them.

Help the patient and his family understand his usual seizure pattern. With most patients it isn't necessary to go to the doctor or emergency room as long as their seizures stay the same. However, they should contact their physician if the seizures worsen in intensity

---

Obtaining a seizure history– discovering the pattern

By Janis L. Morrison, RN

A complete seizure history can point to the causes of a patient's epilepsy. It gives clues as to when seizures are most likely to happen, disarming the fear and feelings of helplessness that arise when seizures strike "out of the blue." When it establishes that the seizure the patient is having now resembles those he's come through before, it gives comfort. When it indicates that the patient is having a new kind of seizure experience, it signals possible danger in the future and the need for reevaluation.

Obviously, such a history can be of great help to a patient with epilepsy, his family, medical personnel at work or school, and health-care workers. To obtain it, ask these questions of your patient and others who have witnessed his seizures:

Does the patient feel or do anything special before a seizure starts? Some patients get nervous, others pace around, let out a little yell, or twitch. If a nurse or friend sees this tip-off, they will know to get ready— maybe by clearing a space, perhaps by helping the patient lie down on the floor.

What happens during a seizure episode? Most patients experience the same type of seizure every time. Have the patient and family tell you everything they can think of. Sometimes—particularly in cases where the patient has absence seizures—this alerts witnesses that behavior they may think simply bizarre is really seizure activity.

How long do seizures last? Any seizure that lasts longer than the time specified on the history can serve as a signal for the patient to seek additional medical help or a reevaluation of the patient's status by the attending physician.

What happens when the seizure is over? You'll want to know whether to expect incontinence, emotional outbursts, or sleepiness. Try to find out whether the patient will benefit from reorientation, a place to lie down, comforting—or just being left alone.

Do seizures occur singly or in groups? Some patients have multiple episodes that can be particularly baffling and frightening if you don't expect them to happen. With this information you can avoid unnecessary trips to the emergency room—which can be demoralizing and economically ruinous for the patient. As long as the patient develops no life-threatening symptoms, such as airway closure, the rule is to let his sei-

THE AUTHOR was education supervisor at a respite care center for patients with mental retardation and cerebral palsy when she originated this interview.

or if they become more frequent.

Encourage the patient to put away feelings of embarrassment or shame at having epilepsy. Epilepsy certainly isn't demonic possession. A person with epilepsy is no more likely than the next person to be mentally incompetent, retarded, or socially inept. People with epilepsy and health professionals must vehemently object when they encoun-

ter such misconceptions from the general public.

With his seizures under control and his sense of self-sufficiency enhanced, the patient is ready for a better quality of life—thanks to you and the care and knowledge you've given him. ■

BIBLIOGRAPHY Adams, R.D. and Victor, M. *Principles of Neurology.* St. Louis: McGraw-Hill Co., 1981. Browne, T.R. and Feldman, R.G. *Epilepsy Diagnosis and Management.* Boston: Little, Brown and Co., 1983. Delgado-Escueta, A.V., Wasterlain, C.G., et al. Status Epilepticus: Mechanisms of Brain Damage and Treatment. *Adv. Neurol.* 34, 1983. Ozuna, J. Psychosocial Aspects of Epilepsy. *Journal of Neurosurgical Nursing,* 11(4):243, 1979. Porter, R.J. *Epilepsy: 100 Elementary Principles.* Philadelphia: W. B. Saunders Co., 1984. Proposal for Revised Clinical and Electroencephalographic Classification of Epileptic Seizures. *Epilepsia* 22:489, 1981. Solomon, G. and Plum, F. *Clinical Management of Seizures: A Guide for the Physician.* W. B. Saunders Co., 1978.

---

zures go for as many as they usually go—but no more.

Are there any other regular patterns involved in the patient's seizures? Given how varied such patterns can be, they may be surprisingly regular. For instance, a patient may have a seizure every day for a week and then none for the next two months. Obviously, the more precise the pattern, the more helpful it is to be aware of it.

Can you think of anything else to tell me? Vague as this question is, it sometimes elicits the most useful answers. For instance, one patient brought out that her seizures tended to occur a few days before her menstrual period. With this knowledge we were able to identify fluid buildup as a contributor to her seizures, and prevent it by making sure she received her diuretic pills at the appropriate times. Her seizures became less frequent, and she was more prepared for them.

Keep a copy of the seizure history at the front of the patient's chart throughout the time he remains in your institution.

I also suggest writing the answers up in terms that laymen can understand, and distributing the history—with the patient's or guardian's permission—to those who are most likely to need the information. Be sure to write the patient's medication dosage and doctor's name on the top, and keep this information current. Doing so will help everyone cope, and ensure understanding and optimal care for your patient.

DIANE SCHAMING, RN, BSN
MAUREEN GORRY, RN, BSN
KIMBERLEY SOROKA, RN
MARY ELLEN CATULLO, RN, BSN

When babies are born with orthopedic problems

The earlier treatment begins, the better the prognosis. Here's how to identify common problems and what to do for your patients and their parents.

DIANE SCHAMING and MAUREEN GORRY are assistant head nurses on the orthopedic unit at Children's Hospital of Pittsburgh. KIMBERLEY SOROKA and MARY ELLEN CATULLO are staff nurses on the unit.
STAFF EDITOR: Sigrid Nagle

A routine physical performed on 2-day-old Melissa Carter uncovered evidence of congenital dislocation, or dysplasia, of the right hip.

Amy and Adam Melville, fraternal twins, were born with clubbed feet. Amy's left foot and both of Adam's turned inward. Amy's was an in utero clubfoot, twisted out of shape by her position in the womb; Adam's problem was congenital.

The prognosis for the infants was excellent. All would walk and run normally as they got older. Melissa and Adam, though, faced months of tedious treatment. Their care would be a constant strain on their parents. Nurses can make this time easier by providing support and education as well as care. Explaining the condition is the first step.

Of every 1,000 newborns, two have a congenital dysplasia of one hip and a third has both hips dislocated. Girls are affected more often than boys.

There are three degrees of displacement, from the mildest—in which the head of the femur sits in the proper location but the acetabulum, or hip socket, has not yet grown large enough to hold the bone securely—to complete displacement of the head of the femur above and behind the acetabulum.

The middle degree of displacement, called subluxation, is the most common. In this case, the head of the femur sits against the rim of the acetabulum, so that the socket is stretched out of shape to accommodate it.

All newborns should be assessed for dysplasia. If diagnosed at birth or shortly thereafter, many infants can escape surgery. If the condition isn't discovered until the child has

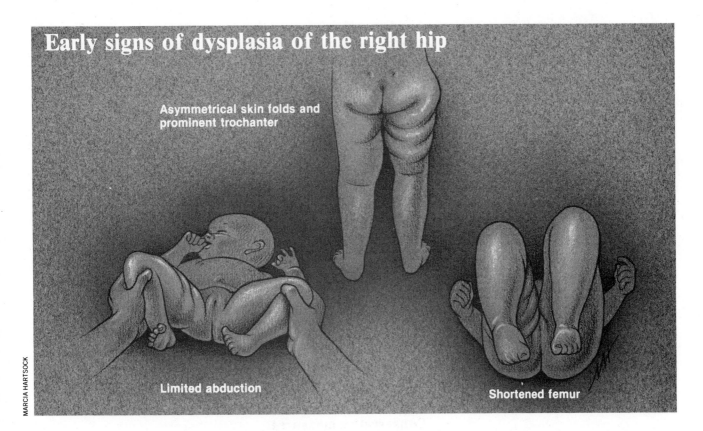

Early signs of dysplasia of the right hip

Asymmetrical skin folds and prominent trochanter

Limited abduction

Shortened femur

MARCIA HARTSOCK

difficulty walking, surgery is almost always necessary.

In Melissa's case, a pediatric nurse practitioner noted that the skin folds over the baby's buttocks and thighs were asymmetrical, the right femur appeared shortened, and the perineum was unusually broad. Alerted to a possible dislocation, the NP tested Melissa's legs for limited abduction—outward movement—and found it in the right leg.

Next, she did the Ortolani test, flexing Melissa's leg and gently moving the thigh first outward and then upward. As she did, she felt the head of the femur slip into the acetabulum. Finally, when the NP pushed the flexed leg down and inward (the Barlow test), she felt it dislocate.

These maneuvers cause little discomfort and no further dislocation. They are nearly always conclusive proof of dysplasia. In this case, an X-ray confirmed a case of subluxation.

Causes and types of clubfoot

Adam's problem, congenital clubfoot, affects one out of every 700 to 1,000 infants—boys twice as often as girls.

Like Adam, most of these children have their heels raised and turned outward, toes turned inward, and soles flexed. This condition is called talipes equinovarus. In most cases the ankle bone, or talus, is deformed, leading to misproportioned ligaments and tendons.

Unlike Adam's, his twin's malformation was not congenital. Amy's was obviously an in utero positional clubfoot because the physician could easily move it into an overcorrected position—

something that is not possible with congenital clubfoot. A foot can also be skewed by a childhood injury or poliomyelitis.

Adam and Amy were promptly scheduled for treatment, since delay would only make correction more difficult.

First steps in stabilizing Melissa's dislocated hip

On the third day of her life, Melissa was fitted with a Pavlik harness. This device, commonly used on infants under six months of age, corrects congenital hip displacement in nine out of 10 cases.

The orthopedic surgeon applied the harness, positioned Melissa's femur, then tightened the straps.

Melissa would be in the harness day and night for three weeks. We showed her parents

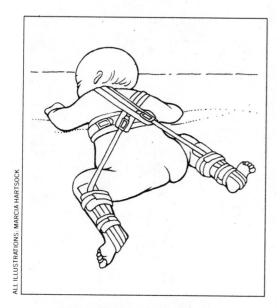

ALL ILLUSTRATIONS: MARCIA HARTSOCK

A Pavlik harness consists of shoulder straps, stirrups, and a chest strap. It is put on both legs even when only one hip is dislocated.

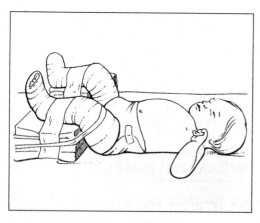

After surgery for clubfoot, infants' legs are placed in bilateral flexed splints taped to sterile towels.

how to put her diaper on right over it. If she fussed, they could hold and comfort her, but under no circumstances were they to remove the apparatus. They were to give her sponge baths, not tub baths, turn her every three or four hours, and watch for signs of skin breakdown.

The surgeon would adjust the harness every week, gradually bringing the femur into normal alignment. The hip usually begins to stabilize in about three days, and by three weeks is very stable. At that point the parents will be able to remove the harness to bathe the baby, but she'll still need to wear it for a few weeks more.

After six weeks in the harness, however, Melissa's hip had not stabilized. She would need more aggressive treatment.

Conservative measures: First resort for clubfoot

When the twins were three days old, the orthopedic surgeon put their clubbed feet into plaster casts that went above the knee so they could not kick them off.

Amy's foot, he reassured her parents, would be completely corrected by a few months of casting. Adam, however, would most likely require surgery—as do 85% of patients with congenital clubfoot. Meanwhile the casts would help straighten his feet and stretch the skin so it would be easier to close incisions later.

The infants' nurses gave the parents an instruction sheet on cast care. They reviewed the procedures with the parents before sending them home, and urged them to call if they had any problems.

Once a week, the doctor saw Amy and Adam in his office. Ev-

ery time, he took off the casts and assessed the feet. Then he straightened them a bit more and applied new casts, a process called serial casting.

At four months Amy's foot was completely corrected. Adam was scheduled for surgery.

Traction and more casting for Melissa's hip

When 6-week-old Melissa was hospitalized, her parents needed as much emotional support as Melissa needed care.

They needed to be reassured that their baby's condition was not their fault, that it did not occur during delivery, and that it generally doesn't run in families. They needed to hear again and again that chances were extremely good that Melissa's hip would develop normally after treatment.

Before performing a reduction under general anesthesia, the child's doctor ordered Bryant's traction—both legs suspended by weights, the buttocks slightly elevated, hips flexed at a 90° angle, and knees fully extended—for a week or two to bring the femoral head fully into position.

The only time Melissa would be released from traction was during feedings, when we would also rub her skin with lotion and assess it for signs of breakdown. Melissa's parents, like most others, ached to rescue her from the traction, to hold and comfort her. We gave them alternatives like stroking her skin or singing to her, but stressed that the more time Melissa spent in traction, the better her chances of getting away with a closed reduction instead of an open one.

Despite everyone's best efforts, however, Melissa did need

an open reduction 10 days later. The surgeon, using fluoroscopy, had realized that he would be unable to center the femoral head perfectly in the acetabulum simply by manipulating it.

He worked through a medial incision, since the head of the femur is easily exposed in an infant under 9 months of age. On an older infant he would have taken an anterior approach.

After positioning the femur and closing the incision, the surgeon put Melissa in a hip spica cast that extended from her nipples to her ankles, with an opening at the perineum. The cast held both hips flexed at approximately a 40° angle, with the legs turned slightly inward.

Melissa was hospitalized for 48 hours postop. During this time she received IV antibiotics to prevent infection. For pain, we started her on 0.1 mg/kg of morphine IV every three or four hours as needed. When she could tolerate fluids we switched her to an acetaminophen with codeine elixir (120 mg acetaminophen and 12 mg codeine in 5 ml). Melissa's doctor ordered 0.5 mg/kg of codeine every three to four hours as needed; some physicians order up to 1.0 mg/kg. Finally, Melissa was put on acetaminophen alone. We also monitored color, warmth, capillary refill time, movement, and sensation in both feet.

Once she began to recover from the surgery and adjust to the cast, Melissa was reasonably comfortable. We told her parents that they could now hold and cuddle her all they wanted. They needed little urging.

Now the biggest challenge for us—and soon for them—would be to keep the cast as free of urine and stool as possible. A

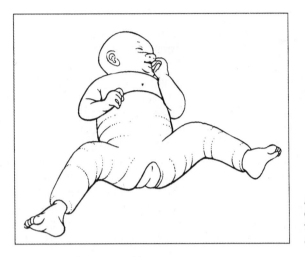

After surgery to correct congenital hip dysplasia, the infant is encased in a hip spica cast.

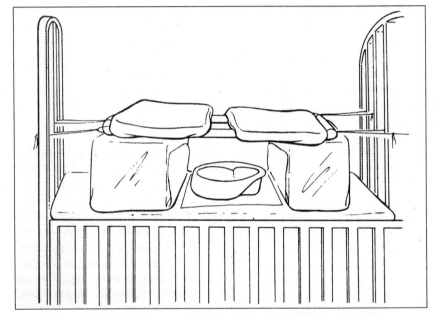

A Bradford frame, which is not available commercially, is used for infants recovering from hip surgery. To make the frame, stretch two pieces of canvas over a rectangle of aluminum tubing, leaving an opening in the middle for the perineum. Cover the canvas with pads and sheets and secure the patient on the frame with a sheet or straps. Then elevate the frame on wooden blocks, with a bedpan underneath the opening. To make the frame stable in the crib, the mattress is removed and a piece of plywood placed over the springs. The frame itself is tied to the bars at the head and foot of the crib.

wet cast will become thin and soft, providing little support.

We've found that a Bradford frame (shown on the preceding page) helps. It serves as both bed and potty. You put the baby, undiapered, on the frame the perineum over its central opening. Then you tuck a piece of plastic wrap, eight to 10 inches long, under the edges of the cast all the way around to cover the area and funnel urine and stool into the bedpan below.

We taught Melissa's parents how to use the frame and gave them our sheet of cast care instructions. We told them that they'd be unable to completely prevent the cast from getting soiled, but that they could minimize the damage by following instructions carefully. For the times when Melissa was not on the frame, we showed them how to tuck a "preemie" diaper into the edges of the cast around the perineum, fastening a larger diaper over the cast to hold the smaller one in place.

They were to give her sponge baths twice a day, each time checking for redness, and turn her every two to three hours, positioning her on her back, stomach, and sides. When the infant was on the frame, we told them, they should make sure that bony prominences and toes rested on well-padded areas.

We also advised smaller and more frequent feeding than usual, since Melissa's enforced inactivity, and the presence of the cast over her stomach, might well decrease her appetite. We instructed them to call if Melissa vomited more than twice in 24 hours—an indication that the cast was too tight in this area.

We knew that the next few weeks would be very stressful for Melissa's parents, so we kept in touch by phone and urged them to call at any time.

Adam's turn comes to undergo surgery

Adam's surgeon made medial, posterior, and lateral incisions to release soft tissue that was causing the boy's feet to turn inward. He didn't perform an osteotomy, which involves shaving the talus, as he might have on an older child, because he hoped that with the ligaments and tendons stretched and a new cast holding the foot in proper position, the bone would now grow normally.

Postop, doctors at our hospital place the infant's feet in long-leg, flexed, anterior-posterior splints secured with biastockinette wrap. Before Adam left the OR, the splints were elevated and taped onto sterile towels, as shown on page 64, so that he couldn't roll over.

We assessed the neurovascular status of Adam's legs every two hours for the first 12 hours postop, then every four hours. Edema is the most common complication of clubfoot repair, so, as with Melissa, we monitored closely for circulatory problems.

At first, Adam fussed even when he was held. We gave pain medication on a schedule similar to Melissa's.

Four days later the worst danger of edema was past. The surgeon put Adam's legs in long, flexed casts, and we prepared him for discharge. After the casts had dried, we petaled all edges with moleskin that had an adhesive backing, something we had done for Melissa, too. We told the parents to keep the child's feet elevated for 48 hours, to prevent swelling. We also taught them how to assess circulation in the toes. Finally, we stressed the importance of keeping the cast clean and dry.

The future for Melissa and Adam

Melissa's cast came off after six weeks. Her hip was perfect. Her surgeon would see her regularly for the next two years. If there were no further problems, she would have full, normal movement of her hips.

Adam's cast was changed after three weeks and removed after six. He would wear plastic dorsiflexion splints at night and during naps for six more months. His parents would perform passive range-of-motion exercises on his feet for 10 to 15 minutes four times a day. The doctor would check his progress every three months for a year, then yearly until he was three or four.

We hoped he would be among the 85% of infants who don't require further surgery. His feet would probably be on the small side and somewhat stiff, but they would undoubtedly take him where he wanted to go. □

BIBLIOGRAPHY

Beaty, J.H. *Campbell's Operative Orthopedics*. St. Louis: C.V. Mosby, 1959. Corbett, D. Information needs of parents of a child in a Pavlik harness. *Orthopaedic Nursing* 7:20, March/April 1988. Cummings, R.J. and Lovell, W.W. Current concepts review of operative treatment of congenital idiopathic club foot. *J. Bone Joint Surg.* 70A:1108, August 1988. Ferguson, A.B., ed. *Orthopedic Surgery in Infancy and Childhood* (5th ed.). Baltimore: Williams and Wilkins, 1981. Hesinger, R.N. *Clinical Symposia* 31/1. Summit, N.J.: CIBA Pharmaceuticals, 1979. Lovell, W.W. and Winter, R.B. *Pediatric Orthopedics* (2nd ed.). Philadelphia: J.B. Lippincott, 1986. Ward, W.T. Personal communications. Whaley, L.F. and Wong, D.L. *Nursing Care of Infants and Children* (3rd ed.). St. Louis: C.V. Mosby, 1987.

UNIT 4
MATERNITY AND
GYNECOLOGIC NURSING

by

Charlotte D. Kain, RNC, EdD

This section covers the health care needs of females from adolescence through late adulthood. Emphasis is placed on the childbearing cycle and the normal neonate, and frequently encountered health care problems.

The unit begins with a review of the anatomy and physiology of the female reproductive system as a basis for understanding the entire childbearing process. Nursing process is emphasized throughout, and nursing diagnoses are used to identify the patient's health care needs and to select nursing interventions.

Nursing process must always be implemented with an awareness of the interrelationship, during childbearing, of the maternal and fetal needs and their manifestations. The nurse needs to keep in mind that interventions for the mother may have an impact on the developing fetus, and vice versa. Medications for maternal conditions may affect the fetus, and fetal distress may require that the mother undergo surgery.

In this unit, a major assertion is that childbearing, for most women, is a normal, healthy life event. Discomforts and complications of childbearing are also covered, and these conditions are presented after the content that reviews the natural progression of events in pregnancy and childbearing. In this manner, the factors that alter pregnancy from a normal life event to a life crisis can be clearly identified.

In addition to childbearing, the unit includes a review of frequently encountered health care conditions of women. These conditions usually involve the reproductive system or its accessory organs, and include normally occurring states, such as menopause, as well as pathologic conditions, such as gynecologic cancer.

Overview of Anatomy and Physiology of the Female Reproductive System

ANATOMY

External Structures

A. *Mons veneris:* rounded, soft, fatty, and loose connective tissue over the symphysis pubis. Dark, curly pubic hair growth in typical triangular shape begins here one to two years before the onset of menstruation.

B. *Labia majora:* lengthwise fatty folds of skin extending from the mons to the perineum that protect the labia minora, the urinary meatus, and the vaginal introitus.

C. *Labia minora:* thinner, lengthwise folds of hairless skin, extending from the clitoris to the fourchette.
   1. Glands in the labia minora lubricate the vulva.
   2. The labia minora are very sensitive because of their rich nerve supply.
   3. The space between the labia minora is called the vestibule.

D. *Clitoris:* small erectile organ located beneath the arch of the pubis, containing more nerve endings than the glans penis; sensitive to temperature and touch; secretes a fatty substance called smegma.

E. *Vestibule:* area formed by the labia minora, clitoris, and fourchette, enclosing the openings to the urethra and vagina, Skene's and Bartholin's glands; easily irritated by chemicals, discharges, or friction.
   1. *Urethra:* external opening to the urinary bladder
   2. *Skene's glands* (also called *paraurethral glands):* secrete a small amount of mucus; especially susceptible to infections
   3. *Bartholin's glands:* located on either side of the vaginal orifice; secrete clear mucus during sexual arousal; susceptible to infection, as well as cyst and abscess formation
   4. *Vaginal orifice* and *hymen:* elastic, partial fold of tissue surrounding opening to the vagina

F. *Fourchette:* thin fold of tissue formed by the merging of the labia majora and labia minora, below the vaginal orifice.

G. *Perineum:* muscular, skin-covered area between vaginal opening and anus.
   1. Underlying the perineum are the paired muscle groups that form the supportive "sling" for the pelvic organs, capable of great distension during the birth process.
   2. An episiotomy can be made in the perineum if necessary to the birth process.

Internal Structures

A. *Fallopian tubes:* paired tubules extending from the cornu of the uterus to the ovaries that serve as the passageway for the ova. Mucosal lining of tubes resembles that of vagina and uterus, therefore infection may extend from lower organs.

B. *Uterus:* hollow, pear-shaped muscular organ, freely movable in pelvic cavity, comprised of *fundus, corpus, isthmus,* and *cervix.* Cervix has internal and external os, separated by the cervical canal. Wall of uterus has three layers.
   1. *Endometrium:* inner layer, highly vascular, shed during menstruation and following delivery
   2. *Myometrium:* middle layer, comprised of smooth muscle fibers running in three directions; expels fetus during birth process, then contracts around blood vessels to prevent hemorrhage
   3. *Parietal peritoneum:* serous outer layer

C. *Ovaries:* oval, almond-sized organs on either side of the uterus that produce ova and hormones.

D. *Vagina:* Muscular, distensible tube connecting perineum and cervix; the birth canal.

The Pelvis

Right and left innominate bones, sacrum, and coccyx form the bony passage through which the baby passes during birth. Relationship between pelvic size/shape and baby may affect labor or make vaginal delivery impossible.

A. Pelvic measurements
   1. True conjugate: from upper margin of symphysis pubis to sacral promontory, should be at least 11 cm; may be obtained by x-ray or ultrasound.
   2. Diagonal conjugate: from lower border of symphysis pubis to sacral promontory; should be 12.5–13 cm; may be obtained by vaginal examination.
   3. Obstetric conjugate: from inner surface of symphysis pubis, slightly below upper border, to sacral promontory, it is the

most important pelvic measurement; can be estimated by subtracting 1.5–2 cm from diagonal conjugate.

4. Intertuberous diameter: measures the outlet between the inner borders of the ischial tuberosities; should be at least 8 cm.

B. Pelvic shapes

1. Android: narrow, heart shaped; male-type pelvis
2. Anthropoid: narrow, oval shaped; resembles ape pelvis
3. Gynecoid: classic female pelvis; wide and well rounded in all directions
4. Platypelloid: wide but flat; may still allow vaginal delivery.

C. Pelvic divisions

1. False pelvis: shallow upper basin of the pelvis; supports the enlarging uterus, but not important obstetrically
2. Linea terminalis: plane dividing upper or false pelvis from lower or true pelvis
3. True pelvis: consists of the pelvic inlet, pelvic cavity, and pelvic outlet. Measurements of true pelvis influence the conduct and progress of labor and delivery.

The Breasts

A. Paired mammary glands on the anterior chest wall, between the second and sixth ribs, comprised of glandular tissue, fat, and connective tissue.

B. Nipple and areola are darker in color than breasts.

C. Responsible for lactation after delivery.

PHYSIOLOGY

Menarche

Onset of the menstrual cycle; puberty.

Menstrual Cycle

A. Complex pituitary/ovarian/uterine interaction.

B. Controls ripening and release of an ovum on a regular basis, and preparation for its fertilization and implantation in a thickened uterine lining (endometrium).

C. When fertilization/implantation do not occur, the endometrium is shed (menstruation), and the cycle begins again, due to follicle-stimulating hormone (FSH) and luteinizing hormone (LH) from the anterior pituitary.

D. Stages of cycle

1. *Menstruation:* first days of cycle when endometrium is shed.
2. *Proliferative phase:* major hormone involved is estrogen, which influences build-up of endometrium; also called *follicular phase.*
3. *Ovulation:* release of ovum, usually 14 days (plus or minus 2) before end of cycle.
4. *Secretory phase:* major hormone is progesterone, which influences myometrium (decreased irritability); also called *luteal phase.*

Menopause (Climacteric)

A. Decline in ovarian function and hormone production.

B. Characterized by menstrual cycle irregularity and, in some women, by vasomotor instability and loss of bone density.

C. See also Menopause, page **431**.

Sexual Response in the Female: Four Phases

A. Excitement phase: vaginal lubrication and vasocongestion of external genitals.

B. Plateau phase: formation of orgasmic platform in vagina.

C. Orgasmic phase: strong rhythmic contractions of vagina and uterus.

D. Resolution phase: cervix dips into seminal pool in vagina; all organs return to previous condition.

The Childbearing Cycle

CONCEPTION

A. The penetration of one ovum (female gamete) by one sperm (male gamete) resulting in a fertilized ovum (zygote).
B. Sex of child is determined at moment of conception by male gamete. If X-bearing male gamete unites with ovum, result is a female child (X + X). If Y-bearing male gamete unites with ovum result, is a male child (X + Y).
C. Usually occurs in the outer third of the fallopian tube.
D. Multiple pregnancies result from
    1. Multiple ovulations and conceptions (dizygotic).
    2. Single ovulation and conception (monozygotic), with an ovum that further divides into two or more; always the same sex; only one chorion.

NIDATION (IMPLANTATION)

A. Burrowing of developing zygote into endometrial lining of uterus.
B. May take 7–10 days after fertilization, while zygote develops to trophoblastic stage.
C. Chorionic villi appear on surface of trophoblast and secrete human chorionic gonadotropin (HCG), which inhibits ovulation during pregnancy by stimulating continuous production of estrogen and progesterone. This secretion of HCG forms the basis of the various tests for pregnancy.

DEVELOPMENTAL STAGES

Fertilized Ovum

A. From conception through first two weeks of pregnancy.
B. Nidation complete by the end of this period.

Embryo

A. From end of second week through end of eighth week (also called period of organogenesis).
B. Critical time in development; embryo most vulnerable to teratogens (harmful substances or conditions), which can result in congenital anomalies.

Fetus

A. From end of eighth week to termination of pregnancy.
B. Continued maturation of already-formed organ systems.

SPECIAL STRUCTURES OF PREGNANCY

Fetal Membranes

A. Arise from the zygote.
B. Inner (amnion) and outer (chorion).
C. Hold the developing fetus as well as the amniotic fluid.

Amniotic Fluid

A. Clear, yellowish fluid surrounding the developing fetus.
B. Average amount 1000 cc.
C. Protects fetus.
    1. Allows free movement.
    2. Maintains temperature.
    3. Provides oral fluid.
D. Can be aspirated and tested for various diseases and abnormalities during pregnancy.

Umbilical Cord

A. Connecting link between fetus and placenta.
B. Contains two arteries and one vein supported by mucoid material (Wharton's jelly) to prevent kinking and knotting.
C. There are no pain receptors in the umbilical cord.

Placenta

A. Transient organ allowing passage of nutrients and waste materials between mother and fetus.
B. Also acts as an endocrine organ and as a protective barrier against some drugs and infectious agents; passage of materials in either direction is effected by
    1. Diffusion: gases, water, electrolytes.
    2. Facilitated transfer: glucose, amino acids, minerals.
    3. Pinocytosis: movement of minute particles (e.g., fats).
    4. Leakage: caused by membrane defect; may allow maternal and fetal blood mixing.

C. Mother also transmits immunoglobin G (IgG) to fetus through placenta, providing limited passive immunity.
D. Hormones produced by the placenta include
　1. HCG: early in pregnancy, responsible for continued action of corpus luteum. Later, is basis of pregnancy tests.
　2. Human chorionic somatomammotropin/human placental lactogen (HCS/HPL): similar to growth hormone; affects maternal insulin production; prepares breasts for lactation.
　3. Estrogen and progesterone: necessary for continuation of pregnancy.

Fetal Circulation

A. Arteries in cord and fetal body carry unoxygenated blood.
B. Veins in cord and in fetal body carry oxygenated blood.
C. Ductus venosus connects umbilical vein and inferior vena cava; closes after birth.
D. Foramen ovale allows blood to flow from right atrium to left atrium, bypassing lungs. Closes functionally at birth because of increased pressure in left atrium; anatomic closure may take several weeks to several months.
E. Ductus arteriosus allows blood flow from pulmonary arteries to aorta, bypassing fetal lungs; closes after delivery.

Fetal Growth and Development

A. Organ systems develop from three primary germ layers.
　1. Ectoderm: outer layer, produces skin, nails, nervous system and tooth enamel.
　2. Mesoderm: middle layer, produces connective tissue, muscles, blood and circulatory system.
　3. Endoderm: inner layer, produces linings of gastrointestinal and respiratory tracts, endocrine glands and auditory canal.
B. Timetable (Table 4.1)
C. Measurement of length of pregnancy
　1. Days: 267–280
　2. Weeks: 40, plus or minus 2
　3. Months (lunar): 10
　4. Months (calendar): 9
　5. Trimesters: 3
D. Estimated due date/estimated date of confinement *(Nägele's Rule)*; see Figure 4.1. This calculation is an estimation only. Most women will deliver within the two weeks before their due date, or in the two weeks after.

- Add 7 days to the first day of the last menstrual period.
- Subtract 3 months
- Add 1 year

Example:

	1st day of LMP:	September 16, 1985.
	Add 7 days =	September 23.
	Subtract 3 months =	June 23.
	Add 1 year =	June 23, 1986 will be estimated due date

Figure 4.1　Nägele's rule.

Table 4.1　Markers in Fetal Development

Date*	Development
4 weeks	All systems in rudimentary form; heart chambers formed and heart is beating. Embryo length about 0.4 cm; weight about 0.4 gm.
8 weeks	Some distinct features in face; head large in proportion to rest of body; some movement. Length about 2.5 cm, weight 2 gm.
12 weeks	Sex distinguishable; ossification in most bones; kidneys secrete urine; able to suck and swallow. Length 6–8 cm, weight 19gm.
16 weeks	More human appearance; earliest movement likely to be felt by mother; meconium in bowel; scalp hair develops. Length 11.5–13.5 cm, weight 100 gm.
20 weeks	Vernix caseosa and lanugo appear; movement usually felt by mother; heart rate audible; bones hardening. Length 16–18.5 cm, weight 300 gm.
24 weeks	Body well proportioned; skin red and wrinkled; hearing established. Length 23 cm, weight 600 gm.
28 weeks	Infant viable, but immature if born at this time. Body less wrinkled; appearance of nails. Length 27 cm, weight 1100 gm.
32 weeks	Subcutaneous fat beginning to deposit; L/S ratio in lungs now 1.2:1; skin smooth and pink. Length 31 cm, weight 1800–2100 gm.
36 weeks	Lanugo disappearing; body usually plump; L/S ratio usually 2:1; definite sleep/wake cycle. Length 35 cm, weight 2200–2900 gm.
40 weeks	Full-term pregnancy. Baby is active, with good muscle tone; strong suck reflex; if male, testes in scrotum; little lanugo. Length 40 cm, weight 3200 gm or more.

*Dates are approximate, but developmental level should have been reached by the end of the time period specified.

PHYSICAL AND PSYCHOLOGIC CHANGES OF PREGNANCY

Reproductive System

A. External structures: enlarged due to increased vascularity.
B. Ovaries
　1. No ovulation during pregnancy
　2. Corpus luteum persists in early pregnancy until development of placenta.
C. Fallopian tubes: elongate as uterus rises in pelvic and abdominal cavities.
D. Vagina
　1. Increased vascularity *(Chadwick's sign)*
　2. Estrogen-induced leukorrhea
　3. Change in pH (less acidic) may favor overgrowth of yeastlike organisms

4. Connective tissue loosens in preparation for distension of labor and delivery.

E. Cervix

1. Softens and loosens in preparation for labor and delivery *(Goodell's sign)*.

2. Mucus production increases, and plug (operculum) is formed as bacterial barricade.

F. Uterus

1. Hypertrophy and hyperplasia of muscle cells

2. Development of fibroelastic tissue that increases ability to contract

3. Shape changes from pearlike to ovoid

4. Rises out of pelvic cavity by 16th week of pregnancy

5. Increased vascularity and softening of isthmus *(Hegar's sign)*

6. Mild contractions *(Braxton Hicks' sign)* beginning in the fourth month through end of pregnancy.

G. Breasts

1. Increased vascularity, sensitivity, and fullness

2. Nipples and areola darken

3. Nipples become more erectile

4. Proliferation of ducts and alveolar tissue

5. Production of colostrum by the second trimester.

Cardiovascular System

A. Blood volume expands as much as 50% to meet demands of new tissue and increased needs of all systems.

B. Progesterone relaxes smooth muscle resulting in vasodilation and accommodation of increased volume.

C. RBC volume increases as much as 30%; may be slight decline in hematocrit as pregnancy progresses because of this relative imbalance.

D. Stroke volume and cardiac output increase.

E. WBCs increase.

F. Greater tendency to coagulation.

G. Blood pressure may drop in early pregnancy; should not rise during last half of pregnancy.

H. Heart rate increases; palpitations possible.

I. Blood flow to uterus and placenta is maximized by left side-lying position.

J. Varicosities may occur in vulva and rectum as well as lower extremities.

Respiratory System

A. Increased vascularity of mucous membranes of this system gives rise to symptoms of nasal and pharyngeal congestion and fullness in the ears.

B. Shape of thorax shortens and widens to accommodate the growing fetus.

C. Slight increase in respiratory rate.

D. Dyspnea may occur at end of third trimester before engagement or "lightening."

Renal System

A. Kidney filtration rate increases as much as 50%.

B. Glucose threshold drops; sodium threshold rises.

C. Water retention increases as pregnancy progresses.

D. Enlarging uterus causes pressure on bladder resulting in frequency of urination, especially during first trimester; later in pregnancy relaxed ureters are displaced laterally, increasing possibility of stasis and infection.

E. Presence of protein (not an expected component of maternal urine) indicates possible renal disease or pregnancy-induced hypertension.

Integumentary System

A. Increased pigmentation of nipples and areolas.

B. Possible appearance of *chloasma* (mask of pregnancy): darkening of areas on forehead and cheekbones.

C. Appearance of *linea nigra*, darkened line bisecting abdomen from symphysis pubis to top of fundus.

D. Striae (stretch marks): separation of underlying connective tissue in breasts, abdomen, thighs, and buttocks; fade after delivery.

E. Greater sweat and sebaceous gland activity.

Musculoskeletal System

A. Alterations in posture and walking gait caused by change in center of gravity as pregnancy progresses.

B. Increased joint mobility as a result of action of ovarian hormone (relaxin) on connective tissue.

C. Possible backache.

D. Occasional cramps in calf may occur with hypocalcemia.

Neurologic System

A. Few changes with a typical pregnancy.

B. Pressure on sciatic nerve may occur later in pregnancy due to fetal position.

Gastrointestinal System

A. Bleeding gums and hypersalivation may occur.

B. Tooth loss due to demineralization should *not* occur.

C. Nausea and vomiting in first trimester due to rising levels of HCG.

D. Appetite usually improves.

E. Strange food combinations or cravings may occur.

F. Progesterone-induced relaxation of muscle tone leads to slow movement of food through GI tract; may result in heartburn.

G. Constipation may occur as water is reabsorbed in large intestine.

H. Emptying time for gallbladder may be prolonged; increased incidence of gallstones.

Endocrine System

A. Pituitary: FSH and LH greatly decreased; oxytocin secreted during labor and after delivery; prolactin responsible for initiation and continuation of lactation.

B. Progesterone secreted by corpus luteum until formation of placenta.

C. Principal source of estrogen is placenta, synthesized from fetal precursors.

D. HCS/HPL produced by placenta; similar to growth hormone, it prepares breasts for lactation; also affects insulin/glucose metabolism. May overstress maternal pancreas.

E. Ovaries secrete relaxin during pregnancy,

F. Slight increase in thyroid activity and basal metabolic rate (BMR).

G. Pancreas may be stressed due to complex interaction of glucose metabolism, HCS/HPL, and cortisol, resulting in diminished effectiveness of insulin, and demand for increased production.

Psychosocial Changes

A. First trimester
1. Mother needs accurate diagnosis of pregnancy.
2. Works through characteristic ambivalence of early pregnancy.
3. Mother is self-centered, baby is "part" of her.
4. Grandparents are usually the first relatives to be told of the pregnancy.

B. Second trimester
1. Mother demonstrates growing realization of baby as separate and needing person.
2. Fantasizes about unborn child.

C. Third trimester
1. "Nesting" activity appears as due date approaches.
2. Desire to be finished with pregnancy.

D. Anxiety over "safe passage" for self and baby through labor and delivery.

E. Reactions of father-to-be may parallel those of mother (e.g., ambivalence, anxiety). Additionally, as mother's pregnancy progresses he may experience similar physical changes.

F. Preparation of siblings varies according to their age and experience.

The Antepartal Period

ASSESSMENT

Determination of Pregnancy

Pregnancy-caused changes in the mother's physical self are the basis for the diagnosis of pregnancy, and are classified as presumptive, probable, or positive.

Presumptive Signs and Symptoms (Subjective)

These changes may be noticed by the mother/health care provider, but are *not* conclusive for pregnancy.
A. Amenorrhea (cessation of menstruation)
B. Nausea and vomiting
C. Urinary frequency
D. Fatigue
E. Breast changes
F. Weight change
G. Skin changes
H. Vaginal changes including leukorrhea
I. Quickening

Probable Signs and Symptoms (Objective)

These changes are usually noted by the health-care provider, but are *still not conclusive* for pregnancy.
A. Uterine enlargement
B. Changes in the uterus and cervix from increased vascularity
C. Ballottement: fetus rebounds against the examiner's hand when pushed gently upwards.
D. Braxton Hicks' contractions: occur early in pregnancy, although not usually sensed by the mother until the third trimester.
E. Laboratory tests for pregnancy
  1. Most tests rely on the presence of HCG in the blood or urine of the woman.
  2. Easy, inexpensive, but may give false readings with any handling error, medications, or detergent residue in laboratory equipment.
  3. Exception is the radioimmunoassay (RIA), which tests for the beta subunit of HCG and is considered to be so accurate as to be diagnostic for pregnancy.
F. Changes in skin pigmentation.

Positive Signs and Symptoms

These signs emanate from the fetus, are noted by the health care provider, and *are conclusive* for pregnancy.
A. Fetal heartbeat: detected as early as eighth week with an electronic device; after 16th week with a more conventional auscultory device.
B. Palpation of fetal outline.
C. Palpation of fetal movements.
D. Demonstration of fetal outline by either ultrasound (after sixth week) or x-ray (after 12th week).

ANALYSIS

Nursing diagnoses for the antepartal period may include
A. Knowledge deficit: information on the following topics needs to be given and reinforced
  1. Danger signals of pregnancy to be reported
  2. Dangerous behaviors during pregnancy (e.g., smoking, using drugs [specially alcohol], use of nonprescription medications)
B. Alteration in nutrition: individualized nutritional information will be needed
C. Activity intolerance: need for additional rest and benefits of a moderate exercise program
D. Anxiety
E. Alteration in bowel elimination, constipation
F. Disturbance in self-concept: body image
G. Alteration in comfort
H. Ineffective individual coping
I. Powerlessness
J. Noncompliance
K. Potential fluid volume deficit

PLANNING AND IMPLEMENTATION

Goals

A. Establish a diagnosis of pregnancy.
B. Gather initial data to form the basis for comparison with data collected as pregnancy progresses.

C. Identify high-risk factors.
D. Propose realistic and necessary interventions.
E. Keep mother and baby in optimum health, providing any needed information.
F. Provide needed information for prepared childbirth.

Interventions

Prenatal Care

A. Time frame
  1. First visit: may be made as soon as woman suspects she is pregnant frequently after first missed period.
  2. Subsequent visits: Every month until the 7th month, every 2 weeks during months 7 and 8, and weekly during the 9th month; more frequent visits are scheduled if problems arise.
B. Conduct of initial visit
  1. Extensive collection of data about patient in all pertinent areas in order to form basis for comparison with data collected on subsequent visits and to screen for any high-risk factors
    a. Menstrual history: menarche, regularity, frequency and duration of flow, last period
    b. Obstetrical history: include sexual history and contraceptive use
    c. Medical history: include past illnesses, surgeries; current use of medications
    d. Family history
    e. Current concerns
  2. Complete physical examination, including internal gynecologic exam, and bimanual exam
  3. Laboratory work, including CBC, urinalysis, Pap test, blood type and Rh, rubella titer, testing for sexually transmitted diseases (STD), other tests as indicated (e.g., TB test)
C. Conduct of subsequent visits
  1. Continue collection of data, especially weight, blood pressure, urine screening for glucose and protein, evaluation of fetal development through auscultation of fetal heart rate (FHR) and palpation of fetal outline, measurement of fundal height as correlation for appropriate progress of pregnancy.
  2. Prepare for any necessary testing.
    a. Have patient void.
    b. Collect baseline data re vital signs.
    c. Collect specimen.
    d. Monitor patient and fetus after procedure.
    e. Provide support to patient.
    f. Document as needed.

Nutrition during Pregnancy

A. Weight gain
  1. Variable, but 25 lb usually appropriate for average woman with single pregnancy.
  2. Woman should have consistent, predictable pattern of weight gain, with only 2–3 lb in first trimester, then average 12 oz gain every week in second and third trimesters.

Table 4.2	Methods of Childbirth
Read method	The so-called "natural" childbirth method. Underlying concept: knowledge diminishes the fear that is key to pain. Classes include information as well as practice in relaxation and abdominal breathing techniques for labor.
Lamaze method	Psychoprophylactic method based on utilization of Pavlovian conditioned response theory. Classes teach replacement of usual response to pain with new, learned responses (breathing, effleurage, relaxation) in order to block recognition of pain and promote positive sense of control in labor.
Bradley method	Husband-coached childbirth. A modification of the Read method emphasizing working in harmony with the body.
Other methods	Hypnosis, yoga, the Wright method, and the Kitzinger method.

  3. Gains mostly reflect maternal tissue in first half of pregnancy, and fetal tissue in second half of pregnancy.
B. Specific nutrient needs
  1. *Calories:* usual addition is 300 kcal/day, but there will be specific guidelines for those beginning pregnancy either over- or underweight.
  2. *Protein:* additional 30 gm/day to ensure intake of 74–76 gm/day; very young pregnant adolescents and those with multiple pregnancies will need more protein.
  3. *Carbohydrates:* intake must be sufficient for energy needs, using fresh fruits and vegetables as much as possible to derive additional fiber benefit; teach to avoid "empty" calories.
  4. *Fats:* high-energy foods, which are needed to carry the fat-soluble vitamins.
  5. *Iron:* needed by mother as well as fetus; reserves usually sufficient for first trimester, supplementation recommended after this time; iron preparations should be taken with source of vitamin C to promote absorption.
  6. *Calcium:* one-third increase needed over prepregnant levels; dairy products most frequent source, with supplementation for those with lactose intolerance.
  7. *Sodium:* contained in most foods; needed in pregnancy; should not be restricted without serious indication.
  8. *Vitamins:* both fat- and water-soluble are needed in pregnancy; essential for tissue growth and development, as well as regulation of metabolism. Generally not synthesized by body, nor stored in large amounts.
C. Dietary supplements: many health care providers supplement the pregnant woman's diet with an iron-fortified multivitamin to ensure essential levels.
D. Special concerns
  1. Religious, ethnic, and cultural practices that influence selection and preparation of foods
  2. Pica (ingestion of nonedible or non-nutritive substances)
  3. Adolescence

4. Economic deprivation
5. Heavy smoking
6. Previous reproductive problems

Education for Parenthood

A. Provision of information about pregnancy, labor and delivery, the postpartum period and lactation.
B. Usually taught in small groups, may be individualized.
C. Topics can be grouped into early and late pregnancy, labor and delivery, and postdelivery/newborn care.
D. Emphasis placed on both physical and psychosocial changes seen in childbearing cycle.
E. Preparation for childbirth: intended to provide knowledge and alternative coping behaviors in order to diminish anxiety and discomfort, and promote cooperation with the birth process; see Table 4.2 for specific methodologies.

Determination of Fetal Status and Risk Factors

A. Fetal diagnostic tests
  1. Used to
    a. Identify or confirm the existence of risk factor(s)
    b. Validate pregnancy
    c. Observe progress of pregnancy
    d. Identify optimum time for induction of labor if indicated
    e. Identify genetic abnormalities
  2. Types
    a. *Chorionic villi sampling (CVS):* earliest test possible on fetal cells; sample obtained by slender catheter passed through cervix to implantation site.
    b. *Ultrasound:* use of sound and returning echo patterns to identify intrabody structures. Useful early in pregnancy to identify gestational sac(s); later uses include assessment of fetal viability, growth patterns, anomalies, fluid volume, uterine anomalies, and adnexal masses. Used as an adjunct to amniocentesis; safe for fetus (no ionizing radiation).
    c. *Amniocentesis:* location and aspiration of amniotic fluid for examination; possible after the 14th week when sufficient amounts are present. Used to identify chromosomal aberrations, sex of fetus, levels of alpha-fetoprotein and other chemicals indicative of neural tube defects and inborn errors of metabolism, gestational age, Rh factor.
    d. *X-ray:* can be used late in pregnancy (after ossification of fetal bones) to confirm position and presentation; not used in early pregnancy to avoid possibility of causing damage to fetus and mother.
    e. *Estriol levels:* chemical index of well-being of fetoplacental unit; determinations possible after 20 weeks, best results after 32 weeks. Mother uses fetal precursors to synthesize estriols in the placenta. Serial determinations yielding rising trend in estriol levels indicate well-functioning fetoplacental unit. Falling levels usually indicate problems. Can be done on 24-hour urine specimen or blood serum.

Table 4.3 Nonstress Test (NST)

Result	Interpretation	Significance
Reactive	2 or more accelerations of 15 beats/min lasting 15 sec or more in 20-min period (associated with each fetal movement)	High-risk pregnancy allowed to continue if twice weekly NSTs are reactive.
Nonreactive	No FHR acceleration, or accelerations less than 15 beats/min or lasting less than 15 sec through fetal movement	Need to attempt to clarify FHR pattern; implement CST and continue external monitoring.
Unsatisfactory	FHR pattern not able to be interpreted	Repeat NST; or do CST.

    f. *L/S ratio:* uses amniotic fluid to ascertain fetal lung maturity through measurement of presence and amounts of the lung surfactants lecithin and sphingomyelin. At 35–36 weeks, ratio is 2:1, indicative of mature levels; once ratio of 2:1 is achieved, newborn less likely to develop respiratory distress syndrome. May be done in laboratory or by "shake" test.
    g. *Creatinine level:* estimates fetal renal maturity and function, uses amniotic fluid.
    h. *Bilirubin level:* high early in pregnancy; drops after 36 weeks gestation; uses amniotic fluid.
    i. Fetal movement count: teach mother to count 2–3 times daily, 30–60 minutes each time; should feel 5–6 movements per counting time. Mother should notify care giver immediately of abrupt change or no movement.
B. Electronic Monitoring
  1. Nonstress test (NST) (see Table 4.3)
    a. Normal fetus produces characteristic FHR pattern changes in response to movement.
    b. In high-risk pregnancies, NST may be used to assess FHR on a frequent basis in order to ascertain fetal well-being.

Table 4.4 Contraction Stress Test (CST)

Result	Interpretation	Significance
Negative	3 contractions, 40–60 sec long, within 10-min period, no late decelerations	Fetus should tolerate labor if it occurs within 1 week.
Positive	Persistent/consistent late decelerations with more than 1/2 contractions	Fetus at increased risk. May need additional testing, may try induction or cesarean birth.
Suspicious	Late decelerations in less than 1/2 contractions	Repeat CST in 24 hr, or other fetal assessment tests.
Unsatisfactory	Inadequate pattern or poor tracing	Same as for suspicious.

2. Contraction stress test (CST) (see Table 4.4)
   a. Based on principle that healthy fetus can withstand decreased oxygen during contraction, but compromised fetus cannot.
   b. Types
      1) nipple-stimulated CST: massage or rolling of one or both nipples to stimulate uterine activity and check effect on FHR.
      2) oxytocin challenge test (OCT): infusion of calibrated dose of IV oxytocin "piggybacked" to main IV line; controlled by infusion pump; amount infused increased every 15–20 minutes until three good uterine contractions are observed within 10-minute period.

EVALUATION

A. Maternal/fetal assessment data remain within acceptable limits; fetus maintains growth and development pattern appropriate to gestational age (evidenced by maternal weight gain, normal increments in fundal height, fetal activity level, other antepartal tests).
B. No complications of pregnancy are evident.
   1. Pregnant woman receives prenatal care (initial and subsequent visits).
   2. Maternal blood pressure, weight gain, and other lab test findings are within normal range.
C. Pregnant woman/family have received adequate educational instruction.
   1. Pregnant woman/family express understanding of childbirth experience and begin transition to role of parenting.
   2. Any necessary testing procedures carried out completely and correctly; patient/fetus in stable condition.

COMPLICATIONS OF PREGNANCY

Pregnancy can be complicated by situations unique to childbearing (e.g., placental bleeding), or by long-standing conditions predating pregnancy and continuing into the childbearing process (e.g., age, socioeconomic status, cardiac problems); for common complications of pregnancy, see Table 4.5.

General Nursing Responsibilities

A. Teach danger signals of pregnancy early in prenatal period so that patient is aware of what needs to be reported to health care provider on an immediate basis (see Table 4.6).
B. Be aware that early teaching allows the patient to participate in the identification and reporting of symptoms that can indicate a problem in her pregnancy.
C. Early recognition and reporting of danger signals usually results in diminishing the risk, and controlling the severity of maternal/fetal complications.
D. Interventions are specific for the individual risks.

Table 4.5	Common Discomforts During Pregnancy	
Discomfort	**Trimester**	**Intervention**
Morning sickness	First	Eat dry carbohydrate in AM; avoid fried, odorous, and greasy foods; small meals rather than large.
Fatigue	First	Rest frequently, as needed.
Urinary frequency	First, end of third	Kegel exercises, perineal pad for leakage.
Heartburn	Second, third	Small meals, bland foods, antacids if ordered.
Constipation	Second, third	Sufficient fluids, foods high in roughage, regular bowel habits. No laxatives unless ordered, including mineral oil.
Hemorrhoids	Third	Avoid constipation; promote regular bowel habits.
Varicosities	Third	Avoid crossing legs and long periods of sitting or standing; rest with feet and hips elevated; avoid elastic garters and other constrictive clothing.
Backache	Third	Use good posture and body mechanics; low-heeled shoes; exercises to strengthen back muscles.
Insomnia	Third	Conscious relaxation; supportive pillows as needed; warm shower before retiring.
Leg cramps	Third	Flex toes toward knees for relief; assure adequate calcium in diet.
Supine hypotensive syndrome	Third	Left side-lying position.
Vaginal discharge	Second	Correct personal hygiene, refer to physician. Do not douche.
Skin changes, dryness, itching	All	Interventions are symptomatic; cool baths, lotions, oils as indicated.

E. Evaluation centers around whether or not the risk was controlled or eliminated, and how the maternal/fetal reaction was controlled.

First Trimester Bleeding Complications

Abortion

A. General information
   1. Loss of pregnancy before viability of fetus; may be spontaneous, therapeutic, or elective (for additional information on therapeutic and elective abortions see Control of Fertility, page 427.)
   2. Types
      a. Threatened abortion

Table 4.6 Danger Signals of Pregnancy

- Any bleeding from vagina
- Gush of fluid from vagina (clear, not urine)
- Regular contractions occurring before due date
- Severe headaches or changes in vision
- Epigastric pain
- Vomiting that persists and is severe
- Change in fetal activity patterns
- Temperature elevation, chills, or "sick" feeling indicative of infection
- Swelling in upper body, especially face and fingers

      1) cervix closed
      2) some bleeding and contractions
      3) fetus not expelled
   b. Inevitable
      1) cervix open
      2) heavier bleeding and stronger contractions
      3) loss of fetus usually not avoidable
   c. Incomplete
      1) expulsion of fetus incomplete
      2) membranes or placenta retained
   d. Complete: all products of conception expelled
   e. Missed: fetus dies in uterus, but is not expelled.
   f. Habitual
      1) three pregnancies in a row culminating in spontaneous abortion
      2) may indicate need for investigation into underlying causes.

B. Assessment findings
  1. Vaginal bleeding (observing carefully for accurate determination of amount, saving all perineal pads)
  2. Contractions, pelvic cramping, backache
  3. Lowered hemoglobin if blood loss significant
  4. Passage of fetus/tissue

C. Nursing interventions
  1. Save all tissue passed.
  2. Keep patient at rest and teach reason for bedrest.
  3. Prepare patient for surgical intervention (D&C or suction evacuation) if needed (see also Therapeutic Abortion, page 404).
  4. Provide discharge teaching re limited activities and coitus after bleeding ceases.
  5. Observe reaction of mother and others, provide emotional support, and give opportunity to express feelings of grief and loss.

Incompetent Cervical Os (Premature Dilation of Cervix)

A. General information: painless condition in which the cervix dilates without uterine contractions and allows passage of the fetus; usually the result of prior cervical trauma.
B. Medical management: may be treated surgically by cerclage (placement of fascia or artificial material to constrict the cervix in a "purse-string" manner). When patient goes into

labor, choice of removal of suture and vaginal delivery, or cesarean birth.
C. Assessment findings
  1. History of repeated, relatively painless abortions
  2. Early and progressive effacement and dilation of cervix
  3. Bulging of membranes through cervical os
D. Nursing interventions
  1. Continue observation for contractions, rupture of membranes, and monitor fetal heart tones.
  2. Position patient to minimize pressure on cervix.

Ectopic Pregnancy

A. General information
  1. Any gestation outside the uterine cavity
  2. Most frequent in the fallopian tubes, where the tissue is incapable of the growth needed to accommodate pregnancy, so rupture of the site usually occurs before 12 weeks.
  3. Any condition that diminishes the tubal lumen may predispose a woman to ectopic pregnancy.
B. Assessment findings
  1. History of missed periods and symptoms of early pregnancy
  2. Abdominal pain, may be localized to one side
  3. Rigid, tender abdomen; sometimes abnormal pelvic mass
  4. Bleeding; if severe may lead to shock
  5. Low hemoglobin and hematocrit, rising white cell count
  6. HCG titers usually lower than in intrauterine pregnancy
C. Nursing interventions
  1. Prepare patient for surgery (removal of affected tube and sometimes ovary).
  2. Institute measures to control/treat shock if hemorrhage severe; continue to monitor postoperatively.
  3. Allow patient to express feelings about loss of pregnancy and concerns about future pregnancies.

Hydatidiform Mole (Gestational Trophoblastic Disease)

A. General information
  1. Proliferation of trophoblasts; embryo dies. Unusual chromosomal patterns seen. The chorionic villi change into a mass of clear, fluid-filled, grapelike vessels.
  2. More common in Orient than elsewhere
  3. Cause essentially unknown
B. Assessment findings
  1. Size of uterus disproportionate to length of pregnancy
  2. High levels of HCG with excessive nausea and vomiting
  3. Dark red to brownish vaginal bleeding after 12th week
  4. Anemia often accompanies bleeding
  5. Symptoms of preeclampsia before usual time of onset
  6. No fetal heart sounds or palpation of fetal parts
  7. Ultrasound shows no fetal skeleton
C. Nursing interventions
  1. Provide pre- and postoperative care for evacuation of uterus.
  2. Teach contraceptive use so that pregnancy is delayed for at

least one year.

3. Teach patient need for follow-up lab work to detect rising HCG levels indicative of choriocarcinoma.
4. Provide emotional support for loss of pregnancy.

Second Trimester Bleeding Complications

There are few unique causes of bleeding in the second trimester. Bleeding may be a late manifestation of condition usually seen in first trimester, such as spontaneous abortion or incompetent cervical os.

Third Trimester Bleeding Complications

Placental problems are the most frequent cause of bleeding in the third trimester.

Placenta Previa

A. General information
   1. Low implantation of the placenta so that it overlays some or all of the internal cervical os.
   2. Cause uncertain, but uterine factors (poor vascularity, fibroid tumors, multiple pregnancies) may be involved.
   3. Amount of cervical os involved classifies placenta previa as marginal, partial, or complete.
B. Assessment findings
   1. Bright red vaginal bleeding after seventh month of pregnancy is cardinal indicator. Bleeding may be intermittent, in gushes, or continuous.
   2. Uterus remains soft.
   3. FHR usually stable unless maternal shock present.
   4. Vaginal examination can result in severe bleeding and should only be undertaken if fetus is mature enough to be born or if recurring hemorrhage demands immediate delivery.
C. Nursing interventions
   1. Ensure complete bedrest.
   2. Maintain sterile conditions for any invasive procedures (including vaginal examination).
   3. Make provision for emergency cesarean birth *(double set-up procedure)*.
   4. Continue to monitor maternal/fetal vital signs.
   5. Measure blood loss carefully.
   6. Assess uterine tone regularly.

Abruptio Placentae

A. General information
   1. Separation of placenta from part or all of normal implantation site, usually accompanied by pain
   2. Usually occurs after 20th week of pregnancy
   3. Seen frequently in women with hypertension, previous abruptio placentae, late pregnancies, and multigravidas, but cause essentially unknown
B. Assessment findings
   1. Painful vaginal bleeding
   2. Tender, boardlike uterus
   3. Slow or absent fetal heart tones
   4. Additional signs of shock

C. Nursing interventions
   1. Ensure bedrest.
   2. Check maternal/fetal vital signs frequently.
   3. Prepare for IV infusions of fluids/blood as indicated.
   4. Monitor urinary output.
   5. Anticipate coagulation problems.
   6. Provide support to parents as outlook for fetus is poor.
   7. Prepare for emergency surgery as indicated.

Hyperemesis Gravidarum

A. General information
   1. Excess nausea and vomiting of early pregnancy leads to dehydration and electrolyte disturbances, especially acidosis.
   2. Causes may include multiple pregnancy, psychologic instability, hydatidiform mole, or may be unknown.
B. Assessment findings
   1. Nausea and vomiting, progressing to retching between meals
   2. Weight loss
C. Nursing interventions
   1. Be nonjudgmental in acceptance of condition; explore patient's response to pregnancy.
   2. Put hospitalized patient in a pleasant, airy room.
   3. Administer IV fluids, monitor I&O.
   4. Provide mouth care.
   6. Monitor progression to solid foods as ordered; observe amounts presented, ingested, and retained.
   7. Restrict visitors if indicated.
   8. Encourage verbalization of feelings about condition.

Toxemias of Pregnancy

General Information

A. Refers to condition unique to pregnancy where vasospastic hypertension is accompanied by proteinuria and edema.
   1. Probable cause: gradual loss of normal pregnancy-related resistance to angiotensin II.
   2. May also be related to decreased production of some vasodilating prostaglandins.
B. Usually appears between 20th and 24th week of pregnancy and disappears after 42nd week.
C. Other terms include *pregnancy-induced hypertension (PIH)* and *metabolic disease of late pregnancy.*
D. Cause essentially unknown, but incidence is high in primigravidas, multiple pregnancies, hydatidiform mole, poor nutrition, essential hypertension; familial tendency.
E. Occurs in 5%–7% of all pregnant women.
F. Condition may be classified relative to symptoms as
   1. Preeclampsia, mild or severe.
   2. Eclampsia.
G. Classic triad of symptoms includes edema/weight gain, hypertension, and proteinuria. Eclampsia includes convulsions and coma.
H. Possible life-threatening complication: HELLP syndrome (*h*emolysis, *e*levated *l*iver enzymes, *l*owered *p*latelets).
I. Only known cure is delivery

Mild Preeclampsia

A. Assessment findings
1. Appearance of symptoms between 20th and 24th week of pregnancy
2. Blood pressure of 140/90 or +30/+15 mm Hg on two consecutive occasions at least 6 hours apart
3. Sudden weight gain (+3 lb/month in second trimester; +1 lb/week in third trimester; or +4.5 lb/week at any time)
4. Slight generalized edema, especially of hands and face
5. Proteinuria of 300 mg/liter in a 24-hour specimen (+1)
B. Nursing interventions
1. Promote bedrest as long as signs of edema or proteinuria are minimal, preferably lying on left side.
2. Provide well-balanced diet with adequate protein and roughage.
3. Explain need for close follow-up, weekly or twice-weekly visits to physician.

Severe Preeclampsia

A. Medical management: magnesium sulfate
1. Magnesium sulfate acts upon the myoneural junction, diminishing neuromuscular transmission.
2. It promotes maternal vasodilation, better tissue perfusion, and has anticonvulsant effect.
3. Nursing responsibilities
   a. Monitor patient's respirations, blood pressure, and reflexes, as well as urinary output frequently.
   b. Administer medications either IV or IM.
4. Antidote for excess levels of magnesium sulfate is calcium gluconate or calcium chloride.
B. Assessment findings
1. Headaches, epigastric pain, nausea and vomiting, visual disturbances, irritability
2. Blood pressure of 150–160/100–110
3. Increased edema and weight gain
4. Proteinuria (5 gm/24 hours) (4+)
C. Nursing interventions
1. Promote complete bedrest, lying on left side.
2. Carefully monitor maternal/fetal vital signs.
3. Monitor I&O, results of laboratory tests.
4. Take daily weights.
5. Do daily fundoscopic examination.
6. Institute seizure precautions.
   a. Restrict visitors.
   b. Minimize all stimuli.
   c. Monitor for hyperreflexia.
   d. Administer sedatives as ordered.
7. Insruct patient about appropriate diet.
8. Continue to monitor 24–48 hours postdelivery.
9. Administer medications as ordered; vasodilator of choice usually hydralazine (Apresoline).

Eclampsia

A. Medical management (see Severe Preeclampsia).
B. Assessment findings

1. Increased hypertension precedes convulsion followed by hypotension and collapse.
2. Coma may ensue.
3. Labor may begin, putting fetus in great jeopardy.
4. Convulsion may recur.
C. Nursing interventions
1. Minimize all stimuli.
   a. Darken room.
   b. Limit visitors.
   c. Use padded bedsides and bedrails.
2. Check vital signs and lab values frequently.
3. Have airway, oxygen, and suction equipment available.
4. Administer medications as ordered.
5. Continue observations 24–48 hours postpartum.

PRE- AND CO-EXISTING DISEASES OF PREGNANCY

Cardiac Conditions

General Information

A. May be the result of congenital heart disease or the sequelae of rheumatic fever/heart disease.
B. May affect pregnancy, but are definitely affected by pregnancy.
C. Classification
1. Class 1: no limitation of activity
2. Class 2: slight limitation of activity
3. Class 3: considerable limitation of activity
4. Class 4: symptoms present even at rest

Prenatal Period

A. Assessment findings
1. Evidence of cardiac decompensation especially when blood volume peaks (weeks 28–32)
2. Cough and dyspnea
3. Edema
4. Heart murmurs
5. Palpitations
6. Rales
B. Nursing interventions
1. Promote frequent rest periods and adequate sleep.
2. Teach patient to recognize and report signs of infection.
3. Compare vital signs to baseline and normal values expected during pregnancy.
4. Assess for factors increasing stress on heart (e.g., anxiety and activity level).
5. Reinforce and promote compliance with physician's plan of care.
6. Teach danger signals for individual patient.

Intrapartal Period

A. Medical management: patient is frequently delivered with use of forceps to shorten "pushing" stage of labor.
B. Nursing interventions

1. Check vital signs every 15 minutes or more frequently if indicated.
2. Check FHR every 15 minutes.
3. Monitor patient's response to stress of labor and watch for signs of decompensation.
4. Administer oxygen and pain medication as ordered, usually PRN.
5. Position patient in sidelying or low semi-Fowler's position.
6. Provide calm atmosphere.

Postpartal Period

A. Nursing interventions
   1. Monitor vital signs, any bleeding, I&O, lab test values, daily weight, rest and diet.
   2. Promote bedrest in appropriate position (see Intrapartal Period above).
   3. Assist with activities of daily living (ADL) as needed.
   4. Prevent infection.
   5. Facilitate nonstressful mother/baby interactions.
   6. Help mother plan for rest and activity patterns at home, as well as household help if indicated.

Endocrine Conditions

Diabetes Mellitus

A. General information
   1. Chronic disease caused by improper metabolic interaction of carbohydrates, fats, proteins, and insulin.
   2. Interaction of pregnancy and diabetes may cause serious complications of pregnancy.
   3. Classifications of diabetes mellitus (see also Unit 2, page 173)
      a. Type 1: formerly called juvenile-onset or insulin-dependent diabetes; onset before age 40
      b. Type 2: formerly called maturity-onset or non-insulin-dependent; onset after age 40
      c. Type 3: formerly called gestational; onset during pregnancy; reversal after termination of pregnancy
      d. Type 4: formerly called secondary; occurs after pancreatic infections or endocrine disorders.
   4. Significance of diabetes in pregnancy
      a. Interaction of estrogen, progesterone, HCS/HPL, and cortisol raise maternal resistance to insulin (ability to use glucose at the cellular level).
      b. If the pancreas cannot respond by producing additional insulin, excess glucose moves across placenta to fetus, where fetal insulin metabolizes it, and acts as growth hormone, promoting macrosomia.
      c. Maternal insulin levels need to be carefully monitored during pregnancy to avoid widely fluctuating levels of blood glucose.
      d. Dose may drop during first trimester, then rise during second and third trimesters.
      e. Higher incidence of fetal anomalies and postdelivery complications in infant of diabetic mother (IDM) (see also page 423).

B. Assessment findings: signs of hyperglycemia
   1. Polyuria
   2. Polydipsia
   3. Weight loss
   4. Polyphagia
   5. Elevated glucose levels in blood and urine

C. Nursing interventions
   1. Assess status of mother and baby frequently.
      a. Monitor carefully fluids, calories, glucose, and insulin during labor and delivery.
      b. Continue careful observation in postdelivery period.
   2. Teach patient the effects and interactions of diabetes and pregnancy and signs of hyper- and hypoglycemia.
   3. Teach patient how to control diabetes in pregnancy, advise of changes that need to be made in nutrition and activity patterns to promote normal glucose levels and prevent complications.
   4. Advise patient of increased risk of infection and how to avoid it.
   5. Observe and report any signs of preeclampsia.
   6. Monitor fetal status throughout pregnancy.

Renal Conditions

Urinary Tract Infections (UTI)

A. General information
   1. Affect 10% of all pregnant women.
   2. Dilated, flaccid, and displaced ureters are a frequent site.
   3. *E. coli* are the usual cause.
   4. May cause premature labor if severe or untreated.

B. Assessment findings
   1. Frequency and urgency of urination
   2. Suprapubic pain
   3. Flank pain (if kidney involved)
   4. Hematuria
   5. Pyuria
   6. Fever and chills

C. Nursing interventions
   1. Encourage high fluid intake.
   2. Provide warm baths to relieve discomfort and promote perineal hygiene.
   3. Administer and monitor intake of prescribed medications (antibiotics, urinary analgesics).
   4. Stress good bladder-emptying schedule.
   5. Monitor for signs of premature labor from severe or untreated infection.

Other Infections

A. General information
   1. Pregnancy is not a prevention against pre- or coexisting infections.
   2. *T*oxoplasmosis, *r*ubella, *c*ytomegalovirus, and *h*erpes (*TORCH infections*) are especially devastating to the fetus, causing abortions, malformations, and even fetal death.
   3. Rubella titer is assessed during early prenatal visit. If mother is deficient in rubella antibodies (less than 1:8 titer), rubella virus vaccine is recommended in immediate postpartum period.

B. General nursing interventions
1. Instruct the pregnant woman in signs and symptoms that indicate infection, especially fever, chills, sore throat, localized pain, or rash.
2. Caution pregnant women to avoid obviously infected persons and other sources of infection, as danger exists for the fetus in all maternal infections.
3. May affect delivery options.

Other Conditions of Risk in Pregnancy

Adolescence

A. General information
1. Pregnancy is a condition of both physical and psychologic risk.
2. Adolescent is frequently undernourished and not yet completely matured either physically or psychosocially.
3. Adolescent is uniquely unsuited for the stresses of pregnancy.
4. Frequency of serious complications increases in adolescent pregnancy, particularly toxemia, and low-birth-weight infants.
B. Nursing interventions
1. Encourage adequate prenatal care.
2. Provide health teaching to prepare for pregnancy, labor and delivery, and motherhood.
3. Provide nutritional counseling.
4. Teach coping skills for labor and delivery.
5. Teach child care skills.

Disseminated Intravascular Coagulation (DIC)

A. General information
1. Also known as *consumptive coagulopathy*
2. A diffuse, pathologic form of clotting, secondary to underlying disease/pathology.
3. Occurs in critical maternity problems such as abruptio placenta, dead fetus syndrome, amniotic fluid embolism, preeclampsia/eclampsia, hydatidiform mole, and hemorrhagic shock
4. Mechanism
   a. Precoagulant substances released in the blood trigger microthrombosis in peripheral vessels and paradoxical consumption of circulating clotting factors.
   b. Fibrin split products accumulate, further interfering with the clotting process.
   c. Platelet and fibrinogen levels drop.
B. Assessment findings
1. Bleeding may range from massive, unanticipated blood loss to localized bleeding (purpura and petechiae)
2. Presence of special maternity problems
3. Prolonged prothrombin and partial thromboplastin times
C. Nursing interventions
1. Assist with medical management of underlying condition.
2. Administer blood component therapy (whole blood, packed cells, fresh frozen plasma, cryoprecipitate) as ordered.

3. Observe for signs of insidious bleeding (oozing IV site, petechiae, lowered hematocrit).
4. Institute nursing measures for severe bleeding/shock if needed.
5. Provide emotional support to patient and family as needed.

Anemia

A. General information
1. Low red cell count may be underlying condition
2. May or may not be exacerbated by physiologic hemodilution of pregnancy
3. Most common medical disorder of pregnancy
B. Assessment findings
1. Patient is pale, tired, short of breath, dizzy.
2. Hgb is less than 11 gm/dl; Hct less than 37%.
C. Nursing interventions
1. Encourage intake of foods with high iron content.
2. Monitor iron supplementation.
3. Teach sequelae of iron ingestion.
4. Assess need for parenteral iron.

SAMPLE QUESTIONS

Mary G. is 22 years old and has missed two of her regular menstrual periods. Her doctor confirms an early, intrauterine pregnancy. She is married and works as a salesperson in a local department store. This is her first pregnancy.

1. To determine Mary's expected due date, which of the following assessments is MOST important?
   o 1. Dates of first menstrual period
   o 2. Date of last intercourse
   o 3. Dates of last menstrual period
   o 4. Age at menarche.

2. During Mary's seventh month, she complains of backache. You teach her to
   o 1. sleep on a soft mattress.
   o 2. walk barefoot at least once/day.
   o 3. perform Kegel exercises once/day.
   o 4. wear low-heeled shoes.

Anne T. is hospitalized for the treatment of severe preeclampsia.

3. Which of the following represents an unusual finding for this condition?
   o 1. Convulsions
   o 2. Blood pressure 160/100
   o 3. Proteinuria 3+
   o 4. Generalized edema

4. The selection of a room for Anne is crucial. You place her
   o 1. in the room next to the elevator.
   o 2. in the room farthest from the nursing station.
   o 3. in the quietest room on the floor.
   o 4. in the labor suite.

Labor and Delivery

OVERVIEW

Five Factors of Labor (Five *P*s)

Passenger

The size, presentation, and position of the fetus.

A. Fetal head (Figure 4.2)

1. Usually the largest part of the baby, it has profound effect on birthing process.
2. Bones of skull are joined by membranous sutures, which allow for overlapping or "molding" of cranial bones during birth process.
3. *Anterior* and *posterior fontanels* are the points of intersection for the sutures, and are important landmarks.
   a. Anterior fontanel is larger, diamond-shaped, and closes about 18 months of age.
   b. Posterior fontanel is smaller, triangular, and usually closes about 3 months of age.
4. Fontanels are used as landmarks for internal examinations during labor to determine position of fetus.

B. Fetal shoulders: may be manipulated during delivery to allow passage of one shoulder at a time.

C. Presentation: that part of the fetus which first enters the pelvis in the birth process (Figure 4.3). Types of presentation are

1. Cephalic: head is presenting part; usually vertex *(occiput)*, which is most favorable for birth. Head is flexed with chin on chest.
2. Breech: buttocks or lower extremities present first. Types are
   a. Frank: thighs flexed, legs extended on anterior body surface, buttocks presenting
   b. Full or complete: thighs and legs flexed, buttocks and feet presenting (baby in squatting position)
   c. Footling: one or both feet are presenting
3. Shoulder: presenting part is the scapula, and baby is in horizontal or transverse position. Cesarean birth indicated.

D. Position: relationship of reference point on fetal presenting part to maternal bony pelvis (Figure 4.4)

1. Maternal bony pelvis divided into four quadrants (right and left anterior, right and left posterior). Relationship is expressed in a three-letter abbreviation: maternal side (R or L) first, next the fetal presentation, and last the maternal quadrant (A or P). Most common positions are

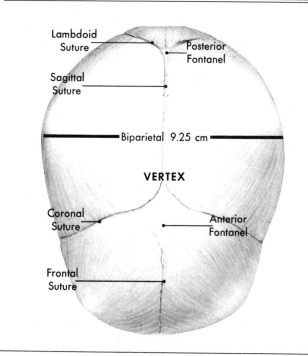

Figure 4.2 The fetal head.
(Reprinted with permission of Ross Laboratories, Columbus, OH, from Clinical Education Aid #13.)

a. LOA (left occiput anterior): fetal occiput is on maternal left side and toward front, face is down. This is a favorable delivery position.

b. ROA (right occiput anterior): fetal occiput on maternal right side toward front, face is down. This is a favorable delivery position.

c. LOP (left occiput posterior): fetal occiput is on maternal left side and toward back, face is up. Mother experiences much back discomfort during labor; labor may be slowed; rotation usually occurs before labor to anterior position, or health care provider may rotate at time of delivery.

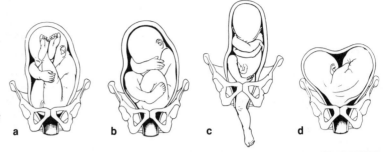

Figure 4.3 Malpresentations.
  a. Frank breech.
  b. Full or complete breech.
  c. Footling.
  d. Shoulder.
  (Reprinted with permission of Ross Laboratories, Columbus, OH, from Clinical Education Aid #18.)

d. ROP (right occiput posterior): fetal occiput is on maternal right side and toward back, face is up. Presents problems similar to LOP.

2. Assessment of fetal position can be made by
  a. *Leopold's maneuvers:* external palpation of maternal abdomen to determine fetal contours or outlines. Maternal obesity, excess amniotic fluid, or uterine tumors may make palpation less accurate.
  b. Vaginal examination: location of sutures and fontanels and determination of relationship to maternal bony pelvis.
  c. Rectal examination: virtually completely replaced by vaginal examination nowadays.
  d. Auscultation of fetal heart tones and determination of quadrant of maternal abdomen where best heard.

Passageway

Shape and measurement of maternal pelvis and distensibility of birth canal (see also Overview of Anatomy and Physiology, page 381).

A. Engagement: fetal presenting part enters true pelvis (inlet). May occur two weeks before labor in primipara; usually occurs at beginning of labor for multipara.

B. Station: measurement of how far the presenting part has descended into the pelvis. Referrant is ischial spines, palpated through lateral vaginal walls.
  1. When presenting part is at ischial spines, station is 0.
  2. If presenting part above ischial spines, station expressed as a negative number (e.g., -1, -2).
  3. If presenting part below ischial spines, station expressed as a positive number (e.g., +1, +2).
  4. "High" or "floating" are terms used to denote unengaged

presenting part.

C. Soft tissue (cervix, vagina): stretches and dilates under the force of contractions to accommodate the passage of the fetus.

Powers

Forces of labor, acting in concert, to expel fetus and placenta. Major forces are

A. Uterine contractions (involuntary)
  1. Frequency: timed from the beginning of one contraction to the begining of the next
  2. Regularity: discernible pattern; better established as pregnancy progresses
  3. Intensity: strength of contraction; a relative assessment without the use of a monitor. May be determined by the "depressability" of the uterus during a contraction. Described as mild, moderate, or strong.
  4. Duration: length of contraction. Contractions lasting more than 90 seconds without a subsequent period of uterine relaxation may have severe implications for the fetus and should be reported.

B. Voluntary bearing down efforts
  1. After full dilation of the cervix, the mother can use her abdominal muscles to help expel the fetus.
  2. These efforts are similar to those for defecation, but the mother is pushing out the fetus from the birth canal.
  3. Contraction of levator ani muscles

Placenta

A. As the placenta usually forms in the fundus of the uterus, it seldom interferes with the progress of labor.

B. A low-lying, marginal, partial, or complete placenta previa

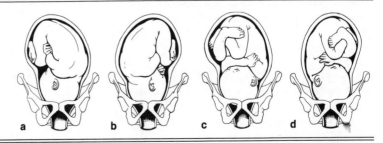

Figure 4.4 Positions.
  a. LOA. **b.** ROA.
  c. LOP. **d.** ROP.
  (Reprinted with permission of Ross Laboratories, Columbus, OH, from Clinical Education Aid #18.)

may require medical intervention to complete the birth process (see also Placenta Previa and Abruptio Placentae, page **392**).

Psychologic Response

A woman who is relaxed, aware, and participating in the birth process usually has a shorter, less intense labor (see also Preparation for Childbirth, page **389**).

The Labor Process

Causes

Actual cause unknown. Factors involved include
A. Progressive uterine distension
B. Increasing intrauterine pressure
C. Aging of the placenta
D. Changes in levels of estrogen, progesterone, and prostaglandins
E. Increasing myometrial irritability

Mechanisms (Vertex Presentation)

A. Engagement
   1. The biparietal diameter of the head passes the pelvic inlet.
   2. The head is fixed in the pelvis.
B. Descent: progress of the presenting part through the pelvis
C. Flexion: chin flexed more firmly onto chest by pressure on fetal head from maternal soft tissues (cervix, vaginal walls, pelvic floor)
D. Internal rotation
   1. Fetal skull rotates along axis from transverse to anteroposterior at pelvic outlet.
   2. Head passes the midpelvis.
E. Extension: head passes under the symphysis pubis and is delivered, occiput first, followed by face and chin.
F. External rotation: head rotates to full alignment with back and shoulders for shoulder delivery mechanisms.
G. *When entire body of baby has emerged from mother's body, birth is complete. This time is recorded as the time of birth.*

Stages of Labor

A. Definitions
   1. Stage 1: from onset of labor until full dilation of cervix
      a. Latent phase: from 0–4 cm
      b. Active phase: 4–8 cm
      c. Transition: 8–10 cm
   2. Stage 2: from full dilation of cervix to birth of baby
   3. Stage 3: from birth of baby to expulsion of placenta
   4. Stage 4: time after birth (usually 1–2 hours) of immediate recovery
B. Cervical changes in first stage of labor
   1. Effacement
      a. Shortening and thinning of cervix
      b. In primipara, effacement is usually well advanced before dilation begins; in a multipara, both effacement and dilation progress together.
   2. Dilation

   a. Enlargement or widening of the cervical os and canal
   b. Full dilation is considered 10 cm.

Duration of Labor

A. Depends on
   1. Regular, progressive uterine contractions
   2. Progressive effacement and dilation of cervix
   3. Progressive descent of presenting part
B. Average length
   1. Primipara
      a. Stage 1: 12–13 hours
      b. Stage 2: 1 hour
      c. Stage 3: 3–4 minutes
      d. Stage 4: 1–2 hours
   2. Multipara
      a. Stage 1: 8 hours
      b. Stage 2: 20 minutes
      c. Stage 3: 4–5 minutes
      d. Stage 4: 1–2 hours

ASSESSMENT DURING LABOR

Fetal Assessment

Auscultation

Auscultate FHR at least every 15 minutes during first stage and every 5 minutes during second stage.
A. Normal range 120–160 beats/minute
B. Best recorded during the 30 seconds immediately following a contraction

Palpation

Assess intensity of contraction by manual palpation of uterine fundus.
A. Mild: tense fundus, but can be indented with fingertips
B. Moderate: firm fundus, difficult to indent with fingertips
C. Strong: very firm fundus, cannot indent with fingertips

Electronic Fetal Monitoring

A. Placement of ultrasound transducer and tocotransducer to record fetal heartbeat and uterine contractions and display them on special graph paper for comparison and identification of normal and abnormal patterns.
B. Can be applied externally to mother's abdomen, or internally, within uterus.
   1. External application
      a. Less precise information collected
      b. May be affected by maternal movements
      c. Can be easily implemented and widely used
      d. Little danger associated with use
   2. Internal application
      a. More precise information collected
      b. Cervix must be dilated and membranes ruptured to be utilized
      c. Physician applies transducers
      d. Sterile technique must be maintained during

application to reduce risk of intrauterine infection

C. Pattern recognition

   1. Nurse is responsible for assessing FHR patterns, implementing appropriate nursing interventions, and reporting suspicious patterns to physician.

   2. Baseline FHR: 120–160, when uterus is not contracting.

   3. Variability is normal, indicative of intact nervous system.

   4. Tachycardia

     a. FHR more than 160 beats/minute lasting longer than 10 minutes.

     b. May have multiple causes.

     c. Oxygen may be administered.

   5. Bradycardia

     a. FHR less than 120 beats/minute lasting longer than 10 minutes.

     b. May have multiple causes.

     c. Oxygen may be administered.

   6. Early deceleration

     a. Deceleration of FHR begins early in contraction, stays within normal range, returns to baseline by end of contraction.

     b. Believed to be the result of compression of fetal head against cervix.

     c. Not an ominous pattern, no nursing interventions required.

   7. Late deceleration

     a. Deceleration of FHR begins late in contraction; exceeds 20 beats/minute; does not return to baseline by end of contraction.

     b. Pattern exists when five occur in a row.

     c. Believed to be the result of uteroplacental insufficiency.

     d. An ominous pattern

     e. Nurse should change maternal position, administer oxygen, discontinue any oxytocin infusion, prepare for early or immediate delivery if pattern remains uncorrected.

   8. Variable deceleration

     a. Onset of deceleration not related to uterine contraction

     b. Swings in FHR abrupt and dramatic, return to baseline frequently rapid

     c. Believed to be the result of compression of the umbilical cord

     d. Although not an ominous pattern, continued nursing assessment required.

     e. Nurse should change maternal position to relieve pressure on cord; if no improvement seen, administer oxygen, discontinue oxytocin if infusing, prepare patient for vaginal exam to assess for prolpased cord (see also Prolapsed Umbilical Cord).

     f. If cord is prolapsed, elevate presenting part off cord; do not attempt to replace cord.

     g. Cesarean delivery will be needed.

Maternal Assessment

Premonitory Assessment

A. Physiologic changes preceding labor

   1. Lightening (engagement): occurs up to two weeks before labor in primipara; at beginning of labor for multipara.

   2. Braxton Hicks' contractions: may become more noticeable; may play a part in ripening of cervix.

   3. Easier respirations from decreased pressure on diaphragm

   4. Frequent urination, from increased pressure on bladder

   5. Restlessness/poor sleeping patterns

True vs False Labor

A. True labor

   1. Contractions increased in frequency, intensity, and duration

   2. Progressive cervical changes

   3. Bloody show

   4. Progressive fetal descent

   5. Walking intensifies contractions.

   6. Discomfort begins in back then radiates to abdomen.

B. False labor

   1. Irregular, inefficient contractions not causing the progressive changes associated with true labor

   2. No bloody show

   3. Discomfort primarily in abdomen, may be relieved by walking

   4. Need to assess patient over period of time to differentiate from true labor

FIRST STAGE OF LABOR

Latent Phase (0 – 4 cm)

Assessment

A. Contractions: frequency, intensity, duration

B. Membranes: intact or ruptured, color of fluid

C. Bloody show

D. Time of onset

E. Cervical changes

F. Time of last ingestion of food

G. FHR every 15 minutes; immediately after rupture of membranes

H. Maternal vital signs

   1. Temperature every 2 hours if membranes ruptured, every 4 hours if intact

   2. Pulse and respirations every 4 hours or PRN as indicated

   3. Blood pressure every half hour or PRN as indicated

I. Is bedrest indicated or mandated

J. Progress of descent (station)

K. Patient's knowledge of labor process

L. Patient's affect

Analysis

Nursing diagnoses for the latent phase of first stage of labor may include

A. Anxiety

B. Ineffective breathing pattern

C. Alteration in comfort: pain

D. Knowledge deficit

Planning and Implementation

A. Goals
   1. Complete all admission procedures.
   2. Labor will progress normally.
   3. Mother/fetus will tolerate latent phase successfully.
B. Interventions
   1. Administer perineal prep/enema if ordered.
   2. Assess vital signs, blood pressure, fetal heart, contractions, bloody show, cervical changes, descent of fetus as scheduled.
   3. Maintain bedrest if indicated or required.
   4. Reinforce/teach breathing techniques as needed.
   5. Support laboring woman/couple based on their needs.
   6. Maintain schedule for voiding every 2 hours.
   7. Apply external fetal monitoring if indicated or ordered.

Evaluation

A. Admission procedures complete
B. Progress through latent stage normal, cervix dilated
C. Mother/fetus tolerate latent phase well, mother as comfortable as possible, vital signs normal, FHR maintained in response to contractions

Active Phase (4–8 cm)

Assessment

A. Cervical changes
B. Bloody show
C. Membranes
D. Progress of descent
E. Maternal/fetal vital signs
F. Patient's affect

Analysis

Nursing diagnoses for the active phase of first stage of labor may include
A. Ineffective individual coping
B. Alteration in oral mucous membranes
C. Knowledge deficit

Planning and Implementation

A. Goals
   1. Progress will be normal through active phase.
   2. Mother/fetus will successfully complete active phase.
B. Interventions
   1. Continue to observe labor progress.
   2. Reinforce/teach breathing techniques as needed.
   3. Position patient for maximum comfort, left side-lying if possible.
   4. Support patient/couple as mother becomes more involved in labor.
   5. Administer analgesia if ordered or indicated.
   6. Assist with anesthesia if given and monitor maternal/fetal vital signs.
   7. Provide ice chips or clear fluids for mother to drink if allowed/desired.

8. Keep patient/couple informed as labor progresses.
9. With posterior position, apply sacral counterpressure, or have father do so.

Evaluation

A. Labor progressing through active phase, dilation progressing
B. Mother/fetus tolerating labor appropriately
C. No complications observed

Transition (8–10 cm)

Assessment

A. Progress of labor
B. Cervical changes
C. Maternal mood changes: if irritable or aggressive may be tiring or unable to cope
D. Signs of nausea, vomiting, trembling, crying
E. Maternal/fetal vital signs
F. Breathing patterns, may be hyperventilating
G. Urge to bear down with contractions

Analysis

Nursing diagnoses for the transition phase of first stage of labor may include
A. Ineffective breathing pattern
B. Powerlessness

Planning and Implementation

A. Goals
   1. Labor will continue to progress through transition.
   2. Mother/fetus will tolerate process well.
   3. Complications will be avoided.
B. Interventions
   1. Continue observation of labor progress, maternal/fetal vital signs.
   2. Give mother positive support if tired or discouraged.
   3. Accept behavioral changes of mother.
   4. Promote appropriate breathing patterns to prevent hyperventilation.
   5. If hyperventilation present, have mother rebreathe expelled carbon dioxide to reverse respiratory alkalosis.
   6. Discourage pushing efforts until cervix is completely dilated, then assist with pushing.
   7. Observe for signs of delivery.

Evaluation

A. Mother/fetus progressed through transition
B. No complications observed
C. Mother/fetus ready for second stage of labor

SECOND STAGE OF LABOR

Assessment

A. Signs of imminent delivery

B. Progress of descent
C. Maternal/fetal vital signs
D. Maternal pushing efforts
E. Vaginal distension
F. Bulging of perineum
G. Crowning
H. Birth of baby

Analysis

Nursing diagnoses for the second stage of labor may include
A. Potential for injury
B. Noncompliance related to exhaustion

Planning and Implementation

A. Goals
  1. Safe delivery of living, uninjured fetus.
  2. Mother will be comfortable after tolerating delivery.
B. Interventions
  1. If necessary, transfer mother carefully to delivery table or birthing chair; support legs equally to prevent/minimize strain on ligaments.
  2. Carefully position mother on delivery table, in delivery chair, or birthing bed to prevent popliteal vein pressure.
  3. Help mother use handles to pull on as she bears down with contractions.
  4. Clean vulva and perineum to prepare for delivery.
  5. Continue observation of maternal/fetal vital signs.
  6. Encourage mother in sustained pushes with each contraction.
  7. Support father's participation if in delivery area.
  8. Catheterize mother's bladder if indicated.
  9. Keep mother informed of delivery progress.
  10. Note time of delivery of baby.

Evaluation

A. Delivery of healthy viable fetus
B. Mother comfortable after procedure
C. No complications during procedure

THIRD STAGE OF LABOR

Assessment

A. Signs of placental separation
  1. Gush of blood
  2. Lengthening of cord
  3. Change in shape of uterus (discoid to globular)
B. Completeness of placenta
C. Status of mother/baby constant for first critical 1–2 hours
  1. Baby's Apgar scores (see Table 4.7)
  2. Blood pressure, pulse, respirations, lochia, fundal status of mother

Analysis

Nursing diagnoses for the third stage of labor may include

Table 4.7   Apgar Scoring

Category	0	1	2	Score
Heart rate	Absent	<100	>100	_____
Respiratory effort	Absent	Slow, irregular	Good cry	_____
Muscle tone	Absent/limp	Some flexion	Active motion	_____
Reflex irritability	No response	Grimace	Cry	_____
Color	Blue, pale	Body pink, extremities blue	All pink	_____
			Total Score	_____

A. Alteration in comfort: pain
B. Potential fluid volume deficit

Planning and Implementation

A. Goals
  1. Placenta will be delivered without complications.
  2. Maternal blood loss will be minimized.
  3. Mother will tolerate procedures well.
B. Interventions
  1. Palpate fundus immediately after delivery of placenta; massage gently if not firm.
  2. Palpate fundus at least every 15 minutes.
  3. Observe lochia for color and amount.
  4. Inspect perineum.
  5. Assist with maternal hygiene as needed.
    a. Clean gown.
    b. Warm blanket.
    c. Clean perineal pads.
  6. Offer fluids as indicated.
  7. Promote beginning relationship with baby and parents through touch and privacy.
  8. Administer medications as ordered/needed.

Evaluation

A. Placenta delivered without complications
B. Minimal maternal blood loss
C. Mother tolerated procedure well

FOURTH STAGE OF LABOR

Assessment

A. Fundal firmness, position
B. Lochia: color, amount
C. Perineum
D. Vital signs
E. IV if running
F. Infant's heart rate, airway, color, muscle tone, reflexes, warmth, activity state
G. Bonding/family integration

Analysis

Nursing diagnoses for the fourth stage of labor may include
A. Alteration in comfort: pain
B. Potential fluid volume deficit

Planning and Implementation

A. Goal: critical first hour(s) after delivery will pass without complication for mother/baby.
B. Interventions
  1. Palpate fundus every 15 minutes for first hour; massage gently if not firm.
  2. Check mother's blood pressure, pulse, respirations every 15 minutes for first hour or until stable.
  3. Check lochia for color and amount every 15 minutes for first hour.
  4. Inspect perineum every 15 minutes for first hour.
  5. Apply ice to perineum if ordered.
  6. Encourage mother to void, particularly if fundus not firm, or displaced.
     a. Use nursing techniques to encourage voiding.
     b. If patient unable to void, get order for catheterization.
     c. Measure first voiding.
  7. Encourage early bonding through breast-feeding if desired.

Evaluation

A. Mother's vital signs stable, fundus and lochia within normal limits
B. Evidence of bonding; parents cuddle, touch, talk to baby
C. No complications observed for mother or baby during crucial time

COMPLICATIONS OF LABOR AND DELIVERY

Premature Labor

A. General information
  1. Labor that occurs before the end of the 37th week of pregnancy.
  2. Cause is frequently unknown, but the following conditions are associated with premature labor
     a. Cervical incompetence
     b. Preeclampsia/eclampsia
     c. Maternal injury
     d. Infection
     e. Multiple births
     f. Placental disorders
B. Medical management
  1. Unless labor is irreversible, or a condition exists in which the mother or fetus would be jeopardized by the continuation of the pregnancy, or the membranes have ruptured, the usual medical intervention is to attempt to arrest the premature labor (tocolysis).
  2. Medications used in the treatment of premature labor
     a. Ritodrine hydrochloride (Yutopar): only drug currently approved by FDA for tocolysis.
        1) beta sympathomimetic that relaxes smooth muscle in the uterus, the vascular system, and the bronchi.
        2) usually results in the interruption of the premature labor, but additionally leads to widening maternal pulse pressure and possible pulmonary edema, especially if given with corticosteroids.
        3) usually administered IV initially, added to a normal saline infusion and controlled by an infusion pump.
        4) IV administration is recommended for at least 12–24 hours at the lowest effective dose to eliminate uterine contractions. IV administration schedule
           a) .05 mg/minute, increasing by .05 mg/minute at 10-minute intervals until maximum of .35 mg/min is reached.
           b) treat at least 12–24 hours.
        5) PO administration should be initiated ½ hour before the IV infusion is discontinued. PO administration schedule: 20 mg q2h for first 24 hours, then 10–20 mg q2h during day, q4h at night.
        6) side effects include maternal tachycardia, diarrhea, hyperglycemia, hypokalemia, fetal tachycardia, and neonatal hypoglycemia.
        7) beta-blocking agent (propranolol [Inderal]) should be on hand to reverse actions of ritodrine if needed.
        8) dosage individualized based on patient response (i.e., action on labor; reaction of mother and fetus).
     b. Magnesium sulfate
        1) used far more frequently in the treatment of preclampsia/eclampsia, magnesium sulfate can be used in the treatment of premature labor.
        2) major effect is to interrupt activity at the myoneural junction to help arrest premature labor.
     c. Ethanol
        1) used only infrequently nowadays because of danger of raised alcohol levels in the fetus
        2) administered IV, often resulting in an inebriated mother and affected fetus.
        3) administered IV, often resulting in an inebriated mother and affected fetus.
     d. Isoxsuprine HCl (Vasodilan) and terbutaline sulfate (Brethine) have also been utilized with success in the treatment of premature labor.
  3. When premature labor cannot or should not be arrested and fetal lung maturity needs to be improved, the use of betamethasone (Celestone) can improve the L/S ratio of lung surfactants. It is administered IM to the mother, usually twice daily for 2 days, then weekly until 34 weeks gestation.

C. Nursing interventions
  1. Keep patient at rest, on left side.
  2. Maintain continuous maternal/fetal monitoring.
     a. Maternal/fetal vital signs every 10 minutes; be alert for abrupt changes.
     b. Monitor maternal I&O.
     c. Monitor urine for glucose and ketones.
     d. Watch cardiac and respiratoty status carefully.
     e. Evaluate lab test results carefully.

3. Administer drugs as ordered/indicated.
   a. Ritodrine hydrochloride (see also Medical Management of Premature Labor)
      1) position patient on left side as much as possible.
      2) apply external fetal monitor.
      3) complete maternal/fetal assessment before each increase in dosage rate.
      4) Special maternal assessments include respiratory status, blood pressure, pulse, I&O, lab values.
      5) notify physician of significant changes.
      6) support patient through stressful period of treatment and uncertainty.
      7) teach patient necessity of continuing oral medication at home if discharged.
   b. Magnesium sulfate: carefully monitor respirations, reflexes, and urinary output (see also Severe Preeclampsia, page **393**).
4. Keep patient informed of all progress/changes.
5. Identify side effects/complications as early as possible.
6. Carry out activities designed to keep patient comfortable.

Postmature/Prolonged Pregnancy

A. General information
   1. Defined as those pregnancies lasting beyond the end of the 42nd week
   2. Fetal jeopardy may exist because of the decreased efficiency of the placenta after the 42nd week, resulting in increased risk of hypoxia and fetal weight loss.
   3. Decreased amounts of vernix also allow the drying of the fetal skin, resulting in a dry, parchmentlike skin condition.
B. Medical management
   1. Directed toward ascertaining precise fetal gestational age and condition, and determining fetal ability to tolerate labor
   2. Induction of labor and possibly cesarean birth
C. Assessment findings
   1. Measurements of fetal gestational age for fetal maturity (see Fetal Diagnostic Tests, page **389**)
D. Nursing interventions
   1. Perform continual monitoring of maternal/fetal vital signs.
   2. Support mother through all testing and labor.
   3. Prepare mother for possible emergency interventions.

Prolapsed Umbilical Cord

A. General information
   1. Displacement of cord in a downward direction, near or ahead of the presenting part, or into the vagina
   2. May occur when membranes rupture, or with ensuing contractions
   3. Associated with breech presentations, unengaged presentations, and premature labors
   4. **Obstetric emergency: if compression of the cord occurs, fetal hypoxia may result in CNS damage or death.**
B. Assessment findings: vaginal exam identifies cord prolapse into vagina

C. Nursing interventions
   1. Check fetal heart tones immediately when membranes rupture, and again after next contraction, or within 5 minutes; report decelerations.
   2. If fetal bradycardia, perform vaginal examination and check for prolapsed cord.
   3. **If cord prolapsed into vagina, exert upward pressure against presenting part to lift part off cord, reducing pressure on cord.**
   4. Get help to move mother into a position where gravity assists in getting presenting part off cord (knee-chest position or severe Trendelenburg's).
   5. Administer oxygen, and prepare for immediate cesarean birth.
   6. If cord protrudes outside vagina, cover with sterile gauze moistened with sterile saline while carrying out above tasks. Do not attempt to replace cord.
   7. Notify physician.

Premature Rupture of Membranes

A. General information
   1. Loss of amniotic fluid, prior to term, unconnected with labor
   2. Dangers associated with this event are prolapsed cord, infection, and the potential need for premature delivery.
B. Assessment findings
   1. Report from mother/family of discharge of fluid
   2. pH of vaginal fluid will differentiate between amniotic fluid (alkaline) and urine or purulent discharge (acidic).
C. Nursing interventions
   1. Monitor maternal/fetal vital signs on continuous basis.
   2. Calculate gestational age.
   3. Observe for signs of infection and for signs of onset of labor.
      a. If signs of infection present, administer antibiotics as ordered and prepare for immediate delivery.
      b. If no maternal infection, induction of labor may be delayed.
   4. Observe and record color, odor, amount of amniotic fluid.
   5. Examine mother for signs of prolapsed cord.
   6. Provide explanations of procedures and findings, and support mother/family.
   7. Prepare mother/family for early birth if indicated.

Fetal Distress

A. General information: common contributing factors are
   1. Cord compression.
   2. Placental abnormalities.
   3. Preexisting maternal disease.
B. Assessment findings
   1. Decelerations in FHR
   2. Meconium-stained amniotic fluid with a vertex presentation
   3. Fetal scalp blood sampling (may be needed for a definitive diagnosis)
C. Nursing interventions
   1. Check FHR on appropriate basis, institute fetal monitoring

if not already in use.

2. Conduct vaginal exam for presentation and position.
3. Place mother on left side, administer oxygen, check for prolapsed cord, notify physician.
4. Support mother and family.
5. Prepare for emergency birth if indicated.

Dystocia

A. General information
 1. Any labor/delivery that is prolonged or difficult
 2. Usually results from a change in the interrelationships among the 5 Ps (factors in labor/delivery): *p*assenger, *p*assage, *p*owers, *p*lacenta, and *p*syche of mother.
 3. Frequently seen causes include
    a. Disproportion between fetal presentation (usually the head) and maternal pelvis (cephalopelvic disproportion [CPD]).
       1) if disproportion is minimal, vaginal birth may be attempted if fetal injuries can be minimized or eliminated.
       2) cesarean birth needed if disproportion is great.
    b. Problems with presentation
       1) any presentation unfavorable for delivery (e.g., breech, shoulder, face, transverse lie)
       2) posterior presentation that does not rotate, or cannot be rotated with ease.
       3) cesarean birth is the usual intervention.
    c. Problems with maternal soft tissue
       1) a full bladder may impede the progress of labor, as can myomata uteri, cervical edema, scar tissue, and congenital anomalies.
       2) emptying the bladder may allow labor to continue; the other conditions may necessitate cesarean birth.
    d. Dysfunctional uterine contractions
       1) contractions may be too weak, too short, too far apart.
       2) progress of labor is affected; progressive dilation, effacement, and descent do not occur in the expected pattern.
       3) classification
          a) primary: inefficient pattern present from beginning of labor; usually a prolonged latent phase.
          b) secondary: efficient pattern that changes to inefficient or stops; may occur in any stage.
B. Assessment findings
 1. Progress of labor slower than expected rate of dilation, effacement, descent for specific patient
 2. Length of labor prolonged
 3. Maternal exhaustion/distress
 4. Fetal distress
C. Nursing interventions
 1. Individualized as to cause.
 2. Provide comfort measures for patient.
 3. Provide clear, supportive descriptions of all actions taken.
 4. Administer analgesia if ordered/indicated.

Table 4.8   **Emergency Delivery of an Infant**

If you have to deliver the baby yourself

- Assess the patient's affect and ability to understand directions, as well as other resources available (other physicians, nurses, auxiliary personnel).
- Stay with patient at all times; mother must not be left alone if delivery is imminent.
- Do not prevent birth of baby.
- Maintain sterile environment if possible.
- Rupture membranes if necessary.
- Support baby's head as it emerges, preventing too-rapid delivery with gentle pressure.
- Check for nuchal cord, slip over head if possible.
- Use gentle aspiration with bulb syringe to remove blood and mucus from nose and mouth.
- Deliver shoulders after external rotation, asking mother to push gently if needed.
- Provide support for baby's body as it is delivered.
- Hold baby in head-down position to facilitate drainage of secretions.
- Promote cry by gently rubbing over back and soles of feet.
- Dry to prevent heat loss.
- Place baby on mother's abdomen.
- Check for signs of placental separation.
- Check mother for excess bleeding; massage uterus PRN.
- Hold placenta as it is delivered.
- Cut cord when pulsations cease, if cord clamp is available; if no clamps, leave intact.
- Wrap baby in dry blanket, give to mother; put to breast if possible.
- Check mother for fundal firmness and excess bleeding.
- Record all pertinent data.
- Comfort mother and family as needed.

---

5. Prepare oxytocin infusion for induction of labor if ordered.
6. Monitor mother/fetus continuously.
7. Prepare for cesarean birth if needed.

Precipitous Labor and Delivery

A. General information
 1. Labor of less than 3 hours
 2. Emergency delivery without patient's physician or midwife
B. Assessment findings
 1. As labor is progressing quickly, assessment may need to be done rapidly.
 2. Patient may have history of previous precipitous labor and delivery.
 3. Desire to push
 4. Observe status of membranes, perineal area for bulging, and for signs of bleeding.
C. Nursing interventions (see Table 4.8)

Amniotic Fluid Embolism

A. General information

1. Escape of amniotic fluid into the maternal circulation, usually in conjunction with a pattern of hypertonic, intense uterine contractions, either naturally or oxytocin induced.

2. **Obstetric emergency: may be fatal to the mother and to the baby.**

B. Assessment findings

1. Sudden onset of respiratory distress, hypotension, chest pain, signs of shock

2. Bleeding (DIC)

3. Cyanosis

4. Pulmonary edema

C. Nursing interventions

1. Initiate emergency life support activities for mother.
   a. Administer oxygen.
   b. Utilize CPR in case of cardiac arrest.

2. Establish IV line for blood transfusion and monitoring of CVP.

3. Administer medications to control bleeding as ordered.

4. Prepare for emergency birth of baby.

5. Keep patient/family informed as possible.

Induction of Labor

A. General information: deliberate stimulation of uterine contractions before the normal occurrence of labor.

B. Medical management: may be accomplished by

1. Amniotomy (the deliberate rupture of membranes)

2. Oxytocins, usually Pitocin

3. Prostaglandin gel (PGE$_2$)

C. Assessment findings

1. Indications for use
   a. Postmature pregnancy
   b. Preeclampsia/eclampsia
   c. Diabetes
   d. Premature rupture of membranes

2. Condition of fetus: mature, engaged vertex fetus in no distress

3. Condition of mother: cervix "ripe" for induction, no CPD

D. Nursing interventions

1. Explain all procedures to patient.

2. Prepare appropriate equipment and medications.
   a. Amniotomy: a small tear made in amniotic membrane as part of sterile vaginal exam
      1) explain sensations to patient.
      2) check FHR immediately before and after procedure; marked changes may indicate prolapsed cord (see page 403).
      3) additional care as for woman with premature rupture of membranes (page 403).
   b. Oxytocin (Pitocin): IV administration, "piggybacked" to main IV
      1) usual dilution 10 u/1000 cc fluid, delivered via infusion pump for greatest accuracy in controlling dosage

2) usual administration rate is 1–2 mU/min, increased no more than 1–2 mU/min at 10-minute intervals until regular pattern of appropriate contractions is established (every 2–3 minutes, lasting less than 90 seconds).

3. Know that continuous monitoring and accurate assessments are essential.
   a. Apply external continuous fetal monitoring equipment.
   b. Monitor maternal condition on a continuous basis: blood pressure, pulse, progress of labor.

4. Discontinue oxytocin infusion when
   a. Fetal distress is noted.
   b. Hypertonic contractions occur.
   c. Signs of other obstetric complications (hemorrhage/shock, abruptio placenta, amniotic fluid embolism) appear.

5. Notify physician of any untoward reactions.

ANALGESIA AND ANESTHESIA

Analgesia for Labor

General Information

A. Definition: the easing of pain or discomfort by the administration of medication that blocks pain recognition or the raising of the pain recognition threshold.

B. Sources of pain/discomfort

1. First stage of labor: stretching of cervix and uterine contractions

2. Second stage of labor: stretching of birth canal and perineum

C. Examples of medications used systemically for labor analgesia

1. Sedatives: help to relieve anxiety; may use secobarbital (Seconal), sodium pentobarbital (Nembutal), phenobarbital.

2. Narcotic analgesics: help to relieve pain; may use morphine, meperidine (Demerol), pentazocine (Talwin).

3. Narcotic antagonists: given to reverse narcotic depression of mother or baby; may use naloxone (Narcan), levallorphan (Lorfan).

4. Analgesic potentiating drugs: given to raise desired effect of analgesic without raising dose of analgesic drug; may use promethazine (Phenergan), promazine (Sparine), propiomazine (Largon), hydroxyzine (Vistaril)

D. Medication administration

1. IV: the preferred route; allows for smaller doses, better control of administration, better prediction of action.

2. IM: still widely used; needs larger dose, absorption may be delayed or erratic.

3. SC: used occasionally for small doses of nonirritating drugs.

Assessment

A. Patient's perception of pain/discomfort

B. Baseline vital signs for later comparison

C. Known allergies
D. Current status of labor: medications best given in active phase of first stage of labor
E. Time of previous doses of medications

Analysis

Nursing diagnoses for labor analgesia may include
A. Alteration in comfort: pain
B. Ineffective individual coping

Planning and Implementation

A. Goals
  1. Medication will relieve maternal discomfort.
  2. Maternal comfort will be achieved with least effect of medication on fetus.
B. Interventions
  1. Administer medications on schedule to maximize maternal effect and minimize fetal effect.
  2. Continue to observe maternal/fetal vital signs for side effects.
  3. Explain to patient that she must remain in bed with side rails up.
  4. Record accurately drug used, time, amount, route, site, and patient response.

Evaluation

A. Medication exerts intended effect.
B. Mother reports positive response to medication.
C. Fetus shows no ill effects from medication.
D. Labor is not affected by medication.

Anesthesia for Labor and Delivery

General information

A. Removal of pain perception by the administration of medication to interrupt the transmission of nerve impulses to the brain.
B. May be administered by inhalation, IV, or regional routes.
C. All methods of labor and delivery anesthesia have their drawbacks, no one method is perfect.
D. Types of labor and delivery anesthesia
  1. Inhalation: mother inhales controlled concentration of gaseous medication.
    a. Administered by trained personnel only
    b. Methoxyflurane (Penthrane) and nitrous oxide commonly used
    c. Dangers include regurgitation and aspiration, uterine relaxation and hemorrhage postdelivery.
  2. IV: rarely used in uncomplicated vaginal deliveries; may be used for cesarean birth (as induction anesthesia).
    a. Administered by trained personnel only
    b. Sodium pentothal commonly used
  3. Regional: medication introduced to specific area to block pain impulses
    a. Always administered by skilled personnel
    b. Medications used include tetracaine (Pontocaine),

lidocaine, bupivacaine (Marcaine), mepivacaine (Carbocaine)
  c. May block nerve at the root or in a peripheral area
    1) nerve root blocks
      a) *lumbar epidural:* may be given intermittently during labor, or at time of delivery; medication is injected over dura through lumbar interspace; absorption of drug is slower, with less hypotension; patient should have no postspinal headache.
      b) *caudal:* may be given intermittently through labor, or at time of delivery; medication is injected through sacral hiatus into peridural space; patient should have no postspinal headache
      c) *subarachnoid (low spinal, saddle block):* given when delivery is imminent; medication is injected into spinal fluid; mother may experience postdelivery headache; keep flat for at least 6–8 hours postspinal and encourage oral fluids postdelivery to facilitate reversal of headache.
    2) peripheral nerve blocks
      a) *paracervical:* instillation of medication into cervix; rarely used during labor because of effect on fetus; useful only in first stage of labor.
      b) *pudendal:* medication injected transvaginally to affect pudendal nerve as it passes behind ischial spines on either side of vagina; useful for delivery and episiotomy if needed.
      c) *perineal (local):* injected into the perineum at the time of delivery in order to perform an episiotomy

Assessment

A. Status of labor progress
B. Maternal/fetal vital signs
C. Allergies
D. Effects of medication on patient (she may need help pushing)
E. Level of anesthesia
F. Return of sensation after anesthesia

Analysis

Nursing diagnoses for anesthesia during labor and delivery may include
A. Impaired physical mobility
B. Potential alteration in tissue perfusion

Planning and Implementation

A. Goals
  1. Pain relief will be obtained.
  2. Healthy maternal/fetal status will be maintained.
B. Interventions
  1. Assist patient to empty bladder.
  2. Assist patient to assume appropriate position.

a. Inhalation anesthesia: supine with wedge under right hip to displace gravid uterus off inferior vena cava
b. Pudendal and perineal: on back or left side
c. Other regional types: on left side or sitting up
3. Check maternal blood pressure and fetal heart rate every 3–5 minutes until stable, then every 15 minutes or PRN.
4. If blood pressure drops, turn patient on left side, administer oxygen, and notify physician.

Evaluation

A. Patient experiences expected pain relief.
B. Fetus exhibits no untoward effects, FHTs remain relatively stable.
C. Labor and delivery carried out as expected.
D. Patient's vital signs remain within normal limits.

OPERATIVE OBSTETRICAL PROCEDURES

Episiotomy

A. General information
1. Incision made in the perineum to enlarge the vaginal opening for delivery
2. Patient usually anesthetized in some manner
3. Types
  a. Midline or median: from posterior vaginal opening through center of perineum toward anal sphincter.
    1) most frequently used
    2) easily done, least discomfort for patient
    3) danger of extension into anal sphincter
  b. Mediolateral: begins at posterior vaginal opening but angles off to left or right at 45 degree angle.
    1) done when need for additional enlargement of vaginal opening is a possibility
    2) mediolateral episiotomy usually more uncomfortable than median
4. Advantages of episiotomy are
  a. Tearing of perineum prevented
  b. Second stage of labor shortened
  c. Stretching of perineal muscles minimized
5. Those opposed to episiotomies argue
  a. Kegel exercises can prepare the perineum to stretch for delivery.
  b. Lacerations may occur anyway.
6. Side-lying delivery minimizes the strain on the perineum and may, if used, reduce incidence of episiotomies.
B. Nursing interventions
1. Apply ice packs to perineal area in first 8 hours to help alleviate pain and swelling.
2. Help promote healing with hot sitz baths.
3. Observe episiotomy site for signs of infection or hematoma.
4. Instruct patient about perineal hygiene.

Forceps Delivery

A. General information
1. Obstetrician's use of special spoon-shaped instruments to effect the delivery of the baby and shorten the second stage of labor
2. Types
  a. Low or outlet: presenting part at vaginal introitus
  b. Mid forceps: presenting part is at or below ischial spines; often a difficult procedure.
  c. High forceps: presenting part above ischial spines. *This procedure has been replaced by cesarean birth.*
3. Requirements for application of forceps
  a. Fully dilated cervix
  b. Presenting part engaged
  c. Vertex or face presentation
  d. Ruptured membranes
  e. No pelvic contractures or disproportions
  f. Bowel and bladder emptied
4. Situations necessitating use
  a. Maternal exhaustion
  b. Fetal distress
  c. Failure of internal rotation
  d. Nerve root anesthesia (patient cannot push)
  e. Maternal heart disease
  f. Poor descent of fetus through birth canal
B. Nursing interventions
1. Anticipate request for forceps if possible.
2. Monitor FHTs continuously.
3. Explain procedure to patient if awake, advise mother/family about possible presence of slight bruising that will go away.

Cesarean Birth

General Information

A. Delivery of the baby through an incision into the abdominal wall and uterus
B. Indications
1. Cephalopelvic disproportion (most frequent reason)
2. Fetal distress
3. Breech presentation, especially in a primipara
4. Placenta previa/placenta abruptio
5. Prolapsed cord
6. Ineffective uterine contractions
7. Maternal diabetes
8. Malpresentations
9. Multiple births
10. Previous cesarean births
11. Other obstetric emergencies and conditions
C. Types
1. Classic: vertical incisions made into both abdomen and uterus
  a. Used when rapid delivery is important, as in fetal distress, prolapsed cord, placenta abruptio
  b. Maternal bleeding greater with this method
2. Low cervical/low segment: transverse incisions made in

abdomen (above pubic hairline) and in uterus

 a. Most common method used

 b. Procedure may take longer than classic because of need to deflect bladder, but blood loss is lessened and adhesions are fewer.

 c. Vaginal birth after this type of cesarean birth is a possibility.

Preoperative

A. Assessment

 1. Maternal/fetal responses to labor

 2. Indications for cesarean birth

 3. Blood and urine test results

B. Analysis: nursing diagnoses for the preoperative phase of cesarean birth may include

 1. Fear

 2. Knowledge deficit

 3. Powerlessness

 4. Disturbance in self-concept

C. Planning and Implementation

 1. Goals

  a. Patient prepared for surgery carefully and competently.

  b. Patient will have procedures explained to her.

 2. Interventions

  a. Shave/prep abdomen and pubic area.

  b. Insert retention catheter into bladder.

  c. Administer preoperative medications as ordered.

  d. Explain all procedures to patient.

  e. Provide emotional support to patient/family as needed.

  f. Complete all preoperative charting responsibilities.

D. Evaluation

 1. Patient adequately prepared for surgery

 2. Patient understands all procedures

Postoperative

A. Assessment

 1. Maternal vital signs

 2. Observation of incision for signs of infection

 3. I&O

 4. Level of consciousness/return of sensation

 5. Fundal firmness and location

 6. Lochia: color, amount, clots, odor

B. Analysis: nursing diagnoses postoperatively for cesarean birth may include

 1. Alteration in comfort: pain

 2. Potential fluid volume deficit

 3. Potential alteration in parenting

C. Planning and Implementation

 1. Goals

  a. Healing will be promoted.

  b. Bonding between mother/couple and baby will be promoted.

  c. No complications will ensue.

 2. Interventions

  a. Implement general postsurgical care (see page **32**),

and general postpartum care (see pages **411–413**).

  b. Assist patient with self-care as needed.

  c. Assist mother with baby care and handling as needed.

  d. Encourage patient to verbalize reaction to all events.

  e. Reinforce any special discharge instructions from physician.

D. Evaluation

 1. Mother and baby tolerated procedures well

 2. No postoperative complications or infection

 3. Maternal/newborn bonding occurring

SAMPLE QUESTIONS

Jane S. is a gravida 1, in the active phase of stage 1 labor. The fetal position is LOA.

5. When Jane's membranes rupture, the nurse should expect to see

 ○ 1. a large amount of bloody fluid

 ○ 2. a moderate amount of clear to straw-colored fluid

 ○ 3. a small amount of greenish fluid

 ○ 4. a small segment of the umbilical cord

6. When Jane's membranes rupture, the nurse's first action should be to

 ○ 1. notify the physician

 ○ 2. measure the amount of fluid

 ○ 3. count the fetal heart rate

 ○ 4. perform a vaginal examination

Mary W.'s baby has just been delivered, and he weighs 9 lb 10 oz. After the delivery, the nurse notices that Mary is chilly and that her fundus has relaxed. She administers the oxytocin that the physician orders.

7. She knows that it has had the expected effect when she

 ○ 1. hears Mary state that she feels warmer now

 ○ 2. sees Mary fall asleep

 ○ 3. hears the baby cry

 ○ 4. feels the uterus become firm

8. Mary had a midline episiotomy performed at delivery. The primary purpose of the episiotomy is to

 ○ 1. allow forceps to be applied

 ○ 2. enlarge the vaginal opening

 ○ 3. eliminate the possibility of lacerations

 ○ 4. eliminate the need for cesarean birth

The Postpartum Period

OVERVIEW

Physical Changes of the Postpartum Period

A. The postpartum period is defined as that period of time, usually six weeks, in which the mother's body experiences anatomic and physiologic changes that reverse the body's adaptation to pregnancy; may also be called *involution*.

B. Begins with the delivery of the placenta and ends when all body systems are returned to, or nearly to, their prepregnant state.

C. May or may not include the return of the ovulatory/menstrual cycle.

Specific Body System Changes

Reproductive System

A. Uterus: a rapid reversal in size
  1. Palpated after delivery below the umbilicus, the uterus regresses approximately 1 fingerbreadth (1 cm) per day until, by the end of the second week postpartum it is a pelvic organ and cannot be palpated through the abdominal wall.
  2. The process is accomplished by cell size reduction.
  3. The endometrial surface is sloughed off as *lochia*, in three stages
      a. *Lochia rubra:* dark red color, days 1–3 after delivery; consists of blood, and cellular debris from decidua.
      b. *Lochia serosa:* pinkish brown, days 4–10; mostly serum, some blood, tissue debris.
      c. *Lochia alba:* yellowish white, days 11–21; mostly leukocytes, with decidua, epithelial cells, mucus.
  4. Lochia has a particular, musty odor. Foul-smelling lochia, however, may indicate infection. Some small clots may be normal immediately after delivery, large clots signify the need for close investigation.
  5. The placental site heals by means of exfoliative shedding, a process that allows the upward growth of the new endometrium and the prevention of scar tissue at the old placental site. This process may take six weeks.

B. Cervix
  1. Flabby immediately after delivery; closes slowly.
  2. Admits one fingertip by the end of one week after delivery.
  3. Shape of external os changed by delivery from round to slitlike opening.

C. Vagina
  1. Edematous after delivery
  2. May have small lacerations
  3. Smooth-walled for 3–4 weeks, then rugae reappear
  4. Hypoestrogenic until ovulation and menstruation resume

D. Ovulation/menstruation
  1. First cycle is usually anovulatory.
  2. If not lactating, menses may resume in 4–6 weeks.
  3. If lactating, menses less predictable; may resume in 12–24 weeks.

E. Breasts
  1. Nonlactating woman
      a. Prolactin levels fall rapidly.
      b. May still secrete colostrum for 2–3 days.
      c. Engorgement of breast tissue resulting from temporary congestion of veins and lymphatic circulation occurs on third day, lasts 24–36 hours, usually resolves spontaneously.
      d. Patient should wear tight bra to compress ducts and use cold applications to reduce swelling.
  2. Lactating woman
      a. High level of prolactin immediately after delivery of placenta continued by frequent contact with nursing baby.
      b. Initial secretion is colostrum, with increasing amounts of true breast milk appearing between 48–96 hours.
      c. Milk "let-down" reflex caused by oxytocin from posterior pituitary released by sucking.
      d. Successful lactation results from the complex interaction of infant sucking reflexes, and maternal production and let-down of milk.

Abdominal Wall/Skin

A. May need six weeks to reestablish good muscle tone.

B. Stretch marks gradually disappear or fade to silvery appearance.

Cardiovascular System

A. Normal blood loss in delivery of single infant is less than

500 cc.

B. Hematocrit usually returns to prepregnancy value within 4–6 weeks.

C. WBC count increases.

D. Increased clotting factors remain for several weeks leaving woman at risk for problems with thrombi.

E. Varicosities regress.

Urinary System

A. May have difficulty voiding in immediate postpartum period as a result of urethral edema.

B. Voiding reflex may be altered.

C. Marked diuresis begins within 12 hours of delivery; increases volume of urinary output as well as perspiration loss.

D. Lactosuria may be seen in nursing mothers

E. Many women will show slight proteinuria during first 1–2 days of involution.

Gastrointestinal System

A. Mother usually hungry after delivery; good appetite is expected.

B. May still experience constipation from lack of muscle tone in abdomen and intestinal tract, and perineal soreness.

Other

All other systems experience normal and rapid regression to prepregnancy status.

POSTPARTAL PSYCHOSOCIAL CHANGES

Adaptation to Parenthood

Motor Skills

New parents must learn new physical skills to care for infant (e.g., feeding, holding, burping, changing diapers, skin care).

Attachment Skills

A. *Bonding:* the development of a caring relationship with the baby. Behaviors include
  1. "Claiming": identifying the ways in which the baby looks or acts like members of the family.
  2. "Identification": establishing the baby's unique nature (assigning the baby his or her own name).
  3. Attachment is facilitated by positive feedback between baby and caregivers.

B. Sensual responses enhance adaptation to parenthood.
  1. Touch: from fingertip, to open palm, to enfolding; touch is an important communication with the baby.
  2. Eye-to-eye contact: a cultural activity that helps to form a trusting relationshsip.
  3. Voice: parents await the baby's first cry; babies respond to the higher-pitched voice that parents use in talking to the baby.
  4. Odor: babies quickly identify their own mother's breast milk by odor.

5. Entrainment: babies move in rhythm to patterns of adult speech.

6. Biorhythm: babies respond to maternal heartbeats.

Maternal Adjustment

Takes place in three phases

Dependent

A. 1–2 days after delivery

B. Mother's needs predominate; mother passive and dependent.

C. Mother needs to talk about labor and delivery experiences to integrate them into the fabric of her life.

D. Mother may need help with everyday activities, as well as child care.

E. Also called "taking-in" phase.

Dependent/Independent

A. By third day mother begins to reassert herself.

B. Identifies own needs, especially for teaching and help with own and baby's needs.

C. Some emotional lability, may cry "for no reason."

D. Mother requires reassurance that she can perform tasks of motherhood.

E. Also called "taking-hold" phase.

Independent

A. Usually evident by fifth or sixth week

B. Shows pattern of life-style that includes new baby but still focuses on entire family as unit.

C. Reestablishment of husband-wife bond seen in this period.

D. Mother may still feel tired and overwhelmed by responsibility and conflicting demands on her time and energies.

E. Also called "letting-go" phase.

ASSESSMENT

Physical

A. Vital signs
  1. Individual protocol until stable, then at least once every 8 hours.
  2. Temperature over 100.4°F (37.8°C) after first 24 hours, lasting more than 48 hours, indicative of infection.

B. Fundus
  1. Should be firm, in midline, slightly below umbilicus immediately after delivery.
  2. After 12 hours should rise to level of umbilicus, or 1 cm above.
  3. Should regress 1 cm/day thereafter until end of second week.
  4. Assessment should always be done with patient's bladder empty.

C. Lochia: color, amount, clots, odor

D. Perineum
  1. Healing of episiotomy

2. Hematoma formation
3. Development of hemorrhoids
E. Breasts: firmness, condition of nipples
F. Elimination patterns: voiding, flatus, bowels
G. Legs: pain, warmth, tenderness indicating thrombosis
H. Perform foot dorsiflexion (Homan's sign).

Psychosocial Adjustment

A. Overall emotional status of parents
B. Parent's knowledge of infant needs
C. Previous experience of parents
D. Physical condition of infant
E. Ethnocultural background and financial status of parents
F. Additional family support available to parents

ANALYSIS

Nursing diagnoses for the postpartum period may include
A. Alteration in bowel elimination: constipation
B. Knowledge deficit
C. Self-care deficit
D. Alteration in pattern of urinary elimination
E. Alteration in family process
F. Potential alteration in parenting
G. Disturbance in self-concept: role performance

PLANNING AND IMPLEMENTATION

Goals

A. Involution and return to prepregnancy state will be accomplished without complication.
B. Parental role(s) will be successfully assumed.
C. New baby will be successfully integrated into family structure.
D. Successful infant feeding patterns (bottle- or breast-feeding) will be established.

Interventions

Physical Care

A. Assess mother according to individual needs during first critical hours after delivery; implement nursing interventions as needed.
B. Implement routine postpartum care after first hours.
  1. Administer medications as ordered (e.g., antilactational, oxytocins, analgesics).
  2. Teach perineal care.
  3. Perform other care as needed (e.g., heat, cold applications).
  4. Measure first voiding for sufficiency, observe I&O for first 24 hours.
  5. Assist with breast-feeding as needed.
C. Encourage measures to promote bowel function: roughage in diet, ambulation, sufficient fluids, attention to urge to defecate. Reassure about integrity of episiotomy.

Adjustment to Parenthood

A. Provide time for parents to be alone with baby in crucial early time after delivery.
B. Identify learning needs of parents.
C. Plan teaching to include both parents where possible.
D. Help parents realize that fatigue is normal at this time.
E. Help parents identify and strengthen their own coping mechanisms.
F. Help parents identify resources available to them.
G. Promote positive self-esteem on part of parents as they learn new role(s).
H. Provide anticipatory guidance for after discharge.
I. Provide information about contraception if requested.
J. Prepare for discharge: reinforce physician's instructions about activities, rest, diet, drugs, exercise, resumption of sexual intercourse, return for postpartum examination.

Infant Feeding

The first year of life is a time of rapid growth and development, necessitating sufficient and appropriate intake of nutrients. The goals of infant nutrition are to provide these nutrients without subjecting the newborn to undue stress.
A. Choices in newborn nutrition
  1. Breast-feeding: also called lactation; provides exact type and distribution of nutrients needed by human newborn in amounts needed.
    a. Initiated by prolactin, which stimulates milk production.
    b. Also affected by oxytocin, which causes "let-down" or delivery of milk to nursing baby.
  2. Formula-feeding (bottle-feeding): utilizes modified cow's milk, goat's milk, or soy formulas as basis for provision of 20 kcal/oz.
    a. Formulas are widely available in ready-to-feed, concentrated, and powdered forms.
    b. They have supplemental vitamins; may also contain added iron.
    c. Concentrated and powdered forms require addition of prescribed amounts of water for appropriate reconstitution.
    d. Sterilization of prepared formulas may be recommended, methods are
      1) terminal heating method: formula and bottles prepared using clean technique; entire batch sterilized at end of preparation
      2) aseptic method: sterile technique and sterile water used to prepare individual bottles and formula
B. Nursing measures to promote successful infant feeding
  1. Assess previous experience and knowledge of process of infant feeding.
  2. Demonstrate how to hold baby for breast-feeding and for feeding with formula.
  3. Show how to burp baby.
  4. Allow time for practice with selected feeding method.
  5. Provide positive reinforcement for successful actions.
  6. Give written instructions for at-home reference.

7. Help parents identify progress and pleasure in feeding infant.
8. If bottle-feeding, demonstrate how to prepare formula using approriate method.
9. If breast-feeding, assess breasts for tenderness or discomfort, and examine nipples for cracks, bleeding, soreness, and erectility.
10. Assist mother with preparation: clean hands, comfortable position, support as needed (extra pillows).
11. Bring infant to nurse as soon as possible after delivery.
12. Demonstrate positioning of baby at breast, initiate rooting reflex, place entire nipple and part of areola into baby's mouth, depress fleshy part of breast away from baby's nose if needed.
13. Allow baby to nurse in short frequent periods: 2–3 minutes first day, lengthening gradually to 10 minutes on each side in later days.
14. Help mother release baby from nipple by breaking suction of baby on nipple.
15. Help mother move baby to alternate breast if needed.
16. Remain with mother at each feeding until she feels confident: see also Table 4.9 for additional information on breast-feeding.
17. Assist bottle-feeding mother with suppression of lactation, accomplished through drug therapy or mechanical inhibition.
    a. Mechanical inhibition: usually takes 48–72 hours
       1) snug breast binder for 2–3 days postdelivery
       2) applications of cold (ice packs) and analgesia to relieve discomfort
       3) avoidance of heat or other stimuli to breasts that increase milk production (including breast pumps)
       4) a well-fitting bra until lactation is suppressed
    b. Medications to suppress lactation
       1) most common drugs used to suppress lactation are hormones (estradiol valerate and chlorotrianisene [TACE], which inhibit the secretion of prolactin. As a major side effect of these estrogenlike hormones is an increased risk of thromboembolism, physicians are increasingly relying on mechanical suppression.
       2) bromocriptin (Parlodel) is a newer agent that acts instead by stimulating the production of prolactin-inhibiting factor, reducing the pituitary's production of prolactin. The usual dose and regimen is
          a) 2.5 mg PO twice daily for 14 days, with the initiation of the medication only after maternal blood pressure has stabilized postdelivery.
          b) administering the medication with food also diminishes any nausea the mother may experience.

EVALUATION

A. Involution successfully initiated and progressing without complication

---

Table 4.9	Tips for Successful Breast-feeding
Breast care	Do not use soap on nipples or areola. Expose nipples to air to toughen them. Know how to pump breast milk if necessary and how to store expressed breast milk.
Nutrition	Need for good maternal nutrition while nursing. ▪ Additional 500 kcal/day ▪ 2–3 liters fluid/day. Know that certain foods may make the baby fussy and will need to be avoided.
Comfort	Wear well-fitting bra; use absorbent pads if leaking occurs. Mild uterine cramping during nursing normal in beginning.
Medications	Avoid medications excreted in breast milk (mother should check with physician before taking any drug while nursing). Birth control pills should not be taken while nursing (decreases milk production).
Sources of help	Inform mother of community support groups available for nursing mothers.

B. Parents begin to assume new role behaviors and identities
C. Beginning integration of newborn into family structure; bonding established
D. Infant feeding techniques mastered; infant growing and developing appropriately
E. Parents comfortable about infant care techniques and can demonstrate knowledge

COMPLICATIONS OF THE POSTPARTUM PERIOD

Postpartum Hemorrhage

A. General Information
   1. A major cause of maternal death
   2. Loss of more than 500 cc blood at the time of delivery or immediately thereafter is considered postpartum hemorrhage.
   3. Major causes include
      a. Uterine atony: loss of muscle tone in the uterus; may be the result of overdistension (large baby, multiple pregnancy, polyhydramnios), overmassage, maternal exhaustion, inhalation anesthesia.
      b. Laceration of the birth canal (cervix, vagina, labia, perineum)
      c. Retained placental fragments or incomplete expulsion of placenta (usually the cause of late postpartum hemorrhage)
      d. Placenta accreta: penetration of the myometrium by the trophoblast, resulting in abnormal adherence of the placenta to the uterine wall. Rare; requires manual removal of the placenta.
B. Assessment findings
   1. "Boggy" uterus, relaxed state indicating atony

2. If uterus is firm with excess bleeding, may indicate lacerations.
3. Dark red blood, with clots
   a. Large amounts with atony
   b. Steady trickle with lacerations
4. Hemorrhage immediately after delivery with atony or lacerations
5. With retained placental fragments, delay of up to two weeks
6. With severe blood loss, signs and symptoms of shock

C. Nursing interventions
1. Identify patients at risk for condition.
2. Monitor fundus frequently if bleeding occurs; when stable, every 15 minutes for 1 hour, then at appropriate intervals.
3. Monitor maternal vitals signs for indications of shock.
4. Administer medications, IV fluids as ordered.
5. Measure I&O.
6. Remain with patient for support and explanation of procedures.
7. Keep patient warm.
8. Prepare for patient's return to delivery room if needed for repair of laceration or removal of placental fragment.
9. Monitor for signs of clotting defects with major loss of blood (see Disseminated Intravascular Coagulation, page 94).

Thrombophlebitis

A. General information
1. Formation of a thrombus when a vein wall is inflamed
2. May be seen in the veins of the legs or pelvis
3. May result from injury, infection, or the normal increase in circulating clotting factors in the pregnant and newly-delivered woman.

B. Assessment findings
1. Pain/discomfort in area of thrombus (legs, pelvis, abdomen)
2. If in the leg, pain, edema, redness over affected area
3. Elevated temperature and chills
4. Peripheral pulses may be decreased
5. Positive Homan's sign
6. If in a deep vein, leg may be cool and pale.

C. Nursing interventions
1. Maintain bedrest, with leg elevated on pillow. *Knee gatch on bed never raised.*
2. Apply moist heat as ordered.
3. Administer analgesics as ordered.
4. Provide bed cradle to keep sheets off leg.
5. Administer anticoagulant therapy as ordered (usually heparin), and observe patient for signs of bleeding.
6. Apply elastic support hose if ordered, with daily inspection of legs with hose removed.
7. Teach patient *not* to massage legs.
8. Allow patient to express fears and reactions to condition.
9. Observe patient for signs of pulmonary embolism.
10. Continue to bring baby to mother for feeding and interaction.

Subinvolution

A. General information
1. Failure of the uterus to revert to prepregnant state through gradual reduction in size and placement
2. May be caused by infection, retained placental fragments, or tumors in the uterus

B. Assessment findings
1. Uterus remains enlarged
2. Fundus higher in the abdomen than anticipated
3. Lochia not progressed from rubra to serosa to alba
4. If caused by infection, possible leukorrhea and backache

C. Nursing interventions
1. Teach patient to recognize unusual bleeding patterns.
2. Teach patient usual pattern of uterine involution.
3. Instruct patient to report abnormal bleeding to physician.
4. Administer oxytocic medications if ordered.

Postpartum Infection

A. General information
1. Any infection of the reproductive tract, associated with giving birth, usually occurring within 10 days of the birth
2. Predisposing factors include
   a. Prolonged rupture of membranes
   b. Cesarean birth
   c. Trauma during birth process
   d. Maternal anemia
   e. Retained placental fragments
3. Infection may be localized or systemic.

B. Assessment findings
1. Temperature of 100.4°F (37.8°C) or more for 2 consecutive days, excluding the first 24 hours
2. Abdominal, perineal, or pelvic pain
3. Foul-smelling vaginal discharge
4. Burning sensation with urination
5. Chills, malaise
6. Rapid pulse and respirations
7. Elevated WBC count (may be normal for postpartum initially), positive culture/sensitivity report for causative organism

C. Nursing interventions
1. Force fluids: patient may need more than 3 liters/day.
2. Administer antibiotics and other medications as ordered.
3. Treat symptoms as they arise (e.g., warm sitz bath for infection in episiotomy).
4. Encourage high-calorie, high-protein diet to promote tissue healing.
5. Position patient in semi- to high-Fowler's to promote drainage and prevent reflux higher into reproductive tract.
6. Support mother if isolated from baby.

Mastitis

A. General information
1. Infection of the breast, usually unilateral
2. Frequently caused by cracked nipples in the nursing mother

3. Causative organism usually hemolytic *S. aureus*
4. If untreated, may result in breast abscess.
B. Assessment findings
   1. Redness, tenderness, or hardened area in the breast
   2. Maternal chills, malaise
   3. Elevated vitals signs, especially temperature and pulse
C. Nursing interventions
   1. Teach/stress importance of handwashing to nursing mother, and wash own hands before touching patient's breast.
   2. Have patient wear well-fitting bra for support.
   3. Administer antibiotics as ordered.
   4. Apply ice if ordered.
   5. Help patient with milk expression on regular basis if nursing is interrupted.

Urinary Tract Infection

A. General information: may be caused postpartally by coliform bacteria, coupled with bladder trauma during the delivery, or a break in technique during catheterization.
B. Assessment findings
   1. Pain in the suprapubic area or at the costovertebral angle
   2. Fever
   3. Burning, urgency, frequency on urination
   4. Increased WBC count and hematuria
   5. Urine culture positive for causative organism
C. Nursing interventions
   1. Check status of bladder frequently in postpartum patient.
   2. Use nursing measures to encourage patient to void.
   3. Force fluids: may need minimum of 3 liters/day.
   4. Catheterize patient if ordered, using sterile technique.
   5. Administer medications as ordered.
   6. Monitor status of progress through continuing lab tests.
   7. Support mother with explanations of interventions.
   8. No need for baby to be separated from mother.

SAMPLE QUESTIONS

Gerry C. and her roommate, Anne B., each delivered a child two days ago. Gerry is breast-feeding; Anne using formula.

9. Which of the following instructions can the nurse give to both mothers?
   o 1. Wear a good, well-supporting bra.
   o 2. Apply warm compresses to breast if too full.
   o 3. Apply cold compresses to breast if too full.
   o 4. Do not apply any soap to your nipples.

10. Because this is Gerry's third child, the nurse should not be surprised if Gerry complains of
   o 1. chest pain.
   o 2. afterbirth cramps.
   o 3. burning on urination.
   o 4. chills.

11. Connie A. delivered a male infant yesterday. While caring for her on her first postpartum day, which of the following behaviors would you expect?
   o 1. Asking specific questions about home care of the infant
   o 2. Concern about when her bowels will move
   o 3. Frequent crying spells for unexplained reasons
   o 4. Acceptance of the nurse's suggestions about personal care

12. Because this is Connie's first child, which of the following goals is most appropriate?
   o 1. Early discharge for mother and baby
   o 2. Rapid adaptation to role of parent
   o 3. Effective education of both parents
   o 4. Minimal need for expression of negative feelings

The Newborn

PHYSIOLOGIC STATUS OF THE NEWBORN

Circulatory

A. Umbilical vein and ductus venosus close immediately after cord is clamped.

B. Foramen ovale closes functionally as respirations are established, but anatomic or permanent closure may take several months.

C. Ductus arteriosus closes with establishment of respiratory function.

D. Heart rate averages 140 beats/minute at birth, with changes noted during sleep and activity.

E. Heart murmurs may be heard; usually have little clinical significance.

F. Average blood pressure is 78/42 mm Hg.

G. Peripheral circulation established slowly; may have mottled (blue/white) appearance for 24 hours.

H. RBC count high immediately after birth, then falls after first week; possible physiologic anemia of infancy.

I. Absence of normal flora in intestine of newborn results in low levels of vitamin K; prophylactic dose of vitamin K given on first day of life.

Respiratory

A. "Thoracic squeeze" in vaginal delivery helps drain fluids from respiratory tract; remainder of fluid absorbed across alveolar membranes into capillaries.

B. Adequate levels of surfactants (lecithin and sphingomyelin) assure mature lung function; prevent alveolar collapse and respiratory distress syndrome.

C. Normal respiratory rate is 30–60 breaths/minute with short periods of apnea; change noted during sleep or activity.

D. Newborns are obligate nose breathers.

E. Chest and abdomen rise simultaneously; no seesaw breathing.

Renal

A. Urine present in bladder at birth, but newborn may not void for first 12–24 hours; later pattern is 6–10 voidings/day, indicative of sufficient fluid intake.

B. Urine is pale and straw colored; initial voidings may leave brick-red spots on diaper from passage of uric acid crystals in urine.

C. Infant unable to concentrate urine for first three months of life.

Digestive

A. Newborn has full cheeks due to well-developed sucking pads.

B. Little saliva is produced.

C. Hard palate should be intact; small raised white areas on palate (Epstein's pearls) are normal.

D. Newborn cannot move food from lips to pharynx; nipple needs to be inserted well into mouth.

E. Circumoral pallor may appear while sucking.

F. Newborn is capable of digesting simple carbohydrates and protein but has difficulty with fats.

G. Immature cardiac sphincter may allow reflux of food when burped; place newborn on right side after feeding to prevent regurgitation.

H. Stomach capacity varies; approximately 50–60 cc.

I. First stool is meconium (black, tarry residue from lower intestine); usually passed within 12–24 hours after birth.

J. Transitional stools are thin, and brownish green in color; after three days, milk stools are usually passed—loose and golden-yellow for the breast-fed infant, formed and pale yellow for the formula-fed infant. Stools may vary in number from 1 every feeding to 1–2/day.

K. Feeding patterns vary; newborn may nurse vigorously immediately after birth, or may need as long as several days to learn to suck effectively. Provide support and encouragement to new mothers during this time as infant feeding is a very emotional area for new mothers.

Hepatic

A. Liver responsible for changing hemoglobin (from breakdown of RBC) into unconjugated bilirubin, which is further changed into conjugated (water-soluble) bilirubin that can be excreted.

B. Excess unconjugated bilirubin can permeate the sclera and the skin, giving a jaundiced or yellow appearance to these tissues.

C. The liver of a mature infant can maintain the level of unconjugated bilirubin at less than 12 mg/dl. Higher levels indicate a possible dysfunction, and the need for intervention.

D. This physiologic jaundice is considered normal in early newborns. It begins to appear after 24 hours, usually between 48–72 hours (see page **422** for additional information on interventions for physiologic jaundice).

Temperature

A. Heat production in newborn accomplished by
   1. Metabolism of "brown fat," a special structure in newborn that is source of heat.
   2. Increased metabolic rate and activity.
B. Newborn cannot shiver as an adult does to release heat.
C. Newborn's body temperature drops quickly after birth; cold stress occurs easily (see page **417** for interventions to prevent heat loss).
D. Body stabilizes temperature in 8–10 hours if unstressed.
E. Cold stress increases oxygen consumption; may lead to metabolic acidosis and respiratory distress.

Immunologic

A. Newborn has passive acquired immunity from IgG from mother during pregnancy and passage of additional antibodies in colostrum and breast milk.
B. Newborn develops own antibodies during first three months, but is at risk for infection during first six weeks.
C. Ability to develop antibodies develops sequentially (see page **288** for typical immunization schedule).

Neurologic/Sensory

Six States of Consciousness

A. Deep sleep
B. Light sleep: some body movements
C. Drowsy: occasional startle; eyes glazed
D. Quiet alert: few movements, but eyes open and bright
E. Active alert: active, occasionally fussy with much facial movement
F. Crying: much activity, eyes open or closed

Periods of Reactivity

A. First (birth through first ½ hour): newborn alert with good sucking reflex
B. Second (4–8 hours after birth): may regurgitate mucus, pass meconium, and again, suck well.

Sleep Cycle

Newborn usually sleeps 17 hours/day.

Hunger Cycle

Varies, depending on mode of feeding.
A. Breast-fed infant may nurse every 2–3 hours.
B. Bottle-fed infant may be fed every 3–4 hours.

Special Senses

A. Sight: eyes are sensitive to light; newborn will fix and gaze at objects, especially those with black and white, regular patterns, but eye movements are uncoordinated.
B. Hearing: can hear before birth (24 weeks); newborn seems best attuned to human speech and its cadences.
C. Taste: sense of taste established; prefers sweet-tasting fluids; derives satisfaction as well as nourishment from sucking.
D. Smell: sense is developed at birth; newborn can identify own mother's breast milk by odor.
E. Touch: newborn is well prepared to receive tactile messages; mother demonstrates touch progression in initial bonding activities.

ASSESSMENT

Physical Examination

A. Weight
   1. Average between 2750 and 3750 gm (6–8¼ lb) at term
   2. Initial loss of 5%–10% of body weight normal during first few days; should be regained in 1–2 weeks
B. Length: average 45.7–55.9 cm (18–22 in)
C. Head circumference: average 31.7–36.8 cm (12½–14½ in); remeasure after several days if significant molding or caput succedaneum present.
D. Chest circumference: average 1.9 cm (¾ in) less than head
E. Skin
   1. Color usually pink; varies with ethnic background.
   2. Pigmentation increases after birth.
   3. Skin may be dry.
   4. Acrocyanosis of hands and feet normal for 24 hours; may develop "newborn rash" (erythema toxicum neonatorum).
   5. Small amounts of lanugo and vernix caseosa still seen.
F. Fontanels
   1. Anterior: diamond shaped
   2. Posterior: triangular
   3. Should be flat and open.
G. Ears
   1. Should be even with canthi of eyes.
   2. Cartilage should be present and firm.
H. Eyes
   1. May be irritated by silver nitrate instillation, some edema/discharge present.
   2. Color is slate blue.
I. Nodule of tissue present in breasts.
J. Female genitalia
   1. Vernix seen between labia.
   2. Blood-tinged mucoid vaginal discharge (pseudomenstruation) from high levels of circulating maternal hormones.
K. Male genitalia
   1. Testes descended or in inguinal canal
   2. Rugae cover scrotum
   3. Meatus at tip of penis
L. Legs

1. Bowed
2. No click or displacement of head of femur observed when hips flexed and abducted

M. Feet
   1. Flat
   2. Soles covered with creases in fully mature infant

N. Muscle tone
   1. Predominantly flexed
   2. Occasional transient tremors of mouth and chin
   3. Newborn can turn head from side to side in prone position.
   4. Needs head supported when held erect or lifted.

O. Reflexes present at birth
   1. Rooting, sucking, and swallowing
   2. Tonic neck, "fencing" attitude
   3. Grasp: newborn's fingers curl around anything placed in palm.
   4. *Moro reflex:* symmetric and bilateral abduction and extension of arms and hands; thumb and forefinger form a C; the "embrace" reflex.
   5. *Startle reflex:* similar to Moro, but with hands clenched.
   6. *Babinski's sign:* flare of toes when foot stroked from base of heel along lateral edge to great toe.

P. Cry
   1. Loud and vigorous
   2. Heard when infant is hungry, disturbed, or uncomfortable.

Apgar Scoring

A. Used to evaluate the newborn in five specific categories at 1 and 5 minutes after birth (see Table 4.7).
B. The 1-minute score reflects transitional values.
C. The composite score at 5 minutes provides the best direction for the planning of newborn care.
D. Composite score interpretations
   1. 0–4: prognosis for newborn is grave.
   2. 5–7: infant needs specialized, intensive care.
   3. 7 or above: infant should do well in normal newborn nursery.

ANALYSIS

Nursing diagnoses for the normal newborn are related to the potential for dysfunction in transition period and first few days of life.

PLANNING AND IMPLEMENTATION

Goals

A. Newborn will adapt to extrauterine life.
   1. Body temperature will be maintained.
   2. Normal breathing and adequate oxygenation will be established.
   3. Cardiovascular function will be stable.
   4. Nutrition and promotion of growth will be established.

B. Positive parent-infant relationship will be established.
C. Potential dysfunctions will be identified early.
D. Needed interventions will be implemented early.

Interventions

Delivery Room

A. Perform Apgar scoring at 1 and 5 minutes after birth.
B. Perform rapid, overall physical and neurologic exam.
   1. Identify obvious congenital anomalies.
   2. Count vessels in cord.
   3. Identify injuries from birth trauma.
C. Prevent heat loss.
   1. Dry infant immediately after birth.
   2. Wrap newborn warmly, cover head, or place in specially warmed area.
   3. Place newborn on warm surfaces (mother's body) or cover cool surfaces (e.g., scale).
   4. Minimize placement of newborn near cooler areas (windows, outside walls).
D. Maintain established respirations and heartbeat.
E. Identify mother and infant with matching bands.
F. Perform cord clamping if physician has not done so.
G. Allow parents to hold infant, or place in warmed area in Trendelenburg's position to facilitate drainage of mucus.
H. Suction gently PRN.
I. Administer oxygen PRN.
J. Promote bonding through early nursing if mother so desires, or by having parents hold newborn.
K. Transfer to nursery at appropriate time.

Nursery

A. Continue actions to prevent heat loss (temperature may be taken rectally or by axilla).
B. When temperature stabilizes, perform complete physical and neurologic exam.
C. Administer medications as ordered.
   1. Silver nitrate: 1–2 drops in each eye in the conjunctival sac to prevent ophthalmia neonatorum
   2. Vitamin K: prophylactic dose
D. Measure and weigh newborn.
E. After temperature has stabilized, bathe and dress newborn, place in open crib.
F. Institute daily care routine.
   1. Take weight.
   2. Monitor temperature, apical pulse, respirations at least every shift.
   3. Suction PRN.
   4. Bathe daily if ordered.
   5. Give diaper area care after each change.
   6. Maintain continued assessment for anomalies.
   7. Give appropriate care to umbilical cord.
   8. Institute feeding schedule as ordered; may offer sterile water before formula is begun.
   9. Note voidings and stools on daily basis.

G. Assess for physiologic jaundice (see also Hyperbilirubinemia, page **422**).
  1. First manifests in the head area (test by depressing skin over bridge of nose) then progresses to chest (depress skin over sternum).
  2. Early feedings promote excretion of bilirubin in urine and stool, diminishing incidence of jaundice.
  3. Prevention of cold stress in newborn diminishes incidence of jaundice.
  4. Loose, greenish stools and green-tinged urine are normal for these infants; advise mother.
  5. These infants need extra fluids to prevent dehydration and replace fluids being excreted.
  6. Advise parents that breast-fed infants may have increased jaundice.
     a. Breast-feeding may be discontinued for 12–24 hours and/or phototherapy used.
     b. Breast-feeding jaundice may occur after newborn goes home.
H. Provide phototherapy if jaundice is noted (see Hyperbilirubinemia, page **422**).
I. Monitor for pathologic jaundice.
  1. Appears at birth or in the first 24 hours.
  2. Bilirubin levels over 12 mg/dl (see Hyperbilirubinemia, page **422**).
J. Male infants may need circumcision care.
  1. Observe for bleeding.
  2. Note first voiding after circumcision.
  3. Clean area appropriately.
  4. Apply dressing if ordered.
K. Perform phenylketonuria (PKU) test before discharge, usually third day of life.
L. Provide teaching and demonstrations as indicated for parents (e.g., feeding, burping, holding, diapering, bathing).

EVALUATION

A. Newborn progress continually observed, normal vital signs for newborn maintained
B. No dysfunctional patterns discerned
C. No congenital anomalies identified
D. Parents comfortable with infant, have initiated bonding
E. Parents comfortable with newborn care
F. All necessary tests carried out at correct time
G. Evidence for continued growth and development at home is positive.

VARIATIONS FROM NORMAL NEWBORN ASSESSMENT FINDINGS

Some variations from the normal assessment findings in the newborn are not indicative of any disorders; others, however, provide information about likely gestational age or the possibility of the existence of a more serious disorder.

Weight

A. Under 2500 gm (5½ lb): small for gestational age (SGA)
B. Over 4100 gm (9 lb): large for gestational age (LGA)

Length

A. Under 45.7 cm (18 in): SGA
B. Over 55.9 cm (22 in): LGA

Head Circumference

A. Under 31.7 (12½ in): microcephaly/SGA
B. Over 36.8 cm (14½ in): hydrocephaly/LGA

Blood Pressure

A. Variation with activity: normal
B. Major difference between upper and lower extremities: possible aortic coarctation

Pulse

A. Persistently under 120: possible heart block
B. Persistently over 170: possible respiratory distress syndrome (see page **424**)

Temperature

A. Elevated: possible dehydration or infection
B. Temperature falls with low environmental temperature, late in cold stress.

Respirations

A. Under 25/minute: possibly result of maternal analgesia
B. Over 60/minute: possible respiratory distress

Skin

A. Milia (blocked sebaceous glands, usually on nose and chin) are essentially normal.
B. "Stork bites"
  1. Capillary hemangiomas above eyebrows and at base of neck under hairline are essentially normal.
  2. Raised capillary hemangiomas on areas other than face or neck are *not* normal findings.
C. Newborn rash (erythema toxicum neonatorum) is normal.
D. Mongolian spots (darkened areas of pigmentation over sacral area and buttocks) are normal and fade in early childhood.
E. Fingernail scratches are normal.
F. Excess lanugo: possible prematurity
G. Vernix
  1. Absent or scarce: possible postmaturity, especially if green tinged
  2. Excess: prematurity

Head

A. Fontanels
  1. Depressed: dehydration

2. Bulging: increased intracranial pressure
B. Hair: coarse or brittle, possible endocrine disorder
C. Scalp: edema present at birth *(caput succedaneum)* from pressure of cervix against presenting part; crosses suture lines; disappears in 3–4 days without intervention.
D. Skull: collection of blood between a skull bone and its periosteum *(cephalhematoma)* from pressure during delivery; does not cross suture line; appears 12–24 hours after delivery; regresses in 3–6 weeks.
E. Eyes
   1. Edema from silver nitrate not uncommon
   2. Strabismus (occasional crossing of eyes) is normal.
F. Ears
   1. Lack of cartilage: possible prematurity
   2. Low placement: possible kidney disorder or Down's syndrome
G. Nose: copious drainage associated with syphilis
H. Mouth
   1. Thrush: appears as white patches in mouth; candida infection passed from mother during passage through birth canal.
   2. Tongue movement and excess salivation: possible esophageal atresia (see page 333).

Neck

Webbing; masses in muscle

Chest

Milky secretion from breasts (witches milk) is result of maternal hormones; self-limiting.

Cord

Fewer than three vessels may indicate congenital anomalies.

Female genitalia

Pseudomenstruation is normal.

Male genitalia

Misplaced urinary meatus
A. *Epispadias:* on upper surface of penis
B. *Hypospadias:* on under surface of penis

Upper extremities

A. Extra fingers
B. Webbed fingers
C. Asymmetric movement: possible trauma or fracture

Lower extremities

A. Extra toes
B. Webbed toes
C. Congenital hip dysplasia
D. Few creases on soles of feet: prematurity

Spine

Tuft of hair: possible occult spina bifida; assess pilonidal area for fistula.

Anus

Lack of meconium after 48 hours may indicate obstruction.

The High-Risk Infant

OVERVIEW

High-risk infants are those whose incidence of illness or death is increased because of prematurity, dysmaturity, postmaturity, physical problems, or birth complications. They are frequently the result of a high-risk pregnancy.

ASSESSMENT

A. History of high-risk pregnancy or other factor possibly affecting fetal development
B. Apgar scores in the delivery room
C. Head-to-toe assessment of the infant (see Assessment of the Normal Newborn, page 416)
D. Determination of gestational age

ANALYSIS

A. Alteration in respiratory function
B. Alteration in nutrition: less than body requirements
C. Potential impairment of skin integrity
D. Alteration in tissue perfusion
E. Potential alteration in parenting
F. Potential for injury

PLANNING AND IMPLEMENTATION

Goals

A. Needs of infant for physical care will be met.
  1. Oxygen: respiratory functioning will be maintained.
  2. Humidity and warmth: temperature will be regulated and cold stress prevented.
  3. Adequate nutrition will be provided.
  4. Tender handling: newborn will receive proper skin care and positioning.
B. Infection or other complications will be prevented.
C. Normal growth and development will be promoted.
D. Needs of parents for closeness with infant will be met; attachment/bonding will be promoted.

Interventions

A. Constantly monitor infant for subtle changes in condition and intervene promptly when necessary.
B. Conserve infant's energy and decrease physiologic stress.
C. Provide appropriate stimulation for infant growth and development.
D. Allow parents to express their reactions and feelings and assist them in attachment behaviors.
E. Teach parents care of infant in preparation for discharge.

EVALUATION

A. Infant's physical condition stabilized and improved on a steady basis
B. Infant's growth and development steady and appropriate
C. Parents demonstrated acceptance of and comfort with infant's condition
D. Parents demonstrated comfort and confidence with infant care at discharge

HIGH-RISK DISORDERS

The Premature Infant

A. General information
  1. Any infant born before the end of the 37th week of pregnancy
  2. Weight usually less than 2500 gm ($5\frac{1}{2}$ lb)
  3. Causes include
     a. Maternal factors: age, smoking, poor nutrition, placental problems, preeclampsia/eclampsia
     b. Fetal factors: multiple pregnancy, infection
     c. Other: socioeconomic status, environmental exposure to harmful substance
  4. Severity of problems related to level of maturity: the earlier the infant is born, the greater the chance of complications.
  5. Major complicating conditions
     a. Respiratory distress syndrome
     b. Thermoregulatory problems
     c. Conservation of energy

d. Infection

e. Hemorrhage

B. Assessment findings

1. Respiratory system

   a. Insufficient surfactant

   b. Apneic episodes

   c. Retractions, nasal flaring, grunting, seesaw pattern of breathing, cyanosis

   d. Increased respiratory rate

2. Thermoregulation: body temperature fluctuates easily (newborn has less subcutaneous fat and muscle mass).

3. Nutritional status

   a. Poor sucking and swallowing reflexes

   b. Poor gag and cough reflexes

4. Skin: lack of subcutaneous fat; reddened; translucent

5. Drainage from umbilicus/eyes

6. Cardiovascular

   a. Petechiae caused by fragile capillaries and prolonged prothrombin time

   b. Increased bleeding at injection sites

7. Neuromuscular

   a. Poor muscle tone

   b. Weak reflexes

   c. Weak, feeble cry

C. Nursing interventions

1. Maintain respirations at less than 60/minute, check every 1–2 hours.

2. Administer oxygen as ordered; check concentration every 2 hours to avoid retrolental fibroplasia while providing adequate oxygenation.

3. Auscultate breath sounds to assess lung expansion.

4. Encourage breathing with gentle rubbing of back and feet.

5. Suction as needed.

6. Reposition every 1–2 hours for maximum lung expansion and prevention of exhaustion.

7. Monitor blood gases and electrolytes.

8. Maintain thermoneutral body temperature; prevent cold stress.

9. Maintain appropriate humidity level.

10. Monitor for signs of infection; these infants have little antibody production and decreased resistance.

11. Feed according to abilities.

12. Monitor sucking reflex; if poor, gavage feeding indicated. Most preterm infants require at least some gavage feeding as it diminishes the effort required for sucking while improving the caloric intake.

13. Use "preemie" nipple if bottle-feeding.

14. Monitor I&O, weight gain or loss; these infants are easily dehydrated, with poor electrolyte balance.

15. Monitor for hypoglycemia and hyperbilirubinemia.

16. Handle carefully; organize care to minimize disturbances.

17. Provide skin care with special attention to cleanliness and careful positioning to prevent breakdown.

18. Monitor heart rate and pattern at least every 1–2 hours; listen apically for 1 full minute.

19. Monitor potential bleeding sites (umbilicus, injection sites, skin); these infants have lowered clotting factors.

20. Monitor overall growth and development of infant; check weight, length, head circumference.

21. Provide tactile stimulation when caring for or feeding infant.

22. Provide complete explanations for parents.

23. Encourage parental involvement in infant's care.

24. Provide support for parents; refer to self-help group of other parents if necessary.

25. Promote parental confidence with infant care before discharge.

The Dysmature Infant (SGA)

A. General information

1. Birth weight in the lowest 10th percentile at term

2. Causes: discounting heredity, possibly intrauterine growth retardation, infections, malformations

B. Assessment findings

1. Skin: loose and dry, little fat, little muscle mass

2. Small body makes skull look larger than normal

3. Sunken abdomen

4. Thin, dry umbilical cord

5. Little scalp hair

6. Wide skull sutures

7. Respiratory distress; may have had hypoxic episodes in utero

8. Hypoglycemia

9. Tremors

10. Weak cry

11. Lethargic

12. Cool to touch

C. Nursing interventions

1. Care of SGA infant is similar in many instances to care of preterm infant.

2. Tailor high-level nursing care to meet specific needs of infant with regard to functioning of all body systems, psychologic growth and development, parental support and teaching, and prevention of complications.

The Postmature Infant

A. General information

1. Born after the completion of 42 weeks of pregnancy

2. Problems caused by progressively less efficient actions of placenta

B. Assessment findings

1. Skin

   a. Vernix and lanugo completely disappeared

   b. Dry, cracked, parchmentlike appearance to skin

   c. Color: yellow to green from meconium staining

2. Depleted subcutaneous fat; old looking

3. Hard nails extending beyond fingertips

4. Signs of birth injury or poor tolerance of birth process

C. Nursing interventions

1. Nursing care of the postmature infant has many characteristics in common with the care given to the premature infant.

2. Design high-level nursing care to identify the infant's

specific physical and psychologic needs; monitor functioning of all body systems, growth and development, parental support and teaching, and prevention of complications.

SPECIAL CONDITIONS IN THE NEONATE

Hyperbilirubinemia

A. General information
1. Elevated serum level of bilirubin in the newborn results in jaundice, or yellow color of body tissues.
2. In physiologic jaundice, average increase from 2 mg/dl in cord blood to 6 mg/dl by 72 hours; not exceeding 12 mg/dl
3. Level at which a newborn will sustain damage to body cells (especially brain cells) from high concentrations of bilirubin is termed pathologic.
4. May result from immaturity of liver, Rh or ABO incompatibility, infection, birth trauma with subsequent bleeding (cephalhematoma), maternal diabetes, hypothermia, medications.
5. Breast milk hormone, pregnanedial, is also thought to contribute to hyperbilirubinemia by inhibiting the conjugation of bilirubin.
6. Major complication is *kernicterus* (brain damage caused by high levels of unconjugated bilirubin).
B. Assessment findings
1. Pathologic jaundice usually appears early, up to 24 hours after birth; represents a process ongoing before birth.
2. Usual pattern of progression is from head to feet. Blanch skin over bony area or look at conjunctiva and buccal membranes in dark-skinned infants.
3. Pallor
4. Dark, concentrated urine
5. Behavior changes (irritability, lethargy)
6. Polycythemia
7. Increased serum bilirubin (direct, indirect, and total) ·
C. Nursing interventions
1. Identify conditions predisposing to hyperbilirubinemia.
2. Prevent progression or complications of jaundice.
3. Assess jaundice levels (visually, lab tests) as needed.
4. Prevent conditions which contribute to development of hyperbilirubinemia (e.g., cold stress, hypoxia, acidosis, hypoglycemia, dehydration, infection).
5. Provide adequate hydration.
6. Implement phototherapy if ordered; exposure of newborn to phototherapy helps to increase conjugation of bilirubin and prevent pathologic levels of bilirubin from developing.
    a. Unclothe infant for maximum skin exposure to light, diaper minimally.
    b. Cover eyes to prevent retinal damage.
    c. Change infant's position every 2 hours for maximum exposure.
    d. Monitor temperature carefully.
    e. Remove from phototherapy for feeding; hold infant to provide human contact.
    f. Provide extra fluids to help excrete bilirubin.

g. Observe skin for signs of irritation.
h. Record phototherapy time.
7. Explain all tests and procedures to parents.
8. Assist with exchange transfusion if ordered.
    a. Keep infant warm and restrained.
    b. Check blood for correct identification, age, and temperature.
    c. Have oxygen and suction equipment available.
    d. Aspirate infant's stomach to prevent vomiting and aspiration.
    e. Obtain baseline vital signs; repeat every 15 minutes throughout procedure.
    f. Monitor amount of transfused blood given via umbilical catheter and time of procedure.
    g. Monitor infant post-transfusion.
        1) assess for bleeding, cold stress, any irregular behavior.
        2) check vital signs.
    h. Keep umbilical cord moist in event of need for further transfusions.
9. Support parents with information on procedures.

Hemolytic Disease of the Newborn (Erythroblastosis Fetalis)

A. General information
1. Characterized by RBC destruction in the newborn, with resultant anemia and hyperbilirubinemia
2. Possibly caused by Rh or ABO incompatibility between the mother and the fetus (antigen/antibody reaction)
3. Mechanisms of Rh incompatibility
    a. Sensitization of Rh-negative woman by transfusion of Rh-positive blood
    b. Sensitization of Rh-negative woman by presence of Rh-positive RBCs from her fetus conceived with Rh-positive man
    c. Approximately 65% of infants conceived by this combination of parents will be Rh positive.
    d. Mother is sensitized by passage of fetal Rh-positive RBCs through placenta, either during pregnancy (break/leak in membrane) or at the time of separation of the placenta after delivery.
    e. This stimulates the mother's immune response system to produce anti-Rh-positive antibodies that attack fetal RBCs and cause hemolysis.
    f. If this sensitization occurs during pregnancy, the fetus is affected in utero; if sensitization occurs at the time of delivery, subsequent pregnancies may be affected.
4. ABO incompatibility
    a. Same underlying mechanism
    b. Mother is blood type O; infant is A, B, or AB.
    c. Reaction in ABO incompatibility is less severe.
B. Rh incompatibility
1. First pregnancy rarely affected
2. Indirect Coombs' test (tests for anti-Rh-positive antibodies in mother's circulation) performed during pregnancy
3. If positive, levels are titrated to determine extent of

maternal sensitization and potential effect on fetus.

4. Direct Coombs' test done on cord blood at delivery to determine presence of anti-Rh-positive antibodies on fetal RBCs.

5. If both indirect and direct Coombs' tests are negative (no formation of anti-Rh-positive antibodies) and infant is Rh positive, then Rh-negative mother can be given Rhogam (Rho[D] human immune globulin) to prevent development of anti-Rh-positive antibodies as the result of sensitization from present (just-terminated) pregnancy.

6. With each pregnancy with a Rh-negative mother and Rh-positive infant and negative direct and indirect Coombs' tests, mother can receive Rhogam to protect future pregnancies.

7. If mother has been sensitized (produced anti-Rh-positive antibodies) Rhogam is not indicated.

8. Rhogam must be injected into unsensitized mother's system within 72 hours of delivery of Rh-positive infant.

C. ABO incompatibility
1. Reaction less severe than with Rh incompatibility
2. First born may be affected because type O mother may have anti-A and anti-B antibodies even before pregnancy.
3. Fetal RBCs with A, B, or AB antigens evoke less severe reaction on part of mother, thus fewer anti-A, anti-B, or anti-AB antibodies are produced.
4. Clinical manifestations of ABO incompatibility are milder and of shorter duration than those of Rh incompatibility.
5. Care must be taken to observe for hemolysis and jaundice.

D. Assessment findings
1. Jaundice and pallor within first 24–36 hours
2. Anemia
3. Erythropoiesis
4. Enlarged placenta
5. Edema and ascites

E. Nursing interventions
1. Determine blood type and Rh early in pregnancy.
2. Determine results of indirect Coombs' test early in pregnancy and again at 28–32 weeks.
3. Determine results of direct Coombs' test on cord blood (type and Rh, hemoglobin and hematocrit).
4. Administer Rhogam IM to mother as ordered.
5. Monitor carefully infants of Rh-negative mothers for jaundice.
6. Implement phototherapy/exchange transfusion for any hyperbilirubinemia (see above).
7. Support parents with explanations and information.

Neonatal Sepsis

A. General information
1. Associated with the presence of pathogenic microorganisms in the blood, especially gram-negative organisms *(E. coli, Aerobacter, Proteus,* and *Klebsiella),* and gram-positive group B beta-hemolytic streptococci.
2. Contributing factors
   a. Prolonged rupture of membranes (more than 24 hours)
   b. Prolonged or difficult labor

c. Maternal infection
d. Infection in hospital personnel
e. Aspiration at birth or later

B. Assessment findings
1. Behavioral changes: lethargy, irritability, poor feeding
2. Frequent periods of apnea
3. Jaundice
4. Low-grade fever
5. Vomiting, diarrhea

C. Nursing interventions
1. Perform cultures as indicated/ordered.
2. Administer antibiotics as ordered.
3. Prevent heat loss.
4. Administer oxygen as indicated.
5. Maintain hydration.
6. Monitor vital signs (temperature, pulse, respirations) frequently.
7. Weigh daily.
8. Stroke back and feet gently to stimulate breathing if infant is apneic.
9. Promote parental attachment and involvement in newborn care.

Hypoglycemia

A. General information
1. Less-than-normal amount of glucose in the blood of the neonate
2. Seen in infants born to diabetic mothers (IDM)
3. These infants are usually LGA (macrosomic) due to high maternal glucose levels that have crossed placenta, stimulating the fetal pancreas to secrete more insulin, which then acts as a growth hormone.
4. At birth, with loss of supply of maternal glucose, newborn may be hypoglycemic.
5. Large size may have caused traumatic vaginal birth, or may have necessitated cesarean birth.
6. Hypoglycemia can also occur in infants who are full term, SGA, post-term, septic, or with any condition that subjects the infant to stress.

B. Assessment findings
1. May be born after 36th week of pregnancy
2. Although LGA, IDMs may be immature/dysmature
3. Higher incidence of congenital anomalies in IDMs
4. General appearance
   a. Puffy body
   b. Enlarged organs
5. Tremors, feeding difficulty, irregular respirations
6. Hypocalcemia and hyperbilirubinemia
7. Respiratory distress
8. Blood glucose levels below 45 mg/dl (20 mg/dl in premature infant) using Dextritix

C. Nursing interventions
1. Provide high-level nursing care similar to that for premature/dysmature infant.

2. Assess blood glucose level at frequent intervals, beginning $\frac{1}{2}$–1 hour after birth.
3. Feed hypoglycemic infant according to nursery protocol (usually glucose water) if suck/swallow reflex present and coordinated.
4. In absence of suck/swallow reflex or if uncoordinated administer IV glucose.

Infant Born to Addicted Mother

A. General information
   1. Substance may be alcohol, heroin, morphine, or any other addictive drug
   2. Mother usually seeks prenatal care only when labor begins, and has frequently taken a dose of addictive substance before seeking help, delaying withdrawal symptoms 12–24 hours.
   3. Withdrawal symptoms in the neonate may be noticed within 24 hours.
B. Assessment findings
   1. Infants born to alcohol-abusing mothers will have facial anomalies, fine-motor dysfunction, genital abnormalities (especially females), and cardiac defects; may be SGA (also called the *fetal alcohol syndrome*).
   2. Hyperirritability and hyperactivity
   3. High-pitched cry common
   4. Respiratory distress, tachypnea, excessive secretions
   5. Vomiting and diarrhea
   6. Elevated temperature
   7. Other signs of withdrawal: sneezing; sweating; yawning; short, nonquiet sleep; frantic sucking
C. Nursing interventions
   1. Reduce external stimuli.
   2. Handle minimally.
   3. Swaddle infant and hold close when handling.
   4. Monitor infant's vital signs.
   5. Suction/resuscitate as required.
   6. Feed frequently, with small amounts.
   7. Measure I&O.
   8. Provide careful skin care.
   9. Administer medications if ordered (may use phenobarbital or paregoric).
   10. Involve parents in care if possible.
   11. Inform parents of infant's condition/progress.

Respiratory Distress Syndrome (RDS)

A. General information
   1. Symptoms (found almost exclusively in the preterm infant) indicate formation of a hyaline membrane in the alveoli of the lungs, causing atelectasis; also known as Hyaline Membrane Disease (HMD).
   2. Deficiency of surfactant (L/S) is implicated in the condition, but underlying cause still unknown.
   3. When premature labor cannot be arrested, betamethasone may be administered to enhance surfactant.
   4. Additional factors: hypoxia, hypothermia, acidosis
   5. Sequelae of RDS may include
      a. Hyperbilirubinemia (see page **422**)

   b. Retrolental fibroplasia: retinal changes, visual impairment and eventually blindness, resulting from too-high oxygen levels during treatment
   c. Bronchopulmonary dysplasia (BPD): damage to the alveolar epithelium of the lungs related to high oxygen concentrations and positive pressure ventilation. May be difficult to wean infant from ventilator, but most recover and have normal x-rays at 6 months to 2 years.
   d. Necrotizing enterocolitis (below).
B. Assessment findings
   1. Respiratory rate of over 60/minute
   2. Retractions, grunting, cyanosis, nasal flaring, chin lag
   3. Increased apical pulse
   4. Hypothermia
   5. Decreased activity level
   6. Elevated levels of carbon dioxide
   7. Metabolic acidosis
   8. X-rays show atelectasis and formation of hyaline membrane in alveoli.
C. Nursing interventions
   1. Maintain infant's body temperature at 97.6°F (36.2°C).
   2. Provide sufficient caloric intake for size, age, and prevention of catabolism (usually IV glucose with gradual increase in feedings); nasogastric tube may be used.
   3. Organize care for minimal handling of infant.
   4. Administer oxygen therapy as ordered.
      a. Monitor oxygen concentration every 2–4 hours; maintain less than 40% concentration if possible.
      b. Oxygen may be administered by hood, nasal prongs, intubation, or mask.
      c. Oxygen may be at atmospheric or increased pressure.
      d. Continuous positive air pressure (CPAP) or positive end-expiratory pressure (PEEP) may be used.
      e. Oxygen should be warmed and humidified.
   5. Monitor infant's blood gases.
   6. If intubated, suction (for less than 5 seconds) PRN using sterile catheter.
   7. Auscultate breath sounds.
   8. Provide chest physiotherapy, postural drainage, and percussion if ordered.
   9. Encourage parental involvement in care (visiting, stroking infant, talking).
   10. Keep parents informed of infant's progress.

Necrotizing Enterocolitis (NEC)

A. General information
   1. An ischemic attack to the intestine resulting in thrombosis and infarction of affected bowel, mucosal ulcerations, pseudomembrane formation, and inflammation
   2. Bacterial action *(E. Coli, Klebsiella)* complicates the process, producing sepsis.
   3. May be precipitated by any event in which blood is shunted away from the intestine to the heart and brain (e.g., fetal distress, low Apgar score, RDS, prematurity, neonatal shock, and asphyxia).
   4. Average age at onset is 4 days.

4. Now that severely ill infants are surviving, NEC is encountered more frequently.
5. May ultimately cause bowel perforation and death.

B. Medical management
  1. Parenteral antibiotics
  2. Gastric decompression
  3. Correction of acidosis and fluid electrolyte imbalances
  4. Surgical removal of the diseased intestine

C. Assessment findings
  1. History indicating high-risk group
  2. Findings related to sepsis
     a. Temperature instability
     b. Apnea, labored respirations
     c. Cardiovascular collapse
     d. Lethargy or irritability
  3. Gastrointestinal symptoms
     a. Abdominal distention and tenderness
     b. Vomiting or increased gastric residual
     c. Poor feeding
     d. Hematest positive stools
     e. X-rays showing air in the bowel wall, adynamic ileus and bowel wall thickening

D. Nursing interventions
  1. Carefully assess infants at risk for early recognition of symptoms.
  2. Discontinue oral feedings, insert nasogastric tube.
  3. Prevent trauma to abdomen by avoiding diapers and planning care for minimal handling.
  4. Maintain acid-base balance by adminstering fluids and electrolytes as ordered.
  5. Administer antibiotics as ordered.
  6. Stroke infant's hands and head and talk to infant as much as possible.
  7. Provide visual and auditory stimulation.
  8. Inform parents of progress and support them in expressing their fears and concerns.

Phenylketonuria (PKU)

A. General information
  1. Inability to metabolize phenylalanine to tyrosine because of an autosomal recessive inherited disorder causing an inborn error of metabolism
  2. Phenylalanine is a composite of almost all proteins; **the danger to the infant is immediate.**
  3. High levels of phenylketones affect brain cells, causing mental retardation.
  4. Initial screening for diagnosis of PKU is made via the Guthrie test, done after the infant has ingested protein for a minimum of 24 hours.
  5. Secondary screening
     a. Done when the infant is about 6 weeks old.
     b. Tests fresh urine with a Phenistix, which changes color.
     c. Parents send in a prepared sheet marking the color.
  6. These tests, mandatory in many states, allow the early diagnosis of the disorder, and dietary interventions to minimize or prevent complications.

B. Assessment findings
  1. Phenylalanine levels greater than 8 mg/dl are diagnostic for PKU.
  2. Newborn appears normal; may be fair with decreased pigmentation.
  3. Untreated PKU can result in failure to thrive, vomiting and eczema; by about 6 months, signs of brain involvement appear.

C. Nursing interventions
  1. Restrict protein intake.
  2. Substitute a low-phenylalanine formula (Lofenalac) for either mother's milk or formula.
  3. Provide special food lists for parents.

SAMPLE QUESTIONS

Baby girl J. was born at 9:15 A.M. At 9:20 A.M. her heart rate was 132 beats/minute, she was crying vigorously, moving all extremities, and only her hands and feet were still slightly blue.

13. The nurse should enter her Apgar score as
    o 1. 7
    o 2. 8
    o 3. 9
    o 4. 10

14. Which of the following findings in Baby girl J. does NOT indicate pathology?
    o 1. Passage of meconium within the first 24 hours
    o 2. Respiratory rate of 70/minute at rest
    o 3. Yellow skin tones at 12 hours of age
    o 4. Bleeding from umbilicus

15. Which nursing action should be included in the care of the infant with a caput succedaneum?
    o 1. Aspiration of the trapped blood under the periosteum
    o 2. Explanation to the parents about the cause/prognosis
    o 3. Gentle rubbing in a circular motion to decrease size
    o 4. Application of cold to reduce size

16. In differentiating physiologic jaundice from pathologic jaundice, which of the following facts is most important?
    o 1. Mother is 37 years of age.
    o 2. Infant is a term newborn.
    o 3. Unconjugated bilirubin level is 6 mg/dl on third day.
    o 4. Appears at 22 hours after birth.

Gynecologic Conditions

FERTILITY AND INFERTILITY

Infertility

General Information

A. Inability to conceive after at least one year of unprotected sexual relations

B. Inability to deliver a live infant after three consecutive pregnancies

C. For the male, inability to impregnate a female partner within the same conditions

D. May be primary (never been pregnant/never impregnated) or secondary (pregnant once, then unable to conceive or carry again)

E. Affects approximately 10%–15% of all couples.

F. Tests for infertility

   1. For the female

      a. Examination of basal body temperature and cervical mucus and identification of time of ovulation

      b. Plasma progesterone level: assesses corpus luteum

      c. Hormone analysis: endocrine function

      d. Endometrial biopsy: receptivity of endometrium

      e. Postcoital test: sperm placement and cervical mucus

      f. Hysterosalpingography: tubal patency/uterine cavity

      g. Rubin's test: tubal patency (uses carbon dioxide)

      h. Pelvic ultrasound: visualization of pelvic tissues

      i. Laparoscopy: visual assessment of pelvic/abdominal organs; performance of minor surgeries

   2. For the male

      a. Sperm analysis: assesses composition, volume, motility, agglutination.

      b. There are fewer assessment tests as well as interventions and successes for male infertility.

Medical Management

A. Infertility of female partner, causes and therapy

   1. Congenital anomalies (absence of organs, improperly formed or abnormal organs): surgical treatment may help in some situations, but cannot replace absent structures.

   2. Irregular/absent ovulation (ovum released irregularly or not at all): endocrine therapy with clomiphene citrate (Clomid)/menotropins (Pergonal) may induce ovulation; risk of ovarian hyperstimulation and release of multiple ova.

   3. Tubal factors (fallopian tubes blocked or scarred from infection, surgery, endometriosis, neoplasms): treatment may include antibiotic therapy, surgery, hysterosalpingogram.

   4. Uterine conditions (endometrium unreceptive, infected): removal of an IUD, antibiotic therapy, or surgery may be helpful.

   5. Vaginal/cervical factors (hostile mucus, sperm allergies, altered Ph due to infection): treatment with antibiotics, proper vaginal hygiene, or artificial insemination may be utilized.

B. Infertility of male partner, causes and therapy

   1. Impotence: may be helped by psychologic counseling/penile implants.

   2. Low/abnormal sperm count (fewer than 20 million/ml semen, low motility, more than 40% abnormal forms): there is no good therapy, use of hormone replacement therapy has had little success.

   3. Varicocele (varicosity within spermatic cord): ligation may be successful.

   4. Infection in any area of the male reproductive system (may affect ability to impregnate): appropriate antibiotic therapy is advised.

   5. Social habits (use of nicotine, alcohol, other drugs; clothes that keep scrotal sac too close to warmth of body): changing these habits may reverse low/absent fertility.

C. Alternatives for infertile couples include

   1. Artificial insemination by husband or donor

   2. In vitro fertilization

   3. Adoption

   4. Surrogate parenting

   5. Embryo transfers

D. Accepting childlessness as a life-style may also be necessary; support groups (e.g., Resolve) may be helpful.

Nursing Interventions

A. Assist with assessment including a complete history, physical exam, lab work and tests for both partners.

B. Monitor psychologic reaction to infertility.
C. Support couple through procedures and tests.
D. Identify any existing abnormalities and provide couple with information about their condition(s).
E. Help couple acknowledge and express their feelings both separately and together.

Control of Fertility

Voluntary prevention of conception through various means, some of which employ devices or medications.

Methods of Conception Control

A. Natural methods
   1. Rhythm
      a. Periodic abstinence from intercourse when ovulating
      b. Uses calculations intended to identify those days of the menstrual cycle when coitus is avoided.
         1) basal body temperature: identification of temperature drop before ovulation, then rise past ovulation; identifies days on which coitus is avoided to avoid conception.
         2) cervical mucus method: identification of changes in cervical mucus; when affected by estrogen and most conducive to penetration by sperm, cervical mucus is clear, stretchy, and slippery; when influenced by progesterone, cervical mucus is thick, cloudy, and sticky and does not allow sperm passage; coitus is avoided during days of estrogen-influenced mucus.
         3) sympto-thermal: combination of basal body temperature and cervical mucus method to increase effectiveness
   2. Coitus interruptus
      a. Withdrawal of the penis from the vagina before ejaculation
      b. Not very safe; pre-ejaculatory fluids from Cowper's glands may contain live, motile sperm.
      c. Demands precise male control.
B. Chemical barriers
   1. Use of foams, creams, jellies, and vaginal suppositories designed to destroy the sperm or limit their motility
   2. Available without a prescription, widely used, especially in conjunction with the diaphragm and the condom
   3. Need to be placed in the vagina before each act of intercourse
   4. Some people may have allergic reaction to the chemicals.
C. Mechanical barriers: diaphragm and condom
   1. Diaphragm: shallow rubber dome fits over cervix, blocking passage of sperm through cervix
      a. Efficiency increased by use of chemical barrier as lubricant
      b. Woman needs to be measured for diaphragm, and refitted after childbirth or weight gain/loss of 10 lb.
      c. Device needs to be left in place 6–8 hours after intercourse.
      d. Woman needs to practice insertion and removal, and to be taught how to check for holes in diaphragm.
   2. Condom: thin stretchable rubber sheath worn over penis during intercourse
      a. Widely available without prescription
      b. Applied with room at tip to accommodate ejaculate
      c. Applied to erect penis before vaginal penetration
      d. Man is instructed to hold on to rim of condom as he withdraws from female to prevent spilling semen.
D. Hormone therapy (oral contraceptives, birth control pills)
   1. Ingestion of estrogen and progesterone on a specific schedule to prevent the release of FSH and LH, thus preventing ovulation and pregnancy
   2. Causes additional tubal, endometrial, and cervical mucus changes.
   3. Available in combined or sequential types
   4. Usually taken beginning on day 5 of the menstrual cycle through day 25, then discontinued
   5. Withdrawal bleeding occurs within 2–3 days.
   6. Contraindications
      a. History of hypertension or vascular disorders
      b. Age over 30
      c. Cigarette smoking
   7. Women using oral contraceptives need to be sure to get sufficient amounts of vitamin B as metabolism of this vitamin is affected.
   8. Minor side effects may include
      a. Weight gain
      b. Breast changes
      c. Headaches
      d. Vaginal spotting
   9. *Report visual changes/disorders immediately.*
E. Intrauterine devices
   1. Placement of plastic or nonreactive device into uterine cavity
   2. Mode of action thought to be the creation of a sterile endometrial inflammation, discourages implantation (nidation).
   3. Does not affect ovulation or conception.
   4. Device is inserted during or just after menstruation, while cervix is slightly open.
   5. May cause cramping and heavy bleeding during menses for several months after insertion.
   6. Tail of IUD hangs into vagina through cervix; woman taught to feel for it before intercourse and after each menses.
   7. A distinct disadvantage is the increased risk of pelvic infection (PID) with use of the IUD.
F. Surgical sterilization
   1. Bilateral tubal ligation in the female to prevent the passage of ova
   2. Bilateral vasectomy in the male to prevent the passage of sperm
   3. Both of these operations should be considered permanent.
   4. Female will still menstruate, but will not conceive.
   5. Male will be incapable of fertilizing his partner after all viable sperm ejaculated from vas deferens (6 weeks or 10 ejaculations).

6. There should be no effect on male capacity for erection or penetration.
7. Hysterectomy also causes permanent sterility in the female.

Nursing Responsibilities in Control of Fertility

A. Assess previous experience of couple or individual.
B. Obtain health history and perform physical examination.
C. Identify present needs for contraception.
D. Determine motivation regarding contraception.
E. Assist the patient/couple in receiving information desired; advise about the various methods available.
F. Assure that patient/couple selects method best suited to their needs.
   1. Support choice of patient/couple as right for them.
   2. Provide time for practice with method chosen, if applicable.
   3. Instruct in side effects/potential complications.
G. Encourage expression of feelings about contraception.

Termination of Pregnancy

General Information

A. Deliberate interruption of a pregnancy in a previable time. Legal in all states since Supreme Court ruling of January 1973, as follows
   1. First trimester: determined by pregnant woman and her physician
   2. Second trimester: determined by pregnant woman and her physician; state can regulate the circumstances to ensure safety.
   3. Third trimester: conditions determined by state law
B. Indications may be physical or psychologic, socioeconomic or genetic.
C. Techniques vary according to trimester.
   1. First trimester: *vacuum extraction* or *dilatation and curettage (D&C)*
      a. Cervix dilated
      b. Products of conception either aspirated or scraped out
      c. Procedure is short, usually well tolerated by patient, and has few complications.
   2. Second trimester
      a. *Saline abortion*
         1) amniotic fluid aspirated from uterus, replaced with same amount 20% saline solution.
         2) contractions begin in 12–24 hours; may be induced by oxytocin (Pitocin).
         3) patient is hospitalized; infection or hypernatremia possible complications.
      b. *Prostaglandins*
         1) injection of prostaglandin into uterus
         2) contractions initiated in under 1 hour
         3) side effects may include nausea and vomiting.
      c. *Hysterotomy*
         1) incision into uterus to remove fetus
         2) may also be used for sterilization.
         3) patient is hospitalized.
         4) care is similar to that for cesarean birth.

3. Third trimester: same as second trimester, if permitted by state law.

Assessment

A. Vaginal bleeding
B. Vital signs
C. Excessive cramping

Analysis

A. Potential fluid volume deficit
B. Potential for injury
C. Potential disturbance in self-concept
D. Knowledge deficit

Planning and Implementation

A. Goals
   1. Recovery from procedure will be free from complications.
   2. Patient will be supported in her decision.
B. Interventions
   1. Explain procedure to patient.
   2. Administer medications as ordered.
   3. Assist with procedure as needed.
   4. Monitor patient carefully during procedure.
   5. Monitor patient postprocedure.
   6. Administer postprocedure medications as ordered (analgesics, antibiotics, oxytocins, Rhogam if mother Rh negative).
   7. Provide contraceptive information as appropriate.

Evaluation

A. Procedure tolerated without complications; vital signs stable, no hemorrhage, products of conception evacuated
B. Patient supported through procedure; emotionally stable

MENSTRUAL DISORDERS

Menstruation is the periodic shedding of the endometrium when there has been no conception. Onset is menarche (age 11–14); cessation is menopause (average age 50).

Assessment

A. Menstrual cycle for symptoms and pattern
B. Patient discomfort with cycles
C. Knowledge base about menses

Analysis

A. Knowledge deficit
B. Alteration in health maintenance
C. Disturbance in self-concept

Planning and Implementation

A. Goals
   1. Patient will receive necessary information.

2. Patient will choose treatment/options best suited to her needs.
B. Interventions
   1. Explain menstrual physiology to patient.
   2. Explain options for treatment to patient.
   3. Provide time for questions.
   4. Reinforce good menstrual hygiene.
   5. Administer medications if ordered.

Evaluation

A. Patient demonstrates knowledge of condition and treatment options.

Specific Disorders

Dysmenorrhea

A. Pain associated with menstruation
B. Usually associated with ovulatory cycles; absent when ovulation suppressed
C. Intensified by stress, cultural factors, and presence of an IUD
D. High levels of prostaglandins found in menstrual flow of women with dysmenorrhea.
E. Treatment may include rest, application of heat, distraction, exercise, analgesia.

Amenorrhea

A. Absence of menstruation
B. Possibly caused by underlying abnormality of endocrine system, stress, rapid weight loss, or strenuous exercise.
C. Treatment is individualized by cause.

Menorrhagia

A. Excessive menstrual flow
B. Possibly caused by endocrine imbalance, uterine tumors, infection
C. Treatment individualized by cause

Metrorrhagia

A. Intercyclic bleeding
B. Frequently the result of a disease process
C. Treatment individualized by cause

Endometriosis

A. Endometrial tissue is found outside the uterus, attached to the ovaries, colon, round ligaments, etc.
B. This tissue reacts to the endocrine stimulation cycle as does the intrauterine endometrium, resulting in inflammation of the extrauterine sites, with pain and fibrosis/scar tissue formation as the eventual result.
C. Actual cause is unknown.
D. May cause dysmenorrhea, dyspareunia, and infertility.
E. Treatment may include the use of oral contraceptives to minimize endometrial buildup or danazol (Danocrine) to suppress menstruation.

F. Pregnancy and lactation may also be recommended as means to suppress menstruation.
G. Surgical intervention (removal of endometrial implants) may be helpful.
H. Hysterectomy and salpingo-oophorectomy are curative.

INFECTIOUS DISORDERS

Sexually Transmitted Diseases (STD)

Infections occurring predominantly in the genital area, and spread by sexual relations.

Assessment

A. Sexual history
B. Physical examination for signs and symptoms of specific disorder

Analysis

A. Knowledge deficit
B. Potential for injury
C. Alteration in health maintenance

Planning and Implementation

A. Goals
   1. Disease process will be identified and treated.
   2. Affected others will be identified and treated.
   3. Complications will be prevented.
B. Interventions
   1. Collect specimens for tests.
   2. Implement isolation technique if indicated.
   3. Teach transmission/prevention techniques.
   4. Assist in case finding.
   5. Administer medications as ordered.
   6. Inform patient of any necessary life-style changes.

Evaluation

A. Patient receiving treatment appropriate to specific disorder, understands treatment regimen.
B. Patient demonstrates knowledge of disease process and transmission.
C. Affected others have been identified and treated.

Specific Disorders

Herpes

A. Genital herpes is caused by herpes simplex virus type 2 (HSV_2).
B. Causes painful vesicles on genitalia, both external and internal.
C. There is no cure.
D. Treatment is symptomatic.
E. If active infection at the end of pregnancy, cesarean birth may be indicated, since virus is lethal to the fetus.

F. Recurrences of the condition may be caused by infection, stress, menses.

G. Acyclovir (Zovirax) is only medication presently approved for HSV$_2$ treatment.

Chlamydia

A. Currently more frequent than gonorrhea

B. Symptoms similar to gonorrhea (cervical/vaginal discharge) or may be asymptomatic

C. Can be transmitted to fetus at birth.

D. Treated with erythromycin

E. If untreated, can lead to pelvic inflammatory disease (PID).

Gonorrhea

A. Caused by *N. gonorrhoeae*

B. Symptoms may include heavy, purulent vaginal discharge, but often asymptomatic in female.

C. May be passed to fetus at time of birth, causing ophthalmia neonatorum and sepsis.

D. Treatment is penicillin; allergic patients may be treated with erythromycin or (if not pregnant) the cephalosporins.

E. All sexual contacts must be treated as well, to prevent "ping-pong" recurrence.

Syphilis

A. Caused by *Treponema pallidum* (spirochete)

B. Crosses placenta after 16th week of pregnancy to infect fetus.

C. Initial symptoms are chancre and lymphadenopathy and may disappear without treatment in 4–6 weeks.

D. Secondary symptoms are rash, malaise, and alopecia and these too may disappear in several weeks without treatment.

E. Tertiary syphilis may recur later in life and affect any organ system, especially cardiovascular and neurologic systems.

F. Diagnosis is made by dark-field exam and serologic tests (VDRL).

G. Treatment is penicillin, or erythromycin if penicillin allergy exists.

Other Genital Infections

Cervical and vaginal infections may be caused by agents other than those associated with STDs. For all female patients with a vaginal infection, nursing actions should include teaching good perineal hygiene.

Trichomonas vaginalis

A. Caused by a protozoan

B. Major symptom is profuse foamy white to greenish discharge that is irritating to genitalia.

C. Treatment is metronidazole (Flagyl) for woman and all sexual partners.

D. Treatment lasts seven days, during which time a condom should be used for intercourse.

E. Alcohol ingestion with Flagyl causes severe gastrointestinal upset.

Candida albicans

A. Caused by a yeast normally found in the vagina.

B. Overgrowth may occur in pregnancy, with diabetes, and steroid or antibiotic therapy.

C. Vaginal examination reveals thick, white, cheesy patches on vaginal walls.

D. Treatment is topical application of clotrimazole (Gyne-Lotrimin), nystatin (Mycostatin), or gentian violet.

E. Candida albicans causes thrush in the newborn by direct contact in the birth canal.

Bacterial Vaginitis

A. Caused by other bacteria invading the vagina

B. Foul or fishy smelling discharge

C. Treatment is specific to causative agent, and usually includes sexual partners for best results.

AIDS (see pages 94–95)

FEMALE REPRODUCTIVE SYSTEM NEOPLASIA

The nursing diagnoses, general goals and interventions, and evaluation for the patient with cancer of the reproductive system are similar to those for any patient with a diagnosis of cancer. Only nursing care specific to the disorder will be discussed here.

Fibrocystic Breast Disease

A. Most common benign breast lesion

B. Cyst(s) may be palpated; surgical biopsy indicated for differential diagnosis.

C. Treatment includes surgical removal of cysts, decreasing or removing caffeine from diet, and danazol (Danocrine) to suppress menses.

Breast Cancer

A. General information
   1. Most common neoplasm in women
   2. Leading cause of death in women age 40–44

B. Medical management
   1. Usually surgical excision; options are simple lumpectomy, simple mastectomy, and radical mastectomy.
   2. Adjuvant treatment with chemotherapy, radiation, and hormone therapy.

C. Assessment findings
   1. Palpation of lump (upper outer quadrant most frequent site) usually first symptom
   2. Skin of breast dimpled
   3. Nipple discharge
   4. Asymmetry of breasts
   5. Surgical biopsy provides definitive diagnosis.

D. Nursing intervenions
   1. Assess breasts for early identification and treatment.
   2. Support patient through recommended/chosen treatment.
   3. Prepare patient for mastectomy if necessary.

Mastectomy

A. General information
   1. Simple mastectomy: removal of breast only, no lymph nodes removed
   2. Radical mastectomy: removal of breast, muscle layer down to chest wall and axillary lymph nodes
B. Nursing interventions
   1. Provide routine pre- and post-op care (see page 31).
   2. Elevate patient's arm on operative side on pillows to minimize edema.
   3. Do not use arm on affected side for blood pressure measurements, IVs, or injections.
   4. Turn only to back and unaffected side.
   5. Monitor patient for bleeding, check under her
   6. Begin range-of-motion exercises immediately on unaffected side.
   7. Start with simple movements on affected side: fingers and hands first, then wrist, elbow, and shoulder movements.
   8. Make abduction the last movement.
   9. Coordinate physical therapy if ordered.
   10. Teach patient about any necessary life-style changes (special care of arm on affected side, monthly breast self-examination on remaining breast, use of prosthesis).
   11. Encourage/arrange visit from support group member.

Cancer of the Cervix

A. Detected by Pap smear, followed by tissue biopsy.
B. Preinvasive conditions may be treated by cryosurgery, laser surgery, cervical conization, or hysterectomy.
C. Invasive conditions are treated by radium therapy and radical hysterectomy.

Cancer of the Uterus

A. May affect endometrium or fundus/corpus
B. Cardinal symptom: abnormal uterine bleeding, either pre- or postmenopause
C. Diagnosis: by endometrial biopsy or fractional curettage; cells washed from uterus under pressure may also be used for diagnosis.
D. Usual intervention: total hysterectomy and bilateral salpingo-oophorectomy
E. Radium therapy and chemotherapy may also be used.

Cancer of the Ovary

A. Etiology unknown
B. Few early symptoms; palpation of ovarian mass is usual first finding.
C. Treatment of choice is surgical removal with total hysterectomy and bilateral salpingo-oophorectomy.
D. Chemotherapy may be used as adjuvant therapy.

Cancer of the Vulva

A. Begins as small, pruritic lesions
B. Diagnosed by biopsy

C. Treatment is either local excision or radical vulvectomy (removal of entire vulva plus superficial and femoral nodes).

Hysterectomy

A. General information
   1. Total hysterectomy: removal of uterine body and cervix only
   2. Subtotal hysterectomy: removal of uterine body leaving cervix in place (seldom performed)
   3. Total abdominal hysterectomy with bilateral salpingo-oophorectomy (TAH-BSO): removal of uterine body, cervix, both ovaries and both fallopian tubes
   4. Radical hysterectomy: removal of uterine body, cervix, connective tissue, part of vagina and pelvic lymph nodes
B. Nursing interventions
   1. Institute routine pre- and post-op care.
   2. Assess for hemorrhage, infection, or other postsurgical complications (e.g., paralytic ileus, thrombophlebitis, pneumonia).
   3. Support woman and family through procedure, encourage expression of feelings and reactions to procedure.
   4. Explain implications of hysterectomy.
      a. No further menses
      b. If ovaries also removed, will have menopause and may need estrogen replacement therapy.
   5. Allow woman (and partner) to verbalize concerns about sexuality postsurgery.
   6. Provide discharge teaching.

MENOPAUSE

The time in a woman's life when menstruation ceases. Fertility also ceases, and symptoms associated with changing hormone levels may occur. Reactions to menopause may be influenced by culture, age at menopause, reproductive and menstrual history, and complications.

Assessment Findings

A. Symptoms related to hormone changes
   1. Vasomotor instability (hot flashes and night sweats)
   2. Emotional disturbances (mood swings, irritability, depression), fatigue, and headache
B. Physical changes include
   1. Atrophy of genitalia
   2. Dyspareunia
   3. Urinary changes (frequency/stress incontinence)
   4. Constipation
   5. Possibly uterine prolapse

Interventions

A. Estrogen replacement therapy (ERT)
   1. Used to control symptoms, especially vasomotor instability and vaginal atrophy, and to prevent osteoporosis
   2. Women with family histories of breast or uterine cancer,

hypertension, thrombophlebitis, or cardiac dysfunction are not good candidates for ERT.

B. Alternatives to ERT include
1. Vitamin E: from dietary sources and supplements
2. Herbs: varied relief with combinations of roots and herbs, such as licorice and dandelion
3. Other medications: Bellergal (phenobarbital, ergotamine tartrate, and belladonna)
4. Kegel exercises for genital atrophy: alternating constriction and relaxation of pubococcygeal muscles (muscles controlling the flow of urine) done at least three times/day
5. Vaginal lubricants for genital atrophy: water-soluble lubricants can diminish dyspareunia.
6. Maintenance of good hydration: at least 8 glasses of water/day.
7. Good perineal hygiene

Complications of Menopause

Osteoporosis

A. Increased porosity of the bone, with increased incidence of spontaneous fractures
B. Other symptoms in the postmenopausal woman include loss of height, back pain, and dowager's hump.
C. Diagnosis by x-ray is not possible until more than 50% of bone mass has already been lost.
D. Decreased bone porosity is inextricably linked with lowered levels of estrogen in the postmenopausal woman. Estrogen plays a part in the absorption of calcium and the stimulation of osteoclasts (new-bone-forming cells).
E. Treatment includes
1. ERT unless contraindicated
2. Supplemental calcium to slow the osteoporotic process (1 gm taken daily at HS)
3. Increased fluid intake (2–3 liters/day will help avoid formation of calculi)
4. High-calcium/high-phosphorus diet with avoidance of excess protein
5. Some exercise on a regular basis

Cystocele/Rectocele

A. Herniations of the anterior and posterior (respectively) walls of the vagina
B. Usually the sequelae of childbirth injuries
C. Herniation allows the bulging of the bladder and the rectum into the vagina.
D. Treatment is surgical repair of these conditions: anterior and posterior *colporrhaphy.*

Prolapse of the Uterus

A. Usually the result of childbirth injuries or relaxation of the cardinal ligaments
B. Allows the uterus to sag backward and downward into the vagina, or outside the body completely.

C. Vaginal hysterectomy is the preferred surgical intervention.
D. If condition does not warrant surgery, the insertion of a *pessary* (supportive device) will help to support and stabilize the uterus.

SAMPLE QUESTIONS

17. In collecting data for a health history of Peggy L., an infertility patient, which of the following findings is most important?
    ○ 1. She is 5 ft 8 in tall and weighs 105 lb
    ○ 2. She has never used any form of contraception
    ○ 3. She has been married for three years
    ○ 4. She has no brothers or sisters

18. The teaching plan for Mary A., who has just been fitted with her first diaphragm, must include
    ○ 1. specific amount of spermicide to be used with diaphragm.
    ○ 2. insertion at least 8 hours before intercourse.
    ○ 3. specific cleaning techniques.
    ○ 4. storage in the refrigerator.

19. Mrs. Jane M. is 64 years old, postmenopausal, and takes calcium supplements on a daily basis. She can reduce the danger of renal calculi by the simple action of
    ○ 1. chewing her calcium tablets rather than swallowing them whole.
    ○ 2. swallowing her calcium tablets with cranberry juice.
    ○ 3. eliminating other sources of calcium from her diet.
    ○ 4. drinking 2–3 quarts of water daily.

20. Mrs. Frances D. is 57 years old and having a routine physical exam. Which of the following assessments would yield critical information as to her postmenopausal status?
    ○ 1. Asking about weight loss of more than 5 lb in the last year
    ○ 2. Asking about her nightly sleep patterns
    ○ 3. Asking about her cultural background
    ○ 4. Asking about her last pregnancy

REFERENCES AND RECOMMENDED READINGS

Bruce, J., & Shearer, S. (1979). *Contraceptives and common sense: Conventional methods reconsidered.* New York: The Population Council.

Bassing, S. (1985). Saving the baby when mom has herpes. *RN, 48*(10), 35–37.

Butnarescu, G., & Tillotson, D. (1983). *Maternity nursing: Theory to practice.* New York: Wiley.

Dodge, J. (1985). When childbirth is a family affair. *RN, 48*(12), 20–21.

Fries, R. (1984). Dodging infectious hazards while you're pregnant. *RN, 47*(11), 50–52.

Holmes J., & Mageira, L. (1987). Maternity nursing. New York: Macmillan.

Jensen, M., & Bobak, I. (1985). *Maternity and gynecologic care; The nurse and the family* (3rd ed.). St. Louis: Mosby.

Johnson, S. (1986). *Nursing assessment and strategies for the family at risk: High risk parenting* (2nd ed.). Philadelphia: Lippincott.

Ladewig, P., et al. (1986). *Essentials of maternal-newborn nursing.* Menlo Park, CA: Addison-Wesley.

Nelson, W., Maxey, L., & Keith, S. (1984). Are we abandoning the AIDS patient? *RN, 47*(7), 18–19.

Olds, S., et al. (1988). Maternal-newborn nursing: A family centered approach (3rd ed.). Menlo Park, CA: Addison-Wesley.

Oxorn, H. (1980). *Human labor and birth* (4th ed.). New York: Appleton-Century-Crofts.

Reeder, S., et al. (1987). *Maternity nursing* (16th ed.). Philadelphia: Lippincott.

Scheideberg, D. (1984). How can you be so sure my baby's dead? *RN, 47*(2), 29–30.

Swearingen, P. (1986). *Manual of nursing therapeutics.* Menlo Park, CA: Addison-Wesley.

Whaley, L., & Wong, D. (1987). Nursing care of infants and children (3rd ed.). St. Louis: Mosby.

Whettam, J. (1984). Update on toxic shock: How to spot it and treat it. *RN, 47*(2), 55, 56, 58, 60.

World population and fertility planning techniques: The next twenty years. Washington, DC: Office of Technology Assessment.

UNIT 4: Reprints

Dealing with third-trimester bleeding

Even slight vaginal bleeding late in a pregnancy can pose
a grave threat to mother and baby. Here's what you need to know
to help them through such a last-minute crisis.

When a woman experiences vaginal bleeding in the third trimester of her pregnancy, two lives may be in danger—the mother's and her unborn infant's. Whether you see the woman first in the hospital, or in some other setting, your actions can play a critical role in determining the outcome. This installment of the **RN** emergency series discusses how to avoid potentially lethal mistakes during assessment and how to prepare the patient for the emergency surgery that may be necessary.

In order to make the proper observations and ask the appropriate questions, you need to know about the three most common causes of third-trimester bleeding:

Placenta previa occurs when the placenta develops in a lower-than-normal position partially or totally covering the cervical os. When so situated, any thinning or dilatation of the cervix can tear it. Placenta previa is characterized by varying amounts of painless, bright red bleeding, usually occurring first around the 34th week of preg-

THE AUTHOR, Carol L. Howe, CNM, DNSc, is an associate professor at the Oregon Health Sciences University in Portland.

Produced by Thom Schwarz, RN

nancy. It's often preceded by "spotting" earlier in the pregnancy.

Abruptio placentae is the premature separation of the placenta from the uterine wall. Separation is accompanied by abdominal pain, uterine irritability, and fetal distress. This condition often accompanies pregnancy-induced hypertension, which may also be called pre-eclampsia or toxemia.

Uterine rupture can occur spontaneously but is usually associated with previous trauma to the uterus—as from cesarean delivery or uterine surgery. It can also be caused by injudicious use of the contraction-producing chemical oxytocin. The rupture causes severe pain and heavy vaginal bleeding. It can lead rapidly to the death of both mother and child.

What—and what not— to do in the field

Should you encounter a patient with vaginal bleeding in a setting outside the hospital, have her lie supine and elevate her feet slightly. This will take some of the pressure off the placenta which may be compressed by the weight of the baby. *Do not attempt to perform a vaginal exam at this time.* Manipulation of the cervix without knowing the cause of the problem can prove disastrous for both mother and child.

Find out first if the patient has experienced aches or cramps that might actually be labor pains, then obtain a history of the bleeding. Find out when it began and whether it was associated with a specific event, such as intercourse, a vaginal examination, a fall, or other trauma. Did it begin with a gush or just spotting? Is the blood dark or bright red? Does it contain any clots? If you can recover those tissue samples, bring them to the ED for examination.

If the patient's anxiety makes it difficult for her to give you an accurate estimate of her blood loss, ask such questions as, "How many pads have you used? Were they soaked or spotted? Is the bleeding as heavy as your period?" When comparing the bleeding to the patient's period, remember to ask whether her menstrual flow is normally heavy or light.

In addition to finding out about blood loss, it's important to take an obstetrical history, including gravidity, parity, last menstrual period, estimated date of confinement, previous ultrasound examinations, and any possible complications. You can take such a history if there's time, but don't let it interfere with your highest priority—getting the patient to the nearest emergency facility.

If the patient has obviously lost a significant amount of blood or shows signs of hemorrhagic shock, call an ambulance immediately. Signs of hemorrhage include confusion, lethargy, agitation, cold, clammy skin, and a rapid, weak, or thready pulse. The patient may also complain of thirst, but she must remain NPO since surgery is a definite possibility.

If the bleeding isn't heavy and the patient shows no sign of shock, you or a family member may be tempted to drive her to the hospital rather than calling an ambulance. This is a risky decision, since the condition of such a patient can deteriorate suddenly and unexpectedly. If you do decide to drive her yourself, have her lie down if possible on the way to the hospital. Use pads or towels to absorb further bleeding, but do not under any circumstances insert a tampon or other object into the vagina. Such insertions may cause additional tearing or perforation of the placenta.

Further evaluation at the hospital
At the hospital, immediately place the patient on bedrest. Check the perineum for bleeding and the presence of clots. To estimate the amount of blood loss, weigh all soiled pads before discarding them.

Every extra gram of weight over the weight of the dry pad indicates approximately one milliliter of blood loss.

Even if there appears to be little bleeding, bear in mind that blood can accumulate retroplacentally. In abruptio placentae, blood may be trapped behind the placenta, resulting in an enlarging uterus. If you suspect this condition, gently measure the height of the fundus with a tape measure and mark it with a pen. Recheck your measurement frequently.

Check vital signs every 15 minutes for signs of hemorrhagic shock, including a weak, rapid pulse, hypotension, and decreased urine output.

In addition to watching for shock, you'll need to assess the patient for less-obvious hemodynamic changes. Look closely, for example, for pallor of the gums or lips. Watch for slow capillary refilling when you compress and then release the earlobe or fingernail beds.

Laboratory studies aren't often helpful in assessing immediate blood loss because they may not show profound changes right away, even in the presence of heavy bleeding. Hematocrit, for example, may not drop significantly for several hours after a hemorrhage.

A most important test is a check for orthostatic hypotension. Take the patient's blood pressure and pulse as she lies supine. Then ask her to stand up or sit upright, and immediately check her vital signs again. If she faints, becomes weak or dizzy, or suffers visual disturbances, or if her blood pressure decreases more than 20 points or her

pulse increases more than 20 beats a minute, she has lost more than 20% of total blood volume—more than the circulatory system can quickly compensate for.

As soon as you finish evaluating the patient's blood loss, notify her physician or, if necessary, obtain the services of the nearest doctor. Summon additional nursing help, too. The likelihood of emergency surgery is high, and rapid preparation requires at least two pairs of skilled hands.

The doctor will undoubtedly want you to insert a large-bore peripheral IV line, insert a urinary catheter, and draw some blood. The IV line—at least 16-gauge—will permit rapid hydration and blood replacement. Once fluid replacement is started, the urinary catheter will enable you to measure urination. The blood should go to the lab for cbc, and typing and cross-matching for two to four units of whole blood for transfusion. Get a clotting profile, too, to rule out disseminated intravascular coagulation or any other clotting disorders.

It's imperative to delay vaginal or rectal examination until the location of the placenta is known. If the placenta lies in front of the presenting part of the fetus, any manipulation of the cervix can turn a serious situation into a catastrophe. Find out whether the patient has had a previous ultrasound examination, which would have determined the location of the placenta. Ultimately, vaginal examination should be left to the physician or a certified nurse midwife.

Closely monitor fetal condition

Any situation that disturbs maternal hemodynamics or disrupts the utero-placental blood flow will take its toll on the fetus. Third-trimester bleeding therefore calls for close fetal monitoring. Electronic monitoring is the ideal method, but you cannot place the internal scalp electrode until placenta previa has been ruled out. Until it has been, continuous auscultation with a Doppler probe is preferable by far to using a traditional obstetric stethoscope. If you get a good pulse, you may want to reassure the mother and father by letting them listen to it.

Pay attention to any significant changes in the baseline fetal heart rate, which should normally be 120 to 160 beats a minute. Periodic changes, especially late decelerations or variables with a slow return to the baseline rate, are particularly ominous. You should call the physician immediately if they occur since delivery may need to be hastened.

Position of the fetus is also important. For instance, if the fetal presenting part is well out of the pelvis or the fetus is in a transverse lie, something, such as the placenta, may be blocking the path out. Easily palpable fetal parts may mean that the infant has been extruded from the uterus after it ruptured. An extremely tense, painful abdomen and uterus can indicate placental bleeding into the myometrium from abruptio placentae.

If a decision for surgery is made, notify the on-call anesthesiologist and OR scrub team to prepare the operating suite. Also summon the patient's pediatrician or the on-call pediatrician to care for the infant after delivery. Obtain the necessary preop information from the patient, and keep her NPO.

Don't neglect emotional support

Although the patient and her family may not know the cause of the third-trimester bleeding, they almost always realize that it has serious implications. They'll be understandably anxious and often quite upset. When possible, allow the husband—or whomever the patient requests—to remain with her to provide emotional support.

The most helpful thing you can do under the circumstances is to remain calm and in control without offering false reassurances that everything will be all right. In fact, everything may be far from all right. In extreme cases, the lives of both the mother and the child may be in danger. What's more, a hysterectomy may be necessary to arrest hemorrhage—a prospect that may be as traumatic for many parents as the loss of the baby.

If the situation is critical, support, comfort, and explanation may have to follow surgery rather than precede it. But these crucial aspects of nursing care must never be neglected, even if they have to be delayed.

Third-trimester vaginal bleeding is always cause for concern. Your astute observations and ability to anticipate the need for intervention can save precious minutes that may be critical to the survival of mother and child. ∎

BIBLIOGRAPHY Grimes, D.A. Estimating vaginal blood loss. *J. Reprod. Med.* 22(4):190, 1979. Howe, C. et al. *Hemorrhage During Late Pregnancy and the Puerperium.* March of Dimes educational module, series 3, module 4, 1984. Oxhorn, H. *Human Labor and Birth* (4th ed.). New York: Appleton-Century-Crofts, 1980.

Helping the patient with vaginitis

Thousands of women suffer chronic discomfort from vaginal infections.
Here's what you can do to help your patients resolve
these frustrating problems—and keep them resolved.
By Deborah Washington, RN, BSN

When it comes to treating vaginitis, relieving the two major complaints—itching and discharge—is only the beginning. To really help these patients, you'll need to make sure that they comply with the full course of treatment and understand their role in preventing recurrence of this all-too-common condition.

Many women avoid seeking treatment until vaginitis becomes chronic or severe, perhaps because they consider the subject too unimportant for medical treatment or too embarrassing to discuss. Such patients need information about the condition, reassurance that it can indeed be remedied, and lots of encouragement to adhere to the treatment regimen.

The key is to gain the patient's trust. Without it, you probably won't get the information you need or the treatment results you hope for. The nurse's response to the patient with vaginitis often affects the patient's own attitude toward

THE AUTHOR is a staff nurse at Cleveland Metropolitan General Hospitals. She wrote this article while a clinical nursing instructor at Magee Women's Hospital in Pittsburgh.

her condition. A supportive, nonjudgmental approach is essential, especially when the suspected route of transmission is sexual intercourse.

Why you can't afford to ignore vaginitis

The symptoms common to vaginitis do not necessarily indicate disease. The vaginal secretions of some women are fairly copious even in the absence of infection. Leukorrhea, a whitish discharge, often occurs immediately before the menarche due to increased production of estrogen. Patients on birth control hormones may experience a similar discharge. Increased vaginal secretions are also common during pregnancy.

This is not to say it's safe to disregard vaginitis. The symptoms may indicate any of a number of conditions—from simple yeast infections to gonorrhea—that require treatment. Nor should the symptoms themselves be dismissed as trivial. Chronic itching can be harder to endure than pain.

Fortunately, vaginitis is easily treatable. You can assure the patient that numerous tablets, vaginal suppositories, and topical preparations are available to relieve her discomfort while destroying the responsible organisms. In addition, teaching the patient that simple preventive measures are likely to thwart future outbreaks can help reassure her that she needn't dread recurrences of the condition for the rest of her life.

The importance of a thorough history

Identification and treatment of vaginitis begin with a careful history. Proceed from the patient's general description of the problem to more specific questioning.

Details about the discharge are important because they often provide a clue to the cause of the problem—though only laboratory tests can determine what organism, if any, is involved. Ask how long the patient has noticed the discharge, whether it's ever appeared before, and if so, how often. Determine the color, consistency, and amount of the discharge, as well as any additional characteristics—whether it's smooth or frothy, odorless or foul smelling.

Because the itching and burning of vaginitis tend to worsen during the menstrual period, ask the patient when her last period occurred and how the symptoms felt then. Find out whether she's experienced any flare-ups at other times, after intercourse, for example.

Painful urination and painful intercourse are other common symptoms about which you should question patients. Patients may fail to connect such symptoms with those for which they're seeking treatment. Also, ask whether the patient has ever been pregnant, and find out what, if any, form of birth control she uses.

The underlying cause of vaginitis is alteration of the normal pH balance of the vagina. A change in the pH of the vagina from its normal slight acidity to a more alkaline pH—as happens during ovulation and after menopause, for example—encourages proliferation of fungi and bacteria. The three types of vaginitis you're most likely to see are candidiasis, trichomoniasis, and nonspecific vaginitis.

The common nuisance of candidiasis

Women presenting with a thick, white, cheesy (caseous) discharge and burning, itching, and localized soreness are probably suffering from candidiasis. This condition is caused by the fungus *Candida albicans* or, less commonly, by *C. tro-*

picalis. Candida infections are also known as monilial infections—after *Monilia*, the genus *candida's* former name—or yeast infections.

If copious, the discharge from candidiasis may cause an itchy rash on the external genitalia. Some victims experience pain during intercourse. Symptoms tend to become exaggerated just before and just after the menstrual period, when the vagina is most alkaline.

Recent research indicates that the incidence of vaginal candidiasis is increasing. Changing sexual mores may be one reason. Some researchers point to the widespread use of antibiotics, which kill normal vaginal flora, permitting yeast overgrowth. Immunosuppression, cytotoxic drugs, diabetes, or pregnancy can also make women susceptible to candidal infections.

C. albicans is part of the normal flora of the skin, mouth, intestinal tract, and vagina. Infections can therefore occur independently of direct contact with an infected person. Even reinfection can take place independently because reservoirs of candida exist in a woman's gastrointestinal tract. Some women, however, do pick up the infection during sexual intercourse, because asymptomatic monilial infections can lie dormant under the foreskins of uncircumcised men.

Candidiasis is generally treated with a vaginal cream or suppository such as nystatin (Korostatin, Mycostatin, Nilstat), clotrimazole (Gyne-Lotrimin), or miconazole (Monistat). Point out to the patient that drainage induced by the medication can stain underpants. Note, too, that tampons absorb internal

meds and should not be used during treatment.

Patient compliance is integral to successful treatment, which often continues well beyond relief of symptoms. You can encourage compliance by explaining that an infection takes time to develop and needs time to go away. Early use of a topical antipruritic preparation can give so much immediate relief that the patient no longer feels a need to continue treatment. Warn her that discontinuing the medication prematurely may induce another flare-up.

Patients with seemingly intractable candidiasis may be harboring two or more of the 18-odd substrains of *C. albicans*. In such cases, more than one drug may be ordered.

The annoying symptoms of trichomoniasis

Trichomoniasis is more likely than candidiasis to be spread by sexual contact and, indeed, is often found with gonorrhea. The infection can also be transmitted by wet washcloths, bathing suits, towels, douche nozzles, and toilet seats. *Trichomonas vaginalis*, the protozoan that causes the disease, can lie dormant indefinitely and stay potent enough to spread while remaining asymptomatic in the carrier. Such factors as emotional stress, lowered resistance, or a change in vaginal pH can bring out *Trichomonas* infections.

Commonly known as "trich," the condition is characterized by a yellow-green, frothy discharge with a strong, foul odor. A severe infection can cause inflammation of the vulva and pain during urination and intercourse. Upon examination, the walls of the vagina may appear inflamed, with red, strawberry-shaped patches that may also be present on the cervix.

The treatment of choice for *Trichomonas* infections is usually metronidazole (Flagyl, Metryl, Protostat, Sātric). The drug may be administered in a single 2-g dose or in three 250-mg doses daily for seven days. The patient should be warned against drinking alcoholic beverages during drug therapy because they can cause headaches, flushing, nausea, vomiting, and abdominal cramps. Pregnant women should not take metronidazole.

Whether or not the patient originally acquired trichomoniasis through sexual contact, she can pass on the infection to a sexual partner. It's therefore important that both partners receive treatment simultaneously to prevent the infection from being passed back and forth indefinitely.

The potential dangers of nonspecific vaginitis

Nonspecific vaginitis, caused by the bacteria *Hemophilus vaginalis* or *Gardnerella vaginalis*, is transmitted primarily through sexual intercourse, although it can also be acquired from towels and toilet seats. According to one recent study, women using IUDs are more likely to develop nonspecific vaginitis than women taking oral contraceptives, although the precise correlation remains unclear.

Nonspecific vaginitis during pregnancy may predispose patients to premature labor and postpartum endometritis. A link between nonspecific vaginitis and mucopurulent cervicitis, which can lead to impairment of fallopian tube function and infertility, has also been noted.

Typical symptoms of nonspecific vaginitis include itching, pain on urination, and pain during intercourse. The characteristic grayish discharge is homogenous, turbid, and foul smelling.

Treatment for *Hemophilus* infections usually involves inserting an applicatorful of sulfa cream (Sultrin, AVC, Triple Sulfa Cream) high in the vagina once a day for six to 14 days. Treatment for women allergic to sulfa drugs consists of inserting a vaginal suppository, such as nitrofurazone (Furacin), twice a day for 10 days. If systemic treatment is necessary, a course of oral antibiotics, such as ampicillin or tetracycline, may be indicated. The usual regimen calls for 250 mg four times a day for 10 days.

Some simple ways to prevent vaginitis

Proper hygiene, adequate rest, and a well-balanced diet, can go far toward preventing vaginitis or its recurrence. Remind patients to wipe the perineum from front to back, to avoid spreading bacteria from the anus to the vagina. Instruct them to change tampons frequently, at least three or four times a day, and to wash their hands before and after every change.

Soap and water are the best means of keeping the vaginal area clean. Warn patients that feminine hygiene sprays and bubble baths can both irritate the vulva and mask odors that might otherwise alert the patient to an incipient infection. Since douching alters the pH balance of the vagina, it should be avoided unless ordered by the physician. The best douching solution is a tablespoon or two of white vinegar in a quart of comfortably warm water. This solution closely mimics normal vaginal pH.

Some soaps are known to trigger vaginal infections for many women. It's therefore wise for women suffering from vaginitis, particularly when it's chronic, to ask their physicians which brands to avoid.

Underpants and pantyhose should have cotton crotches, for optimal ventilation. Tight pants that cut off air flow to the vagina may be fashionable but help create an atmosphere in which bacteria flourish.

Overweight women whose thighs rub together are at risk for vaginal infection since they have less ventilation of the genital area. Telling such women that losing weight could reduce their susceptibility to infection may encourage them to shed excess pounds.

Women who have multiple sex partners are also at high risk for vaginal infection. You may wish to mention this risk to patients without asking whether it applies to them. Follow up by observing that condoms can protect against infection as well as conception.

Kegel exercises, designed to tone the pubococcygeus muscles, can help prevent vaginitis by promoting the passage of vaginal secretions. Instruct the patient to squeeze her buttocks together while drawing in the pelvis and to maintain that position for three seconds. Then have her relax the pubococcygeus muscles for three seconds before beginning the cycle again. She should repeat this procedure several times a day.

To find out whether she's doing the exercises properly, the patient can insert a finger into the vagina while performing them. This will tell her whether or not the muscles are tensing and relaxing. Another test is to stop and start the flow of urine at will. A side benefit of doing Kegel exercises is enhanced sexual pleasure for both the woman and her male partner.

Keep in mind as you teach vaginitis patients that your attitude and encouragement may be as important to their recovery as the factual information you give them. The more convincingly you stress the need for compliance and prevention, and the more comfortable your patients feel with your instructions, the more likely they are to get rid of their vaginitis—and keep it from returning. ∎

Intransigent genital infection? Suspect chlamydiae

BY ELAINE LARSON, RN, PhD, FAAN

One of the nation's most prevalent sexually transmitted diseases has received so little publicity that it is almost unknown. The bacteria involved aren't any you've seen on a hospital lab report. Yet the resulting disease is three times as common as gonorrhea in the U.S., and the most common cause of blindness world-wide. Are you able to name the bacteria that can cause:

- Pneumonia.
- Lower abdominal pain.
- Purulent vaginal discharge.
- Salpingitis, cervicitis, and pelvic inflammatory disease.
- Proctitis and epididymitis.
- Ectopic pregnancy, spontaneous abortion, and sterility.[1, 2]
- Neonatal conjunctivitis.

The answer is chlamydiae, bacteria so small that until recently they were thought to be viruses. These bacteria's growth requirements are so special—they can be grown only in tissue culture and in yolk sacs of embryonated chicks—that they can't be identified by the usual microbiology lab tests. In fact, culture techniques to isolate the organisms, and blood tests to detect antibody titers, are currently available in just a few medical centers.

Diagnosis based on symptoms is also difficult, since chlamydiae can cause subclinical or chronic infections that last for years. In many cases no attempt is even made to diagnose the disease, allowing it to go untreated and spread unhindered.

The following two examples are typical of the estimated 2.5 million cases of chlamydial infection that occur in the U.S. each year.

Ms. J., a 19-year-old primipara, was seen in the women's clinic of a large medical center after experiencing a spontaneous abortion. The pregnancy had appeared normal, although Ms. J. reported that over the past two years she had experienced some lower abdominal pain and slight purulent discharge from the vagina. These symptoms, however, had seemed to resolve without treatment. Because of this history, chlamydial infection was suspected. Serologic tests revealed a high antibody titer for *Chlamydia,* and the spontaneous abortion was attributed to this infection.

Ms. K. brought her two-week-old baby to a pediatric clinic because the child had red, draining eyes. A review of the infant's clinical record showed that silver nitrate (AgNO$_3$) drops had been administered at birth to prevent gonococcal conjunctivitis. Since results of the mother's cervical culture for gonorrhea were negative, the baby's conjunctivitis was attributed to a chlamydial infection.

Cases like these are occurring with increasing frequency. In adults, chlamydial infection is at least three times more common than gonorrhea. About 40% of nongonococcal urethritis (NGU) and 70% of post-gonococcal urethritis is caused by chlamydiae. Chlamydial infection is now the most common cause of neonatal conjunctivitis.

The species of chlamydiae—*C. trachomatis*—that is most common in the U.S. has at least 15 serotypes.* Those labeled D through K are the ones that cause the genital and ocular syndromes that are being increasingly identified in this country today.

Serious complications

Genital chlamydial infections are spread through sexual contact. After an incubation period of two to three weeks, the infected person may have some genital discharge. Asymptomatic infections are, however, common in both sexes. Sequelae can be serious, especially for women of childbearing age. Such problems as salpingitis, cervicitis, and pelvic inflammatory disease may possibly lead to ectopic pregnancy, spontaneous abortion, or sterility. In addition, some investigators suspect that chlamydiae may also cause sterility in men.

Both sexes can also develop extragenital problems such as conjunctivitis, pneumonia, Fitz-Hugh-Curtis syndrome (a perihepatitis associated with both chlamydiae and gonococci), and Reiter's syndrome (a disease charac-

C. trachomatis serotypes L-1. L-2. and L-3 cause lymphogranuloma venereum. a sexually transmitted disease that is uncommon in the U.S. This disease, in rare cases. can result in genital elephantiasis. Serotypes A. B. Ba. and C cause trachoma. a chronic conjunctivitis that's very common in Asia and Africa and the major cause of blindness in the world. About 400 million people currently have trachoma. and approximately 10% of them will eventually be blinded. *C. psittaci.* the other species of chlamydiae. causes psittacosis or ornithosis. uncommon in the U.S

THE AUTHOR *is a Robert Wood Johnson Clinical Nurse Scholar at the University of Pennsylvania in Philadelphia.*

terized by arthritis, urethritis, conjunctivitis, and mucocutaneous lesions). Even contact with infected genital secretions in swimming pools can result in chlamydial conjunctivitis (hence the name "swimming pool conjunctivitis").[3] And passage through an infected birth canal can also cause *C. trachomatis* infection.

If a mother has a genital chlamydial infection, her baby has a 50% chance of developing inclusion conjunctivitis. About one to five babies per 100 live births are affected. Usually the infection is not noted in the hospital and often goes totally unreported. At one to two weeks of age, however, infected babies develop red, draining eyes. In rare cases conjunctival scarring occurs, but usually the infection will resolve itself spontaneously after several weeks.

Chlamydial pneumonia among neonates is more common than whooping cough. Although afebrile, the babies have a cough and diffuse lung involvement. But unless the lung infection is preceded by diagnosed inclusion conjunctivitis, the diagnosis of chlamydial pneumonia may also be missed. For this reason, the exact incidence is unknown. Chlamydiae have also been implicated as a possible cause of otitis media in infants.

Given the difficulties of detection, stemming the epidemic depends on our awareness of the disease. High-risk, sexually active individuals should be screened for chlamydiae, especially if they are pregnant or under treatment for nonspecific NGU. Resistance to treatment of *any* genital or ocular infection gives good reason to suspect the presence of chlamydiae. Pending laboratory confirmation of gonorrhea, for example, patients are often treated with ampicillin or penicillin. Lack of response to this therapy would be highly suggestive.

Long-term therapy

Since a major part of the *Chlamydia* bacterium's life cycle takes place inside human cells (see "Why therapy must be prolonged," at right), the disease is often chronic, and curing it takes time. Tetracycline is the treat-

Chlamydial diseases common in the U.S.

Males
Epididymitis
Proctitis

Females
Cervicitis
Postpartal endometritis
Salpingitis
Vaginitis

All adults
Conjunctivitis
Pelvic inflammatory disease (PID)
Pneumonia
Sterility
Urethritis

Neonates
Inclusion conjunctivitis
Otitis media (possibly)
Pneumonia

Why therapy must be prolonged
Chlamydia's unique life cycle makes for a difficult cure.

Although the small chlamydiae bacteria do produce a toxin, this does not seem to be their main source of virulence. Instead, their pathogenic effects result from the gram-negative-like bacteria's invasion of cells and interference with host-cell synthesis; the bacteria "take over," causing cell death.

Like the viruses they were once mistaken for, chlamydiae are parasites, dependent on host cells for energy and replication. But the unique aspect of the chlamydial growth cycle is that the bacteria can also survive outside of cells and infect new cells. The mature chlamydiae bacteria, called elementary bodies (EBs), survive in extracellular space and induce host cells to engulf and ingest them. Once inside the cells, the bacteria protect themselves from being lysed (killed) by metamorphosing into initial bodies (IBs) after six to eight hours.

The IBs cannot survive outside their hosts, but can reproduce themselves, like all bacteria, by binary fission. The IBs continue to divide, eventually forming huge *inclusion bodies* that can almost completely fill the host cells. (The presence of these characteristic inclusion bodies in conjunctival scrapings or genital secretions is the key to diagnosing chlamydial infection.) In the inclusion bodies, new EBs develop and mature. Within 24 to 48 hours, the host cells rupture and release the newly matured EBs, which, in turn, infect other cells.

Because most of its life cycle is spent inside human cells, the *Chlamydia* bacterium is difficult to destroy. Impress on the patient that therapy must continue a minimum of three weeks so that the bacteria can be eliminated while they're in the vulnerable EB stage, before they enter a host cell.

ment of choice; so far strains of chlamydiae resistant to this drug have not been isolated. But tetracycline is contraindicated for pregnant women and for neonates, because of its mottling effect on fetal and neonatal teeth. In such cases, erythromycin or sulfisoxazole can also be used.

Whatever agent is chosen, therapy must be long-term—at least three

weeks.[1,2] Be sure to impress this point on the patient, as a shorter duration of treatment is likely to fail. The patient who understands the potentially serious complications of continued infection, and why medication must be taken long after symptoms disappear, is more likely to comply with the therapy. Even when therapy is prolonged, however, reinfection is common, since the immune response to chlamydiae is inadequate. In order to prevent reinfection, asymptomatic carriers and sex partners of the patient also need to be treated.

Treating neonatal inclusion conjunctivitis is even more difficult. The silver nitrate used in most hospitals as prophylaxis for conjunctivitis does not seem to be totally effective against chlamydiae. In addition, silver nitrate itself frequently causes chemical conjunctivitis. Several groups have studied the efficacy of topical tetracycline and erythromycin, but results have been inconclusive.

Treatment failures may be due to poor administration of the eye drops or persistent reseeding of eyes with chlamydiae, as well as to antimicrobial ineffectiveness. You can help by making sure that antibacterial eye drops are properly administered to both eyes of the newborn, and by staying alert to any ocular infections that may suggest the presence of these bacteria.

Although there is great need for improved diagnostic and treatment protocols, current knowledge does give us the potential for intervening in this nationwide epidemic. Success depends on our commitment to screening and diagnosis, as well as our ability to convince patients to follow through with therapeutic regimens. In combination, these two ingredients can help stem the damage being caused by these insidious bacteria. ■

REFERENCES **1.** Holmes. K.K. The *chlamydia* epidemic. *JAMA* 245:1718. 1981. **2.** Schacter. J. Chlamydial infections: Parts I. II. III. *New Engl. J. Med.* 298:428. 490. 540. 1981. **3.** Davis. B. et al. *Microbiology.* Hagerstown. Md.: Harper & Row. 1980.

BIBLIOGRAPHY Arya. O.P. et al. Epidemiological and clinical correlates of chlamydial infections of the cervix *Br. J. Vener. Dis.* 57:118. April 1981. Hammerschlag. M.R. et al. Erythromycin ointment for ocular prophylaxis of neonatal chlamydial infections. *JAMA* 244:2291. 1981. Hunter. J.M. et al. *Chlamydia trachomatis* and *Ureaplasma urealyticum* in men attending a sexually transmitted diseases clinic. *Br. J. Vener. Dis.* 57:130. April 1981.

The "other" STDs

AIDS is not the only sexually transmitted disease to have burgeoned in the 1980s. Can you spot the symptoms of the five other much more common STDs? Can you answer the questions that your patients will have about treatment and transmission?

By Priscilla McElhose, RN, BSN, MN

The post-MI patient who breaks out with genital blisters, the trauma patient who develops a urethral discharge, the patient who's admitted for severe pelvic inflammatory disease—all have one thing in common: Each has a sexually transmitted disease.

While AIDS may be the most feared and best publicized STD, it is by no means the most common. In fact, while everyone talks about AIDS, up to one American in 10 has become infected with chlamydia, gonorrhea, syphilis, genital warts, or genital herpes.

The possible consequences of these five most prevalent STDs include sterility, miscarriage, birth defects, and, perhaps, cervical and other genital cancers.

Every nurse has an important part to play in the fight against sexually transmitted diseases. You need to recognize the symptoms and teach infected patients how to

THE AUTHOR, a nurse practitioner, has worked since 1979 at the Sexually Transmitted Disease Clinic at Harborview Medical Center in Seattle.

Produced by Jeanne DiPaola

comply with treatment and take measures to prevent further transmission. You must respond accurately and sensitively to your patient's pressing questions: "Is it curable? How can I tell my partner? Can I still have sex? Will it make me sterile?" The law also requires you to report certain cases of sexually transmitted disease to the health authorities.

Though these five diseases—two bacterial and three viral—are not as dramatic as AIDS, they are equally deserving of your careful attention.

Chlamydia:
The silent menace

Chlamydia, an infection caused by the *Chlamydia trachomatis* bacteria, strikes an estimated three million to five million Americans each year.

Within three weeks after becoming infected, men may experience burning on urination and a white or clear discharge from the penis, indicating urethral infection—or specifically, non-gonococcal urethritis, or NGU.

Women may develop a yellowish endocervical discharge, painful urination, or spotting after intercourse or between menstrual periods. Chlamydial infection of the rectum can produce itching, constipation, slight bleeding, and mucus-covered stools.

Patients who experience such early symptoms might be considered fortunate: Chlamydia's greatest threat by far lies in the fact that it's often asymptomatic.

As a result, the patient feels no need to seek treatment, and the disease may go undiagnosed until a complication sends him to see the physician.

In men that may be epididymitis—inflammation of the sperm ducts that can cause sterility—or Reiter's syndrome, which includes urethritis, conjunctivitis, arthritis, and skin lesions. Women may develop pelvic inflammatory disease (PID), which can result in infertility and increased risk of ectopic pregnancy.

Infants who are born to infected women are at risk. For a complete discussion of how STDs affect infants in utero and at birth, see the box on page 57.

Chlamydia can almost always be cured by a seven-day course of oral antibiotics. Most patients will receive tetracycline 500 mg qid or doxycycline (Doxy-Caps) 100 mg bid. Pregnant women, who should avoid these first-line drugs, may take erythromycin 500 mg four times a day.

Be sure the patient understands that the disease is dangerous even when asymptomatic. Stress the importance of completing the entire course of antibiotics to eradicate all bacteria. And make sure he knows how and when to take the medication. Tell the patient receiving tetracycline, for example, to take the drug one hour before or two hours after meals. Remind him to avoid dairy products, antacids, mineral supplements, and direct sunlight. Advise him to have follow-up cultures taken two to three weeks after finishing the medication.

Explain that chlamydial infections are transmitted only by sexual intercourse, never through casual contact. Encourage the patient to notify all sexual partners within the past three weeks, so they, too, can be treated. Urge abstinence from sex until follow-up cultures are negative and thereafter use of condoms lubricated with a spermicide containing nonoxynol-9 to prevent reinfection from chlamydia and other STDs.*

Gonorrhea: On the rise among heterosexuals

Nearly a million new cases of gonorrhea—or, "clap," as it's called on the street—are reported to public health officials each year. While the disease appears to be declining among homosexual men, it's increasing in all other groups.

Like chlamydia, gonorrhea is caused by bacterial infection. In this case, the infective organism is

*For more information on how to prevent the spread of STDs, see "What you and your patients need to know about safer sex" in the Sept. 1987 issue of **RN**.

a gram-negative diplococcus, *Neisseria gonorrhoeae.*

Most infected men usually develop symptoms of gonococcal urethritis—painful urination and a profuse yellowish discharge from the penis—within two to five days of initial infection. Only about half of infected women develop symptoms, which can include vaginal discharge and burning or pain on urination.

People can also acquire anorectal and pharyngeal gonococcal infections as a result of sexual activity. Anorectal gonorrhea is usually asymptomatic, but patients may experience itching, constipation, or blood or mucus in the stool. Pharyngeal infection occasionally causes sore throat.

Patients who remain untreated are at risk for the same complications as those with chlamydia—PID in women and, infrequently, epididymitis in men—as well as systemic gonorrheal infection, which can result in septicemia, arthritis, or skin lesions.

Preferred treatment for anogenital gonorrhea in women and heterosexual men is either amoxicillin 3 gm PO or ampicillin 3.5 gm PO, plus probenecid 1 gm PO. Since these patients often have concurrent chlamydial infections, they are also put on the seven-day regimen of tetracycline or doxycycline.

Homosexual men, who are more likely to have multisite gonorrheal infections, are given IM penicillin 4.8 million units or ceftriaxone sodium (Rocephin) 125 mg to 250 mg IM. Patients with anogenital infections caused by penicillin-resistant strains of gonorrhea are also given ceftriaxone, and ceftriaxone is used

as a first-line drug in some communities where resistant strains are common. Patients who are allergic to penicillin may well be allergic to ceftriaxone too: They receive spectinomycin 2 gm IM.

Most patients respond to treatment within 12 hours and experience complete resolution of symptoms within three days.

Inform the patient that you're required to report all cases of gonorrhea to public health officials and explain what kind of follow-up is customary in your area. In our community, someone from the department of health contacts each patient, gives information on the prevention of STDs, and asks for help in notifying recent sex partners that they've been exposed.

Instruct patients to avoid sex while they're receiving treatment and to have follow-up cultures taken a week after they've finished their medication.

Urge patients to use condoms to avoid future infection and to seek treatment promptly if symptoms recur. Remind women that they won't always have symptoms and urge them to go for screening if their partners become infected.

Syphilis: Resurgence of an ancient plague

Despite a widely held misconception that syphilis has been all but wiped out in this country, nearly 28,000 new cases were reported last year. The majority of patients are homosexual men. Some experts anticipate, however, that the rising incidence among heterosexuals may return the annual caseload to the 70,000 level of the early 1980s, before fear of AIDS brought about changes in gay sexual activity.

Syphilis, caused by the *Treponema pallidum* bacteria, is characterized by four well-defined stages. Symptoms of the earliest stage, primary syphilis, appear three weeks to 90 days after initial infection. Patients may first notice one or several painless, papular lesions on their genitals, anus, or mouth. The lesions, called chancres, break down into indurated ulcers with firm, raised borders and then disappear again within three weeks. Women with chancres on the cervix may never detect their presence.

After several more weeks or months, patients can progress to secondary syphilis. Its main symptom, which can last two to six weeks, is a skin rash that is highly variable—in fact, it can resemble almost anything.

The next stage, latent syphilis, can last up to 30 years. The patient will have no symptoms, though blood tests will remain positive.

The final stage, tertiary syphilis, can affect the heart and blood vessels, the brain and central nervous system, and occasionally the liver, bones, and skin. Complications in the central nervous system can cause seizures or convulsions; those in the heart can cause death.

Patients with primary, secondary, or early latent syphilis receive a single IM injection of benzathine penicillin G (Bicillin) 2.4 million units. Those who've been in the latent stage for longer than a year are given 7.2 million units IM, divided into three weekly doses. Patients with tertiary syphilis must be hospitalized for a 10-day regimen of IV penicillin G, 10 to 20 million units a day, followed by three weekly IM injections of benzathine penicillin G, 2.4 million units in each dose. Patients who have a history of adverse reaction to penicillin may be given oral tetracycline 500 mg four times a day for 15 to 30 days, depending on the stage of their illness.

With treatment, syphilis is curable at any stage. Up to 10% of patients, however, don't respond to the first round of antibiotics and may require a subsequent course of treatment with higher doses over a longer period of time. It's essential that patients receiving tetracycline understand the importance of adhering to the prolonged regimen, since missing only a few doses increases the chance of drug failure. Urge these patients to obtain repeat blood tests one, six, 12, and 24 months after therapy to be sure of a cure.

Caution all patients with primary or secondary syphilis about the possibility of a Jarisch-Herxheimer reaction, a flu-like syndrome that can develop within four hours of starting antibiotic therapy. Symptoms usually disappear within 24 hours.

Instruct patients with primary syphilis to avoid intercourse until all lesions are healed to keep from infecting their partners. Instruct those with primary and secondary syphilis to notify everyone they've had sex with since becoming infected. After the secondary stage, the disease is no longer contagious. Be sure to tell patients that you must report all cases of syphilis to public health authorities and explain local follow-up procedures.

To help patients avoid future infection, encourage them to check all partners for lesions or rashes. Also stress the importance of seeking prompt medical attention if symptoms recur. Be sure your patients understand that just because lesions clear up without treatment, it does not mean the infection has gone away.

Genital warts: A strong link to cancer

Each year an estimated 400,000 to 600,000 Americans develop genital warts—a disease caused by the human papilloma virus.

Warts—one or more painless, soft, fleshy, growths—usually appear one or two months after exposure, but can take as long as nine months to incubate. Some warts are so small they can be identified only with a colposcopic exam of the cervix and vagina or a Pap smear.

Although much remains to be learned about how the papilloma virus progresses, doctors have observed that the warm, moist environment in the genital area seems to favor wart growth. Outbreaks appear to be exacerbated during pregnancy and in patients with defective immune systems.

Patients with a history of genital warts may be at increased risk for certain types of cancer. The human papilloma virus is associated with up to 90% of cervical malignancies and may play a role in cancers of the vagina, anus, vulva, and penis.

There's no cure for genital warts, and treatments used to resolve symptoms can be uncomfortable and vary in effectiveness. Cryotherapy with liquid nitrogen offers the best combination of effectiveness and freedom from unpleasant effects. Electrocautery, excision, and laser surgery are used, but they're more painful and carry more risk of scarring.

Many doctors treat warts with weekly topical applications of 10% podophyllin in tincture of benzoin. The patient leaves the medication on four to six hours and then washes it off. Podophyllin, however, can be locally or systemically toxic and should not be used extensively on mucosal tissue or during pregnancy. Patients with warts inside the urethra may be given antimetabolites, such as 5-fluorouracil.

If a patient on your unit has genital warts, urge him to visit his doctor or a sex disease clinic after discharge. Tell him that treatment may be needed for up to eight weeks to destroy the growths. All recent sex partners should be examined and female partners should have a Pap smear.

Recommend use of a condom during intercourse while treatment is going on and for several months afterward, when the rate of recurrence is high. Urge female patients to have regular gynecologic exams, including a Pap test, to screen for cervical abnormalities.

Herpes: Discomfort, but not doom

Genital herpes is a disease caused by the herpes simplex virus, types I and II. Each year there are between 400,000 and 600,000 new cases of herpes. Some 20 million people have yearly recurrences.

Primary herpes is characterized by one or more genital blisters that usually appear seven to 10 days after initial infection. The blisters progress to shallow, painful ulcerations that resolve without treatment in about two to four weeks. Other symptoms may include muscle pain, headache, and swollen, tender lymph nodes in the groin.

Symptoms are milder during recurrences than during a primary attack. In fact, patients with histories of childhood cold sores or other non-genital herpes outbreaks usually escape altogether the severe symptoms of primary genital herpes. In recurrences, there are fewer, less painful lesions that heal in a shorter period of time—typically, four to seven days. Between outbreaks, patients are asymptomatic.

The most common complication of genital herpes is the spread of lesions to other sites, usually the mouth, eyes, or cuticles. Rarely, patients with primary herpes can develop central nervous system complications, including stiff neck, headache, intolerance to light, or aseptic meningitis.

Treatment is aimed at speeding resolution of symptoms and reducing the frequency and severity of recurrences. Patients with primary herpes infections receive oral acyclovir (Zovirax) 200 mg five times a day for 10 days. Those suffering a severe recurrence may be given the same regimen, though usually for only five days. For patients with frequent recurrences—six or more a year—the physician may order a continuous regimen of acyclovir 200 mg two to five times a day. Pregnant patients who experience a severe first attack of genital her-

STDs in pregnancy: Effects on the baby

Sexually transmitted organisms can cause a host of serious complications during pregnancy, including miscarriage, premature rupture of the membranes, and premature delivery. The organisms can also be passed to the infant in utero or during delivery, sometimes with devastating results. The effects on the baby differ with each type of infection:

Chlamydia. Infants exposed to chlamydial infection in utero often develop perinatal complications—pneumonia or conjunctivitis, for example.

Gonorrhea. Anal, vaginal, and nasopharyngeal infections are common in infants exposed to gonorrhea in utero. Those exposed during delivery are at risk of ocular infection.

Syphilis. Survival rates are poor for infants born with symptoms of congenital syphilis, which include skeletal abnormalities and defects in the major organ systems. Even those who are asymptomatic at birth can develop complications later, unless they receive treatment.

Genital warts. An infected mother can transmit the virus to her child during vaginal delivery. Symptoms of infection in the newborn include warts on the genitals or in the throat.

Herpes. A mother with active genital herpes at the time of delivery can also pass the virus to her infant. The effects on the child can range from a localized infection of the eyes, skin, or mucous membranes to life-threatening systemic complications, often involving the central nervous system.

To prevent such heartbreaking consequences, women who have STDs should notify their doctor or clinic as soon as they become pregnant. Good, early prenatal care and extra precautions at delivery—in some cases, for example, delivery by Cesarean section—can help reduce the risk of infecting the baby.*

*For more information on how to protect newborns from contracting herpes from their mothers, see "Saving the baby when Mom has herpes" in the Oct. 1985 issue of **RN**.

pes are treated with a topical ointment form of acyclovir, since they must avoid the oral drug.

Suggest other local treatments patients can use at home to supplement drug therapy—such as, frequent washing and drying of genitals with a warm, gentle soap and drying them with a warm hair dryer. Stress the importance of washing hands after using the bathroom to avoid spreading the infection. Patients can also reduce the frequency of recurrences by maintaining their overall health and avoiding stress as much as possible.

Counseling is especially important for patients with herpes. Reassure them that having the disease need not mean the end of their sex lives. Discuss when and how they might tell prospective partners about their disease. You can suggest, for example, that they put off having sex until they know a new partner well enough to discuss

so sensitive an issue. Suggest, too, that they not wait until lovemaking has already been started to initiate the discussion.

Urge patients to avoid sex during outbreaks. During the year after the first outbreak, providing they use condoms to contain shedding virus, patients can have intercourse in the symptom-free periods without too much danger of infecting partners. Subsequently, the rate of viral shedding during symptom-free periods declines, and condoms—though they will maximize safety—may no longer be needed.

If your patient seems unable or unwilling to accept the changes in lifestyle the disease demands, you might want to refer him for psychological counseling. Some communities have support groups for herpes sufferers and hotlines to answer questions about the disease. Find out what services are available in your area and prepare the informa-

tion as a handout to give patients when they're discharged .

Good nursing support is important to all patients with sexually transmitted diseases. By helping them understand the symptoms, treatment, and possible complications of their infection and teaching them how to avoid passing it on to their partners, you can give your patients a much needed feeling of control over their disease—and their lives. ∎

BIBLIOGRAPHY Corey, L. et al. Genital herpes simplex virus infection. *Ann. Intern. Med.* 98:6, June 1983. Handsfield, H.H. et al. *Sexually Transmitted Diseases: Clinical Practice Guidelines*, Seattle: King County Department of Public Health, 1985. Handsfield, H.H. Sexually transmitted diseases. *Hospital Practice*, Jan. 1982. Holmes, K.K. et al. (eds.) *Sexually Transmitted Diseases*, New York: McGraw-Hill, 1984. Holmes, K.K. and Handsfield, H.H. Sexually transmitted diseases. In *Harrison's Principles of Internal Medicine*, Petersdorf, R.G. et al. (eds.), New York: McGraw-Hill, 1983. U.S. Department of Health and Human Services Public Health Service, *Sexually Transmitted Diseases Summary*, Atlanta: Centers for Disease Control, 1986. Wiesner, P.J. Gonorrhea. *Cutis*, March 1981.

When your pregnant patient has diabetes

Each year in this country, nearly 90,000 pregnant women develop diabetes. For these women, good nursing care can make the difference between a happy and a tragic outcome.
By Carolyn Robertson, RN, MSN

Sixty years ago, before synthetic insulin, few diabetic women conceived. Those who did often didn't survive pregnancy.

Today, most diabetic women can have complication-free pregnancies and deliver healthy babies–with extensive monitoring and guidance. Your goal is to help the patient control blood sugar levels in spite of pregnancy-related alterations in nutrient needs and metabolism.

How pregnancy affects blood glucose

Every diabetic woman should consult her doctor before conceiving. Every woman without a history of diabetes should be screened for hyperglycemia or glucose intolerance no later than 28 weeks after she conceives. That's because changes that occur in pregnancy can easily compromise blood sugar control.

A woman needs to eat more, of course, when she's pregnant. In addition, the body increases levels of hormones—including cortisol, estrogen, progesterone, and human placental lactogen—that raise resistance to insulin. Also, from the second trimester on, the placenta manufactures an enzyme that destroys insulin.

With increased food intake and decreased insulin effectiveness, it's easy to see that a diabetic woman needs to intensify her regimen for controlling hyperglycemia during pregnancy. Furthermore, some 5% of nondiabetic women develop diabetes during pregnancy because they fail to produce enough extra insulin to compensate for their body's less efficient use of the hormone. Women with gestational diabetes—that which first appears during pregnancy—must learn im-

mediately to avoid hyperglycemia.

The consequences of failure to adjust can be grave. Hyperglycemia during the first trimester can disrupt fetal organ formation. High blood sugar during the second trimester puts the mother at risk for pyelonephritis and overproduction of amniotic fluid. In the final trimester, hyperglycemia can cause the fetus to develop an overly large pancreas and hyperinsulinemia. These abnormalities can lead to large body size (macrosomia), intrauterine death, neonatal hypoglycemia, respiratory distress syndrome, and electrolyte imbalance.

How to maintain safe glucose levels

To protect the fetus in the crucial first stages of growth, doctors recommend that a diabetic woman delay conception until she has maintained normal blood glucose levels for at least a month. From conception to delivery, all women should keep blood glucose levels at about 80-110 mg/dl.

The primary tool for maintaining blood sugar in this safe range is diet. The typical pregnant diabetic should plan to gain 25-30 pounds by her ninth month. A nutritionist tells her to eat 25-30 cal/kg of her pre-pregnancy weight each day, 40 to 50 percent of it in the form of complex carbohydrates—e.g., vegetables, cereals, breads, grains—and the rest proteins and fats. You should help her select appropriate foods from these groups. Emphasize the need to shun candy, honey, molasses, and other simple carbohydrates. Advise frequent meals—three meals and four snacks a day is

THE AUTHOR is a diabetes clinical nurse specialist at the New York University Medical Center in New York City. She's also an educator and diabetes manager working with a group of endocrinologists in collaborative practice for high-risk diabetics.

Produced by David Anderson

Special tests for the pregnant diabetic

Whenever a woman presents with diabetes, either at her first visit or during the course of her pregnancy, she should receive a complete physical exam and have a special laboratory workup. In addition to the usual prenatal tests, the physician should request renal function studies, including a BUN, and a 24-hour urine for creatinine and protein. She should also have baseline ophthalmologic studies done to detect retinopathy. The physician will also order a glycosylated hemoglobin, which tells what the woman's mean glucose level has been over the past 1-2 months. These exams will be repeated periodically, especially if the woman has had long-standing diabetes.

Fetal surveillance begins in the first trimester. Besides the usual prenatal monitoring of uterine size and fetal position and movement, patients with antecedent diabetes receive biochemical and sonographic evaluations to rule out anomalies. Maternal levels of alphafetoprotein—an antigen normally produced by the fetus— are checked at 15 to 18 weeks to screen for neural tube defects. A fetal echocardiogram is often done at 18 to 20 weeks to assess cardiac structure and function. Clinicians will continue to monitor the fetus via serial sonograms from the second trimester onward.

Physicians begin non-stress testing and measuring serum levels of the hormone estriol in the third trimester because these are indicators of fetal well-being. One or both of these tests will be done several times a week by the 38th week. The doctor may also perform an amniocentesis to determine fetal lung maturity. A lecithin/sphingomyelin ratio of 2.5 to 3.0/1.0 indicates such maturity if the mother is diabetic. However, if phosphatidylglycerol is also present in the amniotic fluid, a lecithin/sphingomylin ratio of 2.0/1.0 indicates fetal lung maturity.

good—to avoid blood sugar swings.

The patient with newly diagnosed gestational diabetes should record everything she eats—how much, when, and where. Review these notes with her to learn how her dietary components affect her blood sugar levels. She can discontinue them when she achieves reliable blood sugar control.

Most pregnant women with antecedent diabetes and many with gestational diabetes must supplement dietary measures with insulin injections. Oral hypoglycemic agents cross the placental barrier and can harm the fetus.

Insulin requirements increase as pregnancy advances. For example, a woman who takes 0.6 units/kg/day before becoming pregnant—a common dose—usually requires 0.7 units/kg/day during the first trimester, 0.8 units/kg/day during the second, and up to 1.0 unit/kg/day at term. Whatever the patient's starting dose, she'll have to taper it up as pregnancy hormones antagonize insulin intake.

Teach the patient to balance insulin injections, meals, and snacks, as explained in "When the patient is also diabetic," **RN**, July 1987.

Normal activity lowers blood sugar levels, but caution against overexercise: The effect of intense activity on the fetus of a diabetic mother is unknown.

Monitor carefully, and react promptly

The patient needs to check her capillary blood sugar levels before breakfast and after each meal. She may need to take additional measurements before each meal and snack when control is inconsistent.

Teach her to use a glucose monitoring device such as Accuchek, or a measuring system—for example, Chemstrips or Glucoscan—and review technique with her when she comes in for clinic visits. Tell her to write down each reading and bring this record to each visit.

Whenever your patient's blood glucose level tops 125 mg/dl, she should call her doctor. The fetus probably won't begin to suffer unless blood sugar goes over 140 mg/dl, but a rising trend needs to be reversed as soon as possible.

Show your patient how to monitor for urinary ketones. She should do this at least once a day. Ketones in the urine means that body tissues aren't receiving enough glucose to function normally. A review of blood glucose tests can indicate the right response. If urinary ketones are present and blood glucose levels are low or normal, the patient needs to eat more carbohydrates. If glucose levels are high, she may need additional insulin.

Teach your patient and her family the symptoms of blood sugar abnormalities. Hyperglycemia causes thirst, nausea, weakness, lethargy, and polyuria. Hypoglycemia causes hunger, nausea, irritability, headache, sweating, and tachycardia. It can also produce neuroglycopenia, which makes the patient insensitive to those symptoms she has.

Hyperglycemia and hypoglyce-mia may be corrected by adjusting dietary intake, insulin dosage, or both. For high blood sugar, the doctor may recommend reducing or omitting one snack. For low blood sugar, he may assign an extra snack—like milk or bread. Discour-age simple sugars unless blood sug-ar falls below 40 mg/dl. These foods can raise levels too high. If severe hypoglycemia occurs with confu-sion or unconsciousness, glucagon should be injected. To learn how to adjust insulin to smooth out a blood sugar peak or valley, see page 21.

You'll have to give all this infor-mation quickly to the woman with gestational diabetes. The sooner she learns about dietary principles, medication regimens, and symp-tom recognition and response, the better for her and her infant.

The diabetic patient needs much emotional support during pregnan-cy. The woman with gestational di-abetes needs even more, as she must learn to cope with an unfore-seen threat to her and her unborn infant. Too, she's disappointed that she must exercise strict self-control at a time when she may have antici-pated a spell of indulgence.

Don't permit the patient to de-spair even if her blood sugar tran-siently rises above 140 mg/dl: In this case the fetus will certainly be stressed, but the stress may not significantly affect development.

When it's time to deliver

Today doctors encourage many dia-betic women to carry their babies to term. They may recommend ear-ly delivery by planned induction or

Fine tuning the insulin regimen

Suppose the patient's capillary blood glucose reading peaks or drops outside of the desired range every afternoon. When dietary modification doesn't solve the prob-lem, you conclude that she needs to adjust an insulin dose—but which one? The decision is complex because the regimen includes several daily injections of overlap-ping short-, medium-, and long-acting preparations. To help you decide correctly, the chart below identifies the specific injections that influence each blood glucose reading throughout the day.

If the blood sugar level is undesirable	Adjust this dose if the patient's regimen is:	
	Mixed split doses of short-acting/medium acting insulin	**Mixed split doses of short-acting/long-acting insulin**
While fasting	Medium-acting insulin taken either before supper or before bed the evening before.	Long-acting insulin taken the morning before.
After breakfast	Short-acting insulin taken before breakfast.	Sort-acting insulin taken before breakfast.
Before lunch	Medium- and short-acting insulin taken before breakfast.	Short-acting insulin taken before breakfast and long-acting insulin taken before supper the day before.
After lunch	Medium-acting insulin taken before breakfast	Short-acting insulin taken before lunch.
Before supper	Medium-acting insulin taken before breakfast.	Short-acting insulin taken before lunch and long-acting insulin taken before supper yesterday.
After supper	Short-acting insulin taken before supper.	Short-acting insulin taken before supper.
Before bedtime	Short-acting insulin taken before supper and medium-acting insulin, (if taken).	Short-acting insulin taken before supper and long-acting insulin taken that morning.

Cesarean section, if the mother has poor control over her blood sugar levels or the infant shows distress.

Doctors prefer to avoid spontaneous delivery when a diabetic has proliferative retinopathy or severe renal or cardiac disease. These complications can lead to retinal hemorrhage, hypertensive crisis, or heart strain if the woman vomits, gags, or performs a Valsalva maneuver during labor or delivery.

When the diabetic patient presents in spontaneous labor, ask when she took her last insulin dose.

For planned inductions and Cesareans, the morning dose of insulin is reduced or witheld and the patient made NPO. Whether delivery is spontaneous or induced, safety depends upon keeping blood glucose levels of 70-100 mg/dl throughout.

To control blood sugar during labor and delivery, the doctor may order an IV line for insulin and glucose. Monitor sugar levels hourly and urinary ketones often. Watch for hypoglycemic symptoms.

Most diabetics need intravenous glucose during labor as the body burns off large amounts of calories to provide energy for contractions. Without enough glucose to fuel contractions, labor may be prolonged.

Monitor the patient closely for 48 to 72 hours after delivery.

How to help after delivery

When gestational diabetes develops during pregnancy, it usually clears up once the placenta is expelled. Some 60% of these patients, however, develop permanent diabetes within 15 years. Fortunately, most can avoid hyperglycemia by diet alone and without the use of medications.

Advise the patient with gestational diabetes to have a follow-up two-hour 75 gm glucose tolerance test six to eight weeks post partum. Inform her that she is at increased risk of this complication during subsequent pregnancies. In addition, encourage her to seek prenatal care early should she conceive again.

Inform her that oral contraceptives, steroids, and thiazide diuretics might lower her glucose tolerance. Encourage her to hold as closely as possible to her ideal body weight, adhere to a healthful, prudent diet, and exercise on a regular basis.

Patients with antecedent diabetes can take as little as 48 hours or as long as a month to revert to their pre-pregnancy insulin needs. Postpartum glucose control is complicated by the new mother's altered sleep and eating patterns. Breastfeeding mothers require more calories—about 500 more a day—and may also need more insulin, per-

Screening for gestational diabetes

Gestational diabetes is so dangerous that the National Diabetes Association and the American College of Obstetrics and Gynecology recommend that all women be screened for it between the 24th and 28th week. Women who are at high risk—because of a previous history of gestational diabetes or spilling sugar in urine, multiple pregnancies, a history of giving birth to infants weighing nine pounds or more, or age 35 or older—should be screened at 16, 24, and 32 weeks.

Urine testing for glycosuria, the easiest test to perform, is not very reliable. The absence of sugar in the urine doesn't preclude an elevated blood sugar level, nor does glycosuria guarantee that the blood sugar level is above normal limits. That's because renal function changes during pregnancy.

Fasting blood sugars provide limited information. Two plasma values above 105 mg/dl are diagnostic of gestational diabetes. However, patients with fasting levels lower than this may still have inadequate post-prandial blood sugar control.

Random blood sugars or unsupervised post-prandial blood sugars are difficult to interpret, because the doctor can't usually know the exact time and carbohydrate content of the patient's last meal.

The 50 gm glucose challenge measures the blood sugar level one hour after the patient drinks a solution containing 50 gm of glucose. If it's above 140 mg/dl, the patient may have diabetes. The doctor then administers a formal three hour 100 gm glucose tolerance test to validate the diagnosis.

The three-hour glucose tolerance test requires careful patient preparation. For three days prior to the test, the patient follows an unrestricted diet that includes a minimum of 150-250 gm/day of carbohydrates, depending on the patient's weight. She then fasts for 10-14 hours, and the doctor measures her fasting blood sugar. If it's above 105 mg/dl, she has gestational diabetes.

Next the patient drinks a solution containing 100 gm of glucose, after which she must remain seated and avoid smoking for three hours. At one, two, and three hours, her blood sugar should be below 190 mg/dl, 160 mg/dl, and 145 mg/dl. If she misses any two of these limits, she has gestational diabetes.

haps 0.7 units/kg/day. Insulin does not cross into breast milk, therefore, the infant shouldn't be affected by the mother's increased insulin requirements. However, if the mother's blood sugar level becomes elevated, so will the glucose content of her breast milk–and this may have long-term adverse consequences for the child.

Frequently, the new mother becomes anxious about her inability to control blood sugar levels tightly. Reassure her that a temporary lapse in glucose control will not present any danger for her. Nonpregnant diabetic women can safely run blood sugar levels 20 to 30 mg/dl higher than pregnant diabetic women.

At each stage of pregnancy, the diabetic patient needs your support and guidance so she can effectively care for herself and her unborn child. ■

BIBLIOGRAPHY American Diabetes Association Workshop: Conference on gestational diabetes, summary and recommendations. *Diabetes Care* 3:499, May 1980. Burrow, G. and Ferri, T., eds. *Medical Complications in Pregnancy.* Philadelphia: W.B. Saunders, Inc., 1982. Jovanovic, L. et al. Effect of euglycemia on the outcome of pregnancy in insulin-dependent diabetic women as compared with normal control subjects. *Am. J. Med.* 71:921, Dec. 1981. Karllson and Kjellmer. Outcome of diabetic pregnancies in relation to the mother's blood sugar level. *Am. J. Obstet. Gynecol.* 112:213, Jan. 15, 1972. O'Sullivan, J. Establishing criteria for gestational diabetes. *Diabetes Care* 3:437, May 1980. Pederson, J. Fetal mortality in diabetics in relation to management during the later part of pregnancy. *Acta Endocrinology* 15:282, March 15, 1954. Peterson, C.M. *Diabetes Management in the 80's.* New York: P.W. Communications, 1982. Seeds, ed. Diabetes in pregnancy. *Clin. Obstet. Gynecol.* 24:1981. Skyler, J.S. et al. Blood glucose control during pregnancy. *Diabetes Care* 3:69, May 1980. Symposium on blood glucose monitoring. *Diabetes Care* 4:392, 1981. U.S. Department of Health and Human Services. *The prevention and treatment of diabetes—A guide for primary care practitioners.* Washington, D.C.: U.S. Government Printing Office, 1983.

Controlling the dangers of epidural analgesia

Epidural pain relief isn't just for OB patients anymore.
Here's what precautions to take when you tend epidural lines.
By Linda Dunajcik, RN, BSN

The practice of administering regional analgesia through an epidural catheter has come a long way since obstetricians first used it 20 years ago to provide pain relief during labor and delivery. Today, many patients receive epidural analgesia to control the pain of thoracic, intra-abdominal, orthopedic, vascular, and other surgical procedures. It's also used for chronic pain.

Epidural analgesia's popularity is easily explained. Properly managed, it provides dependable, long-acting, site-specific pain relief with low doses of drugs. It reduces the threat of systemic side effects—such as respiratory depression—that are usually associated with general anesthesia.

Like many of today's sophisticated medical techniques, however, epidural analgesia leaves very little room for mistakes. You must know the necessary precautions to observe when you assist at the placement of the epidural catheter, and

THE AUTHOR is a med/surg nurse educator at the University of Missouri Hospital and Clinics in Columbia, Mo.

Produced by David Anderson

also when you tend the epidural lines. And you have to teach the patient to alert you to any impending complications.

Placing the catheter, positioning the patient

The anesthesiologist may insert the epidural catheter either in the operating room or at the patient's bedside. He may request the patient to sit up and lean forward, or he may have him lie in a fetal position. Both of these postures extend the spine, widening the spaces between vertebrae.

The physician injects lidocaine into the skin over an intervertebral space, and waits until the medication takes effect—in approximately 15 minutes. Then he inserts an epidural needle and advances it to the epidural space, which is located between the periosteum of the spinal canal and the dura mater of the spinal cord.

He then threads a catheter through the needle 2 to 3 cm into the epidural space. The catheter is anchored with a sterile dressing and tape.

Every caregiver must employ strict sterile technique during the entire procedure to prevent introducing infection into the spinal cord.

The downward course of pain relief

Once the catheter is in place, local anesthetics and narcotics can be given through it.

When local anesthetics come into contact with sensory nerve roots in the epidural space, they block pain impulses. The patient feels no pain in areas served by those nerves.

Narcotics, once introduced into the epidural space, pass through the dura mater to the dorsal horn of the spinal cord. Locking onto opiate receptors there, they block ascending pain impulses, desensitizing the patient from the injection downward. Raising the head of the bed 30° will prevent upward migration of the drug in the spinal cord—and, thus, respiratory depression.

Most often, you'll administer epidural analgesia by continuous infusion. An infusion pump assures even flow of medication, preventing slackenings that may reduce pain relief or surges that can produce complications.

How to set up a continuous infusion

Connect the pump tubing to a micron filter—a catch size of 0.22 microns is good—to intercept undissolved particles. Then connect the tubing to the epidural infusion bag. Purge the line and filter, then attach the line to the catheter.

Label the tubing, the infusion bag, and the front of the pump with tape reading "EPIDURAL." This helps all caregivers avoid confusing the epidural line with other similar-looking intravenous lines. Minimizing the chances of such confusion is crucial: Accidental epidural infusion of IV solutions—such as vasodilators, antibiotics, and chemotherapy agents—could damage or destroy nerve tissue, possibly paralyzing or killing the patient.

Tape over all injection ports connected to the epidural line. This, too, safeguards against accidental injection into the epidural space.

How to administer a continuous infusion

Whenever you give any intravenous or epidural solution to a patient with an epidural line, ask a colleague to confirm the purpose of all lines and double-check that the medication goes into the right one.

Before starting an epidural infusion, make certain the label shows the correct drug, dosage, and expiration date. Confirm the indication of an epidural route, and be sure the solution is preservative-free. Even small amounts of preserva-

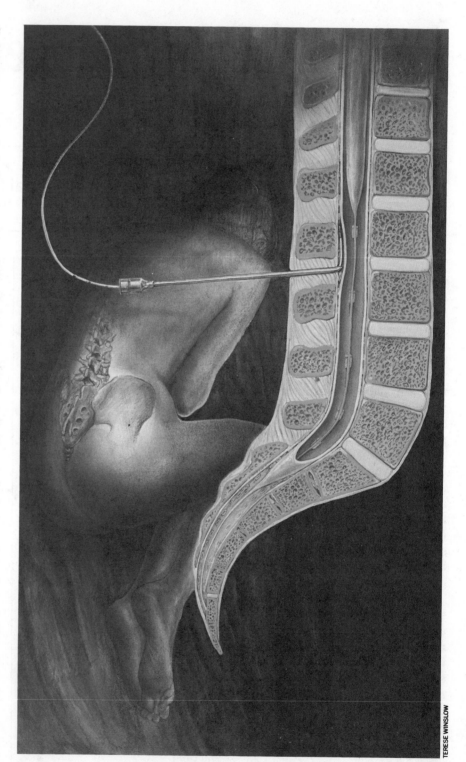

TERESE WINSLOW

How to prevent infection of the epidural site

Exercise strict aseptic technique whenever you handle the epidural catheter, infusion lines, connections, and solutions. Wash your hands with an antiseptic soap and water before assisting with insertion or changing your patient's dressing, solution, or tubing. Use sterile gloves, masks, and drapes during the epidural insertion.

Prior to the insertion, prep the epidural insertion site with an antiseptic (i.e., povidone-iodine) employing gentle friction. After insertion cover the site with a sterile dressing. Transparent occlusive dressings are best because they help in the daily inspection of the site. Change the dressing every 72 hours, or whenever it becomes non-occlusive. Timing and dating the dressing will help you keep track of when the next change is needed.

Change the tubing and filter of continuous infusions every 48 hours. If your filters are effective for only 24 hours, change them daily at the same time you hang a new infusion bag. Once opened, infusion solutions expire in 24 hours.

Assess the epidural site at least daily—every shift is even better. Gently palpate the dressing. If the patient has excessive pain or tenderness or an unexplained fever, inspect the site visually and notify the anesthesiologist.

Don't reconnect lines that have been accidentally disconnected and contaminated. Cap the line and notify your anesthesiologist. Many doctors remove contaminated lines to prevent possible complications of spinal meningitis or abscess.

tive can damage the spinal cord.

To avoid giving an accidental bolus, never purge an epidural line while it's connected to the catheter. A narcotic bolus may flow upward in the spinal cord, and if it gets too high it may cause respiratory depression. Too much local anesthetic will extend the block to large motor nerves, causing temporary paralysis in the area receiving analgesia.

After purging the line, tape all connections to prevent accidental disconnection and contamination of the epidural solution.

Avoid these dangers when giving a bolus

Some hospitals allow nurses to give drugs in bolus through an epidural catheter. Before you do so, check the line placement by gentle aspiration with a sterile syringe. If the epidural catheter is properly positioned, you will not aspirate fluid.

Aspiration of clear fluid may indicate that the catheter has drifted into the intrathecal space. Bloody aspirate may indicate displacement into the vascular system. In either case, don't administer the epidural bolus, but call the anesthesiologist.

How to monitor for problems

If you've used sterile technique and taken precautions to make sure that you're giving the right medication in the right amount through the right line, the patient's epidural analgesia should proceed smoothly.

Nevertheless, you must monitor

for common complications. Teach the patient to notify you if he develops any of the following symptoms:

Headache. If your patient complains of a headache, have him slowly sit up. If the pain becomes more intense as he rises, it's probably a spinal headache. The most likely explanation is that the catheter has punctured the dura, causing a leakage of cerebrospinal fluid. You may confirm this hypothesis by observing clear drainage on the dressing or by aspirating the line for clear fluid.

Fever, nuchal rigidity, mental changes. If you see these signs of systemic infection, meningitis, or spinal abscess, notify the anesthesiologist. He may order antibiotics and discontinue the epidural catheter to prevent the infection from spreading into the epidural space.

Excessive pain or tenderness at the infusion site. Observe and palpate the infusion site every shift for signs of local infection. The anesthesiologist may respond with antibiotics or discontinuation of the catheter.

These complications can strike any patient

You should also assess the patient for signs that he's getting too much medication or getting it in the wrong place. Watch for:

Hypotension. Low blood pressure most commonly occurs as a side effect of local anesthetics. It can also occur when narcotics go into the bloodstream due to intravascular catheter displacement.

Take blood pressure hourly for the first 24 hours after starting or increasing a continuous infusion, and thereafter every two hours. Take blood presure immediately after giving a bolus of medication, and thereafter every 20 minutes. Continue assessing at regular intervals until the drug's duration of effectiveness is past.*

If the patient's blood pressure falls lower than the anesthesiologist tells you it should—common thresholds for patients without any complicating disease would be 90 systolic or 60 diastolic—notify the doctor. Place the patient's head flat. Elevate his legs and manipulate them through passive range-of-motion exercises to send blood to the vital organs.

The anesthesiologist may order IV fluids to raise the blood pressure. He may order oxygen to avoid hypoxia.

If hypotension is a side effect of a local anesthetic, the doctor may order an intravenous sympathomimetic drug such as ephedrine or mephentermine sulfate (Wyamine sulfate) to reverse it. If it's due to intravascular infusion of a narcotic, he'll remove the catheter.

Respiratory depression. This serious complication usually results from administration of too much narcotic. Occasionally, it results from too much local anesthetic or direct infusion of epidural analgesic doses into the intrathecal space due to a displaced catheter.

Assess your patient's respiratory function each time you take his blood pressure. Check respiratory rate and depth, and look at skin col-

*Duration times of local anesthetics are in the article by Nicholls cited in the bibliography; those of common narcotics are in the article by Leib and Hurtig.

Where epidural narcotics stop pain

Sites of action differ for epidurally administered local anesthetics and narcotics. Local anesthetics cut off pain signals primarily in the dorsal root ganglion, before they enter the spinal cord. Narcotics block pain pathways inside the spinal cord by occupying opiate receptors in the dorsal horn.

Different sites and modes of action give rise to different side effects and potential complications. The anesthetist must take care not to give too much local anesthetic because the excess will spread forward in the epidural space. If the drug blocks outgoing motor signals at the ventral root, severe hypotension and loss of muscle responsiveness can result. Excess narcotic may be carried by the CSF to the respiratory centers of the brain.

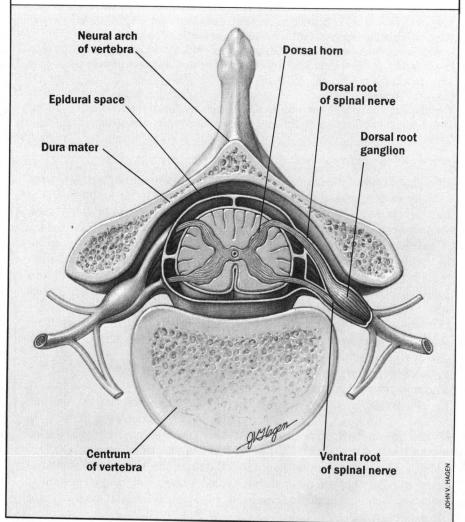

Neural arch of vertebra

Epidural space

Dura mater

Dorsal horn

Dorsal root of spinal nerve

Dorsal root ganglion

Centrum of vertebra

Ventral root of spinal nerve

JOHN V. HAGEN

or. Ask the patient if he's experiencing difficulty breathing. Keep abreast of the results of any blood gas analyses the anesthesiologist may order: An elevated carbon dioxide concentration could be a clue to incipient respiratory depression.

Inform the anesthesiologist of any decline in your patient's respiratory function. If necessary, manually ventilate the patient with an ambu bag and oxygen.

If respiratory depression results from the administration of an epidural narcotic, intravenous naloxone (Narcan) may be ordered. If it follows administration of a local anesthetic, the anesthesiologist may discontinue the drug. He will remove the catheter if its tip has slipped into the intrathecal space. If respiratory paralysis occurs, he will intubate your patient and place him on ventilator assistance until the effects of the drug wear off.

Urine retention. Assess your patient's urine output twice each shift. If it's low and the patient's bladder is distended, try to promote voiding by placing his hand in warm water. If this doesn't work, tell the doctor. He may order subcutaneous bethanechol chloride or catheterization to get flow started.

Numbness or tingling in the lower legs. The patient may experience these symptoms if the epidural catheter rubs against neural tissue. Notify the anesthesiologist, who may remove the catheter.

Beware these effects of local anesthetics

You must be aware of certain potential complications that are much more likely when the patient receives local anesthetics epidurally:

Neurological impairment. Assess this patient for loss of motor ability and insensitivity to touch, pressure, and temperature. These deficits are signs that large motor nerve fibers are being affected—an indication that the dose may be too great.

If your patient has motor weakness, notify the anesthesiologist immediately. He may reduce the dose, or if he finds that there has been displacement into the intrathecal space, he may remove the catheter.

Circumoral tingling, tinnitis, dizziness, blurred vision, tremors, or convulsions. These signs of systemic toxicity are related to accidental intravascular administration of epidural local anesthetics. Convulsions could lead to hypoxia and eventual cardiovascular collapse.

If you suspect systemic toxicity, stop the infusion and notify the anesthesiologist; have a co-worker notify him if you're occupied with providing supportive measures for convulsions. The doctor may order intravenous diazepam and O_2 by face mask for convulsions. He will discontinue the line if it has been displaced intravascularly.

Control side effects from narcotics

Patients who are receiving narcotics epidurally are vulnerable to some special complications in addition to respiratory depression.

Pruritis, nausea, and vomiting. These are common side effects of narcotics. Use clean, lightweight linens to reduce itching. Give diphenydramine (Benadryl) or other antipruritic drugs and antiemetics as ordered. Protect the patient from aspiration by turning him on his side and elevating the head of his bed.

Notify the anesthesiologist if the side effects persist. He may order a continuous low-dosage intravenous infusion of naloxone.

Sending the patient on his way

To protect your patient against falls, check his balance and motor strength before you allow him to walk.

When the time comes to remove the catheter, have the patient flex his back as he did for its placement. Check the catheter closely to make sure that its black tip has come out with the rest of the instrument. If the tip is missing, alert the anesthesiologist as soon as possible. An abandoned tip may move around in the patient's body and cause neural deficits. Surgery may be necessary to get it out.

If you follow all these guidelines closely, your patient should have a safe and pain-free time while in the hospital. ∎

BIBLIOGRAPHY Alberico, J. Breaking the chronic pain cycle. *Am. J. Nurs.* 10:1222, Oct. 1984. Kotelko, D.M. et al. Epidural morphine analgesia after cesarean delivery. *Obstet. Gynecol.* 63:409, March 1984. Bromage, P.R., et al. Epidural narcotics for post-operative analgesia. *Anesth. and Analg.* 59:473, July 1980. Bromage, P.R., et al. Non-respiratory side effects of epidural morphine. *Anesth. and Analg.*, 61:490, June 1982. Nicholls, E.T. et al. Epidural anesthesia for the woman in labor, *Am. J. Nurs.* 10:1826, Oct. 1981. Grinde, J.W. et al. Pain management by epidural analgesia: The challenge for nursing. *Heart and Lung,* 13:105, March 1984. Hurtig, J.B. and Leib, R.A. Epidural and intrathecal narcotics for pain management. *Heart and Lung.* 13:164, March 1985. MacLaughlin, S. Epidural anesthesia for obstetric patients. *JOGN,* 1:9, Jan./Feb. 1981.

The Pill, the patient, and you

The wide array of oral contraceptives on the market means you and your patients need to know all you can to make choices—whether to take, which to take, and when to take.
By Susan A. Orshan, RN,C, MA

"The Pill" is the primary method of birth control for nearly 10 million American women. Chances are, at least one of your patients is taking this medication—and you may be, too. Popular or not, though, it's still controversial, and with good reason. Though oral contraceptives have undergone many refinements over the last 20 years, The Pill still has annoying side effects and is by no means safe for everyone.

Understanding the hormonal changes and how the various types of oral contraceptives affect them will help you make your own choices or counsel patients to better make theirs.

Oral contraceptives: How they work

During the normal menstrual cycle, levels of estrogen and progesterone are constantly changing. Both are at their lowest during menstruation. After that, the estrogen level rises, peaking just before ovulation, and then dropping abruptly afterward. Progesterone, on the other hand, begins its rise after ovulation, peaks just before menstruation, then declines sharply. For conception to occur, the balance of estrogen and progesterone within the cycle must be maintained. Oral contraceptives disrupt the balance by manipulating hormone levels.

Among nearly 60 on the market today, there are just two basic types: the mini-pill, which contains only progesterone, and the combination pill, which adds estrogen.

The mini-pill is slightly less effective: About three women out of 100 taking it will become pregnant in a year, compared with not even one woman per 100 taking the combination pill. The mini-pill is, however, the best alternative for patients who should not take estrogen—heavy smokers over age 35, for example, or women who are subject to vascular or migraine headaches.

For women who can take estrogen, the optimal dosage seems to be 30 mcg to 35 mcg. Below that, there is an extremely high incidence of breakthrough bleeding, while above 50 mcg the occurrence of serious side effects, including stroke, rises sharply. The progesterones found in combination OCs vary from brand to brand not only in amount but in method of action and side effects.

Besides these differences, combination oral contraceptives fall into three separate classifications: monophasic, biphasic, and triphasic. Monophasic OCs contain the same amount of estrogen and progesterone throughout the menstrual cycle. Biphasic and triphasic pills

THE AUTHOR is a member of the adjunct faculty of New York University's Division of Nursing, where she is a doctoral candidate. She is also in private practice as a women's health-care consultant in Hoboken, N.J.
Produced by Sigrid Nagle

were developed to minimize side effects by mimicking the hormonal changes of the normal cycle. At this time there's no evidence that either is superior to the monophasic.

Contraindications and warning signs

Some women shouldn't take oral contraceptives in any form. The reason: Their use is linked to increased risk of several serious conditions, including MI, thromboembolism, stroke, liver tumors, and gallbladder disease. Under no circumstances, then, should a woman with a history of phlebitis, stroke, coronary artery disease, or breast cancer take The Pill. Nor should anyone who has had an estrogen-dependent tumor or liver tumor, or whose liver function is currently impaired. A woman with severe hypertension or diabetes should also find another contraceptive.

Even if a woman has nothing in her history to contraindicate the use of OCs, she should still be aware of the risks. Tell her to contact her physician if she develops any of the following warning signs:

Acute abdominal pain may be a symptom of gallbladder disease, hepatic adenoma, blood clot, or pancreatitis.

Chest pain, shortness of breath, or coughing blood can indicate a blood clot in the lungs or myocardial infarction.

Headaches or blurry vision may be symptoms of hypertension or stroke.

Severe leg pain is a cardinal sign of a blood clot in the leg.

In the publication *Contraceptive Technology 1986-7*, family planning authorities Hatcher, Guest, et al. suggest that the acronym ACHES will help women remember these danger signs. Each letter stands for a susceptible part of the body: A for abdomen, C for chest, H for head, E for eye. Then add an S— for severe leg pain.

Reactions that also need prompt attention include serious depression, jaundice, and breast lumps. The box on the next page lists common, less worrisome side effects.

Interaction with drugs and vitamins

Because The Pill becomes such a part of everyday life, many women forget that it is medication. It affects the absorption of other medications, and vice versa.

The following drugs decrease the effect of The Pill: ampicillin, penicillin V, tetracycline, rifampin (Rifadin, Rimactane; an ingredient in Rifamate), barbiturates, dihydroergotamine (D.H.E. 45), phenytoin (Dilantin) and other antiepileptics, griseofulvin (Fulvicin), neomycin, and sulfamethoxazole (an ingredient in Bactrim, Septra).

OCs, in turn, decrease the effects of insulin and oral hypoglycemics, oral anticoagulants, and guanethidine (Ismelin; an ingredient in Esimil). They prolong the action of meperidine (Demerol).

Taken with oral contraceptives, troleandomycin (TAO) may result in jaundice.

Because of such drug interactions, a woman should inform anyone who prescribes for her that she is on The Pill. The physician may have to adjust the dosage accordingly. Or, the patient may have to use alternate means of contraception while on a particular medication and for several days after.

Anyone on an oral contraceptive should also realize the importance of a balanced diet. OCs increase the risk of some nutritional deficiencies—primarily of folic acid, and vitamins C, B_2, B_6, and B_{12}.

Such nutritional deficiencies may become evident in decreased plasma levels or if the following symptoms develop: bleeding gums or poor wound healing (vitamin C deficiency), inflamed tongue or cheilosis (B_2 deficiency), numbness in the extremities (B_6 deficiency), and fatigue or sore throat (B_{12} or folic acid deficiency).

Since a patient on oral contraceptives has higher blood levels of iron and copper, she doesn't need supplements or a diet rich in these minerals. Not enough research has been done in this area, however, to know whether it may be dangerous to take such supplements.

What to tell your patient

As you're probably aware, oral contraceptives are prepackaged in 21- and 28-day dispensers, and the patient usually begins taking them on the fifth day after menstruation starts. A patient who is on the 21-day type takes one pill a day for three weeks, none for the next seven days—during which menstruation occurs—then begins a new pack on the eighth day.

If she is on a 28-day regimen, she takes a pill every day. The first 21 pills contain hormones; the remaining seven either have inert ingredients and are given for compliance,

Side effects of the pill

Contraception is not the only result of taking The Pill. There are also numerous side effects. Serious complications include thromboembolism, stroke, myocardial infarction, liver tumors, and gallbladder disease. Less serious and in some cases more common side effects are grouped below according to when they may occur.

The patient should report any of these to her doctor. Some can be eliminated simply by changing to an oral contraceptive with a different dose of estrogen or another type of progesterone. For example, some progesterones create an excess of androgen in the system, which may cause severe acne. A woman who develops acne, therefore, may need a pill containing a progesterone without androgenic effects.

All side effects are not unpleasant, however. Oral contraceptive users enjoy a decreased risk of ovarian and endometrial cancers. Many find that they have a lighter menstrual flow, accompanied by less dysmenorrhea and a smaller loss in iron. Additionally, such women are at a lower risk of trichomoniasis or developing toxic shock syndrome or rheumatoid arthritis.

Worse in first three months	Constant over time	Worse over time
Nausea with dizziness	Headaches	Headaches during menstrual week
Blood clots	Anxiety, depression, fatigue	Weight gain
Edema	Decrease in libido	Monilial vaginitis
Breast fullness, tenderness	Acne	Missed menses
Breakthrough bleeding		Chloasma; photodermatitis
Abdominal cramping		Predisposition to gallbladder disease
Suppression of lactation		Hirsutism
Mood swings		Cystic breast changes
		Hypertension
		Myoma growth
		Spider angiomata

Adapted from *Contraceptive Technology 1986-7*.

or contain iron to protect against anemia during menstruation.

Here are some problems you may be asked about:

► Your patient forgets to take a pill: Tell her to take the missed pill the following day, along with the pill for that day. Until her next period she should use an additional means of contraception, or have her partner use a condom.

► She misses two pills in a row: Have her take two pills on the following day, and two on the day after that. Again, backup contraception is in order.

► She misses three or more pills in a row: She has two choices. She can take two pills a day until she is back on schedule, or she can stop using pills altogether and start a new pack on the following Sunday—even if she is bleeding. She needs backup contraception while she is off The Pill and during the first two weeks she's on a new package.

► The patient does not menstruate on schedule: If she's taken all her pills she's probably not pregnant and can continue taking them on the regular schedule.

► Menstruation does not occur and the patient has missed one or more pills during the cycle: There's a possibility that she's pregnant. Tell her to stop taking the pills immediately, phone her physician or nurse practitioner, and use some form of backup contraception.

► The patient experiences vomiting or diarrhea for several days: She may not be absorbing The Pill and should use backup contraception while continuing to take the rest of the pack. If the same problem occurs the following month, she should alert her physician or nurse practitioner.

▶ The patient decides she wants to become pregnant: She should talk with her health-care provider before trying to conceive. Some physicians recommend waiting three months after coming off oral contraceptives before attempting con-

ception. That time span allows the body to settle back into its natural rhythm.

Because taking oral contraceptives can be such a confusing business, your patient is bound to have questions along the way. If you keep this material in mind, you'll be able to help her make informed choices and cope with any of the major and minor problems that may occur. ■

BIBLIOGRAPHY Block, M. and Rulin, M.C. Managing patients on oral contraceptives. *Am. Fam. Physician* 32:154, 1985. Budoff, P.W., Darney, P.D., et al. Prescribing oral contraceptives in 1985. *Patient Care* 19:16, 1985. Dickerson, J. The Pill: a closer look. *Am. J. Nurs.* 83:1393, 1983. Hatcher, R.A., Guest, F., et al. *Contraceptive Technology, 1986-7* (13th ed.) New York, Irvington Publishers, 1986. Ory, H.W. The noncontraceptive health benefits from oral contraceptive use. *Family Planning Perspectives* 14:182, 1982. Veninga, K.S. Effects of oral contraceptives on vitamins B$_6$, B$_{12}$, C, and Folacin. *Journal of Nurse-Midwifery* 29:386, 1984. Webb, J.C. Nutritional effects of oral contraceptive use: a review. *J. Reprod. Med.* 25:150, 1980.

Postpartum depression: Assessing risk, restoring balance

Assessing the new mother's emotional status
is essential, but the full range of care
begins months before the birth.

By Priscilla Busch, RN, CS, EdD, and
Kathleen Perrin, RN, CCRN, MS

In anticipating the birth of a child, few women stop to think that they might be among the three out of four new mothers who suffer from postpartum depression. The majority of these women experience mild to moderate reactions—the baby blues. One in a hundred suffers from severe postpartum psychosis.

Why so many become depressed and some are more severely affected than others isn't clear. Possible causes include hormonal changes due to labor and delivery, physical stress, a history of depression, and unresolved emotional conflicts.

Psychosocial stress also contributes. It can result from changes in a woman's body image or role definition, violated expectations about labor and delivery or the baby's behavior, or a recent life change like the loss of a job or a family move.

Postpartum depression usually passes without treatment. When depression is severe, however, immediate intervention may be essential to prevent abuse or suicide. Nurses can play a key role in helping new mothers get through mild cases of the baby blues and identifying those experiencing or at risk for more severe depression.

Spotting
the baby blues

Since shorter hospital stays allow little time to detect mild depression, which typically develops on the third day postpartum, assessment must begin in the prenatal period. During clinic visits or classes, try to establish how a woman feels about her pregnancy and whether she perceives her partner as loving and supportive. A woman who's ambivalent about the child or worried about her relationship with the father could be headed for trouble and will need close follow-up care.

Postpartum, observe the mother's interactions with her newborn. Does she maintain eye contact? Does she hold the baby close to her body? Is her voice animated and affectionate or flat and devoid of emotion? Is she relaxed and nurturant, fretful and overprotective, or insensitive and neglectful?

The new mother with mild postpartum depression may seem overanxious or hostile. She may complain about the way the baby, her husband, or others in the family are acting and seem ill at ease with the child. During Karen Johnson's first well-baby visit, these were the signs that alerted the pediatric nurse practitioner. A few open-ended questions drew out Karen's feelings.

Married for five years before she became pregnant, Karen continued working as a secretary at a small college until the day before Derek was born. Since she'd managed home and career competently during her pregnancy, Karen expected an easy transition to motherhood. Accustomed to a well-organized, adult environment, she wasn't prepared for her son's sometimes unpredictable timetable. After a few days at home with the baby, Karen found it difficult to complete such

THE AUTHORS are assistant professors in nursing at St. Anselm College in Manchester, N.H.

Produced by Mary-Beth Moriarty, RN, CCRN

simple tasks as changing Derek's diapers. His fussy periods, during which he ignored her conscientious mothering completely, were especially stressful.

To add to her distress, Karen hadn't anticipated her husband's limited response to the baby. Before Derek's birth, Mark and Karen had shared household responsibilities equally. Now there seemed to be a shift toward stereotyped male and female roles.

Mark became more involved with his work. He was preparing for a certification exam and thought his professional advancement was crucial to the family's financial future.

Karen felt isolated from her husband, burdened by the daily demands of infant care, and generally exhausted. The compounded stress brought her to tears several times a day.

Coping with mild depression

The nurse practitioner avoided using pat phrases such as "Wait it out, it will get better." and "Try to get some sleep when you can." Instead, she suggested that Karen join a peer support group—an informal gathering of mothers with infants and toddlers that met twice a week for an hour or so to socialize, share information, and suggest different approaches to child-care problems.

She also recommended an assertiveness workshop where Karen learned techniques that helped her communicate her needs to Mark without arguing. As a result, Mark realized that his role as father was more than breadwinner. He agreed to spend some time each day with the baby before studying for his exam and reclaimed his share of household tasks.

When Karen brought Derek for his three-month visit, the nurse practitioner saw a distinct change. More secure and confident in her role as mother, Karen was preparing to return to work part time.

When the signs are more obvious

Susan Perkins also began to feel down in the dumps after her son Jesse was born, but her occasional tearful spells soon escalated to near-constant crying. Susan displayed other classic signs of moderate depression as well: She ate very little, sometimes went for days without showering or dressing, and awakened every morning around 2:00 a.m. Unable to fall back to sleep, Susan spent the early morning hours wandering around the house or driving in her car.

Susan's husband, Paul, became increasingly concerned and took more responsibility for Jesse's care. He called their pediatrician when Susan told him she didn't love the baby and understood how easy it would be to abuse an infant who took so much and gave so little in return.

Susan needed more structured interventions than Karen Johnson. Based upon his observations of Susan's interactions with her son, the physician made a referral for outpatient care. A pediatric nurse practitioner met with Susan twice a week. The nurse gave her information and support on mothering issues and also provided some informal bolstering for Paul as well.

Despite reassurance from her husband and the nurse practitioner, Susan was convinced that her mothering wasn't good. Although the baby was gaining weight, she thought Jesse wasn't eating well. While trying to help Susan look at her fears, the nurse practitioner discovered a link to the stillbirth of a daughter two years before. Susan had suppressed the event, refusing to speak of the child or visit the grave.

The nurse practitioner referred Susan for psychiatric counseling that helped her begin to resolve these feelings. Six months later her eating and sleeping patterns had returned to normal. Susan also felt more confident about her mothering skills and she began to take a more active role in Jesse's care.

Severe depression: A crisis situation

At first glance, Clarice Williams' case appeared similar to that of Susan Perkins. Since the birth of Yvonne three months before, Clarice had slept and eaten very little. She was disheveled and spent much of her time staring into space or pacing the floor. Her husband, Greg, had taken over responsibility for child care.

A closer assessment revealed severe depression. Increasingly confused, Clarice often muttered to herself. She wouldn't go into the kitchen because she was afraid of knives. She believed that her baby was dead and that her mother controlled her mind.

Clarice was suffering from the most severe form of postpartum depression, which is characterized by psychotic delusions and the threat of violence. Hospitalization was essential.

During the admission interview Clarice spoke of long-standing conflict with her mother. She'd pressured Clarice since childhood to become a businesswoman and community leader like herself. Unrelenting criticism of her daughter's shyness amounted to psychological abuse.

Initial interventions included close observation, protection, and reassurance. The primary nurse assigned to Clarice stressed these points while establishing a trusting relationship with her. Although Clarice's doctor prescribed an antidepressant, suicide was still a risk. Clarice made a verbal contract with her primary nurse: She'd call the nurse if she had thoughts of harming herself.

As Clarice's symptoms improved she started to talk about her feelings toward the baby without self-reproach. When Greg brought the child to see Clarice, her primary nurse supervised the visits and provided a role model for nurturing behavior.

Eight weeks after admission, Clarice was discharged. She was scheduled for weekly outpatient follow-up and renewed her contract to call the nurse if she had thoughts of hurting herself or the baby. Seven months later, although she still needed a great deal of support and assistance, Clarice began to take a more active role in her daughter's care.

Every mother faces a period of adjustment when a child is born, but prenatal classes can ease the strain by offering important facts about newborn care, the needs and responses of infants, and the impact of childbirth on mother and family. Pregnant women are usually most receptive to these lessons during the second trimester, when they typically focus on the unborn child.

After birth, nurses who are familiar with the three levels of postpartum depression can assess new mothers and intervene when appropriate. They can also educate family members and the general public about the symptoms of depression and when to seek help.

Whenever it's needed, education and support from nurses can help new mothers beat the baby blues. ■

BIBLIOGRAPHY. Bibring, G. and Valenstein, A. Psychological aspects of pregnancy. *Clin. Obstet. Gynecol.* 19:357, April 1976. Braverman, J. and Roux, J. Screening for the patient at risk for postpartum depression. *Obstet. Gynecol.* 52:8, Dec. 1978. Dalton, K. *Who is at Risk? Depression after Childbirth.* Cambridge: Oxford University Press, 1980. Handford, P. Postpartum depression: What is it, what helps? *Canadian Nurse* Jan. 1985. Levy, V. The maternity blues in postpartum and postoperative women. *Br. J. Psychiatry* 151:368, Sept. 1987. Saks. Depressed mood during pregnancy and the puerperium: Clinical recognition and implication for clinical practice. *Am. J. Psychiatry* 142:6, June 1985. Stuart, G. and Sundeen, S. *Principles and Practice of Psychiatric Nursing.* St. Louis: C.V. Mosby Co., 1987.

Cruel myths and clinical facts about menopause

Many women approach menopause not knowing what to expect—or expecting the worst. Here's how to help them through this mid-life transition.

By Valerie Ann McKeon, RN, MSN, PhD

Most women live a full third of their lives after menopause. This can be a vibrant time, but myths and misinformation cause many to dread the experience of physical change and the years that follow it.

Nurses are in an ideal position to foster more realistic and positive attitudes. We can replace half-truths with facts about the changes menopause brings and those that it doesn't. With our support, women can move comfortably through this mid-life transition and look to the future with confidence.

Separating fact from fiction

Menopause, defined as the cessation of menses, is considered to have occurred when a year has gone by without a menstrual period. Most American women reach menopause between the ages of 48 and 55; the median age is 51.

Starting in the early 40s, however, more and more of a woman's cycles occur without ovulation. Inter-

THE AUTHOR is an associate professor of nursing at Saint Anselm College in Manchester, N.H.

Produced by Helen Lippman Collins

vals between periods may change as a result, with cycles becoming shorter or longer than usual. As ovarian function continues to decline, menstruation becomes less and less frequent and eventually stops.

The period of waning ovarian function plus the years just after menopause are called the climacteric. During the climacteric, many women experience hot flashes and profuse perspiration, and some begin to have pain during intercourse, the result of increasing thinning and dryness of the vaginal walls. Today, these are recognized as the only symptoms that are directly related to diminishing estrogen levels.

In the past, however, menopause was the scapegoat for almost every imaginable physical and psychological problem, from obesity and palpitations to depression and schizophrenia. Many physical symptoms once linked to menopause are now recognized as part of the aging process.

Psychological problems during the climacteric, many studies have

shown, are far less common than once supposed and not directly related to declining hormone levels. It's true that a woman who gets severe hot flashes at night may lose sleep, which can lead to anxiety or depression. It's not true that declining hormones *cause* anxiety and depression.

Further, mid-life tends to bring not one "change of life" but many. Children leave the nest (or they don't). The world of work welcomes a woman back to a stressful career (or it doesn't). Parents may become dependent, sick, or die. All of these psychosocial changes, plus the added difficulty of aging gracefully in a society that seems to worship youth, sometimes cause emotional distress.

Help promote a positive outlook

If a woman going through menopause tells you she feels fragile, reassure her that she's not going to fall apart. Reaching menopause does not accelerate the gradual aging process that we're all going through. Neither does it indicate

Physiologic changes as a woman ages . . .

In uterine size, shape, and lining

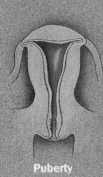
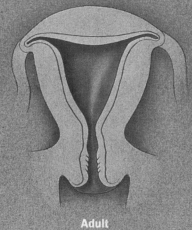
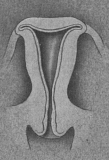

Puberty

Adult
(nulliparous)

Adult
(parous)

Postmenopause

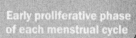
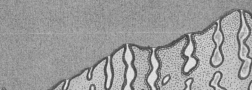
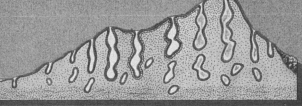
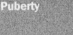
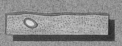

Puberty

Adult

Postmenopause

In vaginal smears and mucosa

Late proliferative phase

Midsecretory phase

Early proliferative phase
of each menstrual cycle

Late secretory phase

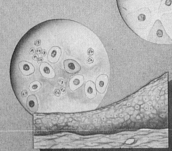
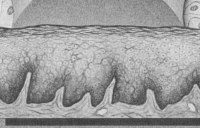
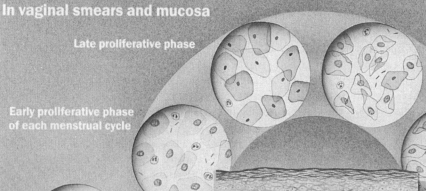
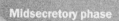
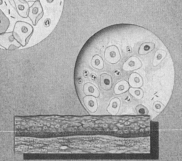

Puberty

Adult

Postmenopause

that a woman is "over the hill."

Change itself can be unsettling, even frightening, but it also offers opportunities for growth. Urge women to use this time to invest in their own well-being.

Finding positive role models is a good way to start. Encourage women to look forward, seeking friends who've passed menopause and continue to be excited about life. Explore attitudes about aging and personal goals, perhaps by using this visualization exercise:

Imagine someone who's nearing menopause and jot down several words to describe her, then do the same for a woman of 60 and a woman of 70. Then picture *yourself* as you would like to be at 50, 60, and 70.

These descriptions are likely to reveal hidden fears and prejudices. Picturing her aging self may help a woman realize she can pick the kind of older person she wants to be.

Remind her that new activities can add richness to life. A more interesting job, a return to school, involvement in a community project or political cause, a healthier lifestyle—are worthy goals at any age.

Good nutrition promotes good health as well as a healthy attitude, so stress a diet rich in fiber, whole grains, and fresh fruits and vegetables and low in fat and cholesterol. If a woman complains of irritability or suffers from headaches, sweating, or frequent feelings of weakness, suggest a hypoglycemic diet: Eliminate refined sugar and flour and eat small meals containing protein five or six times a day.

Exercise also helps to reduce stress, and women who've never been active should be urged to start now. Aerobic exercises such as walking, bicycling, and swimming—done regularly—help control weight and maintain cardiovascular fitness. Competitive sports like golf and tennis offer companionship as well.

Coping with hot flashes

Four out of five women pass menopause without experiencing symptoms severe enough to warrant medical attention, but most suffer at least occasional hot flashes.

A flash is an intense feeling of heat, usually above the waist, often accompanied by beading perspiration. It generally lasts only a few minutes. Some women's faces get red and blotchy, which is why hot flashes are sometimes referred to as flushes.

The flashes may stop after several months or continue for five years or longer. In most cases, flashes are mild and infrequent, but some women may be drenched in perspiration many times each day and night.

Although the exact cause of this discomfort is unknown, the decline in estrogen production is believed to affect the hypothalamus, which controls body temperature. The result is vasomotor instability. The body becomes more sensitive to heat, so that hot flashes and perspiration are merely an attempt to cool off.

Anything that affects body temperature can trigger a flash—from a hot meal or beverage to hot weather, a warm room, an alcoholic drink, spicy foods, or an emotional upset. The best advice, then, is to keep cool both physically and emotionally.

Specific suggestions you can offer: Wear clothing made of cotton or other natural fibers and dress in loose layers. Keep the house cool, and use lightweight blankets at night.

Limit red wine, chocolate, and aged cheeses. They contain tyramine, an amino acid that causes the release of norepinephrine in the hypothalamus, which resets the body's thermostat and triggers a flash.

Try to avoid smoking, caffeine, and excessive alcohol intake, all of which can cause irritability and are thus apt to make hot flashes even worse.

Other tips: Frequent swims and lukewarm showers may stretch the intervals between flashes and make them less intense. When one begins, stand in a cool breeze, use a fan, sip a glass of water or juice, or even imagine a cool, comfortable place.

Compensating for vaginal atrophy

Unlike hot flashes, which stop once the body has adjusted to postmenopausal hormone levels, genital atrophy is progressive. Beginning around the time of menopause and continuing through old age, the vagina gradually loses elasticity and lubrication, and its walls become thinner and more fragile.

Low estrogen levels also reduce the acidity of the urethra and base of the bladder, which lowers resistance to urinary pathogens. Drinking six to eight glasses of water, cranberry juice, or unsweetened citrus juices each day and taking vitamin C tablets can help stave off UTIs. Urinating before and after intercourse helps, too.

Sexual activity is the best way to keep the vagina flexible and elastic. Talk to women about their sexuality and assure them that the notion of the postmenopausal woman as sexless is a fallacy. Menopause marks the end of the ability to bear children, not the ability to give and receive physical love.

If intercourse becomes painful, suggest a water-soluble lubricant such as K-Y Jelly. Petroleum jelly and other oil-based products interfere with natural lubrication.

Warn a woman who's starting menopause that menstrual periods may stop for months and then resume. Pregnancy is a possibility, so birth control should be continued until at least 12 months have gone by without a period. If a woman begins bleeding after a year or more has passed, however, advise her to seek medical attention at once: Postmenopausal bleeding can be a symptom of endometrial cancer.

If vaginal itching is a problem, suggest vitamin E cream. Per-

What to tell women about ERT

Misconceptions about estrogen replacement therapy are almost as widespread as menopause myths. Some women reject ERT for fear of side effects, while others view it as a panacea for aging. Here's what to tell your patients about the benefits and risks:

Women who experience troublesome menopausal symptoms—frequent hot flashes, night sweats severe enough to cause insomnia, or pain during intercourse, for instance—should be encouraged to seek medical care. Short-term ERT is often a safe and effective way to alleviate the distress.

Many doctors also recommend lifetime ERT, starting around the onset of menopause. It slows the bone loss that leads to osteoporosis and may also have beneficial effects on the heart. A number of studies suggest that estrogen increases the level of high density lipoproteins (the "healthy" cholesterol) in the blood and helps the arteries maintain elasticity.

Explain to women considering ERT that carefully monitored short-term therapy poses little risk. Less is known about long-term effects, but you can point out that current regimens include progestin, eliminating the increased risk of uterine cancer that came from taking estrogen alone. It works like this: Estrogen _promotes_ the overgrowth of the endometrium, a condition that can cause endometrial cancer. Progestin _diminishes_ the overgrowth by causing the endometrium to shed. That shedding often results in regular vaginal bleeding similar to a menstrual period, a side effect that's annoying but safe.

Explain, too, that women on ERT do not share the risks of blood clots and stroke faced by women on oral contraceptives. That's because ERT involves a far lower dose of estrogen.

While women requiring treatment for vaginal dryness often use a topical estrogen cream, most others take ERT orally. Though some doctors recommend a continuous dosing regimen, the usual dose is 0.625 mg of estrogen on days one to 25 of the cycle or calendar month and 5 to 10 mg of progestin on the last 10 to 14 days. Common side effects are headaches, nausea, vaginal discharge, fluid retention, swollen breasts, and weight gain. A rise in blood pressure or abnormal vaginal bleeding calls for immediate medical attention.

A new method of administering estrogen, the transdermal estradiol patch, alleviates side effects in some cases. Patches, available in 0.05 or 0.1 mg strength, are worn on the abdomen or another part of the trunk, either continuously or for the first 21 days of the cycle. The patient takes progestin orally on some of those days, usually the first 12.

Though the patch may irritate the skin, it offers other advantages: It's less likely than oral estrogen to cause hypertension or gastric distress. Some women find it easier to use than pills, since it requires changing only twice a week.

The patch delivers a lower dose of estrogen but, in many women, still controls menopausal symptoms. It is not yet known, however, if the patch delivers a high enough dose of estrogen to protect against osteoporosis.

Urge women who are at risk for osteoporosis to discuss long-term therapy with their physicians. That group includes women with light coloring, a slight build, or a family history of osteoporosis.

Other risk factors to consider: early menopause, whether it be natural or through surgical removal of the ovaries, extreme lack of exercise _or_ a history of strenuous exercise accompanied

fumed or deodorant soaps, bubble baths, girdles, pantyhose, and tight pants can all cause irritation. Douching should be done only if a doctor recommends it.

If vaginal discomfort or hot flashes become severe, low-dose estrogen replacement therapy can help. Some physicians favor short-term therapy for symptom relief only. Others recommend long-term

hormone replacement, particularly for women at risk for osteoporosis.

Whether symptoms are mild or severe, menopause is an important transition in every woman's life. Nurses can help women face it with equanimity—and look forward to the years that follow—by providing facts, interventions, and support. ∎

BIBLIOGRAPHY Colls, J. Perimenopausal transition: contemporary perspectives and management alternatives. *NAACOG Update Series* 3, 1984. Greenwood, S. *Menopause, Naturally: Preparing for the Second Half of Life*. San Francisco: Volcano Press, 1984. Hemphill, D. and Kimber, Y. *A Positive Look at Menopause*. Planned Parenthood of Central Missouri, 1982. LaRocco, S. and Polit, D. Women's knowledge about the menopause. *Nurse Res.* 29:10, Jan./Feb. 1980. McKeon, V. Cause of hot flashes. *Nursing* 17:91, July 1987. McKeon, V. Tips for handling hot flashes. *Nursing* 17:124, Sept. 1987. Mead Johnson Laboratories. *For the Woman Approaching Menopause*. Evansville, Ind. 1985. Millette, B. and Hawkins, J. *Women and the Menopause*. Reston, Va.: Reston Publishing Co., 1983. Nurses Association of the American College of Obstetricians and Gynecologists. *Menopause*. Technical Bulletin 10, March 1980. Pederson, B. and Pendelton, E. Menopause: a welcome or dreaded stage of development. *J. Nurse Midwife* 23:45, Fall 1978. Voda, A., Dinnerstein, M., et al., eds. *Changing Perspectives on Menopause*. Austin: University of Texas Press, 1982.

by amenorrhea, excessive drinking, smoking, and prolonged use of corticosteroids or anti-inflammatory drugs.

Although a calcium-rich diet alone will not prevent osteoporosis, women who've habitually consumed little calcium or who have a condition that impairs calcium absorption are at risk as well.

All women on ERT should have regular checkups, including a gynecologic exam, mammogram, and blood pressure check. Any woman who's obese or has a history of hypertension or cardiovascular disease, thrombophlebitis, diabetes, liver disease, seizure disorder, migraine headaches, gallbladder disease, benign breast disease, or cancer requires even closer monitoring. ERT is also not recommended for women whose mothers took diethylstilbestrol (DES) during pregnancy or for anyone who's had estrogen-dependent breast cancer.

BIBLIOGRAPHY *Age Page*. National Institute on Aging, National Institutes of Health. Bethesda, Md., Jan. 1988. Hammond, C. and Maxson, W. Estrogen replacement therapy. *Clin. Obstet Gynaecol.* 29:407, June 1986. Nachtigall, L. and Heilman, J. *Estrogen: the facts can change your life*. New York: Harper and Row, 1986. Practical aspects of estrogen replacement therapy. *Nurses' Drug Alert*. 12:83, Nov. 1988.

Time won't tell if that OB patient's out of danger

This assessment form gives you more than a clock to use in deciding if a patient is ready for discharge to the unit.
By Myrtle Taylor Williams, RN, MSN, and Carolyn Jones Bell, RN, BSN

Deciding when a new mother can be released to the maternity unit can be tricky even for experienced staffers. Many hospitals rely on the clock rather than assessment skills. A patient may be discharged one hour after an easy vaginal delivery, or three hours after a cesarean.

However, this time-oriented approach makes it simple to overlook subtle signs of impending complications. To promote more individualized care, we use the assessment form on the opposite page. Because we serve many high-risk, indigent women who've had little prenatal care, we admit all new mothers to an OB post-anesthesia recovery unit—whether they've had anesthesia or not—for monitoring.

A scoring system to track complications

The chart's most valuable section is the CINNSCORE—an acronym for nine aspects of the patient's condition, from Consciousness to Episiotomy. Every 15 minutes for the first 90 minutes postpartum and every half an hour thereafter, our nurses evaluate the patient and assign a score of 2, 1, or 0 to each CINNSCORE area.

Before the patient can be released, she must have a total CINNSCORE of at least 17 on two consecutive assessments. We also require that her pulse, BP, and respiration be stable across at least five consecutive assessments.

The CINNSCORE lets us assess the following areas:

Consciousness. Depending on the kind of anesthesia the patient has had, as well as her individual ability to overcome its effect, she may be fully awake, arousable, or completely unresponsive.

Involuting uterus. Shortly after delivery, the uterus should begin to contract and become firm. Abdominal massage can speed the process along, but the effect will be temporary as long as placental fragments remain in the uterus.

Nadir fundus. Immediately after delivery the upper part of the uterus, or fundus, is two to three

THE AUTHORS: Ms. Williams, presently the assistant director of nursing resource development at Texas Children's Hospital in Houston, spent five years as a maternal and child health educator at Houston's Jefferson Davis Hospital. Ms. Bell has been the head nurse of the obstetrical recovery room at Jefferson Davis for the past 10 years. She also lectures widely on perinatal care.

Produced by Paul L. Cerrato

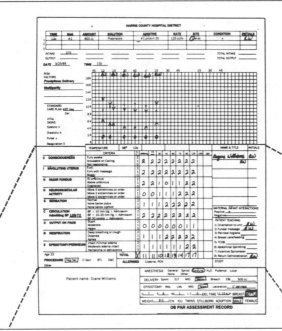

A better way to monitor postpartum status

This assessment form features a unique scoring system, shown in detail below. Calculating a CINNSCORE allows nurses to evaluate newly-delivered mothers on nine clinical parameters—from consciousness and respiration to OB-specific items such as involuting uterus and episiotomy—before releasing them to an OB unit. The form also provides space to record delivery events, patient teaching, risk factors, vital signs, and IV therapy.

	CRITERIA	S C	ARRIVAL	15 min	30	45	60	75	90	120	150	180
	TEMPERATURE 98^8 12p											
C CONSCIOUSNESS	Fully awake / Arousable on Calling / Not responding	2 1 0	2	2	2	2	2	2	2			
I INVOLUTING UTERUS	Firm / Firm with massage / Boggy	2 1 0	2	2	2	2	2	2	2			
N NADIR FUNDUS	At umbilicus / Above umbilicus / Displaced	2 1 0	2	2	1	0	1	1	2	2		
N NEUROMUSCULAR ACTIVITY	Move 4 extremities on order / Move 2 extremities on order / Move 0 extremities on order	2 1 0	0	0	1	1	1	2	2	2		
S SENSATION	Normal / None below pubis / None below xiphoid	2 1 0	1	1	1	2	2	2	2	2		
C CIRCULATION Admitting BP 125/72	BP ± 10 mm Hg ± Admission / BP ± 10-20 mm Hg ± Admission / BP 20 mmHg ± Admission	2 1 0	2	2	2	2	2	2	2			
O OUTPUT ON PADS	Scant / Moderate / Heavy	2 1 0	0	0	0	0	0	0	1	1		
R RESPIRATION	Deep breathing or cough / Dyspnea / Apnea	2 1 0	1	1	1	2	2	2	2			
E EPISIOTOMY/PERINEUM	Intact minimal edema / Moderate edema intact / Hematoma or dehiscence	2 1 0	1	1	1	1	1	1	2	2		
Age 33	**TOTAL**	✕	11	11	10	12	13	14	17	17		

NAME & TITLE: *Regina Williams* RN — INITIALS: RW

PROCEDURE [Vag Del] C-Sect BTL D&C
Other:

ALLERGIES Codeine, PCN

MATERNAL INFANT INTERACTIONS
Positive __+__
Negative _____

PATIENT TEACHING
1) Orientation to unit __RW__
2) Fundal massage __RW__
3) Perineal hygiene _____
4) Breast care/feeding _____
5) TCDB
6) Abdominal Splintting _____
7) Incentive Spirometer
8) Return Demonstration __RW__

STUDY

finger breadths below the umbilicus. (During the first postpartum day it rises to approximately the level of the navel, then drops to its lowest point in the pelvic cavity over the next 10 to 14 days.)

Palpating the abdomen will help determine if the uterus is above the umbilicus or shifted to the side. Either situation may mean that the urinary bladder is distended and pressing against the uterus. If so, getting the patient to urinate may relieve this condition. If a patient's fundus is displaced, she shouldn't be released until the problem is corrected. If it's slightly above the umbilicus, she can be released, providing all other CINNSCORE readings are perfect.

Neuromuscular activity. Assessing the patient's ability to move her legs helps determine whether epidural or spinal anesthesia has worn off. (On rare occasions, it's also possible for an anesthetic given in the lower spinal cord to travel upward and affect the arms as well.) We keep the patient in recovery until it's clear that neuromuscular function is normalizing.

Sensation. Under ordinary circumstances, after epidural or spinal anesthesia there may be some numbness below the waist. Ideally, the patient should be able to move her legs before being released.

Circulation. To leave recovery, an OB patient's blood pressure—one measure of circulatory status—must be within 10 to 20 mm Hg of her BP on admission, assuming that the admission reading was normal. A larger drop in BP could signal hypovolemia.

Output on pads. Lochia rubra,

the earliest postpartum vaginal discharge, is composed of blood and placental fragments. If the patient saturates more than one peripad in an hour, that's reason enough not to release her since it may suggest hemorrhaging. Methylergonovine (Methergine) IM is used to retard bleeding and hasten uterine involution. The drug is contraindicated in patients who have hypertension.

Respiration. Before release, the patient should be breathing normally and able to cough up respiratory secretions. Shortness of breath might indicate lingering anesthetic effects, an embolism, or fluid overload due to overaggressive IV therapy. Occasionally, an epidural anesthetic works its way up the spinal cord and causes persistent apnea, so that the patient has to be put on a respirator.

Episiotomy/perineum. We carefully inspect the incision site for redness, swelling, and tenderness. Patients aren't released if there's evidence of a hematoma or dehiscence. Ideally, a woman who hasn't had an episiotomy should have an intact perineum and only slight edema.

The sample CINNSCORE that's on page 475 shows that patient, Diane Williams, who had an epidural block, was still feeling the anesthetic's effects when she arrived in recovery. Over the next hour and a half, neuromuscular activity, sensation, and breathing scores improved as the anesthesia wore off.

Since an epidural will numb the nerves feeding the urinary bladder, patients often retain urine because they don't feel the need to void. Ms. Williams' fundus was at the umbili-

cus when she got to recovery, but within 45 minutes her bladder became distended, displacing the fundus. The nurse inserted a catheter, as ordered, and the patient was ready for discharge by 2:00 p.m.

An orderly format for other data

In addition to the CINNSCORE, the assessment form allows space for recording other essentials of obstetrical care.

Delivery events. At the bottom of the form we note the kind of anesthesia the patient had, the type of delivery—spontaneous, elective low forceps (ELF), mid-forceps (MID), and so on—and an estimate of blood lost (EBL). The nurse who takes the patient to the recovery room is responsible for recording these data, along with the infant's weight, sex, time of birth, feeding method and type of episiotomy performed: midline (MID) or right or left mediolateral (RML, LML).

A patient who's had general anesthesia, of course, will remain longer in recovery than one who's had a local. Likewise, a serious perineal laceration or excessive blood loss—more than 500 ml for a vaginal delivery—may extend her stay.

We record past birth events—number of pregnancies in a space marked G for gravidity, live births next to P for parity, abortions next to Ab, and live children next to LC.

Risk factors. After each pregnancy, a woman's uterus tends to lose some muscle tone and may involute slowly after delivery, increasing the risk of bleeding. A very rapid delivery may increase that risk too, because the uterus or vagina may tear. Pregnancy-induced hypertension is another danger. The nurse who admits the patient to the RR notes such problems on the assessment form.

Vital signs. Pulse may be somewhat slow right after delivery; blood pressure and respiration rate should be within the normal range. Patients stay in recovery until vital signs are stable, as noted earlier. Any suspicious trends are reported to the physician. For instance, rising pulse and respiration rates and falling blood pressure in a patient who's lost a lot of blood may mean the onset of hypovolemic shock.

The assessment form also provides space for recording I&O, IV infusions, patient teaching, maternal-infant interactions, and allergies. Medications, deep tendon reflexes, and nursing observations are noted on a second page (not shown in our illustration).

Our assessment protocol has served us—and our patients—well in the last seven years. It's helped us individualize postpartum care and consistently meet JCAHO requirements for transfer of patients from recovery. Incorporating the CINNSCORE and other key components of the form into your unit's documentation system might help you do the same. ■

DEBORAH L. RUST, RN,C, MSN
ELIZABETH MYERS KLOPPENBORG, RN, MS

Don't underestimate the lumpectomy patient's needs

*Women who choose
a lumpectomy undergo
a simpler surgical procedure
than those who have
mastectomies, but their need
for nursing care and support
is just as great.*

DEBORAH RUST is an instructor in med/surg nursing at the Christ Hospital School of Nursing, Cincinnati.
ELIZABETH KLOPPENBORG, a former med/surg instructor at Christ Hospital School of Nursing, now works for HealthMark, a medical consulting firm in Charlotte, N.C.

Oncologist Jane DeLuca gently confirmed Eva Smith's fears. The hard lump in the upper outer quadrant of the patient's right breast was cancer. Both women sat silently for several moments.

Dr. DeLuca told Mrs. Smith that the prognosis was good because they had caught the disease early. She promised to do everything she could to bring about a lasting remission.

The first decision was already upon them, the physician continued. Mrs. Smith could choose to have a mastectomy or—because the tumor was well-defined and less than 5 cm, did not involve the nipple, and hadn't metastasized—she could decide to have a lumpectomy.

Mastectomy is the standard intervention. Removal of the entire breast ensures that no neoplastic cells remain in the area, and, of course, cancer cannot recur at the same site.

In a lumpectomy, only the tumor and some surrounding tissue are removed. The rest of the breast is left intact. The final word isn't yet in on the rates of cancer recurrence after lumpectomy, but the news so far is encouraging. In clinical trials reported in 1988, the National Surgical Adjuvant Breast Cancer Project found that lumpectomy followed by radiation therapy produced eight-year disease-free survival rates equal to mastectomy. Other studies have yielded similar results.

Mrs. Smith decided that keeping her breast was worth the slightly greater uncertainty associated with the newer procedure. She was admitted to our hospital. Knowing that the patient is spared the unhappiness of losing a breast is only one among many reasons why caring for women who undergo lumpectomy is so rewarding.

Before surgery:
Ease the patient's anxiety

Although lumpectomy allows a woman to save her breast, it doesn't eliminate the anguish any diagnosis of cancer brings. The nursing staff realized that keeping Mrs. Smith's morale up was one of the most important things we could do for her. Simply letting her talk about her concerns helped. We also informed her early on about the local American Cancer Society's Reach for Recovery program, designed to help women handle their diagnosis and treatment.

The evening before surgery, Mrs. Smith's spirits hit bottom. She was afraid of dying, and anxious about the prospects of prolonged illness and pain. A nurse reminded her that remission in early stage cancer is the rule rather than the exception.

Patients like Mrs. Smith, who

are given a choice of treatments, have the added burden of wondering if they have chosen the right one. The nurse reassured her patient that as far as anyone knows, lumpectomy with radiation is as effective as mastectomy for patients with early stage cancer like hers.

Mrs. Smith also worried about how her breast would look after surgery—and how her husband would react. The nurse calmed her with the information that Dr. DeLuca, like many doctors, discourages lumpectomy unless she thinks the patient's breast is large enough to permit tumor removal without deformity. She encouraged the patient to discuss her concerns frankly with her husband.

By the end of this conversation, Mrs. Smith's spirits had lifted, and she seemed better equipped to deal with the surgery and follow-up therapy.

We prepared her for the next day's happenings. Lumpectomy is performed under general anesthesia. The procedure generally takes between one and two hours.

After the surgery:
Prevent complications

Mrs. Smith returned from surgery wearing a 4 x 4 dressing over her incision and a closed self-suction drain. We checked the dressing and drain every four hours the first day, and once a shift thereafter. At first the drain collected 60-75 cc of bright red fluid per shift. By evening, output became sero-sanguineous, a sign that healing

was beginning. Volume tapered off gradually over three days and the drain was removed.

A lumpectomy procedure usually includes dissection of the axillary lymph node nearest the affected breast. This tissue is then biopsied for signs of cancer. Removal of the node obstructs the flow of lymph in the arm, putting the patient at risk for lymphedema.

To protect Mrs. Smith from this complication, we elevated her right arm on a pillow and checked it frequently for circulatory problems. Assessments included comparing the right arm with the left to see if it was pale or swollen, palpation of radial pulses, limb temperature, and capillary refill time.

We advised Mrs. Smith not to stretch with her arm or do anything painful with it. Tension on the suture line can cause hemorrhage, especially as breast tissue is very vascular. Wearing a bra is usually optional. Mrs. Smith chose not to, because she was afraid the pressure might hurt.

To relieve any pain that was caused by the axillary dissection, we administered IM meperidine (Demerol) immediately postop. Later on that day, Mrs. Smith was switched over to oral analgesics.

Prepare the patient
for home health care

On the first postop day, the nursing staff started teaching Mrs. Smith the self-care skills she would need at home.

The suture line needs to be

cleaned with hydrogen peroxide once a day until the sutures are removed. During cleaning Mrs. Smith would check the incision for redness, warmth, swelling, and drainage. She was told to report any of these to her doctor.

Mrs. Smith had to protect her right arm from injury and infection, both of which can give rise to lymphedema. We advised her to use the left arm for activities such as vacuuming, gardening, and carrying things. We also recommended that she wear a thimble when sewing, use a soft cloth to push back cuticles, and shave her armpits with an electric shaver rather than a razor blade.

Venipunctures, injections, or blood pressure readings should not be done on the affected arm. Also potentially damaging to the limb are harsh chemicals, abrasive compounds, sunburn, and insect bites.

Mrs. Smith learned to recognize signs of infection, including redness, soreness, and swelling. If these developed, she was to keep the arm elevated and call her physician. If she incurred a minor cut or injury, she would immediately wash it with soap and water, apply antibacterial medication, and cover it with a bandage.

To prevent circulatory constriction that might possibly lead to lymphedema, we advised Mrs. Smith to choose loose clothing and to remember to wear her wristwatch and bracelets on her left arm.

Dr. DeLuca would tell Mrs. Smith when these precautions were no longer necessary. That would not be until collateral lymph circulation developed to carry the flow that formerly went through the removed node, possibly about six weeks after the lumpectomy.

Mrs. Smith complained of discomfort from the axillary dissection and skin tightness from the healing incision. With the doctor's permission, we taught her to do the exercises described on the next two pages, which help restore full range of motion.

Any person with a history of breast cancer is at risk for a recurrence. We explained the importance of early detection and taught Mrs. Smith how to examine her own breasts, using the American Cancer Society's guidelines. Dr. DeLuca would continue to follow her condition closely.

The nursing staff also talked to the patient's two adult daughters and sister, tactfully informing them that since a close family member had now been diagnosed with breast cancer they, too, were considered at increased risk for the disease. We taught them how to perform breast self-exam, stressing the importance of doing it once a month.

The entire family needs emotional support

Similar to many lumpectomy patients, Mrs. Smith was still uneasy about her altered body image, and anxious about possible recurrence.

Her family also needed support, especially her husband. He had a reaction that's quite typical in husbands of breast cancer patients: He was afraid that he might cause the cancer to come back if he touched his wife's breasts during lovemaking. We had to assure him that this is impossible.

Mr. Smith's fear that his wife would shortly die was less easily resolved. We encouraged the couple to continue sharing their feelings with each other, and reminded them about the availability of a Reach to Recovery volunteer to provide support and information.

Some women go home as early as the first or second day postlumpectomy. Mrs. Smith, whose drainage tapered off more slowly, was discharged on the fourth postop day. At that time her incision was healing and she had no signs of lymphedema. She showed good understanding of all necessary precautions, and—just as important—confidence that she and her family could cope.

She also had a clinic appointment to start the next stage of her treatment.

Explain radiation therapy and "boosts"

Radiation therapy follows lumpectomy to kill any cancer cells that might have been left behind. Mrs. Smith's treatments started in our outpatient clinic when her sutures had healed, two weeks after her surgery. A nurse from our floor met her at the clinic to explain the procedure and implications.

The entire breast is radiated with a total dose of approximately 5,000 rads. Radiation may

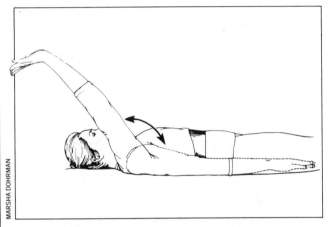

Exercises for recovery

The exercises illustrated here will help you regain full range of motion in your arm. Two others—rotating your head to the left and right, and breathing deeply to let your chest expand—will also help. Do 10 repetitions of each exercise once per day after you return home. Be sure not to continue any exercise movement past the point where it begins to hurt.

MARSHA DOHRMAN

1 Lie in bed with your arm at your side. Then raise your arm straight up and back, as if reaching for the headboard.

2 Lying in bed, clasp your hands behind your head and push your elbows into the mattress.

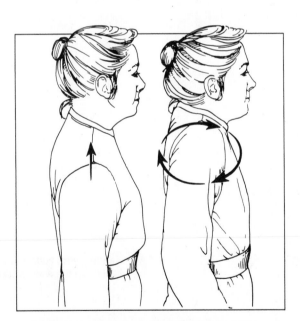

3 Raise your shoulders and rotate them forward, down, and back in a circular motion to loosen your chest, shoulder, and upper back muscles.

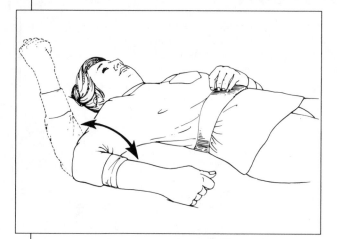

4 With your elbow bent and your arm on the bed at a 90-degree angle to your body, rotate your shoulder forward and bring your forearm down toward your feet, then up.

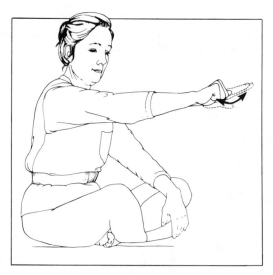

5 With your arm raised, clench and unclench your fist.

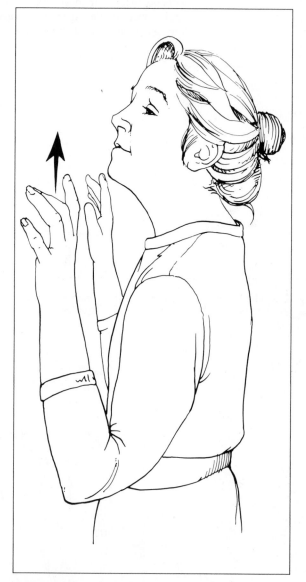

6 Standing with your palm flat against a wall, "walk" up the wall with your fingers.

Adapted from *Radiation Therapy: A Treatment for Early-Stage Breast Cancer*, National Cancer Institute, 1984.

make the skin a little red, rough, or taut during therapy. Patients may be tempted to apply lotions or powders, and need to be warned against it as many contain small amounts of metal that can lead to skin irritation when irradiated. We also cautioned Mrs. Smith to use mild soap, to preserve skin markings used to delineate treatment areas, and to keep the treated area out of the sun. (For more information, see "Radiation therapy: Saving your patient's skin" in the June 1989 issue of **RN**.)

Patients may feel tired after treatments because the body expends energy to metabolize the cells destroyed by radiation. The staff advised Mrs. Smith to conserve energy and to eat a high-protein, high-calorie diet.

Initial radiation is followed two weeks later with another "boost" radiation. This extra exposure is sometimes done on an outpatient basis using an electron beam. In Mrs. Smith's case, however, Dr. DeLuca preferred to implant radioactive iridium (IR-192) seeds in the site where the tumor had been.

The patient receives local anesthesia for iridium implantation. The implant doesn't harm the patient's normal tissues, but good judgment dictates minimizing others' exposure to the radiation. Therefore, no nurse provides bedside care for more than 20 minutes per shift. Visitors may remain near the patient for no more than 20 minutes per day. We placed a lead shield in Mrs. Smith's room, and we and her husband visited with her from behind it.

The implants are removed and the patient discharged after two or three days.

Prepare the patient for chemo side effects

Two and a half months after that awful day in Dr. DeLuca's office, Mrs. Smith had completed lumpectomy and radiation. Her spirits were high and her strength good. Now she had only one treatment hurdle left to clear.

Dr. DeLuca adheres to the latest National Cancer Institute guidelines that recommend chemotherapy for all women following lumpectomy or mastectomy. Previously, many doctors administered chemotherapy only when lymph nodes tested positive for cancer.

The chemotherapy drugs most often prescribed are cyclophosphamide (Cytoxan), methotrexate (Folex. Mexate), fluorouracil (Adrucil, 5-FU), and doxorubicin (Adriamycin). It's important to prepare your patient for unpleasant side effects such as nausea, vomiting, and temporary hair loss. Other possible reactions include decreased WBC and platelet count, nervous system disturbances, hemorrhagic cystitis, inflamed mucous membranes, and heart arrhythmias (see "Chemo: A nurse's guide to action, administration, and side effects" in last month's **RN**).

A patient whose white cell count goes below 1,000 is at high risk for infection. To decrease her exposure to pathogens, we told Mrs. Smith to avoid crowds and people with colds and other contagious infections. We also

In early trials, lumpectomy followed by radiation therapy produced survival rates as high as mastectomy.

taught her to watch out for any signs of infection, such as fever, chills, and cough, and to report them to the physician. Even a low fever is significant in a patient with a reduced white cell count.

If platelets fall below 50,000, indicating thrombocytopenia, a patient needs to take precautions to avoid bleeding. We reminded Mrs. Smith to use an electric shaver to prevent accidental cuts, and we recommended foam-tipped tooth cleaners or alcohol-free mouthwash instead of a toothbrush. We explained the importance of a high-fiber diet and stool softeners to prevent constipation and possible rectal bleeding, and instructed her to observe her urine and stools for blood. Subcutaneous or intramuscular injections, rectal temperatures, enemas, and suppositories are to be avoided, also.

In addition to other forms of chemotherapy, the National

Cancer Institute recommends hormone therapy after lumpectomy for women with estrogen- or progesterone-dependent cancer. Therefore, because Mrs. Smith's tumor was found to contain estrogen receptors, she was given tamoxifen (Nolvadex), an antiestrogen drug. Side effects are relatively mild, mostly hot flashes.

Six years later, Dr. DeLuca still sees Eva Smith every six months. Thus far, she has found no signs of new cancer. After each examination, Mrs. Smith comes to visit the nurses who cared for her. She simply wants to share her joy in being alive with us.

As lumpectomy continues to show favorable results in treating early breast cancer, more patients like Eva Smith will select this option. Like all patients with breast cancer, they'll benefit greatly from your expertise and support. □

BIBLIOGRAPHY

Bader, J., Lippman, M., et al. Preliminary report of the NCI early breast cancer study: A prospective randomized comparison of lumpectomy and radiation to mastectomy for stage I and II breast cancer. *Int. J. Radiat. Oncol. Biol. Phys.* 13:160, 1987. Baeza, M.R., Sole, J., et al. Conservative treatment of early breast cancer. *Int. J. Radiat. Oncol. Biol. Phys.* 14:669, 1988. Eich, S.J. Promising early breast cancer treatment—without mastectomy. *Cancer Nurs.* 8:51, 1985. Fallowfield, L.J., Baum, M., and Maguire, G.P. Effects of breast conservation on psychological morbidity associated with diagnosis and treatment of early breast cancer. *BMJ* 293:1331, 1986. Fisher, B., Bauer, M., et al. Five year results of randomized clinical trial comparing total mastectomy and segmental mastectomy with or without radiation in the treatment of breast cancer. *N. Engl. J. Med.* 312:665, 1985. Fisher, B., Redmond, C., et al. Eight-year results of a randomized clinical trial comparing total mastectomy and lumpectomy with or without irradiation in the treatment of breast cancer. *N. Engl. J. Med.* 320:822, 1989.

The pros and cons of circumcision

Circumcision is still the nation's
most frequently performed
surgical procedure, yet
it's becoming more and
more controversial. Here's
what to tell parents.
By Lee Rothberg, RN

All parents should make an informed decision about circumcising their sons, yet many don't.

Unless they think to question the obstetrician or the pediatrician prior to delivery, the subject often doesn't come up until after the baby is born. Then, hounded by relatives, friends, physicians, and nurses, they must make their choice under pressure.

You can help them make the right choice for their child. Make sure they're familiar with the arguments for and against circumcision, and let them know what their decision will entail.

Why circumsize the baby?

Circumcision is routine in the U.S., despite findings by the American Academy of Pediatrics that it's

THE AUTHOR, a former OB/GYN nurse, is a member of the editorial board of *The Woman's Newspaper* in Princeton, N.J., and writes frequently on health issues.

generally unnecessary. The strongest arguments in favor of circumcision are, in fact, cultural not medical. Let's review those arguments.

Religious. Some religions dictate that male infants be circumcised. Parents who embrace these religions will usually be aware of the procedures they must follow for the circumcision ritual.

Psychological. An often-heard argument involves the so-called "locker-room syndrome." Its proponents claim that adolescent boys will make fun of their uncircumcised peers. Such teasing, it's said, can be traumatic because adolescence is not a time when a boy wants to be different—in any way—from his classmates.

Nor, it is thought, will he want to be different from his father, who is probably circumcised.

Rumor has it that uncircumcised men experience more sexual pleasure than those who are circum-

cised. Actual research studies, however, indicate that there's no difference.

Medical. Infant circumcision is sometimes viewed as a preventive measure, since anywhere from 2% to 10% of uncircumcised adult males must undergo the procedure for medical reasons. These include recurrent infections of the glans and foreskin, phimosis—the inability to retract the foreskin from the glans of the penis, or paraphimosis—the inability to push the retracted foreskin back over the glans.

Some researchers claim that the female sexual partners of uncircumcised men develop more frequent vaginal infections than the partners of circumcised men. The clinical evidence here is contradictory, but circumcision does make it easier to clean the glans and avoid infection.

When parents don't want to circumsize

The main reason parents give for not circumcising their sons is the desire to avoid unnecessary surgery. Others simply don't like to tamper with nature when there is no compelling reason to do so. Still others believe that circumcision causes the infant deep-seated psychological harm.

Despite the position taken by the American Academy of Pediatrics, there is little popular support for parents who decide against circumcision. You'll have to go out of your way to reassure such parents that they've made a good choice. You also need to tell them how to care for their son's uncircumcised penis.

Parents of uncircumcised boys are often told to "retract the foreskin and clean the glans." This advice is inappropriate. The foreskin and glans develop from the same embryonic tissue, and, in most boys, the foreskin doesn't separate from the glans until somewhere between the ages of three and six. At birth the foreskin may be slightly retractable, but it's rarely fully so. Trying to force back the foreskin can cause it to tear and may lead to infection.

Once the child has reached the age of three, it's all right for parents to try to retract the foreskin during his bath. They should hold the shaft of the penis with the thumb and index finger and *gently* pull the skin of the shaft back toward the child's abdomen. If they meet any resistance or if the child displays any signs of discomfort, however, they should stop. They can try the procedure again in a few months.

Most complications of the uncircumcised penis result, in fact, from forcible retraction of the foreskin. Phimosis usually develops when fibrotic tissue forms at the site of small tears at the edge of the foreskin. Paraphimosis often occurs when a barely retractable foreskin is forced back. Edema results, preventing the return of the foreskin to its normal position over the glans.

Posthitis (inflammation of the foreskin), balanitis (inflammation of the glans), or balanoposthitis (a combination of both) is most often seen in older boys and adults who don't practice good hygiene. If par-

ents make penile hygiene a part of the daily routine early in life, their sons will learn how to care for themselves and should have few, if any, problems.

What's involved in circumcision

Circumcision is usually performed by the mother's obstetrician. With the child restrained, the physician cleans the penis and surrounding area with an anti-bacterial solution. He then slits the infant's foreskin or draws it over a cone and places a special surgical clamp on it to close off the blood vessels. After that he removes about one centimeter of the foreskin. He applies Vaseline gauze after the procedure to reduce irritation.

Parents may ask you whether the procedure is painful. It's best to be honest and tell them that if circumcision is done without local anesthesia, the baby will have some discomfort. Until recently, physicians have been reluctant to administer anesthesia because of possible side effects, but its use is becoming more common.

As with any minor surgery, circumcision isn't 100% safe. Hemorrhage, infection, and trauma to the penis can occur. Pressure dressings, antibiotics, or sutures may be needed if any of these complications arise.

Another risk is that adhesions may develop. The glans can adhere to the skin of the penile shaft where the foreskin was removed. The penis becomes tethered, trapping bacteria and smegma, a secretion of the sebaceous glands.

Several precautions can mini-

mize these risks. To begin with, newborns shouldn't be circumcised in the first 24 hours of life. The chance of bleeding during this period is higher than when the infant is a little older.

Circumcision should never be performed on an infant with a family history of bleeding disorders or hemophilia, nor should it be performed if the mother takes anticoagulants or aspirin. Premature infants are not candidates for the procedure until they are considered strong enough to undergo it. Infants born with any abnormality of the glans, foreskin, or urethral meatus, such as epispadias or hypospadias, should not be circumcised until they have been evaluated by a urologist. If he decides the procedure is appropriate, he will probably perform it himself, using the foreskin to repair the abnormality.

How to care for the site

In the period immediately following the circumcision, check the infant hourly for bleeding, swelling, redness, or pus. Be sure to change the child's diaper frequently and apply fresh Vaseline gauze to the penis with each diaper change. When the parents are ready to take their son home, tell them to do the same.

Also instruct the parents to observe the circumcision site for any signs of infection, such as swelling, redness, or pus. Sometimes, a yellow or gray exudate will form as the site heals. This is normal and shouldn't be mistaken for pus. The circumcision site should heal within a week.

Beginning approximately two weeks after the circumcision and continuing for eight weeks, the parents should gently retract the skin of the shaft from the glans during the baby's daily bath. Doing so will help prevent the formation of adhesions.

By sharing your knowledge of this procedure, you can help parents make a truly informed decision. Then, whatever their choice, give them your support. They need to feel they've done the right thing for their son. ■

BIBLIOGRAPHY *Circumcision: a personal choice.* Washington, D.C.: American College of Obstetrics and Gynecology, 1984. Boyce, W.T. Care of the foreskin. *Pediatrics in review* 5:26, July 1983. Brunner, L. and Suddarth, D. *The Lippincott manual of nursing practice.* Philadelphia: J.B. Lippincott Co., 1978. DeMoya, D. and DeMoya, A. Preventing adhesions from circumcision. *RN* 48:75, June 1985. Gibbons, M.B. Circumcision: the controversy continues. *Pediatric Nursing* 10:103, March/April 1984. Herrera, A.J., Hsu, H.S., et al. The role of parental information in the incidence of circumcision. *Pediatrics* 70:597, Oct. 1982. Williamson, P. and Williamson, M. Psychological stress reduction by a local anesthetic during newborn circumcision. *Pediatrics* 71:36, Jan. 1983.

UNIT 5:
PSYCHIATRIC-MENTAL HEALTH NURSING

by

Jeanne Gelman, RN, MSN

An important aspect of professional nursing is the use of therapeutic intervention for clients who are experiencing emotional distress. A client does not have to have a psychiatric diagnosis to be in emotional distress, and often clients and their families may respond to illness or injury with anxiety and fear that can be manifested in a variety of behaviors. The principles of psychiatric-mental health nursing and therapeutic interventions can be applied to any client, family, or group in need.

To plan appropriate interventions, nurses need to have an understanding and knowledge of personality development and other theories to analyze behaviors of the client or others. Theories, principles, and treatment modalities are the *science* of psychiatric-mental health nursing.

The manner the nurse selects to use the science of mental health nursing is based in part on that nurse's personal attributes. Personal experiences, the ability to implement principles and theories, and the willingness to use therapeutic communication constitute the art of psychiatric-mental health nursing. This creative aspect of each nurse is the therapeutic use of self involved in planning and implementing effective nursing interventions for dealing with clients who are experiencing emotional distress.

The following principles of psychiatric-mental health nursing help form the basis of the therapeutic use of self.

- Be aware of your own feelings and responses.
- Maintain objectivity while being aware of your own needs.
- Use empathy (recognizing/identifing somewhat with client's emotions to understand behavior) not sympathy (close identification/duplication of client's emotions).
- Focus on the needs of the client, not on your own needs; be consistent and trustworthy.
- Accept clients as they are, be nonjudgmental.
- Recognize that emotions influence behaviors.
- Observe a client's behaviors to analyze needs/problems.

- Accept client's need to use defenses/behaviors to deal with emotional distress.
- Accept client's negative emotions.
- Avoid verbal reprimands, physical force, giving advice, or imposing your own values on clients.
- Avoid intimate relationships while maintaining a caring attitude.
- Assess clients in the context of their social/cultural group.
- Teach/explain on client's level of capability.
- Treat clients with respect, caring, and compassion.

Asking yourself, "What is this client's need at this time?" can assist you to determine the best response to questions.

Overview of Psychiatric-Mental Health Nursing

THEORETICAL BASIS

Medical-biologic Model

A. Emotional distress is viewed as illness.

B. Symptoms can be classified to determine a psychiatric diagnosis.

C. DSM III R*
1. Description of disorders
2. Criteria (behaviors) that must be met for diagnosis to be made
3. Axis: the dimensions and factors included when assessing a client with a mental disorder
   a. I and II: clinical syndromes (e.g., bipolar, antisocial personality, mental retardation)
   b. III: physical disorders and symptoms (e.g., cystic fibrosis, hypertension)
   c. IV: psychosocial stressors: acute and long-term severity of stressors
   d. V: functioning of client, rating of symptoms and their effect on activities of daily living (ADL) or violence to self/others

D. Diagnosed psychiatric illnesses are within the realm of medical practice and have a particular course, prognosis, and treatment regimen.

E. Treatment can include psychotropic drugs, electroconvulsive therapy (ECT), hospitalization, and psychotherapy.

F. There is no proven cause, but theory is that biochemical/genetic factors play a part in the development of mental illness. Theories with schizophrenia and affective disorders include
1. Genetic: increased risk when close relative (e.g., parent, sibling) has disorder
2. Possible link to neurotransmitter activity

Psychodynamic/Psychoanalytic Model (Freud)

A. Instincts (drives) produce energy.

B. There are genetically determined drives for sex and aggression.

C. Human behavior is determined by past experiences and responses.

---

*American Psychiatric Association. (1987). *Diagnostic and Statistical Manual of Mental Disorders* (4th ed.).

D. All behavior has meaning and can be understood.

E. Emotionally painful experiences/anxiety motivate behavior.

F. Client can change behavior and responses when made aware of the reasons for them.

G. Freud's theory of personality
1. *Id:* present at birth; instinctual drive for pleasure and immediate gratification, unconscious. *Libido* is the sexual and/or aggressive energy (drive). Operates on pleasure principle.
2. *Ego:* develops as sense of self that is distinct from world of reality; conscious, preconscious, and unconscious. Operates on reality principle.
   a. Conscious: awareness of own thoughts and perceptions of reality
   b. Preconscious: knowledge not readily available to conscious awareness but can be brought to awareness with effort (e.g., recalling name of a character in a book)
   c. Unconscious: knowledge that cannot be brought into conscious awareness without interventions such as psychoanalysis, hypnotism, or drugs
   d. Functions of the ego
      1) control and regulate instinctual drives
      2) mediate between id drives and demands of reality; id drives vs superego restrictions
      3) reality testing: evaluate and judge external world
      4) store up experiences in "memory"
      5) direct motor activity and actions
      6) solve problems
      7) use defense mechanisms to protect self
3. *Superego:* develops as person unconsciously incorporates standards and restrictions from parents to guide behaviors, thoughts, and feelings. Conscious awareness of acceptable/unacceptable thoughts, feelings, and actions is "conscience."

H. Freud's psychosexual developmental stages
1. *Oral*
   a. 0-18 months
   b. Pleasure and gratification through mouth
   c. Behaviors: dependency, eating, crying, biting
   d. Distinguishes between self and mother
   e. Develops body image, aggressive drives
2. *Anal*
   a. 18 months-3 years

b. Pleasure through elimination or retention of feces
c. Behaviors: control of holding on or letting go
d. Develops concept of power, punishment, ambivalence, concern with cleanliness or being dirty

3. *Phallic/Oedipal*
   a. 3-6 years
   b. Pleasure through genitals
   c. Behaviors: touching of genitals, erotic attachment to parent of opposite sex
   d. Develops fear of punishment by parent of same sex, guilt, sexual identity

4. *Latency*
   a. 6-12 years
   b. Energy used to gain new skills in social relationships and knowledge
   c. Behaviors: sense of industry and mastery
   d. Learns control over aggressive, destructive impulses
   e. Acquires friends

5. *Genital*
   a. 12-20 years
   b. Sexual pleasure through genitals
   c. Behaviors: becomes independent of parents, responsible for self
   d. Develops sexual identity, ability to love and work

Psychosocial Model (Erikson)

A. Emphasis on psychosocial rather than psychosexual development
B. Developmental stages have goals (tasks).
C. Challenge in each stage is to resolve conflict (e.g., trust vs mistrust).
D. Resolution of conflict prepares individual for next developmental stage.
E. Personality develops according to biologic, psychologic, and social influences
F. Erikson's psychosocial developmental tasks
   1. *Trust vs mistrust*
      a. 0-18 months
      b. Learn to trust others and self vs withdrawal, estrangement
   2. *Autonomy vs shame and doubt*
      a. 18 months-3 years
      b. Learn self-control and the degree one has to control the environment vs compulsive compliance or defiance
   3. *Initiative vs guilt*
      a. 3-5 years
      b. Learn to influence environment, evaluate own behavior vs fear of doing wrong, lack of self-confidence, over-restricting actions
   4. *Industry vs inferiority*
      a. 6-12 years
      b. Creative; develop sense of competency vs sense of inadequacy
   5. *Identity vs role diffusion*
      a. 12-20 years

b. Develop sense of self; preparation, planning for adult roles vs doubts relating to sexual identity, occupation/career
   6. *Intimacy vs isolation*
      a. 18-25 years
      b. Develop intimate relationship with another; commitment to career vs avoidance of choices in relationships, work, or life-style
   7. *Generativity vs stagnation*
      a. 21-45 years
      b. Productive; use of energies to guide next generation vs lack of interests, concern with self needs
   8. *Integrity vs despair*
      a. 45 years to end of life
      b. Relationships extended, belief that own life has been worthwhile vs lack of meaning of one's life, fear of death

Interpersonal Model (Sullivan)

A. Behavior motivated by need to avoid anxiety and satisfy needs
B. Sullivan's developmental tasks
   1. *Infancy*
      a. 0-18 months
      b. Others will satisfy needs
   2. *Childhood*
      a. 18 months-6 years
      b. Learn to delay need gratification
   3. *Juvenile*
      a. 6-9 years
      b. Learn to relate to peers
   4. *Preadolescence*
      a. 9-12 years
      b. Learn to relate to friends of same sex
   5. *Early adolescence*
      a. 12-14 years
      b. Learn independence and how to relate to opposite sex
   6. *Late adolescence*
      a. 14-21 years
      b. Develop intimate relationship with person of opposite sex

Therapeutic Nurse-Client Relationship (Peplau)

A. Based on Sullivan's interpersonal model
B. Therapeutic relationship is between nurse (helper) and client (recipient of care). The goal is to work together to assist client to grow and to resolve problems.
C. Differs from social relationship where both parties form alliance for mutual benefit.
D. Therapeutic use of self
   1. Focus is on client needs but nurse is also aware of own needs.
   2. Self-awareness enables nurse to avoid having own needs influence perception of client.
   3. Determine what client/family needs are at the time.
E. Three phases of nurse-client relationship
   1. *Orientation*

a. Nurse explains relationship to client, defines both nurse's and client's roles.

b. Nurse determines what client expects from the relationship and what can be done for the client.

c. Nurse contracts with client about when and where future meetings will take place.

d. Nurse assesses client and develops a plan of care based on appropriate nursing diagnoses.

e. Limits/termination of relationship are introduced (e.g., "We will be meeting for 30 minutes every morning while you are in the hospital.").

2. *Working phase*

a. Client's problems and needs are identified and explored as nurse and client develop mutual acceptance.

b. Client's dysfunctional symptoms, feelings, or interpersonal relationships are identified.

c. Therapeutic techniques are employed to reduce anxiety and to promote positive change and independence.

d. Goals are evaluated as therapeutic work proceeds, and changed as determined by client's progress.

3. *Termination*

a. Relationship and growth in nurse and client are summarized.

b. Client may become anxious and react with increased dependence, hostility, or withdrawal.

c. These reactions are discussed with client.

d. Feelings of nurse and client concerning termination should be discussed in context of finiteness of relationship.

F. Transference and countertransference

1. *Transference:* occurs when client transfers conflicts/feelings from past to the nurse. *Example:* Client becomes overly dependent, clinging to nurse who represents (unconsciously to client) the nurturing client desires from own mother.

2. *Countertransference:* occurs when nurse responds to client emotionally, as if in a personal, not professional/therapeutic relationship. Countertransference is a normal occurrence, but must be recognized so that supervision or consultation can keep it from undermining the nurse-client relationship. *Example:* Nurse is sarcastic and judgmental to client who has history of drug abuse. Client represents (unconsciously to nurse) the nurse's brother who has abused drugs.

3. Interventions

a. Reflect on reasons for behaviors of client or nurse.

b. Establish therapeutic goals for this relationship.

c. If unable to control these occurrences, transfer client to another nurse.

Human Motivation/Need Model (Maslow)

A. Hierarchy of needs in order of importance

1. Physiologic: oxygen, food, water, sleep, sex

2. Safety: security, protection, freedom from anxiety

3. Love and belonging: freedom from loneliness/alienation

4. Esteem and recognition: freedom from sense of worthlessness, inferiority, and helplessness

5. Self-actualization: aesthetic needs, self-fulfillment, creativity, spirituality

B. Primary needs (oxygen, fluids) need to be met prior to dealing with higher-level needs (esteem, recognition).

C. Focus on provision of positive aspects such as feeling safe, having someone care, affiliation

Behavioral Model (Pavlov, Skinner)

A. Behavior is learned and retained by positive reinforcement.

B. Motivation for behavior is not considered.

C. Behaviors that are not adaptive can be replaced by more adaptive behaviors.

Community Mental Health Model

A. Emotional distress stems from personal and social factors.

1. Family problems (e.g., divorce, single parenthood)

2. Social factors (e.g., unemployment, lack of support groups, changing mores)

B. Health care a right

C. Decreased need for hospitalization, increased community care

D. Collaboration of social and health care services

E. Comprehensive services

1. Emergency care

2. Inpatient/outpatient services

3. Substance-abuse treatment

4. Transitional living arrangements (temporary residence instead of inpatient care)

5. Consultation and education to increase knowledge of mental health

F. Prevention

1. Primary prevention

a. Minimize development of serious emotional distress: promote mental health, identify persons at risk.

b. Anticipate problems such as developmental crises (e.g., birth of first child, midlife crisis, death of spouse).

2. Secondary prevention: early case finding and treatment (drug therapy, outpatient, short-term hospitalization).

3. Tertiary prevention: restore client to optimal functioning; facilitate return of client to home and community by use of social agencies.

NURSING PROCESS

A. Applies to all clients, not only to those with psychiatric diagnosis; incorporates holism.

B. Utilized in a unique manner for psychosocial assessment.

C. Sets goals (with client, whenever possible) that can be measured in behavioral terms (e.g., client will dress self and eat breakfast before 9 A.M.).

D. Uses principles of therapeutic communication for interventions.

E. Evaluates whether, how well goals were met.

Physical Assessment

A. Subjective reporting of health history

B. Objective data (general status and appearance)

1. Age: client's appearance in relation to chronologic age

2. Attire: appropriateness of clothing to age/situation

3. Hygiene: cleanliness and grooming, or lack thereof

4. Physical health: weight, physical distress

5. Psychomotor: posture, movement, activity level
6. Sleep and rest
C. Neurologic assessment/level of consciousness

Mental Status Assessment

Emotional Status Assessment

Observation of mood and affect, noting following aspects
A. Appropriateness
B. Description: flat, sad, smiling, serious
C. Stability
D. Specific feelings and moods

Cognitive Assessment

Evaluation of thought, sensorium, intelligence
A. Intellectual performance
  1. Orientation to person, place, and time
  2. Attention and concentration
  3. Knowledge/educational level
  4. Memory: short and long term
  5. Judgment
  6. Insight into illness
  7. Ability to use abstraction
B. Speech
  1. Amount, volume, clarity
  2. Characteristics: pressured. slow or fast, dull or lively
  3. Echolalia, neologisms
C. Thoughts
  1. Content and clarity
  2. Characteristics: spontaneity, speed, loose associations, blocked, flight of ideas, repetitions

Social/Cultural Considerations

A. Age: assess for developmental tasks and developmental crises, age-related problems.
  1. 0–18 months: development of trust and sense of self, dependency
  2. 18 months–3 years: development of autonomy and beginning self-reliance, toilet training
  3. 3–6 years: development of sexual identity, relationships with peers, adjustment to school
  4. 6–12 years: mastery of skills, beginning self-esteem, identification with others outside family, social relationships
  5. 12–18 years: sense of self solidifies, separation and individuation often follow some disorganization and rebellion, substance abuse
  6. 18–25 years: identification with peer group, setting of personal and career goals to master future
  7. 25–38 years: take place in adult world, commitments made relating to career, marriage, parenthood
  8. 38–65 years: review of past accomplishments; may set new and reasonable goals; midlife crises when present achievements have not met goals set in earlier stages of development

  9. 65/70 to death: loss of friends/spouse, retirement, loss of some social/physical functions
B. Family/community relationships
  1. Role of client in family
  2. Family harmony, family support for or dependency on client
  3. Client's perception of family
  4. Availability of community support groups to client (include government social agencies; religious, ethnic, and volunteer agencies)
C. Socioeconomic group/education
  1. Factors that relate to how client is approached and how client perceives own present state
  2. Determination of level of teaching and need for social services
D. Cultural/spiritual background
  1. Assess behaviors in context of client's culture.
  2. Avoid stereotyping persons as having attributes of their culture/subculture.
  3. Note client's religious/philosophic beliefs.

ANALYSIS

Select nursing diagnoses based on collected data. Decide which is most important. Specific nursing diagnoses will be given when discussing particular disorders, but those nursing diagnoses generally appropriate to the client with psychiatric-mental health disorders include
A. Anxiety
B. Ineffective family coping
C. Ineffective individual coping: denial, defensive, impaired adjustment
D. Decisional conflict
E. Fatigue
F. Fear
G. Hopelessness
H. Potential for injury
I. Knowledge deficit
J. Powerlessness
K. Self-care deficit
L. Disturbance in self-concept: body image (perception of own physical appearance, usually set before adulthood), self-esteem (judgment/comparison of self to own ideal and to others' performance), situational low self-esteem, chronic low self-esteem, role performance (perception of fulfillment of own role in relation to self expectations), personal identity (sense of self)
M. Sleep pattern disturbances
N. Altered thought processes
O. Potential for violence

PLANNING AND IMPLEMENTATION

Goals

A. Client will
  1. Participate in treatment program.
  2. Be oriented to time, place, and person and exhibit reality-based behavior.

3. Recognize reasons for behavior and develop alternative coping mechanisms.
4. Maintain or improve self-care activities.
5. Be protected from harmful behaviors.

B. There will be mutual agreement of nurse and client whenever possible.

C. Short-term goals are set for immediate problems; they should be feasible and within client's capabilities.

D. Long-term goals are related to discharge planning and prevention of recurrence or exacerbation of symptoms.

Interventions

The nurse will use therapeutic intervention and the nurse-client relationship to help the client achieve the goals of therapy. Interventions must be geared to the level of the client's capability, and must relate to the specific problems identified for the individual client, family, or group.

Therapeutic Communication

A. Facilitative: use the following approaches to intervene therapeutically
   1. Silence: client able to think about self/problem; does not feel pressure or obligation to speak.
   2. Offering self: offer to provide comfort to client by presence (*Nurse:* "I'll sit with you." "I'll walk with you.").
   3. Accepting: indicate nonjudgmental acceptance of client and his perceptions by nodding and following what client says.
   4. Giving recognition: indicate to client your awareness of him and his behaviors (*Nurse:* "Good morning, John. You have combed your hair this morning.").
   5. Making observations: verbalize what you perceive (*Nurse:* "I notice that you can't seem to sit still.").
   6. Encouraging description: ask client to verbalize his perception (*Nurse:* "Tell me when you need to get up and walk around." "What is happening to you now?").
   7. Using broad openings: encourage client to introduce topic of conversation (*Nurse:* "Where shall we begin today?" "What are you thinking about?").
   8. Offering general leads: encourage client to continue discussing topic (*Nurse:* "And then?" "Tell me more about that.").
   9. Reflecting: direct client's questions/statements back to encourage expression of ideas and feelings (*Client:* "Do you think I should call my father?" *Nurse:* "What do you want to do?").
   10. Restating: repeat what client has said (*Client:* "I don't want to take the medicine." *Nurse:* "You don't want to take this medication?").
   11. Focusing: encourage client to stay on topic/point (*Nurse:* "You were talking about . . .").
   12. Exploring: encourage client to express feelings or ideas in more depth (*Nurse:* "Tell me more about . . ." "How did you respond to . . .?").
   13. Clarification: encourage client to make idea or feeling more explicit, understandable (*Nurse:* "I don't understand what you mean. Could you explain it to me?").
   14. Presenting reality: report events/situations as they really are (*Client:* "I don't get to talk to my doctor." *Nurse:* "I saw your doctor talking to you this morning.").
   15. Translating into feelings: encourage client to verbalize feelings expressed in another way (*Client:* "I will never get better." *Nurse:* "You sound rather hopeless and helpless.").
   16. Suggesting collaboration: offer to work with client toward goal (*Client:* "I fail at everything I try." *Nurse:* "Maybe we can figure out something together so that you can accomplish something you want to do.").

B. Ineffective communication styles: the following nontherapeutic approaches tend to block therapeutic communication and are sometimes used by nurses to avoid becoming involved with client's emotional distress; often a protective action on part of nurse.
   1. Reassuring: telling client there is no need to worry or be anxious (*Client:* "I'm nervous about this test." *Nurse:* "Everything will be all right.").
   2. Advising: telling client what you believe should be done (*Client:* "I am going to . . ." *Nurse:* "Why don't you do . . . instead?" or "I think you should do . . .").
   3. Requesting explanation: asking client to provide reasons for his feelings/behavior. The use of "why" questions should be avoided (*Nurse:* "Why do you feel, think, or act, this way?").
   4. Stereotypical response: replying to client with meaningless clichés (*Client:* "I hate being in the hospital." *Nurse:* "There's good and bad about everything.").
   5. Belittling feelings: minimizing or making light of client's distress or discomfort (*Client:* "I'm so depressed about . . ." *Nurse:* "Everyone feels sad at times.").
   6. Defending: protecting person or institutions (*Client:* "Ms. Jones is a rotten nurse." *Nurse:* "Ms. Jones is one of our best nurses.").
   7. Approving: giving approval to client's behavior or opinion (*Client:* "I'm going to change my attitude." *Nurse:* "That's good.").
   8. Disapproving: telling client certain behavior or opinions do not meet your approval (*Client:* "I am going to sign myself out of here." *Nurse:* "I'd rather you wouldn't do that.").
   9. Agreeing: letting client know that you think, feel alike; nurse verbalizes agreement.
   10. Disagreeing: letting client know that you do not agree; telling client that you do not believe he is right.
   11. Probing: questioning client about a topic he has indicated he does not want to discuss.
   12. Denial: refusing to recognize client's perception (*Client:* "I am a hopeless case." *Nurse:* "You are not hopeless. There is always hope.").
   13. Changing topic: letting client know you do not want to discuss a problem by introducing a new topic (*Client:* "I am a hopeless case." *Nurse:* "It's time to fill out your menu.").

Group Therapy

A. Groups of clients with one (or more) therapist meet to alleviate client problems in

  1. Interpersonal relations/communication
  2. Coping with particular stressors (e.g., ostomy groups)
  3. Self-understanding
B. Purposes
  1. Increase self-awareness
  2. Improve interpersonal relationships
  3. Make changes in behavior
  4. Deal with particular stressors
C. Stages of group development
  1. Beginning stage
    a. Anxiety in new situation
    b. Information given
    c. Group norms established
  2. Middle stage
    a. Group cohesiveness
    b. Members confronting each other
    c. Reliance on group member leading to self-reliance
    d. Sense of trust established
  3. Termination stage
    a. Individual member may leave abruptly.
    b. Group decides work is done.
    c. Ambivalence felt about termination.
    d. Ideally, group members have met goals.
D. Role of the nurse
  1. Explain purpose and rules of group
  2. Introduce group members
  3. Promote group cohesiveness
  4. Focus on problems of group and group process
  5. Encourage participation
  6. Role model
  7. Facilitate communication
  8. Set limits

Family Therapy

A. Client is whole family, although a family member may be "identified client."
B. Purposes
  1. Improve relationships among family members
  2. Promote family function
  3. Resolve family problem(s)
C. Process
  1. Problem(s) are identified by each family member.
  2. Members discuss their involvement in problem(s).
  3. Members discuss how problem(s) affect them.
  4. Members explore ways each of them can help resolve problem(s).
D. Role of the nurse
  1. Assess interactions among family members
  2. Make observations to family members
  3. Encourage expression of feelings by family members to one another
  4. Assists family in resolving problems

Milieu Therapy

A. Total environment (milieu) has an effect on individual's behavior, including

  1. Physical environment (i.e., cleanliness, noise, colors, fresh air, light)
  2. Relationships of staff to staff, staff to clients, and client to clients
  3. Atmosphere of safety, caring, mutual respect (e.g., client-run community meeting, community-set standards for behaviors)
B. Purposes
  1. Improve client's behavior
  2. Involve client in decision making of unit
  3. Increase client's sense of autonomy
  4. Increase communication among clients and between clients and staff
  5. Set structure of unit and behavioral limits
  6. Form a sense of community
C. Role of the nurse
  1. Involve clients in decision making
  2. Promote involvement of all staff
  3. Promote development of social skills of individual clients (e.g., nurse serves as role model)
  4. Encourage sense of community in staff and clients

Crisis Intervention

A. Client cannot resolve problem with usual problem-solving skills. Problem is so serious that functioning (homeostasis) is threatened. Crisis can be developmental (e.g., birth of first child) or situational (e.g., home destroyed by fire). Generally lasts for a few days, but can continue for weeks; is usually limited to 6 weeks.
B. Purposes
  1. Support client during time of crisis
  2. Resolution of crisis
  3. Restore client at least to precrisis level of functioning
  4. Allow client to attain higher level of functioning through acquiring greater skill in problem solving
C. Process
  1. Crisis event occurs: client unable to solve problem.
  2. Increase in level of client's anxiety.
  3. Client may use trial and error approach.
  4. If problem unresolved, anxiety escalates and client seeks help
D. Role of the nurse
  1. Assess client's perception of problem: realistic/distorted
  2. Determine situational supports (e.g., family, neighbors, agencies)
  3. Explore previous coping behaviors of client
  4. Offer support in resolving crisis
  5. Enlist help of situational supports
  6. Help client develop new, more effective coping behaviors
  7. Convey hope to client that crisis can be resolved
  8. Work with client as he resolves crisis

Behavior Modification

A. Based on theory that all behavior is learned as a result of positive reinforcement. Behaviors can be changed by substituting new behaviors.

B. Purpose: change unacceptable or maladaptive behaviors

C. Process

1. Determine the unacceptable behavior.
2. Identify more adaptive behavior to replace the unacceptable behavior.
3. Apply learning principles.
   a. Respond to unacceptable behavior by negative reinforcement (punishment) or by withholding positive reinforcement (ignore behavior).
   b. Determine what client views as reward.
4. When desired behavior occurs, present positive reinforcement (reward).
5. Consistently reward desired behavior.
6. Consistently respond to unacceptable behavior with negative reinforcement/ignoring behavior.

D. Types

1. *Counter conditioning:* specific stimulus evokes a maladaptive response that is replaced with a more adaptive response.
2. *Systematic desensitization*
   a. Expose to small amount of stimulus while ensuring relaxation (client cannot be anxious and relaxed at same time).
   b. Continue relaxing client while increasing amount of stimulus.
   c. Fear response to stimulus is eventually extinguished.
3. *Token economy:* tokens (rewards such as candy) are used to reinforce desired behaviors.

Psychotropic Medications

A variety of agents are used to control disordered thinking, anxiety and mood disorders. Effects, side effects, and nursing implications are summarized with each disorder.

EVALUATION

A. How well have goals been met? If not met, why not?

1. Review prior steps of nursing process.
   a. Do you need more assessment data?
   b. Were nursing diagnoses prioritized?
   c. Were goals feasible and measurable?
   d. Were interventions appropriate?
2. Revise goals as necessary.

B. Client

1. Enrolled/participates in appropriate treatment program.
2. Expresses concerns/needs and develops a therapeutic relationship with nurse.
3. Identifies causes for behavior; learns and uses alternative coping mechanisms.
4. Demonstrates ability to care for self at optimum level and to identify areas where assistance is needed.
5. Does not engage in harmful behaviors; shows increased ability to control destructive impulses.

C. Client's behavior demonstrates optimal orientation to reality (e.g., can state name, place); interacts appropriately with others.

BEHAVIORS RELATED TO EMOTIONAL DISTRESS

Anxiety

A. General information

1. One of the most important concepts in psychiatric-mental health nursing.
2. Anxiety is present in almost every instance where clients are experiencing emotional distress/have a diagnosed psychiatric illness.
3. Experienced as a sense of emotional or physical distress as the individual responds to an unknown threat or thwarting of unmet needs.
4. The ego protects itself from the effects of anxiety by the use of defense mechanisms (see Table 5.1).
5. Physiologic responses are related to autonomic nervous system response and to level of anxiety.
   a. Subjective: client experiences feelings of tension, need to act, uneasiness, distress, and apprehension or fear.
   b. Objective: client exhibits restlessness, inability to concentrate, tension, dilated pupils, changes in vital signs (usually increased by sympathetic nervous system response, may be decreased by parasympathetic reactions).
6. Anxiety can be viewed positively (motivates us to change and grow) or negatively (interferes with problem-solving ability and affects functioning).
   a. *Trait anxiety:* individual's normal level of anxiety. Some people are usually rather intense while others are more relaxed; may be related to genetic predisposition/early experiences (repressed conflicts).
   b. *State anxiety:* change in person's anxiety level in response to stressors (environmental or any internal threat to the ego).
7. Levels of anxiety
   a. *Mild:* increased awareness; ability to problem solve, learn; increase in perceptual field; minimal muscle tension
   b. *Moderate:* optimal level for learning, perceptual field narrows to pay attention to particular details, increased tension to solve problems or meet challenges
   c. *Severe:* sympathetic nervous system (flight/fight response); increase in blood pressure, pulse, and respirations; narrowed perceptual field, fixed vision, dilated pupils, can perceive scattered details or only one detail; difficulty in problem solving
   d. *Panic:* decrease in vital signs (release of sympathetic response), distorted perceptual field, inability to solve problems, disorganized behavior, feelings of helplessness/terror

B. Nursing interventions

1. Determine the level of client's anxiety by assessing verbal and nonverbal behaviors and physiologic symptoms.

2. Determine cause(s) of anxiety with client, if possible.
3. Encourage client to move from affective (feeling) mode to cognitive (thinking) behavior (e.g., ask client, "What are you thinking?"). Stay with client. Reduce anxiety by remaining calm yourself; use silence, or speak slowly and softly.
4. Help client recognize own anxious behavior.
5. Provide outlets (e.g., talking, psychomotor activity, crying, tasks).
6. Provide support and encourage client to find way to cope with anxiety.
7. In panic state nurse must make decisions.
   a. Do not leave client alone.
   b. Encourage ventilation of thoughts and feelings.
   c. Use firm voice and give short, explicit directions (e.g., "Sit in this chair. I will sit here next to you.").
   d. Engage client in motor activity to reduce tension (e.g., "We can take a brisk walk around the day room. Let's go.").

Defense Mechanisms

Usually unconscious processes used by ego to defend itself from anxiety and threats (see Table 5.1).

Disorders of Perception

Occur with increased anxiety, disordered thinking/impaired reality testing

A. *Illusions*
   1. General information: stimulus in the environment is misperceived (e.g., car backfiring is perceived as a gunshot; a bathrobe in an open closet is perceived as a person in the closet); may be visual, auditory, tactile, gustatory, olfactory.
   2. Nursing intervention: show/explain stimulus to client to promote reality testing.
B. *Delusions*
   1. General information: fixed, false set of beliefs that are real to client.
      a. Grandiose: false belief that client has power, wealth, or status or is famous person
      b. Persecutory: false belief that client is the object of another's harassment or harmful intent
      c. Somatic: false belief that client has some physical/physiologic defect
   2. Nursing interventions
      a. Avoid arguing; client cannot be convinced, even with evidence, that the belief is false.
      b. Determine client's need (grandiose delusion may indicate low self-esteem; provide opportunities to succeed at task that will enhance self-concept).
      c. Reduce anxiety to encourage decreased need to use delusions.
      d. Accept client's need for delusion, present (but do not insist that client accept) reality.
      e. After therapeutic relationship has been established, you can express doubt about delusions to client.
      f. Direct client's attention to nondelusional, nonthreatening topics (e.g., current events, client's hobbies or interests).

C. *Ideas of reference*
   1. General information: belief that events or behaviors of others relate to self (e.g., telephone rings in nurse's station, client believes "they" are calling for him; two nurses are talking and laughing, client believes nurses are talking/laughing at him.)
   2. Nursing interventions are the same as for delusions.
D. *Hallucinations*
   1. General information: sensory perceptions that have no stimulus in environment; most common hallucinations are auditory and visual (e.g., hearing voices; seeing persons, animals, objects).
   2. Nursing interventions
      a. Encourage client to describe hallucination.
      b. Accept that this is a real experience for client.
      c. Present reality.
      d. Example: nurse sees client in listening attitude or responding to auditory hallucinations. *Nurse:* "You seem to be listening/talking." *Client:* "The voices are telling me to hurt myself." *Nurse:* "I don't hear the voices. Tell me what the voices are saying to you."

Withdrawal

A. General information: withdrawal from social interaction by not talking, walking away, turning away, sleeping or feigning sleep
B. Nursing interventions
   1. Use silence.
   2. Offer self.
   3. Discuss nonthreatening topics that will not provoke increased anxiety.
   4. Be consistent; keep promises, promote trust.

Hostility and Aggression

A. General information
   1. Hostile behavior: responding to nurse with anger, insults, threats
   2. Assaultive behavior: attempting to physically harm others
   3. Usually nurse is not real object of client's anger, but is convenient target for angry feelings/verbalizations.
B. Nursing interventions
   1. Hostility
      a. Recognize own response of anger or defensiveness.
      b. Determine source of client's anger.
      c. Accept angry feelings.
      d. Attempt to have client verbalize feelings and channel into acceptable behaviors.
   2. Physical aggression/assaultive behaviors (client may act on increased anxiety by throwing objects or attempt to physically harm others)
      a. Assess for increased anxiety.
      b. Attempt to have client verbalize feelings.
      c. Talk client down.
      d. Obtain help if client becomes assaultive.

Table 5.1   Defense Mechanisms

Type	Characteristics	Examples
Denial	Refusal to acknowledge a part of reality	A client on strict bedrest is walking down the hall; shows refusal to acknowledge need to stay in bed because of illness. A client states admission to the mental hospital is for reasons other than mental illness.
Repression	Threatening thoughts are pushed into the unconscious, anxiety and other symptoms are observed; client unable to have conscious awareness of conflicts or events that are source of anxiety.	"I don't know why I have to wash my hands all the time, I just have to."
Suppression	Consciously putting a threatening/distressing thought out of one's awareness.	A nurse must study for the NCLEX, but she has had a heated argument with her boyfriend. She decides to not think about the problem until she finishes studying, then she will attempt to resolve it.
Rationalization	Developing an acceptable, justifiable (to self) reason for behavior	A friend tells you that he has been in an automobile accident because the car skidded on wet leaves in the road; you return to the scene of the accident, but there are no leaves; friend admits to you and to self that he was probably driving too fast.
Reaction-formation	Engaging in behavior that is opposite of true desires	A man has an unconscious desire to view x-rated films; he circulates a petition to close the theatre where such films are shown.
Sublimation	Anxiety channeled into socially acceptable behavior	A student is upset because she received a failing grade on a test; she knows that she will feel better if she goes jogging and goes out to run a few miles.
Compensation	Making up for a deficit by success in another area	A young man who cannot make any varsity teams becomes the chess champion in his school.
Projection	Placing own undesirable trait onto another; blaming others for own difficulty	A student who would like to cheat on an exam states that other students are trying to cheat; a paranoid client claims that the FBI had him committed to the mental hospital.
Displacement	Directing feelings about one object/person toward a less threatening object/person	The head nurse reprimands you; you do not argue even though you do not agree with her reprimand; when you return home that evening you are hostile towards your roommate.
Identification	Taking onto oneself the traits of others that one admires	You greatly admire the clinical specialist in your hospital; unconsciously you begin to use the approaches she uses with clients.
Introjection	Symbolic incorporation of another into one's own personality	John becomes depressed when his father dies; John's feelings are directed to the mental image he has of his father.
Conversion	Anxiety converted into a physical symptom that is motor or sensory in nature	A young woman unconsciously desires to strike her mother; she develops sudden paralysis of her arms.
Symbolization	Representing an idea or object by a substitute object or sign.	A man who was spurned by a librarian develops a dislike of books and reading.
Dissociation	Separation or splitting off of one aspect of mental process from conscious awareness.	A student who prides herself on being prompt does not recall the times that she arrived late for class.
Undoing	Behavior that is opposite of earlier unacceptable behavior or thought	Joan tells an ethnic joke to a coworker, Sally; Sally, a member of that ethnic group, is offended; the following week Joan offers to work the weekend for Sally.
Regression	Behavior that reflects an earlier level of development. Adults hospitalized with serious illnesses sometimes will engage in regressive behaviors.	When a new baby is brought home, 5-year-old Billy begins to wet his pants although he had not done this for the past 2½ years.

Self-mutilation

A. General information: behaviors cause physical injury but are not motivated by the desire to die.

B. Nursing interventions
1. Assess for suicide risk.
2. Offer support.
3. Protect client from carrying out self-mutilation actions.
4. Remove objects that can be used for self-harm.
5. Observe for changes in behaviors and attitudes.

Suicide

A. General information
1. Ideation: verbalization of wish to die (overt or disguised)
2. Gestures: engaging in nonlethal behaviors (e.g., superficial scratches, ingestion of medication in amounts that are not likely to cause serious injury/death)
3. Actions: engaging in behaviors or planning to engage in behaviors that have potential to cause death
4. May or may not be associated with a psychiatric disorder
5. Groups at risk (see Table 5.2)

B. Assessment findings
1. Verbal cues
   a. Overt: "I intend to commit suicide."
   b. Disguised: "I have the answer to my problems."
2. Behavioral cues
   a. Giving away prized possessions
   b. Getting financial affairs in order, making a will
   c. Suicidal ideation/gestures
   d. Indications of hopelessness, depression
   e. Sudden changes in behaviors and attitudes (person suddenly becomes apathetic, depressed; person suddenly becomes alert, positive)

Table 5.2 Groups at Increased Risk for Suicide

- Adolescents
- Elderly
- Terminally ill
- Persons who have experienced loss/stress
- Survivors of persons who have committed suicide
- Depressed persons (when depression begins to lift)
- Alcoholics
- Policemen, physicians, dentists
- Minority groups
- Persons who have attempted suicide previously
- More women attempt suicide; more men complete suicide.

---

3. For lethality assessment, see Table 5.3.

C. Nursing interventions
1. Contract with client to report suicidal attempt.
2. Assess suicide risk.
   a. Ask client if he thinks about, intends to harm himself.
   b. Ask client if he has formulation of plan; if details are worked out, when? where? how?
   c. Check availability of method (e.g., gun, pills).
3. Keep client under constant observation.
4. Remove any objects that can be used in suicide attempt (e.g., shoe laces, sharp objects).
5. Therapeutic intervention
   a. Support aspects of wish to live; clients often ambivalent: wish to live and wish to die.
   b. Use one-to-one nurse/client relationship (let client know you care for him).
   c. Allow client to express feelings of hopelessness, helplessness, worthlessness.
   d. Provide hope.
   e. Provide diversionary activities.
   f. Utilize support groups (e.g., family, clergy).
6. Following a suicide
   a. Encourage survivors to discuss client's death, their feelings and fears.
   b. Provide anticipatory guidance to family who may experience problems at holidays, anniversaries.
   c. Hold staff meetings to ventilate feelings.

Table 5.3 Lethality Assessment

- Plans for suicide: when? where? how?
- Means available: what will be used? is it available to client?
- Lethality of means (e.g., tranquilizers are less lethal when used alone than when combined with alcohol; guns are more lethal than plan to cut wrists)
  - Most lethal: gunshot, hanging, jumping from high places, carbon monoxide, potent poisons (e.g., cyanide)
  - Less lethal: nonprescription drugs, wrist cutting, tranquilizers without CNS depressants
- Possibility of "rescue"
- Support systems available or sense of isolation
- Availability of alcohol or drugs
- Severe/panic level of anxiety
- Hostility
- Disorganized thinking
- Preoccupation with thought of suicide plan

Psychiatric Disorders (DSM III R)

DISORDERS OF INFANCY, CHILDHOOD, AND ADOLESCENCE

Overview

A. A specific group of disorders beginning in infancy, childhood, or adolescence
B. Clients in these age groups may also evidence other disorders such as depression or schizophrenia.
C. Intellectual, behavioral, and/or emotional dysfunction of the young client also has an effect on the family, which may require nursing intervention.

Assessment

Newborn/Infants

A. Maturation
B. Developmental level
C. Sensorimotor capabilities
D. Bonding
E. Response to cuddling

Children/Adolescents

A. Motor skills
B. Communication abilities
C. Vocational/academic skills
D. Social and behavioral problems
E. Behavioral changes
F. Growth and development: physical/emotional
G. Self-concept
H. Knowledge of disorder

Parents/Family

A. Response to infant/child/adolescent with disorder
B. Guilt, sense of loss
C. Sibling jealousy/resentment
D. Knowledge of disorder
E. Expectations
F. Plans for future (home care/institutionalization)

Analysis

Nursing diagnoses for a child/family with a psychiatric-mental health disorder may include
A. Client
  1. Anxiety
  2. Altered bowel/urinary elimination
  3. Ineffective individual coping
  4. Potential for injury
  5. Knowledge deficit
  6. Self-care deficit
  7. Disturbance in self-concept
  8. Sensory-perceptual alterations
  9. Sexual dysfunction
  10. Potential for violence
B. Parents/family
  1. Anxiety
  2. Ineffective family coping
  3. Altered family process
  4. Anticipatory grieving
  5. Knowledge deficit
  6. Altered parenting

Planning and Implementaion

Goals

A. Client will
  1. Communicate thoughts and feelings about self-concept.
  2. Perform tasks at optimal level of capability.
  3. Develop trusting relationship with care givers.
B. Parents/family will
  1. Communicate feelings and responses to child and to disorder.
  2. Demonstrate knowledge of disorder.
  3. Formulate plans for child's care.

Interventions

A. Client
  1. Establish a therapeutic relationship by accepting client and client's limitations.
  2. Promote communication by use of therapeutic techniques, play therapy.

3. Encourage independence in task performance with guidance and support.

B. Parents/family
   1. Promote communication by accepting family responses.
   2. Provide information about disorder.
   3. Contact appropriate person/agency for consultation with family about care and assistance with the child.

Evaluation

Client

A. Demonstrates trust in care givers.
B. Relates feelings about self verbally or symbolically.
C. Performs activities of daily living (ADL) and tasks at optimal level.

Parents/family

A. Relate positive/negative responses to child.
B. Demonstrate understanding of disorder and child's potential.
C. With consultant, formulate a plan for child's care.

Specific Disorders

Mental Retardation

A. General information
   1. Significant subaverage intelligence resulting in maladaptive behaviors with onset before age of 18 years
   2. Etiology
      a. 25% biologic
         1) chromosomal (e.g., Down's syndrome)
         2) metabolic (e.g., PKU)
         3) usually diagnosed at birth or in early years
      b. Remaining 75% of unknown etiology
         1) may be related to social or nutritional deprivation, genetic factors
         2) may not be diagnosed until the child starts school
   3. Degrees of retardation
      a. Mild mental retardation (IQ 50–70)
         1) 80% of cases
         2) educable to 6th grade level
         3) able to become self-supporting
      b. Moderate mental retardation (IQ 35–49)
         1) 12% of cases
         2) educable to 2nd grade level
         3) able to perform skills but will need supervision at work
      c. Severe mental retardation (IQ 20–34)
         1) 7% of cases
         2) may learn to talk/communicate
         3) able to perform simple tasks and elementary hygiene
      d. Profound mental retardation (IQ below 20)
         1) less than 1% of cases
         2) some speech/communication possible
B. Assessment findings
   1. Intellectual impairment (determine degree)
   2. Sensorimotor impairment

3. Communication, social, behavioral impairment
4. Lack of self-esteem and poor self-image
5. Sense of loss, guilt, nonacceptance or unrealistic expectations on part of parents/family

C. Nursing interventions
   1. Promote optimal functioning in ADL and feelings of accomplishment, self-worth.
   2. Provide opportunities for client/family to communicate thoughts, feelings.
   3. Provide positive reinforcement for every success.
   4. Accept client's limitations and set goals accordingly.
   5. Provide support and information about disorder to family.
   6. Accept family's response to client.

Anxiety Disorders of Childhood/Adolescence

A. General information
   1. *Separation anxiety:* excessive anxiety and worry about being separated from person(s)/places to whom child has become attached (e.g., refusal to leave mother/home to attend school)
   2. *Avoidant disorder:* reluctance to enter social relationships with others, creating an interference with social growth
   3. *Overanxious disorders:* pervasive, unrealistic worry or concern about competency; somatic complaints without physical basis
B. Assessment findings: excessive anxiety related to separation, social interaction, and achievements
C. Nursing intervention: provide information regarding available mental health services for child and family.

Disorders with Physical Manifestations

A. General information
   1. Important to rule out any physiologic cause
   2. Often related to stress or conflict in the family
   3. May affect child's family/social interactions and development
B. Assessment findings
   1. *Enuresis:* urinary incontinence (bed-wetting) after age 5 not caused by physical disorder
   2. *Encopresis:* fecal incontinence after age 4 not caused by physical disorder
   3. *Tics:* involuntary, repetitive movements
   4. *Stuttering:* repetition of sounds, words or frequent hesitations in speaking
C. Nursing interventions
   1. Provide information about the disorders and emphasize that they are treatable.
   2. Determine whether family therapy may be indicated, as well as individual therapy for child.
   3. Offer support and help child/family overcome feelings of shame or guilt.
   4. For enuresis and encopresis, utilize toilet training techniques.
   5. Encourage discussion of client/family response to symptoms.

Infantile Autism

A. General information
 1. Develops prior to 30 months of age.
 2. Child does not relate to people, but may become attached to objects.
 3. This is a rare disorder, may have a physiologic basis.
 4. More common in upper socioeconomic groups.
 5. Chronic disorder, more than $^2/_3$ of these children remain severely handicapped and dependent on care givers.
 6. Special education is necessary.
 7. Family may choose institutionalization for optimum care.
B. Assessment findings
 1. Infant not responsive to cuddling; may even show an aversion to being touched
 2. No eye contact or facial responsiveness
 3. Impaired or no verbal communication
 4. Echolalia (repetition of words/phrases spoken by others)
 5. Inability to tolerate change
 6. Ritualistic behavior
 7. Fascination with movement, spinning objects
 8. Labile moods
 9. Unresponsive or overresponsive to stimuli
 10. Potential to develop seizure disorders
C. Nursing interventions
 1. Provide parents/family with support and information about the disorder, opportunities for therapy and education for the child.
 2. Assist child with ADL.
 3. Promote reality testing.
 4. Encourage child to develop a relationship with another person.
 5. Maintain regular schedule for activities.
 6. Provide constant routine for child (place for eating, sitting, sleeping).
 7. Protect child from self-injury.
 8. Provide safe environment.
 9. Institute seizure precautions if necessary.

Pervasive Developmental Disorder

A. General information
 1. Develops after 30 months but before 12 years of age
 2. Rare disorder, more commonly found in males
 3. Chronic disorder, children usually unable to function independently
 4. Special education and institutional care may be necessary.
B. Assessment findings
 1. Gross and sustained impairment in social relationships
 2. Excessive anxiety, panic attacks
 3. Labile moods
 4. Resistance to change
 5. Posturing, walking on tiptoe
 6. Unresponsiveness or overresponsiveness to stimuli
 7. Potential for self-mutilation
C. Nursing interventions: same as for Infantile Autism.

Eating Disorders

A. General information
 1. Gross disturbances in eating behaviors
 2. *Pica:* persistent eating of substances such as plaster, paint, or sand
 3. *Bulimia:* binge eating; the ingestion of large amounts of food in short time, often followed by self-induced vomiting. May be accompanied by affective disorders and fear of being unable to stop this behavior. Manifested by fluctuations in weight caused by binges of eating and fasting.
 4. *Anorexia nervosa:* refusal to eat or aberration in eating patterns resulting in severe emaciation that can be life threatening. Characterized by a fear of becoming fat, and a body-image disturbance where clients claim to feel fat even when extremely thin. This disorder is most common (95%) in adolescent and young adult females. There is a mortality rate of 15%–20%.
B. Assessment findings (anorexia nervosa)
 1. History of high activity and achievement in academics, athletics
 2. Social withdrawal and poor family and individual coping skills
 3. Preoccupation with being thin; inability to recognize degree of own emaciation (distorted body image)
 4. Weight loss of 25% or more of original body weight
 5. Amenorrhea
 6. Electrolyte imbalance
 7. Depression
C. Nursing interventions
 1. Monitor vital signs.
 2. Measure I&O.
 3. Weigh client 3 times/week at the same time (check to be sure client has not hidden heavy objects when being weighed, weigh in hospital gown).
 4. Set limits on time allotted for eating.
 5. Record amount eaten.
 6. Stay with client during meals, focusing on client, not on food.
 7. Accompany client to bathroom for at least ½ hour after eating to prevent self-induced vomiting.
 8. Individual/family therapy may be necessary.
 9. Encourage client to express feelings.
 10. Help client to set realistic goal for self and to reduce need for being perfect.
 11. Encourage client to discuss own body image; present reality; do not argue with client.
 12. Teach relaxation techniques.
 13. Help client identify interests and positive aspects of self.

SAMPLE QUESTIONS

1. Eddie, 6 years old, has been diagnosed with enuresis after tests revealed no organic cause of bed wetting. Eddie's mother

is upset and blames the problem on his father. "It's all his father's fault!" Your initial response is
- ○ 1. Why do you say that?
- ○ 2. It's usually nobody's fault.
- ○ 3. You seem really upset by this.
- ○ 4. Why are you blaming Eddie's father?

2. Kara, 17 years old, is admitted with anorexia nervosa. You have been assigned to sit with her while she eats her dinner. Kara says to you, "My primary nurse trusts me. I don't see why you don't." Your best response is
- ○ 1. I do trust you, but I was assigned to be with you.
- ○ 2. It sounds as if you are manipulating me.
- ○ 3. OK. When I return, you should have eaten everything.
- ○ 4. Who is your primary nurse?

ORGANIC MENTAL DISORDERS (OMD)

Overview

A. A group of disorders with a known or presumed etiology
B. Frequently manifest as dementia or delirium
C. May be substance induced (drugs or alcohol) or caused by a disease process; etiology may be unknown.
D. It is important for the nurse to assess behaviors rather than focus on medical diagnoses.
E. Behaviors related to impaired brain functioning may be temporary or permanent, with increasing degeneration and eventual loss of brain function.
F. Not exclusive to old age, may complicate illnesses in any age group.

Types

A. *Organic brain syndrome (OBS):* syndromes that have no reference to etiology such as delirium or dementias.
B. *Delirium*
   1. Manifested by reduced awareness of environment, disorders of perception, thought, speech, and attention deficits.
   2. Usually of brief duration
   3. May occur postoperatively or following head injury, intoxication from drugs/alcohol, acute disease, or injury.
C. *Dementia*
   1. Loss of intellectual abilities resulting in impaired social and occupational functioning
   2. May be temporary, or progressive loss may occur
   3. Found predominantly in elderly
   4. Personality changes are usually an exaggeration of former character traits (e.g., suspicious, nontrusting person becomes paranoid); but alteration can also occur (e.g., formerly neat and orderly person pays no attention to hygiene, becomes sloppy and dirty).
   5. Memory impairment; short-term memory loss may be most obvious.
   6. Organic etiology may be known; conditions include intoxication, infections, tumors, circulatory disorders (cerebral atherosclerosis), trauma, Huntington's chorea, Korsakoff's syndrome, Creutzfeld-Jakob disease, neurosyphilis.
   7. Specific etiology may not be known (e.g., Alzheimer's disease, Pick's disease).
   8. Frequently these clients cannot perform basic ADL.

Assessment

A. Mental status assessment, especially orientation to time and place, memory, and judgment
B. Nutritional status
C. Ability to perform ADL, self-care
D. Presence of confabulation (making up information to fill in memory gaps)
E. Behavioral/social changes
F. Disorders of perception
G. Impaired motor skills, coordination
H. Change in sleep patterns
I. Elimination: constipation/incontinence
J. Family response to client's condition

Analysis

Nursing diagnoses for clients with OMD may include
A. Anxiety
B. Impaired verbal communication
C. Ineffective individual/family coping
D. Altered family process
E. Altered fluid volume
F. Potential for injury
G. Altered nutrition
H. Self-care deficit
I. Disturbance in self-concept
J. Sleep pattern disturbance
K. Altered thought processes
L. Potential for violence

Planning/Implementation

Goals

A. Client will
   1. Be protected from injury.
   2. Retain optimal cognitive function and self-care abilities.
   3. Have fear/anxiety minimized.
   4. Maintain adequate nutrition/hydration.
B. Family will communicate feelings about client.

Interventions

A. Institute safety measures: side rails, frequent checks, restraints only as last resort and for protection of client as ordered by physician.
B. Maintain reality orientation.
   1. Client may not be capable of reality testing.

2. Continue to address client by name.

3. Maintain awareness of client's limitations in this area.

4. Do not tell client to "remember"; severe memory loss may make client incapable of memory.

C. Assist/support with self-care needs; arrange for necessary assistive devices, help with feeding; encourage fluids.

D. Avoid "insight" therapy and discussion of impaired mental functioning as this may increase anxiety.

E. Provide spouse/family with information about client's capabilities.

F. Provide support for spouse/family; encourage continued interaction with client.

Evaluation

A. Client
1. Remains free from injuries.
2. Retains cognitive functions and self-care ability as far as possible; interacts with others appropriately.
3. Maintains appropriate weight.

B. Family
1. Expresses sense of loss or frustration related to client's condition.
2. Continues contact with client.

SAMPLE QUESTIONS

Millie Robertson, aged 74, was recently admitted to a nursing home because of confusion, disorientation, and negativistic behavior.

3. Her family states that Millie is in good health. Millie asks you, "Where am I?" Your best response is
   - ○ 1. Don't worry, Millie. You're safe here.
   - ○ 2. Where do you think you are?
   - ○ 3. What did your family tell you?
   - ○ 4. You're at the community nursing home.

4. Which of the following would be an appropriate strategy in reorienting Millie to where her room is?
   - ○ 1. Place pictures of her family on the bedside stand.
   - ○ 2. Put her name in large letters on her forehead.
   - ○ 3. Remind Millie where her room is.
   - ○ 4. Let the other residents know where Millie's room is.

5. Which activity would you engage Millie in at the nursing home?
   - ○ 1. Reminiscent groups
   - ○ 2. Sing-alongs
   - ○ 3. Discussion groups
   - ○ 4. Exercise class

6. Millie has had difficulty sleeping since admission. Which of the following would be the best intervention?
   - ○ 1. Provide her with a glass of warm milk.
   - ○ 2. Ask the physician for a mild sedative.
   - ○ 3. Do not allow Millie to take naps during the day.
   - ○ 4. Ask her family what they prefer.

SUBSTANCE USE DISORDERS

Overview

A. The use of chemical agents (alcohol and drugs) to change behavior and mood

B. Abuse: continued use despite problems (social, occupational, psychologic) that are caused by substance or continued use in hazardous situations (e.g., operating machinery, driving)

C. Dependence
1. Need for larger amounts (tolerance)
2. Unsuccessful attempts to decrease/discontinue use
3. Inability to function as usual in work, social activities
4. Withdrawal symptoms (psychologic/physical distress when substance is reduced/discontinued)

D. Addiction: compulsive use of a substance; physiologic and psychologic dependence

PSYCHOACTIVE SUBSTANCE-INDUCED ORGANIC MENTAL DISORDERS

The use of substances that result in intoxication or withdrawal syndromes, delirium, hallucinations, delusions, mood disorders

Assessment

A. Determine substance used, amount and time taken, and if combined with other drugs

B. Pupillary changes, changes in vital signs or level of consciousness

C. Presence of dehydration

D. Presence of nutritional and vitamin deficiencies

E. Suicide potential: ideation, gestures

F. Level of anxiety

G. Use of denial/projection

H. Symptoms of overdose (will be drug-specific; see Table 5.4)

I. Drug-use patterns: what, when, why substances are used

Analysis

Nursing diagnoses for clients with a psychoactive substance abuse disorder may include

A. Anxiety

B. Ineffective individual/family coping

C. Fear

D. Altered fluid volume

E. Potential for injury

F. Altered nutrition

G. Self-care deficit

H. Disturbance in self-concept

I. Sensory-perceptual alterations

J. Sleep pattern disturbance

K. Altered thought processes

L. Potential for violence

Planning and Intervention

Goals

Client will

A. Be protected from injury.

B. Receive adequate hydration and nutrition.

C. Terminate use of substance being abused without withdrawal symptoms; emergency care will be provided if symptoms cannot be avoided.

D. Have decreased feelings of anxiety.

E. Receive information and consider help for substance-abuse disorder.

Interventions

A. Assess drug use pattern: identity, recent use, and frequency of use of prescription and nonprescription drugs, other substances (e.g., alcohol, nicotine).

B. Support client during acute phase of detoxification or withdrawal.
1. Stay with client; reassure that current manifestations are temporary.
2. Monitor vital signs, level of consciousness.
3. Institute suicide precautions.
4. Administer medications (to prevent withdrawal) as ordered.
5. If patient is experiencing panic, talk down, possibly with assistance of family/friends.
6. If client is hallucinating, reinforce reality, speak in a calm voice.
7. Confront client's use of denial.
8. Monitor your own responses of sympathy/anger.
9. Be aware of transference/countertransference.
10. Maintain course of action in plan of care; client must follow plan.
11. Involve staff in negotiating care plan revisions.

C. Rehabilitation/longer-term care
1. Provide nonthreatening environment.
2. Set limits on unacceptable behavior.
3. Provide adequate diet and fluids.
4. Provide information relating to substance abuse and rehabilitation programs.

Evaluation

A. Client experienced no injury.

B. Vital signs are stable.

C. Withdrawal proceeded without symptoms; client remains drug/alcohol free.

D. Client can discuss substance-abuse problem and requests or agrees to consider rehabilitation/therapy for problem.

Specific Disorders

Alcohol Abuse/Dependence

A. General information
1. Alcohol is a legal substance and there are millions of social drinkers.
2. Alcohol is classified as a central nervous system depressant.
3. Alcohol abuse/dependence is a major problem in this country with over 10 million adults identified as alcoholics.
4. Only approximately 5% of alcoholics are the "skid row" type.
5. Incidence is increasing in women and adolescents.

6. Considered a disease that can be arrested, but not cured.
7. Important to assess history of alcohol consumption for clients admitted to hospital for non-alcohol-related disorders, because they may go into withdrawal.
8. Socioeconomic as well as a physiologic problem, resulting in increased health care costs and loss of productivity if ability to maintain a job is impaired.
9. Alcohol used with other substances (barbiturates, antianxiety drugs) may have lethal consequences.
10. Long-term use may result in loss of health (gastritis, cirrhosis, hepatitis, malnutrition, cardiac and neural disorders) and life (suicide, automobile accidents).
11. Directly related problems include withdrawal, delirium tremens and alcohol-related dementia
   a. *Withdrawal*
   1) alcohol consumption reduced/discontinued following continuous consumption for many days or longer
   2) withdrawal is progressive and has four stages:
   I: at least 8 hours after last drink; symptoms include mild tremors, tachycardia, increased blood pressure, diaphoresis, nervousness
   II: gross tremors, hyperactivity, profound confusion, loss of appetite, insomnia, weakness, disorientation, illusions, auditory and visual hallucinations
   III: 12–48 hours after last drink: symptoms include (in addition to those found in I and II) severe hallucinations, grand mal seizures
   IV: 3–5 days after last drink: delirium tremens, confusion, agitation, severe psychomotor activity, hallucinations, insomnia, tachycardia
   3) withdrawal may last less than a week or may evolve into alcohol withdrawal delirium (delirium tremens).
   b. *Delirium tremens (DTs)*
   1) history of alcohol abuse usually for more than 5 years
   2) may be preceded by seizures
   3) symptoms occur 2–3 days after alcohol reduced/discontinued.
   4) signs include tachycardia, increased blood pressure, agitation, delusions, hallucinations.
   c. *Alcohol hallucinosis:* hallucinations only
   d. *Alcohol-related dementia:* caused by poor nutrition
   1) thiamine deficiency results in *Korsakoff's dementia/psychosis;* symptoms include chronic disorientation, confabulation.
   2) Korsakoff's psychosis is sometimes preceded by *Wernicke's encephalopathy.* Confusion and ataxia are predominant symptoms.
   3) large doses of thiamine may prevent the development of Korsakoff's psychosis.

B. Medical management
1. Vitamin and nutritional therapy
2. Antianxiety drugs (sedatives, tranquilizers)
3. Disulfiram (Antabuse)
   a. Produces unpleasant reaction (thirst, sweating, palpitations, vomiting, dyspnea, respiratory and

cardiac failure) when taken with alcohol.
b. 500 mg/day for 1–2 weeks; usual maintenance dose is 250 mg/day.
c. Duration of action is $\frac{1}{2}$ to several hours; no alcohol should be taken at least 12 hours before taking drug.
d. Increases effects of antianxiety drugs and oral anticoagulants.
e. Side effects include headache, dry mouth, somnolence, flushing.
f. Nursing responsibilities
  1) teach client the nature of severe reaction and importance of avoiding all alcohol (including cough medicine, foods prepared with alcohol, etc.).
  2) teach client to carry an identification card in case of accidental alcohol ingestion.
  3) monitor effects of antianxiety drugs if being taken at the same time.
  4) monitor for bleeding if taking oral anticoagulants.
4. High doses of chlordiazepoxide (Librium) to control withdrawal in acute detoxification.
C. Assessment findings
  1. Dependent personality; often using denial as a defense mechanism
  2. Tendency to minimize and underreport amount of alcohol consumed
  3. Intoxication: blood alcohol level 0.15 (150 mg alcohol/100 cc blood)
  4. Signs of impaired judgment, motor skills, and slurred speech
  5. Behavior may be boisterous and euphoric or aggressive, or may be depressed and withdrawn
  6. Signs of withdrawal, DTs, or alcohol-related dementias
D. Nursing interventions
  1. Stay with client.
  2. Monitor vital signs.
  3. Observe for tremors, seizures, increased agitation, anxiety, disorders of perception.
  4. Administer medications as ordered; observe effects/side effects of tranquilizers carefully.
  5. If disorders of perception occur, explain that these are part of the withdrawal process.
  6. Provide fluids, adequate nutrition, and quiet environment.
  7. When client is stable, provide information about rehabilitation programs (Alcoholics Anonymous); at this stage client may be willing to consider a program to stop drinking.
  8. Provide information about Alanon (for spouse and adult family members) and Alateen (for children).

Psychoactive Drug Use

A. General information
  1. Drugs abused may be prescription or "street" drugs
  2. Types of drugs frequently abused
    a. Barbiturates, antianxiety drugs, hypnotics
    b. Opioids (narcotics): heroin, morphine, meperidine, methadone, hydromorphone
    c. Amphetamines: amphetamine, dextroamphetamine, methamphetamine (speed), some appetite suppressants
    d. Cocaine, hydrochloride cocaine (crack)
    e. Phencyclidine (PCP)
    f. Hallucinogens: LSD, mescaline, DMT
    g. Cannabis: marijuana, hashish, THC
B. Assessment findings and nursing interventions for overdoses vary with particular drug; see Table 5.4.
C. Polydrug abusers
  1. Common pattern of drug use
  2. Synergistic effect: drugs interact so that effect is greater than if each drug is taken separately
  3. Additive effect: two of more drugs with same action are taken together (e.g., barbiturates with alcohol will result in heavy sedation).

SCHIZOPHRENIC DISORDERS

Overview

A. Characterized by disordered thinking, delusions, hallucinations, depersonalization (feeling of being strange, not oneself), impaired reality testing (psychosis), and impaired interpersonal relationships.
B. Regression to the earliest stages of development is often noted (e.g., incontinence, mutism).
C. Onset is usually in adolescence/early adulthood.
D. Client may be seriously impaired and unable to perform ADL.
E. Etiology is not known; theories include
  1. Genetic: 1% of population; risk approximately 15% with one schizophrenic parent, approximately 30% with two.
  2. Family: double-bind communication; message sent is negated.
  3. Biochemical: increased dopamine activation.
  4. Interaction of predisposing risk and environmental stress.
  5. Psychoanalytic: fragile ego resorts to dysfunctional use of defense mechanisms (e.g., identification, projection).
F. Prior to onset (premorbid) client may have been suspicious, eccentric, or withdrawn.

Classifications

A. *Disorganized:* incoherent; delusions are not organized; social withdrawal; affect blunted, silly, or inappropriate
B. *Catatonic:* psychomotor disturbances
  1. Stupor: mute, little reaction or movements
  2. Excitement: purposeless, excited motor activity
  3. Posturing: voluntary, inappropriate, bizarre postures
C. *Paranoid:* delusions and hallucinations of persecution/grandeur
D. *Undifferentiated:* disorganized behaviors, delusions and hallucinations

Assessment

A. Four As
  1. *Affect:* flat, blunted
  2. *Associative looseness:* verbalizations are disorganized
  3. *Ambivalence:* cannot choose between conflicting emotions

Table 5.4 Commonly Abused Drugs

Drug	Effect	Dependence	Assessment Findings	Overdose	Nursing Interventions for Overdose
Barbiturates					
Antianxiety drugs, hypnotics	Reduction in anxiety, escape from stress	Psychologic at first, then physiologic; withdrawal similar to alcohol withdrawal, to point of delirium. Cross-tolerance to other depressants	Irritability, weight loss, changes in mood or motor coordination	Slurred speech, lethargy, respiratory depression, coma; use combined with alcohol can be lethal	Keep person awake and moving to prevent coma; maintain airway.
Opioids/Narcotics					
Heroin, morphine, meperidine, methadone	Euphoria, dysphoria, and/or apathy	Psychologic dependence rapidly leading to physical; signs of withdrawal: cramps, nausea, vomiting, diarrhea; sleep disturbance, chills and shaking	Pinpoint pupils, mental clouding, lethargy, impaired memory and judgment, evidence of needle tracks, inflamed nasal mucosa if drug is snorted	Depressed consciousness and respirations, dilated pupils with anoxia or polydrug use	Provide emergency support of vital functions. In withdrawal, administer methadone or Narcan as ordered.
Cocaine/crack	Sense of confidence, euphoria, psychomotor hyperactivity followed by "crash"	Psychologic dependence to produce feeling of well-being	Restlessness, weight loss, possible disorders of perception, dilated pupils	High fever, hallucinations, cardiac arrhythmias, increased blood pressure, convulsions, death	Provide emergency support of vital functions and talk down if hallucinating.
Amphetamines					
Amphetamine, dextroamphetamine, methamphetamine	Depressed appetite; increased activity, awareness, sense of well-being	Long-term use or high doses may produce delirium, paranoid-like delusions, withdrawal, depression, fatigue, sleep disturbances	Same as cocaine, plus suicidal ideation	Same as cocaine	Same as cocaine, plus suicide precautions. Observe for increased anxiety to panic, which may potentiate assaultive behavior.
Phencyclidine (PCP)	Euphoria, psychomotor agitation, emotional lability	Not reported	Vomiting, hallucinations, paranoid ideation, agitation	Violent behavior, suicide, respiratory arrest, delirium, coma, increased blood pressure and pulse	Monitor vital signs. Observe for suicidal or assaultive behavior. Provide nonthreatening environment, reality orientation, support.
Hallucinogens					
LSD, mescaline	Disordered perceptions, depersonalization	Not reported	"Bad trip," high anxiety to panic; hallucinations may occur long after drug has been metabolized; flashbacks may produce long-lasting psychotic disorders	Reduced LOC	Same as PCP, plus talk client down.
Cannabis Marijuana, hashish, THC	Euphoria, intense perceptions, relaxation, lethargy	Not reported	Increased pulse rate and appetite; impaired judgment and coordination	Panic reaction, nausea, vomiting, depression and disorders of perception	In panic, talk down. In severe depression, institute suicide precautions.

4. *Autistic thinking:* thoughts on self, extreme withdrawal, unable to relate to outside world
B. Any changes in thoughts, speech, affect
C. Ability to perform self-care activities, nutritional deficits
D. Suicide potential
E. Aggression
F. Regression
G. Impaired communication

Analysis

Nursing diagnoses for clients with schizophrenic disorders may include
A. Anxiety
B. Impaired communication
C. Ineffective individual/family coping
D. Altered fluid volume
E. Potential for injury
F. Altered nutrition
G. Powerlessness
H. Self-care deficit
I. Disturbance in self-concept
J. Sensory-perceptual alteration
K. Sleep pattern disturbance
L. Social isolation
M. Potential for violence

Planning and Implementation

Goals

Client will
A. Develop a trusting/therapeutic relationship with nurse.
B. Be oriented, able to test reality.
C. Be protected from injury.
D. Be able to recognize impending loss of control.
E. Adhere to medication regimen.
F. Participate in activities.
G. Increase ability to care for self.

Interventions

A. Offer self in development of therapeutic relationship.
B. Use silence.
C. Set time for interaction with client.
D. Encourage reality orientation but understand that delusions/hallucinations are real to client.
E. Assist with feeding/dressing as necessary.
F. Check on client frequently, remove potentially harmful objects.
G. Contract with client to tell you when anxiety is becoming so high loss of control is possible.
H. Administer antipsychotic medications as ordered (see Table 5.5 for side effects and dosages); observe for effects.
  1. Reduction of hallucinations, delusions, agitation
  2. Postural hypotension
    a. Obtain baseline blood pressure and monitor sitting/standing.
    b. Client must lie prone for 1 hour following injection.
    c. Teach client to sit up or stand up slowly.
    d. Elevate client's legs while seated.
    e. Withhold drug if systolic pressure drops below 20–30 mm Hg.
  3. Photosensitivity
    a. Advise use of sun screen.
    b. Avoid exposure to sunlight.
  4. Agranulocytosis
    a. Instruct client to report sore throat or fever.
    b. Institute reverse isolation if necessary.
  5. Elimination
    a. Measure I&O.
    b. Check bladder distension.
    c. Keep bowel record.
  6. Sedation
    a. Avoid use of heavy machinery.
    b. Do not drive.
  7. Extrapyramidal symptoms
    a. Dystonic reactions
      1) sudden contractions of face, tongue, extraocular muscles
      2) administer antiparkinson agents prn (e.g., benztropine (Cogentin) 1–8 mg or diphenhydramine (Benadryl) 10–50 mg), which can be given PO or IM for faster relief; trihexyphenidyl (Artane) 3–15 mg PO only can also be used prn.
      3) remain with client; this is a frightening experience and usually occurs when medication is started.
    b. Parkinson syndrome
      1) occurs within 1–3 weeks
      2) tremors, rigid posture, masklike facial appearance
      3) administer antiparkinson agents prn.
    c. Akathisia
      1) motor restlessness
      2) need to keep moving
      3) administer antiparkinson agents.
      4) do not mistake this for agitation and increase antipsychotic medication.
      5) reduce medications to see if symptoms decrease.
      6) determine if movement is under voluntary control.
    d. Tardive dyskinesia
      1) irreversible involuntary movements of tongue, face, extremities
      2) may occur after prolonged use of antipsychotics
    e. Elderly clients should receive doses reduced by one-half to one-third of recommended level.
I. Encourage participation in milieu, group, art, and occupational therapies when client able to tolerate them.

Evaluation

Client
A. Stays with nurse prescribed period of time.
B. Is oriented to reality, can state name, place, date.
C. Can feed/dress self with specified amount of assistance.
D. Has/will not attempt to injure self or others.

Table 5.5   Antipsychotic Medications

Drug	Acute Symptoms	Dosages Maintenance/Day	Range/Day	Profound Side Effects
Chlorpromazine (Thorazine)	25–100 mg IM q1–4h PRN	200–600 mg PO	200–2000 mg PO	Sedation Anticholinergic effects: dry mouth, blurred vision, constipation, urinary retention postural hypotension
Thioridazine (Mellaril)	—	150–300 mg PO	150–800 mg PO	Sedation
Fluphenazine HCl (Prolixin, Permitil)	1.25 mg IM, max 10 mg IM, divided doses	1–5 mg PO	1–10 mg PO	Extrapyramidal effects: dystonic reactions (muscular contractions of tongue, face, throat; opisthotonos); tremors, rigid posture; akathisia (restlessness); tardive dyskinesia
Fluphenazine decanoate/ enanthate (Prolixin, Permitil)	—	25 mg IM q2wk	25–100 mg IM	Extrapyramidal
Trifluoperazine (Stelazine)	1–2 mg IM q4h; 2–4 mg PO, max 10 mg qd	2–4 mg PO	2–10 mg PO	Extrapyramidal
Triflupromazine (Vesprin)	10–75 mg IM	50–150 mg PO/IM	50–150 mg PO/IM	Sedation, hypotension
Perphenazine (Trilafon)	5–10 mg IM q6h, max 30 mg IM qd	16–64 mg PO	12–64 mg PO	Extrapyramidal
Haloperidol (Haldol)	2–10 mg IM in divided doses	2–8 mg PO	6–100 mg PO	Extrapyramidal
Thiothizene (Navane)	8–16 mg IM in divided doses	6–10 mg PO	6–60 mg PO	Extrapyramidal
Loxapine (Loxitane)	—	60–100 mg PO	10–250 mg PO	Extrapyramidal

E. Adheres to medication regimen with minimal side effects.
F. Participates in activities.

SAMPLE QUESTIONS

Ronald, 23 years old, was voluntarily admitted to the inpatient unit with a diagnosis of paranoid schizophrenia.

7. *As you approach Ronald, he says, "If you come any closer, I'll die." This is an example of a(an)*
   ○ 1. hallucination.
   ○ 2. delusion.
   ○ 3. illusion.
   ○ 4. idea of reference.

8. Your best response to this behavior is
   ○ 1. How can I hurt you?
   ○ 2. Ronald, I'm the nurse.
   ○ 3. Tell me more about this.
   ○ 4. That's a silly thing to say.

9. Later that day you notice that Ronald is pacing the halls and is agitated. You hear him say, "Those f____ doctors are trying to commit me to the state hospital." Your continued assessment includes
   ○ 1. clarifying information with the doctor.
   ○ 2. observing Ronald for rising anxiety.
   ○ 3. reviewing history of involuntary commitment.
   ○ 4. checking dosage of prescribed medication.

10. When communicating with a paranoid client, the main principle is to
   ○ 1. use logic and be persistent.
   ○ 2. provide an anxiety-free environment.
   ○ 3. express doubt and do not argue.
   ○ 4. encourage ventilation of anger.

11. An appropriate activity for Ronald to engage in is
   ○ 1. competitive sports.
   ○ 2. Bingo.
   ○ 3. Trivial Pursuit.
   ○ 4. daily walks.

DELUSIONAL (PARANOID) DISORDERS

Overview

A. Reality testing is intact except for delusions of persecution, jealousy, and grandiosity. Ideas of reference and social isolation may also be noted.
B. Onset in middle age or later
C. May be chronic (over 6 months) or acute (less than 6 months)
D. Not due to organic causes; functional disorder
E. Most clients able to perform self-care activities
F. Intellectual and occupational functioning not impaired
G. Social/marital functioning severely impaired
H. Paranoid behavior may be associated with organic mental disorders and schizophrenia.

Classifications

A. *Paranoid disorder:* persistent persecutory, jealous delusions for a least one week
B. *Paranoia:* paranoid disorder that is chronic, above symptoms evident for at least six months
C. *Acute paranoid disorder:* sudden onset of above symptoms related to sudden change in environment

Characteristics

A. Suspiciousness
B. Delusions: grandiose, persecutory, erotic, jealous
C. Haughty, superior manner
D. Severe impairment in social and family relationships; progressive estrangement
E. May be anger, hostility, aggression

Assessment

A. Behavior changes, problems
B. Social functioning
C. Changes in thought processes
D. Delusions
E. Duration

Analysis

Nursing diagnoses for clients with paranoid disorders may include
A. Anxiety
B. Altered self-concept
C. Altered thought processes

Planning and Implementation

Goals

Client will
A. Develop a trusting/therapeutic relationship with nurse.
B. Decrease frequency of delusional content in speech.

Interventions

A. Keep all promises made to client.
B. Present reality but accept client's need for delusions.
C. Schedule brief, frequent interactions.
D. Respect client's privacy, but offer self and encourage interaction.
E. Do not touch client or whisper behind client.

Evaluation

Client
A. Stayed with nurse for specified period of time.
B. Relates realistic appraisal of events.

AFFECTIVE DISORDERS

Overview

A. Characterized by disturbance in mood (affect) that is either depression or elation (mania); occur in a variety of patterns, alone or together (see Figure 5.1). Disturbance is beyond normal range of mood experience by most people.
B. *Bipolar disorder:* components of both depression and elation (formerly called manic-depression)
C. *Cyclothymic disorder:* some symptoms of both mania and depression, often separated by long periods of normal mood
D. *Dysthymic disorder (depressive neurosis):* long-standing symptoms of depression alternating with short periods of normal mood; client usually able to maintain roles in job, school, etc.
E. Etiology is unknown; theories include
  1. Genetic: approximately 7% of general population; risk is 20% if a close relative has depression
  2. Biochmical: alteration in catecholamine (e.g., norepinephrine)
  3. Psychoanalytic: anger turned inward (i.e., anger toward significant other is turned into anger toward self)

Assessment

A. Mood: dysphoric; blue/sad or elated/aggressive
B. Presence of psychomotor agitation, retardation, or hyperactivity
C. Disorders of cognition: narrowed perception and interests, impaired concentration, grandiose delusions, flight of ideas in elation stage
D. Sexual functioning changes
E. Appropriateness of appearance/dress
F. Appetite
G. Potential for suicide

Analysis

Nursing diagnoses for clients with affective disorders may include
A. Altered bowel elimination
B. Impaired communication
C. Ineffective individual coping
D. Potential for injury to self and others
E. Altered nutrition: fluids
F. Self-care deficit
G. Disturbance in self-concept
H. Sleep pattern disturbance
I. Altered thought processes

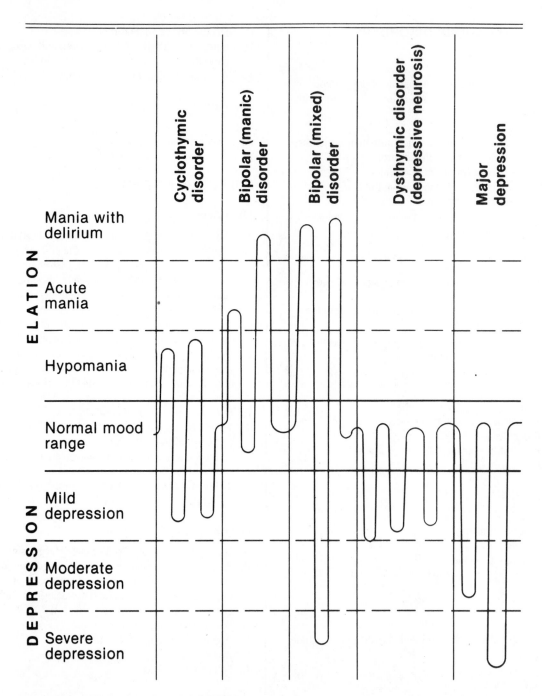

Mania with delirium: persecutory delusions, grandiose delusions, hallucinations

Acute mania: flight of ideas, impulsive behavior, bizarre dress and behavior, distractibility

Hypomania: decreased sleep, inflated self-esteem, increased activity, irritability

Mild depression: sadness, irritability, sleep disorders, social withdrawal, crying and tearful, low energy

Moderate depression: recurring thoughts of suicide, hopelessness, helplessness

Severe depression: delusions, hallucinations, psychomotor retardation and stupor, agitation (in depression with melancholia)

Figure 5.1 Patterns of mood disturbances in affective disorders

Planning and Implementation

Goals

Client will

A. Be protected from injury.

B. Receive adequate rest and sleep.

C. Maintain adequate intake of fluids and nutrients, regular elimination.

D. Develop trusting/therapeutic relationship with nurse.

E. Be oriented to reality.

F. Participate in planned activities.

Interventions

A. Assess for suicide potential.

B. Encourage verbalization of feelings of hopelessness and helplessness.

C. Provide quiet environment for rest and sleep.

D. Provide small, attractive meals; encourage intake of fluids.

E. Maintain bowel record.

F. Use silence and broad openings, focus on client's verbal/nonverbal behaviors.

G. Present reality but accept client's need for delusions.

H. Accept client's negative responses, hostility.

I. Provide activities and tasks to raise client's self-esteem.

J. Assist with self-care as needed.

K. If client is agitated
  1. Work with client on a one-to-one basis.
  2. Walk with client; provide some diversional activity.
  3. Reduce environmental stimuli (e.g., put in a quiet room, dim lights).

Evaluation

Client

A. Has gained or maintained weight.

B. Reports any suicidal ideation.

C. Sleeps a specified number of hours.

D. Can meet own needs for ADL.

E. Has realistic appraisal of self.

Specific Disorders

Bipolar Disorder (Manic Episode)

A. General information
  1. Onset usually before age 30
  2. Characterized by hyperactivity and euphoria that may become sarcasm or hostility

B. Assessment findings
  1. Hyperactivity to the point of physical exhaustion
  2. Flamboyant dress/makeup
  3. Sexual acting out
  4. Impulsive behaviors
  5. Flight of ideas: inability to finish one thought before jumping to another
  6. Loud, domineering, manipulative behavior
  7. Distractibility
  8. Dehydration, nutritional deficits
  9. Delusions of grandeur
  10. Possible short-term depression (risk of suicide)
  11. Hostility, aggression

C. Medical management
  1. Lithium carbonate (Eskalith, Lithane, Lithotabs)
     a. Initial dosage levels: 600 mg tid, to maintain a blood serum level of 1.0–1.5 mEq/liter; blood serum levels should be checked 12 hours after last dose, twice a week.
     b. Maintenance dosage levels: 300 mg tid/qid, to maintain a blood serum level of 0.6–1.2 mEq/liter; checked monthly.
     c. Toxicity when blood levels higher than 2.0 mEq/liter: tremors, nausea and vomiting, thirst, polyuria, coma, seizures, cardiac arrest
  2. Antipsychotics may also be given for hyperactivity, agitation, psychotic behavior. Chlorpromazine (Thorazine) and haloperidol (Haldol) are most commonly used (see Table 5.5).

D. Nursing interventions
  1. Determine what client is attempting to tell you; use active listening.
  2. Assist client in focusing on a topic.
  3. Offer finger foods, high-nutrition foods, and fluids.
  4. Provide quiet environment, decrease stimuli.
  5. Stay with client, use silence.
  6. Remove harmful objects.
  7. Be accepting of hostile statements.
  8. Do not argue with client.
  9. Use distraction to divert client from behaviors that are harmful to self or others.
  10. Administer medications as ordered and observe for effects/side effects.
     a. Teach clients early signs of toxicity.
     b. Maintain fluid and salt intake.
     c. Avoid diuretics.
     d. Monitor lithium blood levels.
  11. Assist in dressing, bathing.

Major Depression

A. General information
  1. Characterized by loss of ambition, lack of interest in activities and sex, low self-esteem, and feelings of boredom and sadness.
  2. Etiology may be physiologic or response to an actual or perceived loss.
  3. These clients are at high risk for suicide, especially when depressed mood begins to lift and/or energy level increases.

B. Medical management
  1. Tricyclic antidepressants: amitriptyline HCl (Elavil), doxepin (Sinequan), imipramine (Tofranil); see Table 5.6
  2. Monoamine oxidase inhibitors (MAOIs): isocarboxazid (Marplan), tranylcypromine (Parnate); see Table 5.6

Table 5.6   Antidepressant Medications

Drug	Dosages Initiating	Maintenance	Side Effects
Tricyclics			
Amitriptyline (Elavil, Endep)	75–100 mg PO	50–100 mg PO at bedtime; 80–100 mg IM in divided doses	Constipation, blurred vision, drowsiness, orthostatic hypotension, urinary retention, dry mouth
Imipramine (Tofranil)	75 mg PO tid	75–100 mg PO	As above
Amoxapine (Asendin)	50–mg PO tid	300 mg PO	As above
Doxepin (Sinequan)	75–1150 mg PO	300 mg PO	As above
Monoamine Oxidase Inhibitors (MAOIs)			
Isocarboxazid (Marplan)	30 mg PO in divided doses	Up to 20 mg PO	As for tricyclics, plus angina, hypoglycemia, hypertensive crisis precipitated by ingestion of foods with tyramine or concurrent use of tricyclics.
Phenalizine (Nardil)	60 mg PO in divided doses	90 mg PO	As above
Tranylcypromine (Parnate)	20 mg PO in divided doses	Up to 30 mg PO	As above

3. ECT

C. Assessment findings

1. Feelings of helplessness, hopelessness, worthlessness
2. Reduction in normal activities or agitation
3. Slowing of body functions/elimination
4. Loss of appetite
5. Inappropriate guilt
6. Self-deprecation, low self-esteem
7. Inability to concentrate, disordered thinking
8. Poor hygiene
9. Slumped posture
10. Crying, ruminating (relates same incident over and over)
11. Dependency
12. Depressed children: possible separation anxiety
13. Elderly clients: possible symptoms of dementia
14. Somatic and persecutory delusions and hallucinations

D. Nursing interventions

1. Monitor I&O.
2. Weigh client regularly.
3. Maintain a schedule of regular appointments.
4. Remove potentially harmful articles.
5. Contract with client to report suicidal ideation, impulses, plans; check client frequently.
6. Assist with dressing, hygiene, and feeding.
7. Encourage discussion of negative/positive aspects of self.
8. Encourage change to more positive topics if self-deprecating thoughts persist.
9. Administer antidepressant medications (see Table 5.6) as ordered.
   a. Tricyclic antidepressants (TCAs)
      1) effectiveness increased by antihistamines, alcohol, benzodiazepines
      2) effectiveness decreased by barbiturates, nicotine, vitamin C
   b. Monoamine oxidase inhibitors (MAOIs)
      1) effectiveness increased with antipsychotic drugs, alcohol, meperidine
      2) avoid foods containing tyramine (e.g., aged cheese, avocados, caffeine, chocolate, sour cream, yogurt); these foods or MAOIs taken with TCAs may result in hypertensive crisis.
   c. Antidepressant medications do not take effect for 2–3 weeks. Encourage client to continue medication even if not feeling better. Be aware of suicide potential during this time.
   d. Warn client not to take any drugs without consulting physician.
10. Assist with ECT as ordered.
    a. Give normal pre-op preparation, including informed consent (see Perioperative Nursing, page 30).
    b. Remove all hairpins, dentures.
    c. Ensure client is wearing loose clothing.
    d. Check vital signs after the procedure.
    e. Assure that any memory loss is temporary.
    f. Assist to room or to care of responsible party if outpatient.

Depression with Melancholia

A. General information: characterized by loss of pleasure in all or most activities

B. Assessment findings

1. Depression worse in the morning
2. Awakens early in the morning, at least 2 hours before normal waking time.
3. Appetite/weight loss
4. Excessive guilt
5. Marked psychomotor activity/retardation

C. Nursing interventions
  1. Institute suicide precautions in clients with agitation (they pose a high suicide risk).
  2. Provide additional interventions as described in Major Depression.

Dysthymic Disorder

A. General information: chronic mood disturbance of at least two years' duration for adults, one year for children
B. Assessment findings
  1. Normal moods for a period of weeks, followed by depression
  2. Insomnia/hypersomnia
  3. Social withdrawal
  4. Loss of interest in activities
  5. Recurrent thoughts of suicide and death
C. Nursing interventions: same as for Major Depression.

NEUROTIC DISORDERS

In DSM III R, the disorders formerly categorized as neurotic disorders are included in Anxiety, Somatoform, and Dissociative Disorders. Reality testing is intact.

ANXIETY DISORDERS

Overview

A. Common element is anxiety, manifested in a variety of behaviors (see also Behaviors Related to Emotional Distress).
B. Therapy relates to reduction of anxiety; when anxiety is reduced, the symptoms will be alleviated.
C. Types include generalized anxiety disorder, panic disorder, phobic disorders, and obsessive-compulsive disorders.

Assessment

A. Level of anxiety: may be to point of panic
B. Vital signs: may be elevated
C. Reality testing: should be intact; can recognize that thoughts are irrational but cannot control them
D. Physical symptoms: no organic basis
E. Memory: possible memory loss or loss of identity
F. Pattern of symptoms: chronic with a pattern of waxing and waning or sudden onset

Analysis

Nursing diagnoses for the client with an anxiety disorder may include
A. Anxiety
B. Fear
C. Ineffective individual coping
D. Powerlessness
E. Disturbance in self-concept

F. Sleep pattern disturbance
G. Altered thought processes

Planning and Implementation

Goals

Client will
A. Develop a trusting/therapeutic relationship with nurse.
B. Recognize causes of anxiety and develop alternative coping mechanisms.
C. Reduce/alleviate symptoms of anxiety.

Interventions

A. Encourage discussion of anxiety and relationship to symptoms.
B. Provide calm, accepting atmosphere.
C. Administer antianxiety medications (for short-term use only) as ordered and monitor effects/side effects.
  1. Diazepam (Valium): 5–20 mg PO daily; 2–10 mg IM or IV daily
  2. Chlordiazepoxide (Librium): 20–100 mg PO daily; 50–100 mg IM or IV daily
  3. Alprazolam (Xanax) 0.75–4 mg PO daily.
  4. Oxazepam (Serax) 30–120 mg PO daily.
  5. Triazolam (Halcion) 0.25–0.5 mg HS.
  6. Side effects
     a. Client may become addicted.
     b. Additive effect with alcohol.
     c. Dizziness may occur when treatment initiated.
     d. Lower doses for elderly client.
     e. Do not stop abruptly; taper doses.
D. Teach patient about self-medication regimen and side effects.

Evaluation

Client
A. Can discuss causes of anxiety with nurse.
B. Demonstrates constructive coping mechanisms and ability to reduce anxiety.
C. Demonstrates knowledge of effects and hazards of antianxiety medications.

Specific Disorders

Phobic Disorders

A. General information
  1. Irrational fears resulting in an avoidance of objects or situations.
  2. Repressed conflicts are projected to outside world and eventually are displaced onto an object or situation.
  3. Client can recognize that fear of these objects/situations is irrational, but cannot control emotional response when confronting or thinking about confronting the particular object/situation.
B. Assessment findings
  1. *Agoraphobia:* most serious phobia; fear of being alone or in public places; may reach point where client panics at thought of being in public places and cannot leave home.

2. *Social phobias:* fear of being in situations where one may be scrutinized and embarrassed by others.

3. *Simple phobias:* irrational fear of specific objects/situations (e.g., snakes, insects, heights, closed places).

C. Nursing interventions

  1. Know that behavior modification and systematic desensitization most commonly used; client cannot be "reasoned" out of behavior.

  2. Do not force contact with feared object/situation, may result in panic.

  3. Administer antianxiety medications (diazepam [Valium], imipramine [Tofranil]) as ordered.

Generalized Anxiety Disorder

A. General information

  1. Persistent anxiety for at least one month

  2. Cannot be controlled by client or displaced, remains free-floating and diffuse

B. Assessment findings

  1. Motor tensions: trembling, muscle aches, jumpiness

  2. Autonomic hyperactivity: sweating, palpitations, dizziness, upset stomach, increased pulse and respirations

  3. Affect: worried and fearful of what might happen

  4. Hyperalert: insomnia, irritability

C. Nursing interventions

  1. Stay with client.

  2. Encourage discussion of anxiety and its source.

  3. Provide calm, relaxing atmosphere.

  4. Administer antianxiety drugs, as ordered.

  5. Observe for effects and side effects.

  6. Monitor vital signs.

  7. Assess for level of anxiety.

Panic Disorder (Acute Anxiety)

A. General information: acute, panic-like attack lasting from a few minutes to an hour.

B. Assessment findings

  1. Sudden onset of intense fear/terror

  2. Symptoms: include dyspnea, palpitations, chest pain, sensation of smothering or choking, faintness, fear of dying, dizziness

  3. When severe, symptoms mimic acute cardiac disease that must be ruled out.

  4. Client may be seen in ER.

C. Nursing interventions: same as for Generalized Anxiety Disorder.

Obsessive-Compulsive Disorder/Neurosis

A. General information

  1. *Obsession*

    a. Recurrent thoughts that client cannot control; often violent, fearful, or doubting in nature (e.g., fear of contamination).

    b. Client cannot keep thoughts from intruding into

consciousness; eventually resorts to defense of undoing (performing ritual behavior).

  2. *Compulsion*

    a. Action (ritual behavior) that serves to reduce tension from obsessive thought

    b. Client may not desire to perform behavior but is unable to stop, as this is the only relief from distress.

    c. May interfere with social/occupational functioning.

B. Nursing interventions

  1. Allow compulsive behavior, but set reasonable limits.

  2. Permit client to complete behavior once started; aggression may result if behavior is not allowed or completed.

  3. Engage client in alternative behaviors (client will not be able to do this alone).

  4. Provide opportunities to perform tasks that meet need for perfectionsim (e.g., stacking and folding linens).

  5. As compulsive behavior decreases, help client to verbalize feelings, concerns.

  6. Help client to make choices, participate in decisions regarding own schedule,

Post-traumatic Stress Disorder (PTSD)

A. General information

  1. Disturbed/disintegrated response to significant trauma

  2. Symptoms occur following crisis event such as war, earthquake, flood, airplane crash, rape or assault.

  3. Reexperiencing of traumatic event in recollections, nightmares

B. Assessment findings

  1. Psychic numbing: not as responsive to persons and events as the traumatic experience

  2. Sleep disturbances (e.g., nightmares)

  3. Avoidance of environment/activities likely to arouse recall of trauma

  4. Symptoms of depression

  5. Possible violent outbursts

  6. Memory impairment

  7. Panic attacks

  8. Substance abuse

C. Nursing interventions

  1. Arrange for individual or group psychotherapy with others who experienced same trauma (e.g., Vietnam war veterans).

  2. Provide crisis counseling, family therapy as needed.

  3. Provide referrals.

SAMPLE QUESTIONS

Lillian, 46 years old, is admitted to the hospital because her family is unable to manage her constant handwashing rituals. Her family reports she washes her hands at least 30 time each day.

12. You notice Lillian's hands are reddened, scaly, and cracked. Your main goal is to

  ○ 1. decrease the number of handwashings a day.

  ○ 2. limit the number of handwashings.

  ○ 3. provide good skin care.

  ○ 4. eliminate the handwashing rituals.

13. The next day, Lillian is scheduled for lab tests. In order to be there on time, your intervention must be to
    o 1. remind Lillian several times of her appointment.
    o 2. limit the number of handwashings.
    o 3. tell her it is her responsibility to be there on time.
    o 4. provide ample time for her to complete her rituals.

14. Which of the following would be an appropriate treatment for Lillian?
    o 1. An unstructured schedule of activities
    o 2. A structured schedule of activities
    o 3. Intense counseling
    o 4. Negative reinforcement every time she performs the ritual.

SOMATOFORM DISORDERS

Overview

A. Anxiety is manifested in somatic (physical) symptoms.
B. There is organic pathology but no organic etiology.
C. Symptoms are real and not under voluntary control of the client.
D. Defense used is somatization or conversion; anxiety is transformed to a physical symptom.

Specific Disorders

Somatization Disorder

A. General information
  1. Multiple, recurrent somatic complaints (fatigue, backache, nausea, menstrual cramps) over many years
  2. No organic etiology for these complaints
B. Assessment findings
  1. Complaints chronic but fluctuating
  2. History of seeking medical attention for many years
  3. Symptoms of anxiety and depression
  4. Somatic complaints may involve any organ system.
C. Nursing interventions
  1. Be aware of own response (irritation/impatience) to client.
  2. Rule out organic basis for current complaints.
  3. Focus on anxiety reduction, not physical symptoms.
  4. Minimize secondary gain.

Conversion Disorder

A. General information
  1. Sudden onset of impairment or loss of motor or sensory function
  2. No physiologic cause
  3. Defenses used are repression and conversion; anxiety is converted to a physical symptom.
  4. Temporal relationship between distressing event and development of symptom (e.g., unconscious desire to hit another may produce paralysis of arm).

5. Primary gain: client is not conscious of conflict, but anxiety is converted to a symptom.
6. Secondary gain: avoidance of anxiety-producing situation; gain support that was not previously provided.
B. Assessment findings
  1. Sudden paralysis, blindness, deafness, etc.
  2. "La belle indifférence": inappropriately calm when describing symptoms
  3. Symptoms not under voluntary control
  4. Usually short term; symptoms will abate as anxiety diminishes.
C. Nursing interventions
  1. Focus on anxiety reduction, not physical symptom.
  2. Use matter-of-fact acceptance of symptom.
  3. Encourage client to discuss conflict.
  4. Do not provide secondary gain by being too attentive.
  5. Provide diversionary activities.

Psychogenic Pain

A. General information: complaint of severe and prolonged pain in absence of supporting physical findings
B. Assessment findings
  1. Pain not relieved by analgesics
  2. Pain not following expected pattern; often severe
  3. Sleep may be interrupted by experience of pain.
C. Nursing interventions: same as for Conversion Disorder.

Hypochondriasis

A. General information
  1. Unrealistic belief of having serious illnesses
  2. Belief persists despite medical reassurance
  3. Defense used is regression.
B. Assessment findings
  1. Preoccupation with bodily functions, which are misinterpreted.
  2. History of seeing many doctors, many diagnostic tests
  3. Dependent behavior: desires/demands great deal of attention.
C. Nursing interventions
  1. Rule out presence of actual disease.
  2. Focus on anxiety not physical symptom.
  3. Set limits on amount of time spent with client.
  4. Reduce anxiety by providing diversionary activities.
  5. Avoid negative response to client's demands by discussing in staff conferences.
  6. Provide client with correct information.

DISSOCIATIVE DISORDERS

Overview

A. Sudden change in client's consciousness, identity, or motor behavior
B. Loss of memory, knowledge of identity, or how individual came to be in a particular place.
C. Defenses are repression and dissociation

Specific Disorders

Psychogenic Amnesia

A. General information: inability to recall information about self with no organic reason
B. Assessment findings
  1. No history of head injury
  2. Retrograde amnesia, may extend far into past
C. Nursing interventions
  1. Rule out organic causes.
  2. Reassure client that his/her identity will be made known to him/her.
  3. Provide safe environment.
  4. Establish nurse-client relationship to reduce anxiety.

Psychogenic Fugue

A. General information
  1. Client travels to strange, often distant place; unaware of how he traveled there, and unable to recall past.
  2. May follow severe psychologic stress.
B. Assessment findings
  1. Memory loss
  2. May have assumed new identity
  3. No recall of fugue state when normal functions return
B. Nursing interventions: same as for Psychogenic Amnesia.

PERSONALITY DISORDERS

Overview

A. Patterns of thinking about self and environment become maladaptive and cause impairment in social or occupational functioning or subjective distress.
B. Usually develop by adolescence.
C. Most common is borderline personality disorder.

Specific Disorders

Borderline Personality Disorder

A. General information: clients are impulsive and unpredictable, have difficulty interacting; characterized by behavior problems
B. Assessment findings
  1. Unstable, intense interpersonal relationships
  2. Impulsive, unpredictable, manipulative behavior; prone to self-harm
  3. Marked mood shifts from anger to dysphoric
  4. Uncertainty about self-image, gender identity, values
  5. Chronic intolerance of being alone, feelings of boredom
  6. Primitive dissociation (splitting): distinct separation of love and hate.
  7. Use of projection and regression.
C. Nursing interventions
  1. Protect from self-mutilation, suicidal gestures.
  2. Establish therapeutic relationship, be aware of own responses to manipulative behaviors.
  3. Maintain objectivity.
  4. Use a calm approach.
  5. Set limits.
  6. Apply plan of care consistently.
  7. Interact with clients when they demonstrate appropriate behavior.
  8. Teach relaxation techniques.

Antisocial Personality Disorder

A. General information
  1. Chronic history of antisocial behaviors (e.g., fighting, stealing, aggressive behaviors, substance abuse, criminal behaviors)
  2. These behaviors usually begin before the age of 15 and continue into adult life.
  3. May be hospitalized for injuries.
B. Assessment findings
  1. Manipulative behavior, may try to obtain special privileges, play one staff member against another
  2. Lack of shame or guilt for behaviors
  3. Insincerity and lying
  4. Impulsive behavior and poor judgment
C. Nursing interventions
  1. Provide model for mature, appropriate behavior.
  2. Observe strict limit setting by all staff.
  3. Monitor own responses to client.
  4. Demonstrate concern, interest in client.
  5. Reinforce positive behaviors (socialization, conforming to limits).
  6. Avoid power struggles.

Psychologic Aspects of Physical Illness

STRESS-RELATED DISORDERS

Overview

A. Actual physiologic change in structure/function of organ or system

B. May be referred to as psychosomatic or psychophysiologic disorders

C. Theorized that client's response to stress is a factor in etiology of disease

D. Stress/anxiety not the sole cause but may be a causative factor in the development/exacerbation of physical symptoms

E. See Table 5.7 for types of disorders with a stress component.

Assessment

A. Health history, family history

B. Physical symptoms

C. Social/cultural considerations

D. Coping behaviors

Analysis

Nursing diagnoses for stress-related disorders may include any nursing diagnosis specific to the physiologic problem as well as

A. Ineffective individual coping

B. Knowledge deficit

C. Disturbance in self-concept

Planning and Implementation

Goals

Client will

A. Receive appropriate treatment for any physical symptoms (e.g., maintenance of blood pressure within normal range).

B. Recognize relationship of stress to physical symptom(s).

C. Acknowledge coping patterns that may affect recurrence of physical symptoms.

D. Recognize relationship of self-concept, self-esteem, role performance to disorder.

E. Develop alternative coping behaviors.

Interventions

A. Provide nursing care specific to physical symptoms.

Table 5.7   Types of Stress-related Disorders

Systems	Examples
Respiratory	Asthma, common cold
Circulatory	Hypertension, migraine headaches
Digestive	Peptic ulcers, colitis
Skin	Hives, dermatitis
Musculoskeletal	Rheumatoid arthritis, chronic backache
Nervous	Fatigue
Endocrine	Dysmenorrhea, diabetes mellitus

B. Establish nurse-client relationship.

C. Encourage discussion of psychosocial problems.

D. Explain relationship of stress to physiologic symptoms.

E. Encourage client to devise alternative coping behaviors, changes in environment, attitude.

F. Role play new behaviors with client.

Evaluation

A. Goals specific to client's physical symptoms have been met.

B. Client
1. Is able to relate stress to physical symptoms.
2. Develops alternative coping behaviors.
3. Engages in role playing of new behaviors.

VICTIMS OF ABUSE

Overview

A. Abuse is physical or sexual assault, emotional abuse or neglect.

B. Victims include children, spouse, elderly or rape victims.

C. Victims are helpless or powerless to prevent the assault on their bodies or personalities.

D. Sometimes victims blame themselves for the assault.

E. The abusers often blame the victims, have poor impulse control, and use their power (physical strength or weapon) to subject victims to their assaults.

Assessment

A. Physical signs of trauma
B. Psychic numbing
C. Dissociation
D. Depression
E. Severe anxiety or panic

Analysis

Nursing diagnoses for victims of abuse may include
A. Anxiety
B. Ineffective individual/family coping
C. Powerlessness

Planning and Implementation

Goals

Client will
A. Receive appropriate treatment for any physiologic problems.
B. Develop a trusting relationship with nurse.
C. Experience a reduction in anxiety.
D. Share experiences and responses with nurse.

Interventions

A. Provide nursing care specific to physiologic problem.
B. Stay with client.
C. Offer support.
D. Employ active listening, broad openings.
E. Notify police when appropriate.
 1. In all cases of suspected child abuse
 2. With rape victim's permission
F. Refer to shelters, social agencies.

Evaluation

A. Goals specific to client's physiologic problems have been met.
B. Client
 1. Is able to share feelings/experiences with nurse.
 2. Develops plan to deal with victim status.

CRITICAL ILLNESS

Overview

A. Individuals in critical life-threatening situations have realistic fears of death or permanent loss of function.
B. Patients and their families may respond to these crises with denial, anger, hostility, withdrawal, guilt, and/or panic.
C. Loss of control and a sense of powerlessness can be overwhelming and detrimental to chance of recovery.

Assessment

A. Physiologic needs (first priority)
B. Anxiety level of patient/family
C. Patient/family fears
D. Coping behaviors of patient/family
E. Social and cultural considerations

Analysis

Nursing diagnoses for the psychologic component of critical illness may include
A. Anxiety
B. Hopelessness
C. Ineffective individual/family coping
D. Knowledge deficit
E. Fear
F. Powerlessness
G. Altered self-concept

Planning and Implementation

Goals

A. Client will
 1. Receive treatment for physiologic problems.
 2. Experience decrease in level of anxiety/fear.
 3. Discuss anxiety/fears with nurse.
B. Family will
 1. Be informed of patient's condition on regular basis.
 2. Discuss anxiety/fears with nurse.
 3. Provide appropriate support to client.

Interventions

A. Provide nursing care specific to physiologic problems.
B. Stay with patient.
C. Explain all procedures slowly, clearly, concisely.
D. Provide opportunities for patient to discuss fears.
E. Provide opportunities for patient to make decisions, have as much control as possible.
F. Encourage family to ask questions.
G. Recognize negative family responses as coping behaviors.
H. Encourage family members to support each other and patient.

Evaluation

A. Goals specific to patient's physiologic status have been met.
B. Patient
 1. Demonstrates a decrease in anxious behaviors.
 2. Is able to express fears verbally.
 3. Has participated in decisions whenever possible.
C. Family members
 1. Have discussed fears.
 2. Demonstrate support for each other and for patient.

SAMPLE QUESTIONS

Tammy, 18 months old, has been admitted for second-degree burns surrounding the genital area. Her mother told you that Tammy grabbed for the hot coffee cup and spilled it on herself.

15. You are required by law to
 ○ 1. testify in court on the injuries.
 ○ 2. report suspected child abuse.
 ○ 3. have the mother arrested.
 ○ 4. refer the mother to counseling.

16. Tammy's mother is 17 years old. In which one of the following would you provide health teaching?
    o 1. Normal growth and development
    o 2. Bonding techniques
    o 3. How to childproof the apartment
    o 4. Parenting skills

Marilyn was returning home from work late and was sexually assaulted. She was brought to the emergency room upset and crying.

17. Your main goal in caring for Marilyn is to
    o 1. assist Marilyn in crisis.
    o 2. notify the policy of the alleged assault.
    o 3. understand Marilyn will have a long recovery period.
    o 4. provide support and comfort.

18. Which of the following is indicative of Marilyn's adjustment to the trauma?
    o 1. She moves to another city.
    o 2. She resumes her work and activities.
    o 3. She takes classes in the martial arts.
    o 4. She remains silent about the assault.

CHRONIC ILLNESS

Overview

A. Chronic illnesses, such as diabetes mellitus, multiple sclerosis, or illnesses/injuries resulting in loss of function or loss of a body part necessitate adaptation to the inherent changes imposed.
B. Clients/families may respond to the losses associated with chronic illness with a variety of behaviors and defenses, including recurrent depression, anger and hostility, denial or acceptance.

Assessment and Analysis

Same as Stress-related Disorders (page 519) as well as
A. Ineffective family coping
B. Potential for self-injury

Planning and Intervention

Goals

A. Client will
    1. Receive appropriate treatment for any physiologic symptoms.
    2. Be able/willing to discuss responses to illness.
    3. Recognize effect of illness on aspects of self-concept.
    4. Develop realistic plans for activities and role functions.
    5. Contract with nurse to report depression/suicidal ideation.
B. Family will
    1. Be able to discuss responses to client illness.
    2. Develop plans to deal with alterations in client's behaviors and functions.

Interventions

A. Provide nursing care specific to physiologic problems.
B. Develop nurse/client relationship through active listening, acceptance of positive and negative client responses.
C. Encourage client to plan activities within present capabilities.
D. Provide information about illness, suggestions for activities.
E. Contract with client to request support in times of depression and to report suicidal ideation.
F. Encourage family members to discuss their response to client's illness.
G. Be accepting and nonjudgmental of negative responses (e.g., anger, hopelessness).
H. Support family efforts to develop plans for their participation in client's care.

Evaluation

A. Client
    1. Receives appropriate treatment for any physiologic problems.
    2. Recognizes/discusses positive and negative responses to illness.
    3. Understands effects of feelings about body image, self-esteem, role function.
    4. Agrees to report depression or suicidal thoughts.
B. Family
    1. Discusses positive and negative responses to client's illness.
    2. Plans/engages in appropriate activities with client.

DEATH AND DYING

Overview

A. One of the most difficult issues in nursing practice
B. Often difficult for nurses to maintain objectivity because of identification and response to death based on own value system and personal experiences

Assessment

A. Stage of dying (Kübler-Ross); see Table 5.8
B. Physical discomfort
C. Emotional reaction (withdrawal, anger, acceptance) and stage of dying
D. Desire to discuss impending death, value of own life
E. Level of consciousness
F. Family needs

Table 5.8   Stages of Dying

1. Denial and isolation
2. Anger
3. Bargaining
4. Depression
5. Acceptance

Analysis

Nursing diagnoses for the dying client may include
A. Anxiety
B. Altered comfort: pain
C. Ineffective individual/family coping
D. Fear
E. Anticipatory grieving
F. Hopelessness
G. Impaired mobility
H. Powerlessness
I. Self-care deficit
J. Social isolation

Planning and Implementation

Goals

A. Client will
1. Be maintained in optimum comfort.
2. Not be alone.
3. Have opportunity to discuss what death means and to progress through stages of dying.
B. Family will have opportunity to be with client as much as they desire.

Interventions

A. Recognize clients/families have own way of dealing with death and dying.
B. Support clients/families as they work through dying process.
C. Accept negative responses from clients/families.
D. Encourage clients/families to discuss feelings related to death and dying.
E. Support staff and seek support for self when dealing with dying client and grieving family.

Evaluation

A. Client is
1. Given and takes opportunity to discuss feelings about impending death and eventually acknowledges inevitable outcome.
2. Comfortable and participates in self-care for as long as possible.
B. Family discusses feelings about loss of loved one.

GRIEF AND MOURNING

Overview

A. Response to loss (person, body part, role)
B. Biologic, psychologic, social implications
C. Affects family system
D. Mourning is process to resolve grief
1. Shock, disbelief are short term
2. Resentment, anger
3. Concentration on loss
a. Possible auditory, visual hallucinations
b. Possible guilt
c. Possible fear of becoming mentally ill

4. Despair, depression
5. Detachment from loss
6. Renewed interest, investment in others/interests

Assessment

A. Weight loss
B. Sleep disturbance
C. Thoughts centered on loss
D. Dependency, withdrawal, anger, guilt
E. Suicide potential

Analysis

A. Ineffective individual/family coping
B. Hopelessness
C. Sleep pattern disturbance
D. Altered thought processes
E. Potential for violence to self

Goals

Client/family will
A. Discuss responses to loss.
B. Resume normal sleeping/eating patterns.
C. Resume ADL as they accept loss.

Interventions

A. Encourage client/family to express feelings.
B. Accept negative feelings/defenses.
C. Employ empathic listening.
D. Explain mourning process and relate to their responses.
E. Refer client/family to support groups.

Evaluation

Client/family
A. Express feelings.
B. Progress through mourning process.
C. Seek necessary support groups.

SAMPLE QUESTIONS

Larry, aged 27, has recently begun experiencing forgetfulness, disorientation, and occasional lapses in memory. Larry, who is gay, was diagnosed with AIDS dementia.

19. Larry's family began sobbing on hearing the diagnosis. The nurse's initial reponse would be
    o 1. You must never give up hope.
    o 2. He was in a high-risk group for AIDS.
    o 3. I can understand your grief.
    o 4. This must be very difficult for you.

20. The primary goal in Larry's care is to
    o 1. enhance the quality of life.
    o 2. teach him about AIDS.
    o 3. discuss his future goals.
    o 4. provide him with comfort and support.

21. One of the major fears experienced by people with AIDS is
    o 1. dying.
    o 2. debilitation.
    o 3. stigma.
    o 4. poverty.

Ethical and Legal Aspects of Psychiatric and Professional Nursing

OVERVIEW

It is important for nurses to recognize that nursing practice is guided by legal restrictions and professional obligations. Legal responsibilities are regulated by state nurse-practice acts, and may vary from state to state. In addition, general standards for the practice of nursing have been developed and published by the American Nurses' Association, who have also developed a code of ethics (see Appendix 3).

Nurses need to be aware of these standards, as well as legal and ethical concepts and principles, since nurses are accountable for their actions in all these areas in their professional role.

Ethical Concepts that Apply to Nursing Practice

A. *Ethics:* rules and principles that guide nursing decisions or conduct in terms of the rightness/wrongness of that decision or action.

B. *Morals:* personally held beliefs, opinions, and attitudes that guide our actions.

C. *Values:* appraisal of what is "good."
   1. Dilemmas may occur when different values conflict.
   2. Example: client's right to refuse treatment may be in conflict with nurse's obligation to benefit client and to carry out treatment.

D. *Ethical dilemma:* a problem in making a decision because there is no clearly correct or right choice. This may result in having to choose an action that violates one principle or value in order to promote another.

E. *Autonomy:* an individual has the right to make his or her own decision regarding treatment and care.

F. *Paternalism:* another person makes decisions about what is right or best for the individual.

G. *Beneficence:* promoting good or doing no harm to another.

H. *Right to know:* right to knowledge necessary or helpful in making an informed decision.

I. *Principle of double effect:* promoting good may involve some expected harm, such as adverse side effects of medication.

J. *Distributive justice:* allocation of goods and services and how or to whom they are distributed.
   1. Equality: everyone receives the same.
   2. Need: greater services go to those with greater needs (e.g.,

critically ill patient receives more intensive nursing care).
   3. Merit: services go to more deserving (used as a criterion for transplant recipients).

Legal Concepts that Apply to Nursing Practice

A. *Standards:* identify the minimal knowledge and conduct expected from a professional practitioner. Standards are applied as they relate to a practitioner's experience and educational preparation. For example, any nurse would be expected to be certain that an ordered medication was being given to the correct patient. However, more complex nursing actions, such as respirator monitoring, would require supervised experience and/or continuing education.

B. *Negligence:* lack of reasonable conduct or care. Omitting an action expected of a prudent person in a particular circumstance is considered negligence, as is committing an action that a prudent person would not.

C. *Malpractice:* professional negligence, misconduct, or unreasonable lack of skill resulting in injury or loss to the recipient of the professional services.

D. *Competence:* ability or qualification to make informed decisions.

E. *Informed consent:* agreement to the performance of a procedure/treatment based on knowledge of facts, risks, and alternatives.
   1. Simple: having capacity to give consent for the treatment or procedure.
   2. Valid: having capacity to give consent and also demonstrating an understanding of the nature of the treatment, expected effects, possible side effects, and alternatives to treatment.

F. *Assault:* unjustifiable threat or attempt to touch or injure another.

G. *Battery:* unlawful touching or injury to another.

H. *Crime:* act that is a violation of duty or breach of law, punishable by the state by fine or imprisonment (see Table 5.9).

I. *Tort:* a legal wrong committed against a person, his or her rights or property; intentional, willfully committed without just cause (see Table 5.9). The person who commits a tort is liable for damages in a civil action.

Table 5.9 Examples of Crimes and Torts

Crimes	Torts
Assault and battery	Assault and battery
Involuntary manslaughter: committing a lawful act that results in the death of a patient	False imprisonment: intentional confinement of a patient without consent
Illegal possession or sale of a controlled substance	Fraud
	Negligence/malpractice: • Medication errors • Carelessness resulting in loss of patient's property • Burns from hot water bottles, heating pads, hot soaks • Failure to prevent falls by not using bed rails • Incompetence in assessing symptoms (shock, chest pain, respiratory distress) • Administering treatment to wrong client

    1. Negligence and malpractice are torts.
    2. Victims of malpractice are entitled to receive monetary awards (damages) to compensate for their injury or loss.
J. *Good Samaritan doctrine:* rescuer is protected from liability when assisting in an emergency situation or rescuing a person from imminent and serious peril, if attempt is not reckless and person's condition is not made worse.

Legal Concepts Related to Psychiatric-Mental Health Nursing

A. *Voluntary commitment:* client consents to hospital admission.
    1. Client must be released when he or she no longer chooses to remain in the hospital.
    2. State laws govern how long a client must remain hospitalized prior to release.
    3. Client has the right to refuse treatment.
B. *Involuntary commitment:* client is hospitalized without consent
    1. Most states require that the client be mentally ill and be a danger to others/self (includes being unable to meet own basic needs such as eating or protection from injury).
    2. In most states the client who has been involuntarily committed may *not* refuse treatment.
C. *Insanity:* a legal term for mental illness where an individual cannot be held responsible for or does not understand the nature of his or her acts.

D. *Insanity defenses:* not guilty by reason of insanity
    1. M'Naghten rule ("right and wrong test"): the accused is not legally responsible for an act if, at the time the act was committed, the person did not, because of mental defect or illness, know the nature of the act or that the act was wrong.
    2. Irresistible impulse: the accused, because of mental illness, did not have the will to resist an impulse to commit the act, even though able to differentiate between right and wrong.
    3. Individuals who commit crimes and successfully plead insanity defenses may be involuntarily committed to psychiatric hospitals under civil commitment laws. There is presently a trend toward finding individuals insane and guilty.
E. *Rights of clients:* rights that each state may grant to its residents committed to a psychiatric hospital
    1. Right to receive treatment and not just be confined
    2. Right to the least restrictive alternative (locked vs unlocked units, inpatient vs outpatient care)
    3. Right to individualized treatment plan and to participation in the development of that plan and to an explanation of the treatment
    4. Right to confidentiality of records
    5. Right to visitors, mail, and use of telephone
    6. Right to refuse to participate in experimental treatments
    7. Right to freedom from seclusion or restraints
    8. Right to an explanation of rights and assertion of grievances

Legal Responsibilities of the Nurse

A nurse is expected to
A. Be responsible for his or her own acts
B. Protect the rights and safety of patients
C. Witness, but not obtain, consent for procedures
D. Document and communicate information regarding patient care and responses
E. Refuse to carry out orders that the nurse knows/believes harmful to the patient
F. Perform acts allowed by that nurse's state nurse-practice act
G. Reveal patient's confidential information only to appropriate persons
H. Perform acts for which the nurse is qualified by either education or experience
I. Witness a will (this is not a legal obligation, but the nurse may choose to do so)
J. Restrain patients only in emergencies to prevent injury to self/others. Patients have the right to be free from unlawful restraint.

REFERENCES AND RECOMMENDED READINGS

Psychiatric-Mental Health Nursing

Abrams, A. (1987). Clinical drug therapy: Rationales for nursing practice (2nd ed.). Philadelphia: Lippincott.

Adams, C., & Macione, A. (Eds.). (1983). Handbook of psychiatric mental health nursing. New York: Wiley.

*Barash, D. (1984). Defusing the violent patient before he explodes. *RN*, *47*(3), 34–37.

Beck, C., Rawlins, R., & Williams, S. (Eds.). (1988). Mental health-psychiatric nursing: A holistic life-cycle approach (2nd ed.). St. Louis: Mosby.

Black, H. (1979). Black's law dictionary. St. Paul, MN: West Publishing.

Cohen, S., & Harris, E. (1981). Mental status assessment. (Reprint #p. 48) New York: American Journal of Nursing Co.

Cook, J., & Fontaine, K. (1987). Essentials of mental health nursing. Menlo Park, CA: Addison-Wesley.

Davis, A., & Aroskar, M. (1983). Ethical dilemmas and nursing practice. Norwalk, CT: Appleton-Century-Crofts.

*Fine, M., & Jenike, M. (1985). ECT: Exploding the myths. *RN*, *48*(9), 58–66.

Haber, J., Hoskins, P., Leach, A., & Sidelau, B. (1987). Comprehensive psychiatric nursing (3rd ed.). New York: McGraw-Hill.

Hinsie, L., & Campbell, R. (1974). Psychiatric dictionary. (4th ed.). New York: Oxford University Press.

Jameton, A. (1984). Nursing practice: The ethical issues. Englewood Cliffs, NJ: Prentice-Hall.

Kneisl, C., & Wilson, H. (1984). Handbook of psychosocial nursing care. Menlo Park, CA: Addison-Wesley.

*Marks, R. (1984). Anorexia and bulimia: Eating habits that can kill. *RN*, *47*(1), 44–47.

*Stevenson, C. (1985). Dealing with drug abusers. *RN*, *48*(4), 37–39.

Wilson, H., & Kneisl, C. (1988). Psychiatric nursing (3rd ed.). Menlo Park, CA: Addison-Wesley.

Legal Issues

Bailey, D. (1984). How careful charting saved my career. *RN*, *47*(11), 15–16.

Bernzweig, E. (1984). Don't cut corners on informed consent. RN, 47(12), 15–16.

Bernzweig, E. (1985). When a nurse doesn't fit the job. *RN*, *48*(1), 13–14.

Bernzweig, E. (1985). The patient who wants help with a will. *RN*, *48*(9), 71–72.

Bernzweig, E. (1985). How communications breakdown can get you sued. *RN*, *48*(12), 47–48.

Collier, J. (1987). When you suspect your patient is a battered wife. *RN*, *50*(5), 222–225.

Guarriello, D. (1984). Can you be sued without a cause? *RN*, *47*(2), 19–23.

Guarriello, D. (1984). When doctor's orders aren't the best medicine. *RN*, *47*(5), 19–20.

Kapp, M. (1985). If you question your patient's competence. RN, 48(10), 59–60.

Kline, P. (1987). Heading off depression in the chronically ill. *RN*, *50*(10), 44–49.

Tammello, A., & Gill, D. (1984). When following orders can cost you your license. *RN*, *47*(7), 13–14.

*Reprints included in 1987 and 1988 editions.

UNIT 5: Reprints

Would your assessment spot a hidden alcoholic?

Uncovering his drinking problem is probably the greatest service you can offer a tight-lipped hospital patient. Overlooking the onset of alcohol withdrawal may be the *last* service you offer him.

By Leonard Goodman, RN

Mary Robertson, a 60-year-old with congestive heart failure, cardiomyopathy, and severe pulmonary edema, is on large doses of diuretics and cardiac medication.

Jon Farrell, once a promising 17-year-old high school athlete, lies paralyzed after an auto accident.

Earl Nelson, 40 years old, is an obese alcoholic suffering from ascites and jaundice. As he emerges from a coma, he becomes combative, tearing his IV line out and demanding to be discharged.

While Mr. Nelson's condition is obvious, the fact is all *three* patients are alcoholics. You'd have had to do a little digging, though, to discover that Mrs. Robertson's cardiac and pulmonary disorders were caused by years of heavy drinking or that Jon Farrell was driving while intoxicated.

The key to recognizing hidden alcoholics is knowing how to take a proper nursing history and physical

THE AUTHOR is health services coordinator for Northwest Treatment Center, a drug and alcohol treatment facility located in Seattle.

Produced by Paul L. Cerrato

exam. Without these skills, odds are your patient's drinking problem will continue to go unnoticed—until severe physical and psychological symptoms become life-threatening.

The physiological effects of alcoholism

Chronic drinking affects a host of organs, but the gastrointestinal system usually breaks down first. Alcohol removes the protective layer of mucin from the stomach wall, exposing its lining to corrosive gastric juices and causing gastritis and possibly ulcers. Never give aspirin to an alcoholic in early recovery. It only exacerbates damage to the stomach lining.

Alcohol may also cause the pancreatic duct to go into spasm where it enters the duodenum. This forces pancreatic enzymes back into the gland, destroying its sensitive tissues and leading to diabetes in some patients. Also be alert to severe abdominal pain and elevated serum amylase readings.

The alcoholic's liver pays a heavy price for detoxifying so much etha-

nol. Initially, excess fat builds up. In time, hepatitis and cirrhosis may occur. Complications of the latter can include lowered resistance to infection, ascites, esophageal varices, poor blood clotting, folic acid deficiency anemia, and hepatic coma. If you suspect liver dysfunction, check the lab sheet for elevated serum levels of bilirubin and the liver enzymes SGOT and SGPT.

Fortunately, cirrhosis affects only 10% of alcoholic patients. Cardiac and neurological problems are more common, including congestive heart failure, peripheral neuropathy, confusion, and ataxia.

The nutritional depletion caused by too much alcohol affects the central nervous system as well. Lack of vitamin B_1, for instance, interferes with the supply of glucose to the brain. That deficiency, along with the direct neurotoxic impact of ethanol, contributes to short-term memory loss, the inability to think abstractly, and difficulty solving everyday problems.

The physical symptoms of chronic alcoholism become most severe during withdrawal. Because ethanol has a very short half-life, withdrawal symptoms usually come on strong and fast. For more on these symptoms, see the discussion of delirium tremens in the box below.

The psychosocial toll taken by alcohol

The psychological effects of alcoholism can be as devastating as the physical. Guilt about neglect of family and job leaves the alcoholic prone to depression and suicide. Alcohol pervades his environment. He develops friendships with other drinkers and most events in his life—from important occasions like the birth of a child, to everyday activities such as watching TV—are "celebrated" with a drink. This preoccupation with alcohol shuts out the patient's family, with spouse and children usually taking on responsibilities that are rightly his.

Alcohol becomes the drinker's closest friend, his most important relationship. At the very time when a patient has lost virtually all control over his drinking habits, he believes he has matters well in hand.

How to spot the problem drinker

A good nursing assessment is the first step toward uncovering this devastating plight, but you'll need an eye as sharp as any detective's.

When examining the skin, look for signs of dehydration, purpura, bruises, and spider nevi—the so-called "W.C. Fields nose." A palpable, tender liver and occult blood in the stool can also provide clues.

Muscle spasms may signal magnesium deficiency, common among chronic drinkers. Muscle wasting is a sign of advanced alcoholism, usually seen in those who've been drinking for decades.

Don't forget to include in your assessment the patient's grooming and the condition of his clothes, sniffing for the smell of liquor and looking for cigarette burns. Keep in mind, though, that many alcoholics

Bringing your patient through the DTs

By Laurie B. Lausé, RN, BSN, MBA

Delirium tremens is an acute psychotic condition that usually comes on 24 to 48 hours after an alcoholic stops drinking. It can, however, take as long as three weeks to develop in some patients; still others develop symptoms while still drinking. Regardless of the time of onset, mortality ranges from 15% to 30% if the DTs are left untreated—often the result of pulmonary and cardiovascular complications.

Symptoms of the DTs include anxiety, shakiness, increasing confusion, sweating, nervousness, forgetfulness, and hallucinations. Because other disorders can mimic it, however, you'll have to do the thorough assessment outlined in the accompanying article to differentiate DTs from conditions such as hypoglycemia or adverse drug reaction.

Once you're convinced that your patient is going through alcohol withdrawal, notify the doctor and get orders to treat the problem.

Which drugs should you administer?

The physician will probably prescribe a tranquilizer such as chlordiazepoxide (Librium) or diazepam (Valium). Some physicians also order phenytoin (Dilantin) to control the seizures that occasionally accompany the DTs. Also check the patient's electrolyte status; magnesium deficiency, for instance, can bring on seizures.

When the physician is prescribing, ask for a prn order so that you can adjust the patient's doses as your follow-up assessments suggest. When drugs are available IV or IM, request the right to give them either way just in case the patient pulls out the IV line.

When adjusting medications, remember that they won't take effect at the normal rate in an alcoholic

THE AUTHOR, formerly head nurse on the gastroenterology unit, is nursing project coordinator at Lee Memorial Hospital in Fort Myers, Fla.

Produced by Paul L. Cerrato

are well-dressed and manicured.

Vital signs are keys, too. The alcoholic will usually have an elevated blood pressure that stays high for some time after admission. A pulse above 100 is also typical, but even more significant is a rising pulse. When it approaches 120, the patient risks life-threatening arrhythmia. Notify the physician and request an order for a tranquilizer such as chlordiazepoxide (Librium) long before it ever gets that high.

Assessing timing and severity of withdrawal

Your job isn't over once you find out that your patient is an alcoholic. You still have to estimate when the withdrawal syndrome that may threaten his life is likely to strike. You'll have to ask the right questions: "Do you drink a lot?" isn't enough. A reply like "Not really" may mean several six-packs of beer a day—or several quarts of whiskey. You'll have to press for exactly how much the patient drinks and how often.

To illustrate—if you were interviewing Mrs. Robertson, the CHF patient you've discovered is an alcoholic—you might ask:

"When did you have your last drink?" You can anticipate the likelihood of a seizure 10 to 20 hours after the last drink. Other major symptoms may take from a day to as long as three weeks to develop.

"How much did you have to drink?" If your patient says "Not very much," pin him down to a specific amount—one drink or five, singles or doubles. The more he's used to consuming, the more severe the withdrawal symptoms are likely to be. If the ER notes say his blood alcohol level is 0.23 mg%, for instance, he's had quite a bit to drink.

"Do you drink every day?" If your patient responds "A couple of times a week," ask which days of the week. These questions help discover not only the amount he consumes, but will help you anticipate the onset of withdrawal. A typical

---

who has hepatic disease. Because the damaged liver processes drugs more slowly than the normal liver, the medication may have a delayed effect. So too, the liver may be unable to detoxify medication quickly enough to prevent a toxic buildup in the tissues.

Thus, it's important not to overmedicate. But you should also avoid undermedicating the patient. Someone who's not combative during your shift may still need medication to control increasing restlessness or tremors.

What kind of nursing care is in order?

Proper management of the DTs requires clear clinical guidelines on charting, standing orders, IVs, prn meds, and the like. When dealing with a patient who is combative, however, discontinue any IVs or tubes that aren't absolutely necessary. Since the patient is more than likely to pull them out, continually replacing them may do him more harm than not having them at all.

You can always restart a line once the patient calms down. When you do, insert it in the upper arm where it will be less accessible to the patient and where it won't get in the way if you need to use arm restraints. Before resorting to restraints, however, try using less restrictive measures, cautiously administering another dose of a prn drug, for instance.

Before restraining a patient, call your supervisor or a security guard to help—for your patient's safety as well as your own. Cloth restraints are adequate for most, but very combative patients may require leather. Regardless of the type used, be sure to get a physician's order within 12 hours of initiating restraints. Once applied, check the skin under the restraints at least every half hour and start range-of-motion exercises. JCAHO regulations also require the patient's needs be attended to every 15 minutes. To that end, make sure the patient is properly fed, bathed, and toileted.

Try to move the patient into a quiet, private room that's near the nurses' station. Remove all personal items that may cause injury. Also take away clothing so he's less likely to leave the unit if he's not in restraints or manages to escape them. Lastly, remember to always speak in a calm, quiet, nonjudgmental manner. Harsh criticism is not only cruel, it can retard the patient's recovery.

BIBLIOGRAPHY Luckermann, J. and Sorensen, K. *Medical-Surgical Nursing*. Philadelphia: W.B. Saunders Co., 1980. Patrick, M., Woods, S., et al. *Medical-Surgical Nursing: Pathophysiological Concepts*. Philadelphia: J.B. Lippincott, 1986.

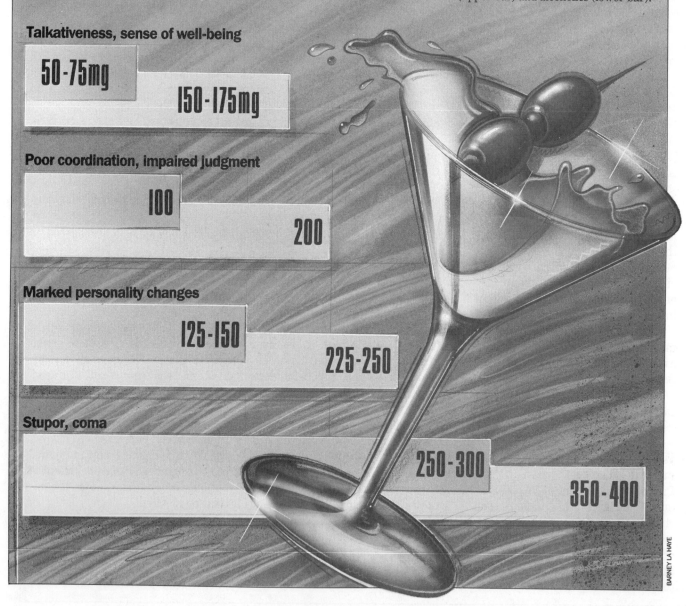

The effects of alcohol

The extent to which alcohol affects a person's behavior depends in part on how much remains in his bloodstream over time—the blood alcohol level. Because an alcoholic has a greater tolerance for alcohol than the social drinker, however, he'll appear to "hold his liquor better." For example, the social drinker will show marked personality changes—say, depression, congeniality, or hostility—with a blood alcohol level of 150 mg%. The alcoholic probably won't be so affected until blood alcohol is 250 mg%. The chart below shows the progressive behavioral changes alcohol brings on and the blood alcohol levels—expressed in mg%—at which they occur in social drinkers (upper bar) and alcoholics (lower bar).

Talkativeness, sense of well-being

50-75mg

150-175mg

Poor coordination, impaired judgment

100

200

Marked personality changes

125-150

225-250

Stupor, coma

250-300

350-400

BARNEY LA HAYE

drinking pattern is to start after work on Wednesday and continue through the weekend. By the following Wednesday, the withdrawal symptoms may be coming on, making the patient very agitated.

"Have you ever seen things that weren't there?" The response "Yes, a couple of times" strongly suggests he's been through the DTs at least once. It can easily happen again.

"Have you ever had a seizure?" "Once, maybe a year ago." If your patient has a history of alcoholic seizures—they're also called rum fits—he's at high risk for a repeat performance.

"Have you ever temporarily lost your memory when you hadn't been drinking?" "You mean a blackout? Yes, I've had them, too." A blackout isn't a drunken stupor, but a bout of amnesia that alcoholics suffer when they're carrying on their everyday affairs. It's a sign of neurological damage.

Treating the hospitalized alcoholic

Benzodiazapines, frequently used to treat the withdrawal syndrome, must be administered cautiously. Impaired hepatic function can prolong drug half-life, increasing the risk of oversedation. To minimize this danger, give only enough medication to make the patient comfortable and keep his pulse down.

Once your patient has made it through withdrawal, the most effective long-term treatment programs call for complete abstinence. Neuroleptics such as chlorpromazine (Thorazine) or haloperidol (Haldol) are contraindicated because the goal of treatment is to help the patient break free from all mind-altering drugs, not just from alcohol.

Once the patient has stopped drinking, psychological counseling can help him in tackling the underlying emotional problems that contributed to his alcoholism.

For long-term therapy, refer the patient to the hospital social worker or substance abuse specialist, if your facility has one, to Alcoholics Anonymous if it doesn't. Also steer family members toward Al-Anon, a support group especially for them.

For a complete listing of the agencies and treatment programs available to alcoholics and their families, consult the *National Directory of Alcoholism and Addiction Treatment Programs* or contact the local chapter of the National Council on Alcoholism.

The hidden alcoholic patient poses a real challenge to your nursing skills. Not only will you have to spot the condition, you'll have to cope with its acute effects, and then help your patient take the first steps toward turning his life around. Through it all, never forget that the person in that bed is not some nameless drunk, but quite possibly the sickest person on your unit. ∎

BIBLIOGRAPHY Crovella, A.C. "When Your Patient's an Alcoholic," *RN*, Feb. 1984. Estes, N.J., Smith-DiJulio, K., and Heinemann, M.E. *Nursing Diagnosis of the Alcoholic Person.* St. Louis: C.V. Mosby Co., 1980. Estes, N.J. and Heinemann, M.E., *Alcoholism: Development, Consequences and Intervention.* St. Louis: C.V. Mosby Co., 1982. Mendelson, J. and Mello, N., eds., *The Diagnosis and Treatment of Alcoholism.* New York: McGraw-Hill, 1985. *National Directory of Alcoholism and Addiction Treatment Programs.* Cleveland: Quantum Press, 1988.

Defusing the violent patient— before he explodes

BY DOROTHY A. BARASH, RN, MSN

Richard slammed down the telephone receiver, began hollering abuses at the other patients in the lounge, and pushed over a chair. A nurse hurried over, stopping a few feet in front of him. "Let's go out to the patio, Richard," she said quietly. "I can see you're feeling angry. I'd like to help." Richard glared at her, pushed over another chair, but then, sullenly, followed her down the hall, mumbling angrily about "that bastard." The situation had come close to erupting into violence. Had it happened on your unit, would you have been able to de-

THE AUTHOR *is associate director of nursing at The Menninger Foundation, in Topeka, Kan.*

Produced by Charlotte Isler
Illustration by Michael Garland

activate it before an outright explosion occurred?

Most nurses worry that they might some day face such an incident, with all its potential danger. And with good reason! A sudden violent outburst by a patient can occur anywhere in a hospital: on a med/surg unit, in the emergency room, and, of course, on a psychiatric unit. So it's important to be prepared psychologically for encounters with a possibly combative patient, as the combination of illness, stress, fear, frustration, and the helplessness that hospitalization entails slowly builds toward a critical mass.

Your first task is to learn to recognize a patient's mounting tension, even if you're busy with another patient or other work. When the aggressive drive

that's present in everyone escalates, for whatever reason, a constructive way to release it must be found, or trouble is inevitable.

Early warning signs

The warning signals are usually obvious. Is a patient angrily slamming the door, or pacing up and down the hall, kicking a wall, or sitting near the nurses' station looking grim and defiant? Is he yelling at another patient, or pushing over furniture, as Richard was in the case above?

He may not even be aware of it, but a patient engaging in such acts is clearly testing you. He wants to see if you notice him, and are reacting to his signals. He's looking for some sign that you're concerned about what he's doing.

Whether conscious of it or not, he's trying to communicate his distress in a nonverbal way, looking for help in regaining the control that's rapidly slipping away from him.

Keep in mind, too, that your patient may well be overreacting to a situation in which he'd normally respond with equanimity, simply because he finds himself in a complex and unfamiliar hospital environment over which he has no control. He may scream at you and others in the unit, for example, although no one has behaved in a provocative manner toward him. Such behavior is especially likely if the patient's family never allowed him, as a child, to vent his anger, so that he was always forced to suppress it.

Your task, then, as soon as you see

Do's and don'ts of dealing with violence

To prevent a crisis

Do:
- Help patient retain his self respect by showing that you understand his concerns.
- Ask how you can help.
- Listen carefully, and watch for nonverbal signals.
- Help patient express his anger by eliciting the real issues.
- Use reality orientation.
- Help patient understand his behavior.
- Remind patient of the consequences of inappropriate behavior.

Don't:
- Promise more than you can actually deliver.
- Imply that he'll be punished for his anger.

If violence seems imminent

Do:
- Try to get patient to talk out his anger.
- Use medication, when possible, instead of physical force.
- Repeat what you want the patient to do, explain your position, offer alternatives.

Don't:
- Approach the patient without backup from other staff members.
- Allow yourself to yell or become aggressive.
- Crowd the patient or attempt to touch him.

When violence erupts

Do:
- Use speed and surprise to secure and carry patient to his room, and restrain him.
- Have a minimum of three persons working together on the restraint team.
- Keep the restrained patient under constant supervision.
- Make it clear that he is not being punished.

Don't:
- Criticize or argue with patient.
- Attempt to reason with a patient whose behavior is due to psychosis street drugs.
- Show your fear.
- Allow other patients to help restrain the violent patient.

that a patient's tension is rising to explosive levels, is to help him find an acceptable way to deal with the frustration, pain, or anger that he's feeling. Start by walking over to him at once and giving him a chance to express his fury verbally. It may not be pleasant for you or the other patients nearby, but it's usually enough to keep the situation from becoming dangerous.

Next, being careful to avoid totally isolating yourself, try to get him away from other patients and bystanders, either back to his own room or to some other quiet area where he can talk to you alone. Tell him that you'd like to know what's bothering him, so he'll realize you understand that he has a reason for being angry, and that you care enough about him to want to help.

Don't take it personally if, in his angry mood, he says things that are demeaning or insulting, either to you or to others. Such insults are actually directed at his illness or other source of anger, rather than at you. Let him see that it's all right for him to be angry in your presence, and that he can successfully release his tension this way without resorting to physical violence. This may well be a new experience for a patient who is used to reacting with violence at home. Seeing that a conflict can be handled peacefully—that he can discharge his angry impulses by talking instead of acting out—will decrease his anxiety.

Special problems

While straightforward talk will be sufficient in most cases, you have to take additional risks into account if there's reason to believe that a patient is psychotic. Paranoid delusions or hallucinations may make such a patient completely opaque to reality. He may hear voices instructing him to strike out, not because he wants to hurt anyone in particular, but in "self defense" against what he perceives to be a hostile environment. Or he may still be angry at someone whom he feels has mistreated him in the past, and contuse you or another staff member or patient with that long-gone offender.

With this type of patient, your most important task is to keep him as oriented to reality as possible. Frequently remind him that he is in the hospital, call him by his name, and keep him aware of who you and others around him are. If he's hallucinating, try to make him understand that the voices urging him on are not real, but a result of his illness. At the same time, encourage him to seek help by talking with staff members whenever he hears such voices. Making him aware of it when his behavior is bizarre will help him learn to separate fantasy from reality, and gradually increase his ability to distinguish between them.

Organic dysfunctions

It's not only psychotic patients who pose special problems. Temporary *organic* derangements can turn sane persons into apparent "maniacs." A hypoglycemic patient, for example, may suddenly become an aggressive, incoherent opponent. Even if he's not wearing a diabetic's ID bracelet, extreme diaphoresis and slurred, unrecognizable speech should tip you off. Rapid restraint and IV injection of 50 gm of 50% dextrose solution usually return these patients to normal.

Jibberish or impaired speech can also result from head injury. If no one can provide a history of cranial trauma, assessing the patient's neurological function for signs of head injury is essential. The patient may have to be restrained even before such assessment. If there's reason to suspect head injury, don't administer any drug that might otherwise be given to quiet the patient; it could prove lethal.

Violent behavior can also stem from delirium tremens. If you suspect this, place your hands in front of the patient as if you're holding a string. If he says he sees the nonexistent string, he's hallucinating—a positive "string sign." Drug intoxication is also a cause of "temporary insanity." Horizontal nystagmus is a sign of phenytoin intoxication. Vertical nystagmus is a sign of PCP or ketamine intoxication, usually the former. Besides the extreme agitation that PCP causes, it eliminates the sense of pain, imparting a false sense of invulnerability.

When all else fails: restraining the violent patient

When violence seems unavoidable, speed, surprise, and sufficient manpower are essential to secure a patient before he, or anyone around him, is hurt. The four-person carry will enable you to get a patient to his room and into restraints safely.

To restrain the patient, apply a waist belt and put cuffs on each wrist. One cuff hasp attaches to the waist belt; another hasp attaches to the strap that's secured to the bed. This allows the patient to keep his arms at his sides. Next, apply a cuff to each ankle and secure both to the bed with one strap.

The patient in restraints is helpless, so it's essential to provide constant supervision, ensuring that no other patient attacks him or that he can't manage to hurt himself. Check extremities frequently for evidence of adequate circulation, and look for skin burns from the sheets if the patient is still attempting to resist. Take measures to prevent aspiration, as well. If a patient is in restraints for more than three hours, allow him to sit up and deep breathe.

Once he has quieted down, you can remove the leg cuffs and, with his arms still cuffed to the waist strap, allow him to use the bathroom. A staff member of the same sex should accompany him, since he cannot protect himself from a fall. Release one arm at mealtime so the patient can feed himself, again with the supervision and help of a staff member.

The patient who continues to struggle, despite restraints, may well need medication to tranquilize or sedate him. Whether or not you have to wait for drugs to be ordered and take effect, make sure the patient is given time, once he does calm down, to discuss the feelings and events leading up to the incident.

"Neutralized" aggression

Never criticize or argue with a patient during a potentially violent incident. Doing so merely challenges his self esteem, and is likely to increase his tension. Instead, support whatever ability he has to stay calm, cooperative, and in control. Give him enough space, too: Keeping your distance will keep *him* from feeling trapped. He'll feel less physically threatened, and therefore less compelled to strike out at you in "self defense."

Approaching the patient calmly and reasonably is the best way to neutralize his aggressive instincts. If *you* appear uncertain or afraid, your fear may immobilize you *and* increase the patient's already dangerous tension. Try to appear calm even if you don't feel it. Use direct, simple statements to let the patient know what you want him to do, whether it's putting down a weapon or going off to a less public area. Your firm voice and expression of confidence can provide the extra measure of stability and control he needs to stay in control himself.

If a patient becomes aggressive repeatedly, he may need to be given, on a temporary basis, tranquilizers or antipsychotics that reduce tension, anxiety, and delusional thinking. Such medications can relieve the intensity of his feelings and allow him to see his conflicts more objectively, making him more willing to accept your help. As he's able to begin dealing with his feelings, with psychotherapy if necessary, the drug regimen can be gradually reduced until he can function adequately without it.

It's possible, of course, that a patient may lose control despite your best preventive efforts. When an assault seems imminent, quick, coordinated action is essential to bring the situation under control before anyone is hurt. At such times, staff feelings run high too, so a well-rehearsed plan for dealing with both potential and actual violence is vital.

On each unit, for each shift, all staff members should be drilled in working as a restraint team. Each should be able to function as team leader, so that whoever has had the best rapport with a specific patient can assume that leadership role. Although the team's first objective is to calm the patient *without* physical intervention, it's very important that all staff members know how to secure, carry, and restrain combative persons.

As a matter of policy, especially on psych units, both patients and staff should be made aware of just what will happen if a patient loses control. This not only reflects concern for everyone in the unit, but also increases the *staff's* feelings of security when violence threatens.

The guiding principle for restraint teams is that dealing with violence is, above all, a group effort. Staff members should *never* try to cope by themselves with a patient who is out of control. If physical restraint *should* become necessary, at least three—and usually four or five—people are needed for effective action.

Techniques of control

Before resorting to restraints, however, you still may be able to talk a patient down. If you're the team leader, approach the patient, with the other team members backing you, and tell the patient clearly that he's out of control. Explain that he will not be allowed to break furniture, or hurt himself or others. Give him a chance to participate in the decision that must be made. Say firmly, "We are going to help you control yourself. Can you go to your room by yourself so you can calm down, or should we help you by using restraints for a while?"

Maintain eye contact with the patient as you're speaking, but remember to keep your distance. Raise your voice if you must to be heard, but don't shout or act aggressively. Stay calm and firm, even if the patient becomes more excited. There's a good chance that once he feels overpowered by the presence of the entire team, he'll get a grip on himself and go to his room. Be sure not to touch him, even if he continues to threaten you or others. Allow him to save face by verbalizing his anger.

Don't attempt to use reason, however, when a patient is out of control, and already violent due to psychosis or the effects of drugs. Use the elements of speed and surprise to quickly secure him, get him to his room, and apply restraints (see "When all else fails," above). There are no halfway measures in such circumstances.

While you're applying restraints, reassure the patient that he's not being punished, that he won't be hurt, and that he'll be released as soon as he regains control of himself. When he does calm down, take time to discuss with him the events and feelings leading up to the incident. This can be a therapeutic experience for him, and may prevent repetitions. Take some time, too, to review, with other staff members, how the incident arose. Look for staff actions that inadvertently may have led the patient to feel threatened; perhaps such external factors can be eliminated or modified.

Certainly, you have more than enough care to provide in the normal course of your shift without having to cope with violence as well. But, like it or not, you have to remember that the danger of violence exists in any setting in which patients are in pain, under stress, and feeling frustrated. It's up to you to defuse outbursts in the making, by recognizing the early signals of mounting tension. And, if you *can't* help a patient regain control with only your verbal intervention, it's essential that you be prepared to apply restraints in a skilled, nonpunitive way. The safety of everyone—patients, staff, and yourself—may depend on it. ■

KATHLEEN RYAN FLETCHER, RN,C, MSN, GNP

Restraints should be a last resort

Physical and chemical restraints aren't the only— or the safest—way of calming an agitated or a disruptive patient.

KATHLEEN FLETCHER is an assistant professor at the University of Virginia School of Nursing, Charlottesville, Va. She also works as a staff nurse at Elder Care Gardens, a nursing home in the same city.
STAFF EDITOR: Sigrid Nagle

Isaac Ingram, 86 years old, was admitted to the urology unit with benign prostatic hypertrophy. He was alert, oriented, cooperative, and knowledgeable about the surgical procedure he was about to undergo. Several hours postop, however, the evening nurse found him acutely confused and agitated. She administered an oral dose of diazepam (Valium) and applied waist and wrist restraints.

When the night nurse entered his room on midnight rounds, he was pulling at the restraints and crying for his mother. In response to her touch, he told her that she had no right to tie him up like a dog.

This distressing scenario will be familiar to med/surg nurses everywhere. Nurses report that although they dislike using restraints and feel guilty doing so, they often believe they have no alternative—particularly if the unit is short-staffed.

Are they right? Let's examine the situation: What type of patient is typically restrained, and why? What kinds of restraints are used? How well do they work? What are the alternatives to restraints?

Who is most likely to be restrained?
What types of restraints are used?

Any patient who is confused, agitated, or disruptive is a candidate for restraints, but research indicates that an elderly patient is eight times more likely to be restrained than a younger one. In fact, one older patient in five is physically restrained during a hospital stay. These restraints include cloth devices secured at the waist or wrists, geriatric chairs with their locking trays, and side rails.

Chemical, or pharmacologic, restraints are also in common use. A review of med/surg patients on several hospital units showed that practically half received at least one psychotropic drug during their stay—a sleeping pill, antidepressant, antipsychotic, or antianxiety drug. In some cases the purpose may not have been to restrain, but these medications tend to inhibit behavior nonetheless.

Frequently, as was the case with Mr. Ingram, physical and chemical restraints are used at the same time.

The purpose of the restraints is generally rationalized as benign: to protect the delirious patient from falling out of bed, the Alzheimer's patient from wandering, or the restless postop patient from pulling out his IV or NG tubing. In reality, the nurse may not have time to work out another solution or may be afraid of legal action should the patient sustain an injury while unrestrained.

In any case, the effects of restraints are problematic.

Problems range from backward vests
to pressure sores and dehydration

As a geriatric nurse practitioner with years of nursing home experience, I know that it's not unusual for staff members to apply mechanical devices improperly. They may tie wrist restraints too tightly, for example, causing friction burns, skin tears, abrasions, bruises, and impaired circulation (you should be able to fit two fingers between the restraint and the patient's wrist).

They sometimes put safety vests on backwards. I know of several facilities in which this incorrect technique has been used for so long it's become the norm. But if the patient slides down in the bed or chair and the restraint draws upward, the result may be an occluded airway. Patients have suffocated in improperly applied vest restraints.

Instead of feeling safe, patients often feel trapped or punished: They wonder what they did to deserve such inhuman treatment. Rather than becoming less agitated, they may become more so. Several studies show that the risk of falls and injuries actually increases because of this agitation: A patient in a chest Posey may become so upset that he tips over his wheelchair; another, confronted with side rails, may try to climb over them and fall.

The immobility that restraints impose is hazardous as well. A contracture can occur within as little as 48 hours. Pressure sores develop when the patient cannot adjust position and, as often happens, the staff is less than punctual about turning. With prolonged inactivity, muscles weaken and tendons shrink.

Dehydration is another concern. A restrained patient cannot reach for a glass of water, and staff members may neglect to encourage fluid intake. Functional incontinence may occur when the patient can't get to the bathroom.

Chemical restraints have additional risks. Since the half-life of drugs is generally increased in older patients, their effect is prolonged. Even low doses of diazepam, one of the most frequently prescribed antianxiety drugs, can result in an overdose if it's given too often. People experience less restorative deep sleep as they age, and barbiturates can exacerbate the problem. Antidepressants not only have side effects but alter the effects of other drugs, such as tranquilizers, anticholinergics, and anticonvulsants.

The antipsychotic haloperidol (Haldol), frequently used today on med/surg units, can cause more behavioral problems than it cures. Its effects include fatigue, increased agitation and restlessness, muscle weakness, and orthostatic hypotension.

Older patients, in fact, have three to five times as many adverse reactions to therapeutic drugs as younger patients do.

All of this should lead us to use restraints as seldom and cautiously as possible.

What choices are available?

We have a number of good alternatives. However, implementing them often requires more time and thought than physically restraining or sedating the patient.

First you need to discover, if possible, the cause of the problem. Is the patient agitated, noisy, combative? He may be in pain. He may be frustrated because he's having difficulty making his needs understood. The noise level on the floor may be upsetting him.

Is he confused? Finding himself in an unfamiliar environment with unfamiliar faces can be profoundly disorienting, and medications often compound the problem—as can electrolyte imbalances and infection.

Does he tend to wander off— or does he just need to move around?

Is he fall prone? His ears may be impacted with wax, disturbing his balance. Or the environment, rather than the patient, may be at fault. Hospitals are notorious for small, cluttered rooms, slippery floors, and poor lighting. (The article that follows this one discusses some

nursing research on falls and a program to combat them.)

You may be able to calm an agitated patient by talking to him soothingly, or playing quiet music, or offering him warm fluids. Look in on him often, so that he gets used to you and begins to trust you. Reassure him that his problems are important to you and that you'll do your best to resolve them. Remind him gently that there are less disruptive ways of asking for assistance.

Perhaps a family member can sit with the patient until he's calmer. If noise is a problem, see if you can find him a quieter room. A night light will help orient him as well as making the room safer to move around in.

Try to find a safe, circumscribed area in which a restless patient can get some exercise, perhaps an enclosed courtyard or a wraparound type of corridor. Expending physical energy often has a calming effect. If a patient tends to get lost because every entrance in your facility looks the same, hang a big sign by his door, or a colorful ribbon.

Finally, keep in mind that most instances of agitation and confusion are short-lived and will resolve without mechanical or chemical intervention.

When the alternatives don't work

Of course, there will be times when restraints of some sort are the only solution. At these times it will help if your facility has a written policy on their use— something that goes well beyond the usual physician's standing order. The policy should stipulate that only one type of restraint be used at first and emphasize the need to select the least restrictive method that fits the patient's condition.

For example, you shouldn't give a pharmacologic restraint to a patient on multiple medications or one who is scheduled for some form of exercise within a few hours. Here you might decide on a vest restraint—but only a vest restraint. When you do use medication, wait and see what its effects are before you consider additional measures.

Initial documentation should detail the reason for the restraint, the ineffectiveness of alternative strategies attempted first, the type, date, and time of the intervention, and the patient's response.

If possible, involve the patient and his family in the decision. Some patients do feel more secure when a restraint is in place, and occasionally even request one!

Explain why you are applying the restraint and assure the patient that you will take it off as soon as possible.

Check to see that there is follow-up documentation on every shift, noting frequency of observation and the condition of the patient's skin, as well as the number of times staff members offered food, fluids, and toileting assistance.

Be sure to remove physical restraints every two hours, and perform active or passive range-of-motion exercises before replacing them.

Keep in mind that with chemical restraints such as haloperidol, thioridazine (Mellaril), or chlorpromazine (Thorazine), intermittent dosing is recommended. Also, when restraints are used for an extended period it's in the patient's best interest to have an interdisciplinary team re-evaluate the need for them periodically.

A protocol that covers these points will not only benefit your patient but also protect you legally. Nurses have been charged with violating their patients' rights, invading their privacy, and denying due process by applying restraints—just as they have been charged with failure to apply restraints.

A different scenario for Mr. Ingram

Clearly, there were other ways of handling Mr. Ingram's problem. Indeed, though his mind was not clear when his night nurse looked in on him, his accusation was, and it shouldn't have been ignored.

His night nurse could have rectified the situation by proceeding as follows:'

Having decided—correctly—that the recent anesthesia, sleep deprivation, and anxiety were the likely culprits, she should have removed the restraints, repositioned him, and then given him a back rub and something warm to drink. While doing so, she should have reoriented him

by talking with him about where he was and what had been happening to him.

If he was still agitated, she could have tried bringing him out to the nurses' station for a short time in a geriatric chair. Only if all else failed should she have considered the continued use of restraints.

In all probability, however, Mr. Ingram would have drifted off to sleep after his warm drink and back rub. Had his evening nurse been more sensitive to his needs, he could have done that hours earlier.

Restraints should be your last line of defense, not the first thing you reach for when you need to calm a patient. □

BIBLIOGRAPHY

Dube, A. and Mitchell, E. Accidental strangulation from vest restraints. *JAMA* 256:2725, Nov. 21, 1986. Evans, L. and Strumps, N. Tying down the elderly: A review of the literature on physical restraints. *J. Am. Geriatr. Soc.* 37:65, Jan. 1987. Foreman, M. Acute confusional states in hospitalized elderly: A research dilemma. *Nurs. Res.* 35:34, Jan./Feb. 1986. Frengley, J.D. and Mion, L.C. Incidence of physical restraints on acute general medical units. *J. Am. Geriatr. Soc.* 34:565, Aug. 1986. McHutchion, E. and Morse, J. Releasing restraints: A nursing dilemma. *Journal of Gerontological Nursing* 15:16, Feb. 1989. Morrison, J., Crinklaw-Wiancko, D., et al. Formulating a restraint use policy. *J. Nurs. Adm.* 17:39, March 1987. Ratzen, R.M. The use of physical force. *Postgrad. Med.* 81:125, Jan. 1987. Robbins, L., Boyko, E., et al. Binding the elderly: A prospective study of the use of mechanical restraints in an acute care hospital. *J. Am. Geriat. Soc.* 35:290, April 1987. Struble, L.M. and Sivertsen, L. Agitation: Behaviors in confused elderly patients. *Journal of Gerontological Nursing* 13:40, Nov. 1987.

Exploding the myths

Despite the controversy surrounding electroconvulsive therapy, it is effective for certain patients.
Here are the facts about ECT and tips to help you ensure patient safety.

By Marin Fine, RN, MS, CS, and Michael A. Jenike, MD

Electro Shock

Electroconvulsive therapy—"shock treatment"—has received a lot of bad press, and many people inside and outside the health-care field oppose its use. Yet ECT, the electrical induction of grand-mal seizures, is considered a safe and effective treatment for severe depression in certain patients. Since some of those patients might be your patients, you should know the facts about ECT and understand the nursing care involved.

Introduced in 1938, ECT was for many years a primary treatment for schizophrenia and depression. Its popularity began to decline, however, with the introduction of antipsychotic and antidepressant drugs in the 1950s. Although these drugs aren't always as effective as ECT in treating severe depression, they're easier to use and generally far less frightening to patients and their families.

Which patients benefit from ECT?

Nevertheless, ECT remains a useful therapeutic tool for certain groups of patients. Severely depressed elderly persons often benefit from ECT, especially if they have chronic physical diseases that preclude the use of antidepressant drugs with anticholinergic, cardiotoxic, and hypotensive effects.

Many depressed patients, especially those with psychotic symptoms, don't respond to medication but do respond to shock therapy. In one study, remission of symptoms occurred in 80% to 85% of people treated with ECT after an unsuccessful trial with drug therapy. In fact, ECT has been found to be consistently 10% to 20% more effective than tricyclic antidepressants and monoamine oxidase inhibitors.

ECT may be the only feasible treatment for severely depressed patients in need of quick relief—pregnant women, for example, or patients who exhibit self-destructive behavior, such as suicide attempts or refusal to eat. It can take four to six weeks to determine whether drugs help these patients. That's time enough for a fetus to suffer harm from the drugs or for a self-destructive patient to do himself injury. ECT usually begins to exert beneficial effects within one week of

THE AUTHORS: Ms. Fine is head nurse of the inpatient psychiatric service at Massachusetts General Hospital in Boston. Dr. Jenike is director of the inpatient psychiatric service.

Produced by Debra Brewin-Wilson, RN, MSN

treatment. It sometimes yields dramatic results, as the following case demonstrates.

One patient's experience with ECT

The day before her hospitalization, 77-year-old Amelia Armstrong's mental status changed drastically. Generally quiet and easy-going, Amelia became emotionally labile, began talking non-stop about religion, and developed psychotic symptoms, including hallucinations and paranoia. An extensive medical work-up revealed no abnormalities except for an EEG that showed temporal slowing. But within two days, Amelia became catatonic—she was mute, barely responsive to painful stimuli, and had to be fed through a nasogastric tube.

On her third day in the hospital, Amelia was transferred to the psychiatric service. A psychiatric consultant contacted a close relative of Amelia's and learned that Amelia had a history of depression. The consultant concluded that Amelia's catatonia was an extreme manifestation of depression. He recommended emergency ECT.

After seven shock treatments, Amelia's condition improved—she began eating, drinking, and walking without assistance. Soon she was discharged from the hospital on a maintenance drug.

Why controversy still rages

Despite its benefits for patients like Amelia, ECT remains controversial. In 1982, a group of former mental patients and their supporters succeeded in getting the procedure banned in Berkeley, Calif., before an injunction blocked implementation of the law.

Such strong feelings about ECT may stem from the fact that no one knows exactly how it works. Moreover, the treatment has been abused. There have been cases where ECT was used as punishment rather than therapy.

It's also been given to patients who probably don't benefit from it. People with personality disorders, for example, sometimes receive ECT even though there's no indication that it helps them unless they're depressed as well. Recognizing such abuses, the American Psychiatric Association is trying to have ECT devices reclassified under the Federal Food and Drug Safety Law, which would bring them under closer scrutiny.

Limiting ECT's side effects

Although ECT is relatively safe, the electrical stimulus used to induce the seizure causes some side effects, such as confusion, temporary amnesia, and slowing of electrical impulses in the brain.

Some patients have complained of mild memory loss for months or even years after ECT, but studies, including objective memory testing, haven't documented any significant or irreversible pathologic changes in the brain. Most ECT patients studied don't believe persistent memory deficits are a major problem.

Refinements of techniques for delivering ECT—using low-energy wave forms to induce the seizure and only one electrode to transmit

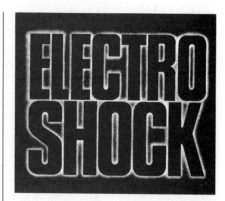

the current—have reduced the incidence of side effects without decreasing therapeutic efficacy. Administration of anticholinergic premedication, short-acting barbiturates for anesthesia, oxygen, and muscle relaxants decrease the risk of injury or discomfort to the patient.

ECT is usually given once every other day, three times a week, for a total of six to 10 sessions. Significant confusion, memory loss, or behavioral changes tend to occur as the number of treatments increases. When these side effects occur, the interval between treatments may be extended.

Which patients are at risk from ECT?

Although it stimulates a seizure, ECT. doesn't cause seizure disorders, and it can be safely used in patients with pre-existing disorders of this type. There are, in fact, no absolute contraindications to ECT. The usual mortality rate is about one in every 10,000 patients treated.

A few conditions are associated with a higher morbidity and mortality rate, however. They include recent myocardial infarction or stroke, severe hypertension, and the presence of an intracerebral mass. ECT should be delayed in patients with these conditions until they've received proper medical management and had ample time to recover. Appropriate premedication and close monitoring can decrease the risks if ECT is urgently needed in any of these cases.

The nurse's role in ECT

The nurse's involvement in ECT is crucial to a successful outcome. Prior to and during a course of therapy, you should assess and document some parameters that reflect the patient's mental and physical status. These include his sleep habits, appetite, bowel habits, energy level, interpersonal relationships, interest in his surroundings, and activity level. Provide the patient and his family with opportunities to ask questions and express their concerns about ECT. Be prepared, too, for questions from other patients if they learn that a fellow patient is receiving ECT.

It will also be your responsibility to make sure that the pretreatment protocol is followed according to the routine outlined in your hospital's procedure manual. Document pre-ECT vital signs and mental status. An ECG, CBC, and X-rays may be required prior to treatment. The consent form, medication list, and preoperative checklist must be completed and are usually attached to the chart.

To decrease the risk of aspiration during the treatment, the patient receives nothing by mouth for at least four hours prior to ECT. Patients scheduled for a morning treatment are usually kept NPO after midnight. A sedative may be given before the procedure to help relax the patient, and atropine will be given to decrease bronchial secretions, which could block the airway.

Following ECT, monitor the patient's condition and ensure his safety. He may be confused for a few hours after treatment, and you may have to reorient him as well as protect him from falling or otherwise injuring himself. Make sure he stays in bed, with the side rails up, until he's fully awake. After the confusion passes, you can encourage the patient to resume his usual activities. If the treatment's been done on an outpatient basis, someone else should drive the patient home. Notify the physician if the patient's clinical status deteriorates or deviates from what would be expected.

You'll also have to tell the patient about any medications he'll be taking. As many as 70% of ECT-treated patients relapse within one year if no maintenance drug is given after the course of ECT. This figure decreases to 10% to 20% with such medication. At Massachusetts General Hospital, the MAO inhibitor tranylcypromine (Parnate) is the drug most often used for maintenance therapy. This drug is well-tolerated by most patients.

Patients on tranylcypromine—and any other MAO inhibitor—should avoid eating foods containing tyramine. These foods include aged cheese, yogurt, wine, beer, ale, vanilla, chocolate, yeast, soy sauce, raisins, sour cream, monosodium glutamate, and dried fish. The liver normally neutralizes tyramine, but MAO inhibitors block this action, allowing the chemical to remain in the circulation. As a result, norepinephrine is released and overstimulates the sympathetic nervous system, causing hypertension.

The most-often-reported side effects from the drug itself are insomnia and orthostatic hypotension. Tell the patient that taking the last dose by 4 p.m. usually prevents insomnia, while measures such as slow position changes can reduce orthostatic hypotension.

ECT remains an effective tool for treating severe depression. It's not only faster, it's more effective than drugs for treating certain types of patients. Health-care professionals owe it to the thousands of patients like Amelia Armstrong who could benefit from ECT to educate their colleagues and the public about this useful therapy. ∎

BIBLIOGRAPHY American Psychiatric Association Task Force on ECT. *Task Force Report #14.* Washington, D.C.: American Psychiatric Association, 1978. Fraser, R.M. and Glass, I.B. Recovery from ECT in elderly patients. *Br. J. Psychiatry* 133:524, December 1978. Fraser, R.M. and Glass, I.B. Unilateral and bilateral ECT in elderly patients. *Acta Psychiatr. Scand.* 62:13, July 1980. Hughes, J., Barraclough, B.M., and Reeve, W. Are patients shocked by ECT? *J. R. Soc. Med.* 74:283, April 1981. Jenike, M.A. Electoconvulsive therapy. In *Massachusetts General Hospital Topics in Geriatrics.* Littleton, Mass.: Wright-PSG 1:37, February 1983. Jenike, M.A. Electroconvulsive therapy: What are the facts? *Geriatrics* 38:33, April 1983. Mandel, M.R. Indications for electroconvulsive therapy in treatment of depression. In *Massachusetts General Hospital Handbook of General Hospital Psychiatry,* Hackett, T.P. and Cassem, N.H., eds. St. Louis: The C.V. Mosby Co., 1978. Scovern, A.W. and Kilmann, P.R. Status of ECT: a review of the outcome literature. *Psychol. Bull.* 87:260, March 1980. Weiner, R.D. The role of electroconvulsive therapy in the treatment of depression in the elderly. *J. Am. Geriatr. Soc.* 30:710, November 1982.

Heading off depression in the chronically ill

A patient who's seriously ill has plenty of reason to be depressed.
If you recognize the symptoms and intervene promptly,
you can spare him unnecessary misery—and maybe save his life.
By Priscilla M. Kline, RN, MSN, and Cynthia C. Chernecky, RN, MN

Jack Winters, a 42-year-old construction worker, was enduring his fourth hospitalization for lymphoma. Financial worries compounded the misery caused by his disease. He'd had to quit his job and fretted constantly that he could no longer support his family. "I'm not worth much to anyone anymore," he told one of his nurses.

Gradually, he paid less and less attention to his grooming. "What's the point of shaving?" he'd say. "My beard will grow back tomorrow, even though nothing else in my body works right."

Then one evening, Mr. Winters removed his IV line and took an overdose of sleeping pills. He survived, but his suicide attempt left his nurses badly shaken. As they agonized over how they might have prevented it, they realized they'd overlooked a number of classic signs that indicated the depth of Mr. Winters' depression.

THE AUTHORS are assistant professors at Clemson University College of Nursing in South Carolina. Ms. Chernecky is on leave to pursue doctoral studies at Case Western University.

Produced by Paul L. Cerrato

Virtually any patient who has a serious illness runs a high risk of developing depression. If severe, depression can drive a patient to suicide. Before that happens, though, he's likely to send out a number of distress signals. If you respond appropriately, you can usually head off problems before they cause a crisis.

The chart on the following page describes the classic symptoms of depression. Be especially alert for such signs when the patient's illness is first diagnosed, when he's hospitalized for treatment, and when his illness suddenly worsens.

When assessing a patient for severe depression, look for *patterns* of behavior. An isolated incident suggesting one symptom or another may not necessarily be cause for alarm. By checking the record of a patient's prior hospitalizations you can sometimes establish whether his behavior is part of a pattern.

Dealing with decreased self-esteem

Serious illness can make even the simplest tasks seem a burden, often leaving the patient with a sense of failure and worthlessness. Help your patient set realistic goals, whether for physical activity or for his dealings with family members and financial matters. You may want to ask someone from the social services department to talk to the patient.

To build Mr. Winters' self-esteem after his suicide attempt, his nurses went out of their way to help him recognize even his minor accomplishments. They tried to spend time with him consistently, even if it was only a few minutes each day. Their actions told Mr. Winters that he was a worthwhile human being. So did the fact that they were patient with his sarcasm and periods of moodiness. In time, he realized that they saw and appreciated the person behind the offensive behavior.

Overcoming feelings of powerlessness

A hospitalized patient cannot avoid some feelings of powerlessness

How depressed is your patient?

The symptoms of depression appear in different guises according to their severity. The examples below can help you assess how far your patient's depression has progressed.

Symptom	Mild	Moderate	Severe
Decreased self-esteem	"I'm not good for anything today." Delayed grooming and poor hygiene.	"I'm not worth anything anymore." No attempt at grooming. Minimal hygiene.	"I'd be better off dead."
Hidden anger	Frequent sarcasm or a "suffering in silence" attitude.	Refusal to speak out in situations that might normally provoke an angry response—e.g., the patient says nothing when a treatment is rescheduled and interferes with visiting hours.	Apathy, serious withdrawal, and failure to express anger when the situation clearly warrants it—e.g., a treatment is cancelled and the patient is kept waiting without being told.
Guilt	"If I'd taken better care of myself, I might have discovered my disease while it could be treated more effectively."	"It's the bad things I've done that have caused my illness."	"This is God's way of punishing me for my sins," or "Now even my family is suffering for my sins."
Ambivalence	"I don't know which treatment to choose." Expressing one set of feelings one day and opposite feelings the next day.	Refusal of a treatment the patient initially agreed to.	Expressing the wish to live while refusing to cooperate in treatment or expressing readiness to die while clinging to every new remedy.
Feelings of powerlessness	"I can't understand how my body could do this to me," or "What's the use, I can't keep up my strength."	"Nothing I do makes any difference anymore."	Complete withdrawal. Failure to take any action on one's own behalf.
Dependency	Allowing a nurse to do more than is obviously necessary, but only for a day or two.	Expecting a nurse to feed, do range-of-motion exercises, assist to bathroom, etc., on a continuous basis.	Complete passivity.
Hopelessness	"I can't seem to do anything right today."	"Nothing seems to be worthwhile now."	"What is there to live for? My family will be better off without me."
Suicidal behavior	Thoughts of suicide, which patient admits to when asked. Some reluctance or ambivalence regarding treatment.	Serious contemplation of suicide and presence of a suicide plan. Failure to cooperate in treatment.	Suicide attempt.

since his disease and the regimented hospital environment dominate so many aspects of his life. You can help your patient minimize those feelings by showing him what aspects of his daily routine he can control.

Explain the various treatment alternatives available, so that he can make informed, intelligent choices about his therapy. Allowing him some degree of control over his daily schedule—for example, the ebb and flow of visitors—will also help to increase his feelings of independence.

Defusing hidden anger

A sense of powerlessness can fuel the patient's anger. As depression deepens, the patient may turn that anger against himself. Helping a patient deal with anger can be difficult because it's often unexpressed or camouflaged. Moreover, nurses sometimes shy away from uncovering anger since it's so unpleasant to handle once unleashed.

There's little reason to fear your patient's anger as long as you can teach him to express it without letting yourself become its target. To this end, create a climate that conveys the fact that you accept anger as a normal emotion. One way to do this is with statements such as, "If I were told I had to have this treatment or die, I'd be furious."

Suggest that the patient keep a "gripe pad" at his bedside. Have him record every complaint, no matter how trivial. Once a day, review it with him, letting him vent his hostilities.

Some patients can dissipate their pent-up rage by exercising. Physical therapy, range-of-motion exercises, or even punching a pillow can serve this purpose when the patient's condition precludes other forms of physical activity.

Relieving the burden of guilt

Many patients feel guilty because they imagine they've brought their diseases on themselves. Providing the patient with accurate information about the causes of his disorder can help relieve such guilt. For example, Mr. Winters' nurses explained the physiology of lymphoma and emphasized that there was no medical evidence to suggest his cancer had been caused by his lifestyle.

If the patient worries about causing hardship to his family, encouraging more open communication may help ease his mind. Once Mr. Winters' family realized how concerned he was about the loss of his job, they were able to reassure him that they loved and needed him regardless of his ability to work.

Beyond such measures, the best way you can help patients relieve guilt is to be a good listener.

Helping to resolve ambivalence

Another common symptom of depression is ambivalence, which shows up as indecisiveness and self-contradiction. The first step in helping a patient who's indecisive about his treatment is to accept his right to choose or reject whatever therapy you're administering. He'll never resolve his ambivalence if you don't provide an emotional climate in which he can openly express it. To do that, you'll need to be an uncritical listener. Don't let your beliefs about proper therapy interfere with your counseling.

Sometimes, just letting the patient know that ambivalence is a normal response to illness is enough to resolve the problem.

Reducing excessive dependency

A certain amount of dependency is necessary if a patient is to benefit from your nursing care. But when depression-induced passivity leads the patient to rely too heavily on your services, you should make it clear—gently but firmly—that he's capable of doing more for himself. Statements such as "Try to wash your face while I adjust the blinds to keep the sun out of your eyes" or "I think you're ready to get out of bed by yourself, but I'll be here in case you need me" let the patient know you're not abandoning him but still expect him to help himself.

Drawing hope from hopelessness

As his depression deepens, the patient may drift into a state of hopelessness. This dangerous symptom is closely related to loss of self-esteem and powerlessness.

One way to counteract despair is to help the patient redefine his expectations. For example, a patient who can't expect recovery can at least hope to be free of pain during the final stages of his illness. Try to replace complete hopelessness with a small yet realistic hope.

Encourage your patient to look less to the future and to appreciate the present. Give him an opportunity to talk over the possible meaning of his illness and its impact on his life. If he wants further spiritual counseling, arrange it.

Heading off suicidal behavior

When hopelessness and feelings of powerlessness are compounded by anger, some patients become self-destructive. Mr. Winters' suicide attempt was his ultimate effort to exert some measure of control over his life. Bolstering a patient's self-esteem and instilling a sense of control can help defuse such self-

destructive thinking. You may also need to refer the patient for psychiatric counseling.

Dealing with a suicidal patient requires that you deal with your own beliefs about the patient's right to take his life. If you find that your feelings interfere with effective care of the patient, you may have to remove yourself from the case.

Seriously ill patients have compelling reasons to be depressed, and relieving that depression may be no simple matter. Counseling may be necessary, but you can usu-

ally help them yourself before the situation gets out of hand. ■

BIBLIOGRAPHY Kline, P.M. Reactive depression in the client with cancer. In *Critical Nursing Care of the Client with Cancer.* Chernecky, C. and Ramsey, P., eds. East Norwalk, Conn.: Appleton-Century-Crofts, 1984. Krouse, H.J. and Krouse, J.H. Cancer as crisis—the critical elements of adjustment. *Nursing Research* 31:96, March/April 1982. Levine, P.M. et al. Mental disorders in cancer patients: A study of 100 psychiatric referrals. *Cancer* 42:1385, 1978. Louhivouri, K.A. and Hakama, M. Risk of suicide among cancer patients. *American Journal of Epidemiology* 109:59, 1979. Maxwell, M.B. Cancer and suicide. *Cancer Nursing* 3:33, Feb. 1980. Whitlock, F.A. Suicide, cancer, and depression. *British Journal of Psychiatry* 132: 269, 1978. Wilson, H.S. and Kneisl, C.R. *Psychiatric Nursing.* Menlo Park, Calif.: Addison-Wesley, 1983.

JULIE McARTHUR, RN, BSN

AIDS dementia
Your assessment can make all the difference

Three people in 10 who have AIDS will develop dementia. Your astute assessment can help them get the care they need in time to make a difference in their lives.

JULIE McARTHUR is the clinical coordinator of the SHARE neuropsychological study at Johns Hopkins University, Baltimore. SHARE researchers are investigating the long-term neurologic manifestations of HIV infection in 1,200 homosexual men.

Douglas, 37 years old, can't remember where he is supposed to meet his best friend. Lately he's also been struggling to find the right words to express himself. He's given up reading the newspaper because it takes him an hour to finish the front page. Douglas wonders if he's losing his mind. He's frightened and doesn't know what to do.

Betty, 32, lies in bed awake but oblivious to her surroundings. Three months ago she was friendly and talkative; now she doesn't recognize her visitors and utters only a few phrases.

Both patients suffer from the most common neurologic effect of HIV infection—AIDS dementia complex.

About 1.5 million Americans harbor the HIV virus. However, not all of them will develop this syndrome. The long-term Multicenter AIDS Cohort Study reveals no evidence of cognitive decline in infected individuals who are asymptomatic. The outlook is not as bright, though, when the infection progresses. Approximately 30% of people with AIDS and 5% of those with symptoms of AIDS-related complex, like diarrhea, fatigue, fever, weight loss, generalized lymphadenopathy, and thrush, eventually develop clinically significant dementia.

Proper treatment depends on distinguishing AIDS dementia from other conditions—for example, depression and opportunistic neurologic infections—that can produce very similar changes. When AIDS dementia strikes, your skillful assessment and prompt intervention can make a difference.

Symptoms of dementia: A triad of subtle changes

The syndrome usually occurs in patients who are profoundly immunosuppressed and have had one or more opportunistic infections. The first symptoms to show up are subtle differences in three areas—cognition, behavior, and motor function—that worsen with time. The patient is generally the first one to notice the major cognitive symptoms of memory impairment, poor concentration, and slowed thought processes.

Like Douglas, a patient may complain that he has trouble remembering appointments or telephone numbers. Others cannot complete routine tasks. For some, the power of concentration is so impaired that conversations and dialogue on television are difficult for them to follow.

Family and friends, on the other hand, are often the first to spot behavioral and personality changes. Typically, they'll tell you the patient seems less animated, that he's "lost his sparkle." Such a patient appears withdrawn and answers questions slowly. It's only the rare individual who develops psychosis with agitated confusion or hallucinations.

Motor dysfunction usually occurs after cognitive and personality changes. The lower rather than the upper extremities are most frequently affected. For example, Betty complained of weakness in her legs and walked unsteadily when she was first hospitalized. As in many patients who have AIDS dementia complex, these symptoms were the result of HIV-related damage to the posterior and lateral columns of the thoracic spinal cord.

Diagnosing dementia: A process of elimination

Your initial assessment not only helps narrow the diagnosis, but also serves as a baseline for evaluating changes in the patient's mental status later. Take a careful history from the patient, family, and significant others.

The interview should include the following key observations and questions:

▶ What is the patient's general appearance? Does he exhibit any mood changes? Does the patient seem apathetic? Is his behavior appropriate?

▶ Does the patient have problems with concentration or speed of thought? Is he attentive or does his mind wander?

▶ Does the patient have trouble remembering appointments or finding things? Can he complete routine tasks? Follow three-step commands?

▶ Are there speech difficulties, such as slurring or difficulty finding words? Is the patient less verbal than usual?

▶ Is the gait steady? Does the patient use a cane, walker, or other supportive device? Does he have any new weakness in the arms or legs?

▶ Is the patient slower or clumsier than usual? Can he execute smooth, rapid, alternating movements such as tapping his fingers?

▶ Has he ever had uncontrolled movements of the limbs, or any seizures?

▶ Has the patient ever been treated for abnormal oxygen, glucose, or electrolyte levels?

▶ Is there a history of drug or alcohol use? Acute intoxication may produce apathy, delirium, hallucinations, and agitation, as well as decreased cognitive and motor function. Years of drug and alcohol use can cause many of the same symptoms as AIDS dementia plus tremors, abnormal gait, spastic weakness, and seizures. Patients going through withdrawal may become agitated or combative, and have hallucinations or seizures. Those who have previously relied on drugs and alcohol to cope with stress may exhibit inappropriate and even primitive behaviors when they are drug-free.

▶ Does the patient have a history of depression or other preexisting emotional condition? Discriminating between depression and dementia is the most difficult—and probably the most important—determination to be made. Mislabeling a clinically depressed individual as demented will impede the appropriate treatment with antidepressants and psychotherapy or supportive counseling. It will also unnecessarily alarm patients who are already vulnerable because of their HIV status.

A misdiagnosis of depression can have serious consequences for the patient who does suffer from dementia. The inappropriate use of antidepressants or sedatives can provoke or exaggerate delirium.

A three-step approach establishes a diagnosis of AIDS dementia. First, HIV infection is confirmed by Western Blot.

Next, identify the characteristic signs and symptoms of AIDS dementia and stage the disease according to its severity. A thorough neurologic exam and cognitive testing establish the degree of impairment. Testing emphasizes memory storage and retrieval, psychomotor speed, and visual-constructional abilities.

Many practitioners utilize the staging scheme outlined on the following page. Developed at the Memorial Sloan-Kettering Center, criteria for each stage focus on functional disability rather than particular neurologic signs.

Finally, other conditions that produce similar symptoms are excluded as the cause of the patient's problem. You'll find a full list of conditions that can mimic AIDS dementia on page 40.

Checking arterial blood gases and blood chemistries helps rule out hypoxia, hypoglycemia, and electrolyte imbalances. Magnetic resonance imaging (MRI) and lumbar puncture can eliminate opportunistic infections and tumors of the central nervous system as possible causes. MRI also documents thinning of the deep white matter in the brain and cortical atrophy—characteristic changes in patients with AIDS dementia.

Clinical staging of AIDS dementia

Stage	Characteristics
Stage 0: Normal	Normal mental and motor function.
Stage 0.5: Equivocal/subclinical	Mild signs (snout response, slowed ocular or extremity movements) may be present. Gait and strength are normal. Able to work and perform activities of daily living.
Stage 1: Mild	Able to perform all but the more demanding aspects of work or ADL but with impaired intelligence or motor ability.
Stage 2: Moderate	Able to perform basic self-care but not to work or handle the more demanding aspects of daily life. Ambulatory, but may require an assistive device.
Stage 3: Severe	Major intellectual incapacity (cannot follow news or personal events, cannot sustain complex conversation) or motor disability. Needs assistance to walk, walks slowly, uses legs and arms clumsily.
Stage 4: End stage	Nearly vegetative. Intellectual and social comprehension and speech are rudimentary. Nearly or completely mute. Paraparesis or paraplegia with urinary and fecal incontinence.

Source: *Memorial Sloan-Kettering Center.*

What to expect when dementia strikes

The speed with which AIDS dementia exacts its toll varies, for unclear reasons. Like Betty, most patients develop moderate to severe dementia about three months after symptoms first appear. A metabolic condition or other systemic illness may punctuate the course of the dementia and possibly advance it more rapidly. Patients who are free from serious systemic illness

Conditions that mimic AIDS dementia

Acute drug intoxication
Ataxia from long-term alcohol use
Cerebral toxoplasmosis
CNS infection
Convulsive disorder
Cryptococcal meningitis
Depression
Drug or alcohol withdrawal
Electrolyte imbalance
Hypoglycemia
Hypoxia
Lymphoma
Neurosyphilis
Organic brain syndrome from long-term drug or alcohol use
Personality disorder

may remain productive for up to two years.

Though early symptoms may vary, the picture for the late stage of AIDS dementia is fairly consistent. Cognitive ability deteriorates until only rudimentary social and intellectual function remains. The patient lies in bed, staring vacantly. He exhibits little spontaneous movement and eventually becomes mute.

Inevitably the patient loses bowel and bladder control. Motor abnormalities at this stage of the syndrome are paraplegia, quadriplegia, and spastic weakness. During the terminal stage, some patients can have tremors, myoclonus—uncontrollable muscle contractions—and generalized seizures.

Drugs offer hope and fight symptoms

Researchers continue to look for effective therapy to battle AIDS dementia. Since it is believed that HIV infection rather than secondary infections causes the syndrome, attention has focused on drugs that act directly on the virus. So far, medical treatment for AIDS dementia has been limited to the antiviral agent zidovudine (Retrovir), which crosses the blood-brain barrier and thus is effective in the central nervous system. (You'll find a detailed discussion of this antiviral agent in "Zidovudine: Flawed champion against AIDS" in the January 1989 issue of **RN**.)

Studies with small numbers of patients with AIDS dementia show that those who received zidovudine improved clinically and performed better on neuropsychological tests. In addition, continuous infusion of the drug has reversed neuropsychological impairment in some children. Encouraging as these findings are, whether zidovudine will permanently reverse AIDS dementia or restore cognitive function in advanced cases remains unclear.

Other medications are used to combat specific symptoms. Patients with a depressive component to their illness receive antidepressants. Since patients with AIDS dementia are especially sensitive to these drugs, expect to begin treatment with smaller than usual doses that are gradually increased to reach the de-

sired effect. The usual regimen is 10 to 20 mg of nortriptyline (Pamelor) at bedtime. Tricyclic antidepressants like nortriptyline are safer than other types of antidepressants for these patients because they have less extreme anticholinergic effects. Nevertheless, you will need to monitor drug levels and observe patients closely for anticholinergic side effects like dry mouth, urinary retention, blurred vision, mental excitement, and confusion.

As the disease progresses and psychomotor retardation grows to be more of a problem, the CNS stimulant methylphenidate (Ritalin) may be prescribed to improve motivation. You'll give 5 to 10 mg of this drug every morning. So far, Ritalin therapy has been more effective for moderate than for severe dementia. Major side effects include seizures, overexcitability, nervousness, and appetite suppression.

Although most patients with AIDS dementia grow quieter and more withdrawn as their disease progresses, a few do hallucinate and become combative or agitated. They may receive neuroleptics such as haloperidol (Haldol). Again, you'll start by giving a smaller than usual dose (probably 0.5 to 1 mg) and increase it slowly to achieve the desired effect.

Coping with dementia: Nurses make a difference

A patient who is newly diagnosed as having mild dementia

faces many issues and decisions. He'll be concerned about working, driving, and living independently as long as possible. Reassure him that you'll work with him and enlist the aid of other professionals when necessary to help him achieve his goals.

But explain that, if he hasn't done so already, now is the time to make critical decisions he may not be able to make later on. The patient and family should discuss life support. If possible, arrange a conference with the patient, spouse or lover, and physician so that everyone involved in his care will have a clear understanding of the patient's wishes.

Legal decisions should also be made now. Urge the patient to designate power of attorney and to write both a will and a living will. Preparing ahead of time will spare the family the pain of making difficult decisions and also help prevent legal entanglements over financial arrangements or distribution of assets later.

Patient education. Teach the patient and his family what they may expect as dementia progresses and how to cope at each stage. Mildly demented patients are quickly frustrated. Suggest easy, practical methods for dealing with minor memory and concentration problems. For example, if a patient finds it difficult to concentrate for extended periods, have him break a task down into parts. The patient can finish one component and take a break before moving on to the next part of the task. Encourage patients to keep lists to help jog their memories. If buttons and laces make dressing a problem, suggest sweatshirts and slip-on shoes.

Setting up achievable, short-term goals that the patient, his nurse, and family can work on will also help his self-esteem. For instance, if a patient can no longer walk even short distances without feeling tired and unstable, teach him how to use a walker, then set a distance he can reach and have him keep practicing.

As the patient's dementia advances, a structured environment will help reduce confusion. Daily activities should follow a regular routine. Post a schedule in an obvious spot—a bulletin board or refrigerator door. Objects should always be kept in the same place. Use clocks and calendars to orient the patient to time and place.

Safety is a vital concern. Keep passageways clear of obstacles and eliminate scatter rugs to help prevent falls. If the patient has problems with coordination or balance, guard rails across the stairs and safety bars in the bathroom may be called for.

The patient may also need supervision to smoke or use the stove. Lower the temperature setting on the hot water heater to avoid burns.

Teach the patient's family how to assess changes in his condition. Stress the importance of reporting their findings. Worsening apathy, for example, could signal the necessity for Ritalin therapy.

Enlist the aid of community health-care professionals early on. A visiting nurse can monitor drug therapy and provide ongoing assessment and instruction. Social workers can help with health insurance and disability claims, applications for public assistance, transportation for outpatients who can no longer drive, and transfers to residential care facilities.

Emotional support. The emotional and psychosocial needs of patient and family can be tremendous. The social worker or visiting nurse can put them in touch with local support and self-help groups and make arrangements for therapy.

In the final stage of his illness, the patient may find comfort in little things—having a picture of a loved one in sight or listening to a favorite tape. Maintaining comfort and dignity are goals to strive for at this time.

Family members and lovers—often dealing with their own diagnosis or fear of diagnosis—will also have strong needs for emotional support as the patient's death approaches. Bereavement counselors and clergy should be on hand to help them cope with their loss.

This is also a very stressful time for the nurse. Feelings of anger and helplessness are common when caring for young people with such a devastating disease. Nurses working with these patients need support, too. Get involved with a support group, talk to friends, and, if necessary, see a counselor.

Regrettably, nurses will continue to be challenged by patients who have AIDS and its resulting dementia. By 1991, an estimated 145,000 people will be living with AIDS—about 44,000 will also have dementia. Your ability to remain alert, honest, flexible, creative, and even humorous will be crucial when caring for these very sick and cognitively impaired people. □

BIBLIOGRAPHY

Green, J. and Kocsis, A. Counselling patients with AIDS-related encephalopathy. *J. R. Coll. Physicians Lond.* 22:166, July 1988. Levy, R., Bredesen, D., and Rosenblum, M. Neurological manifestations of the acquired immunodeficiency syndrome (AIDS): Experience at UCSF and review of the literature. *J. Neurosurg.* 62:475, April 1985. McArthur, J. Neurologic manifestations of AIDS. *Medicine* 66:407, 1987. McArthur, J., Cohen, B., et al. Low prevalence of neurological and neuropsychological abnormalities in otherwise healthy HIV-1 infected individuals. *Ann. Neurol.* 26:601, 1989. Navia, B., Jordan, B., and Price, R. The AIDS dementia complex: I. Clinical features. *Ann. Neurol.* 19:517, June 1986. Navia, B. and Price, R. Dementia complicating AIDS. *Psych. Ann.* 16:158, January 1986. Navia, B. and Price, R. The acquired immunodeficiency syndrome dementia complex as the presenting or sole manifestation of human immunodeficiency virus infection. *Arch. Neurol.* 44:65, January 1987. Petito, C., Navia, B., et al. Vacuolar myelopathy pathologically resembling subacute combined degeneration in patients with the acquired immunodeficiency syndrome. *N. Engl. J. Med.* 312:874, April 4, 1985. Pizzo, P., Eddy, J., et al. Effect of continuous intravenous infusion of zidovudine (AZT) in children with symptomatic HIV infection. *N. Engl. J. Med.* 391:889, Oct. 6, 1988. Price, R., Sidtis, J., and Rosenblum, M. AIDS dementia complex: Some current questions. *Ann. Neurol. (supp.)* 23:S27, 1988. Price, R. and Brew, B. AIDS commentary. *J. Infect. Dis.* 158:1079, December 1988. Selnes, O., Miller, E., et al. HIV-1 infections: No evidence of cognitive decline during the asymptomatic stages. *Neurology* (in press). Vogt, M. and Hirsch, M. Prospects for the prevention and therapy of infections with the human immunodeficiency virus. *Rev. Infect. Dis.* 8:991, 1986. Yarchoan, R., Thomas, R., et al. Long-term administration of 3'-azido-2', 3'-dideoxythymidine to patients with AIDS-related neurological disease. *Ann. Neurol. (supp.)* 23:S82, 1988.

UNIT 6
QUESTIONS AND ANSWERS

by

Anne R. Waldman, RN,C, MSN
Holly Hillman, RN, MSN
Charlotte D. Kain, RN,C, EdD
Constance O. Kolva, RN, MSN
Marie T. O'Toole, RN, MSN
Janice Selekman, RN, DNSc

This section contains two 90-question tests similar in structure and content to those you will find on the NCLEX-RN examination. At the end of each section are the correct answers, the rationales for the correct answers, and the Phases of the Nursing Process, the Categories of Client Needs, and the Cognitive Level for each question.

Following the directions for test taking described in Unit 1. Allow 90 minutes for each Practice Test. The following codes are used in the answers and rationales to categorize the test items.

NL = PHASES OF THE NURSING PROCESS
A = Assessment
An = Analysis
P = Planning
I = Implementation
E = Evaluation

CN = CLIENT NEED
I   = Safe, Effective Care Environment
II = Physiologic Integrity
III = Psychologic Integrity
IV = Health Promotion/Maintenance

CL = COGNITIVE LEVEL
K = Knowledge
C = Comprehension
Ap = Application
An = Analysis

The following sample answer should help you understand how to interpret these codes.

ANSWER		RATIONALE	NP	CN	CL
#1	4	Hemorrhagic reactions are a result of banked blood that is low in platelets and coagulation factors.	An	II	C

The elements are as follows:

#1 is the question or item number in the test; 4 is the correct answer.

The rationale explains the correct answer.

The phase of the nursing process is analysis.

The category of cognitive level is physiologic integrity.

The cognitive level is comprehension.

Practice Test 1

Mr. Tim Santoro, age 56, has had a significant problem with alcohol abuse for the past 15 years. His wife brings him to the Emergency Department because of increasing confusion and the coughing of blood. His medical diagnosis is cirrhosis of the liver. He has ascites and esophageal varices.

1. Assessment of Mr. Santoro would reveal all of the following changes EXCEPT
   o 1. bulging flanks.
   o 2. protruding umbilicus.
   o 3. abdominal distension.
   o 4. bluish discoloration of the umbilicus.

2. The major dietary treatment for ascites calls for
   o 1. high protein.
   o 2. increased potassium.
   o 3. restricted fluids.
   o 4. restricted sodium.

3. Which laboratory value would the nurse expect to find in Mr. Santoro as a result of liver failure?
   o 1. Decreased serum creatinine
   o 2. Decreased sodium
   o 3. Increased ammonia
   o 4. Increased calcium

Mr. Santoro begins to experience severe GI bleeding.

4. The plan of care to meet Mr. Santoro's fluid needs should include, as a priority, strategies for
   o 1. accommodating his frequent need for the bedpan.
   o 2. maintaining the gastric pH.
   o 3. monitoring vital signs on an hourly basis.
   o 4. rapid blood and fluid administration.

A Sengstaken-Blakemore tube is inserted in an effort to stop the bleeding.

5. After the Sengstaken-Blakemore tube is inserted, Mr. Santoro has difficulty breathing. Based on this information, the FIRST action the nurse should take is to
   o 1. deflate the esophageal balloon.
   o 2. encourage him to take deep breaths.
   o 3. monitor his vital signs.
   o 4. notify the physician.

Michael Kirby, age 2, is admitted to the hospital with cystic fibrosis. As a result of malabsorption, he is small for his age.

6. What dietary suggestions can the nurse recommend to Michael's mother to enhance his growth?
   o 1. Low-fat, low-residue, and high-potassium diet
   o 2. Low-carbohydrate, soft diet with no sugar products
   o 3. High-carbohydrate, high-fat diet, with extra water between meals.
   o 4. High-protein, high-calorie meals with skimmed milk shakes between meals.

7. Mrs. Kirby asks why Michael has cystic fibrosis. The nurse explains that cystic fibrosis
   o 1. develops due to meconium ileus at birth.
   o 2. is an autosomal recessive genetic defect.
   o 3. occurs during embryologic development.
   o 4. results from chromosomal nondysjunction that occurred at conception.

Because of home commitments, Mrs. Kirby cannnot stay overnight with Michael.

8. The nurse recommends that she
   o 1. leave something of hers with Michael and tell him she'll be back in the morning.
   o 2. leave while he is in the playroom.
   o 3. leave after he has fallen asleep.
   o 4. tell him she'll be back in a few minutes after she has dinner.

Mrs. Kirby tells the nurse that the family is planning their first summer vacation with Michael. She wants to know if there are any special precautions needed because of his cystic fibrosis.

9. Mrs. Kirby will need to know that children with cystic fibrosis are particularly susceptible to
   o 1. severe sunburn.
   o 2. infectious diarrhea.
   o 3. heat prostration.
   o 4. respiratory allergies.

Mrs. Susan List, age 28, comes to the prenatal clinic because she thinks she might be pregnant. She tells the nurse that her menstrual periods are irregular but, since her last menses seven weeks ago, she's noticed some physiologic changes in her body.

10. Which finding should the nurse expect when assessing Mrs. List for a PROBABLE sign of pregnancy?
    ○ 1. Morning sickness
    ○ 2. Urinary frequency
    ○ 3. Auscultation of fetal heart tones
    ○ 4. A positive urine pregnancy test

11. Mrs. List tells the nurse that the first day of her last normal menstrual period was June l5th. Using Nägele's rule, her baby should be due about
    ○ 1. March 8th.
    ○ 2. March l5th.
    ○ 3. March 22nd.
    ○ 4. March 29th.

When Mrs. List returns for her six-month visit, she reports that she is having a problem with constipation.

12. To minimize this condition, the nurse should instruct her to
    ○ 1. increase her fluid intake to 3 liters/day.
    ○ 2. request a prescription for a laxative from her physician.
    ○ 3. stop taking her iron supplements.
    ○ 4. take 2 tbsp of mineral oil daily.

Mrs. List has been working as a salesperson throughout her pregnancy and would like to continue working until the middle of her ninth month. At her eight-month visit, she weighs l50 lb, is 5 ft 6 in tall and reports that her back hurts at the end of the day.

13. What advice should the nurse give to increase Mrs. List's comfort level?
    ○ 1. Lose weight
    ○ 2. Quit her job
    ○ 3. Rest with her legs elevated at all times
    ○ 4. Wear low heeled shoes

Mrs. List is admitted to the hospital in labor. Vaginal examination reveals that she is 8 cm dilated.

14. At this point in her labor, which of the following statements would the nurse expect her to make?
    ○ 1. I can't decide what to name my baby.
    ○ 2. It feels good to push with each contraction.
    ○ 3. Take your hand off my stomach when I have a contraction.
    ○ 4. This isn't as bad as I expected.

15. In order to support Mrs. List during this phase of her labor, the nurse should
    ○ 1. leave her alone most of the time.
    ○ 2. offer her a back rub during contractions.
    ○ 3. offer her sips of oral fluids.
    ○ 4. provide her with warm blankets.

16. Mrs. List is placed on an external fetal monitor. The nurse notices that the fetal heart rate is erratic during contractions but returns to baseline at the end of each contraction. This should be recorded as
    ○ 1. early decelerations.
    ○ 2. variable decelerations.
    ○ 3. late decelerations.
    ○ 4. fetal distress.

17. After observing the fetal heart rate pattern in question #l6, the nurse should
    ○ 1. apply an oxygen mask.
    ○ 2. change Mrs. List's position to left side lying.
    ○ 3. get Mrs. List out of bed and walk her around.
    ○ 4. move Mrs. List to the delivery room.

During delivery, a mediolateral episiotomy is performed and Mrs. List delivers a 7 lb 8 oz girl.

18. To detect postpartum complications in Mrs. List as soon as possible, the nurse should be particularly alert for all of the following EXCEPT
    ○ 1. a foul lochial odor.
    ○ 2. discomfort while sitting.
    ○ 3. ecchymosis and edema of the perineum.
    ○ 4. separation of the episiotomy wound edges.

19. On the second day postpartum, the nurse asks Mrs. List to describe her vaginal bleeding. The nurse should expect her to say that it is
    ○ 1. red and moderate.
    ○ 2. red with clots.
    ○ 3. scant and brown.
    ○ 4. thin and white.

Mrs. List is going to breast-feed her baby.

20. What is the best indication that the let-down reflex has been achieved in a nursing mother?
    ○ 1. Increased prolactin levels
    ○ 2. Milk dripping from the opposite breast
    ○ 3. Progressive weight gain in the infant
    ○ 4. Relief of breast engorgement

21. To prevent cracked nipples while she is breast-feeding, Mrs. List should be taught to
    ○ 1. apply lanolin prior to feedings.
    ○ 2. nurse at least 20 minutes on each breast the first day.
    ○ 3. use plastic bra liners.
    ○ 4. wash her nipples with water only.

22. What is the best indication that the breast-fed baby is digesting the breast milk properly?
    ○ 1. The baby does not experience colic.
    ○ 2. The baby passes dark green, pasty stools.
    ○ 3. The baby passes soft, golden-yellow stools.
    ○ 4. The baby sleeps for several hours after each feeding.

Mr. Jim Wald, age 46, is on the verge of losing his job because of a drinking problem. He voluntarily enters an alcohol detoxification program.

23. The most important information for Mr. Wald to accurately relate to the staff when admitted for detoxification is the amount, type, and
    - o 1. time(s) of substance(s) taken over the past 24 hours.
    - o 2. frequency of substance(s) taken over the past week.
    - o 3. frequency of substance(s) taken over the past two weeks.
    - o 4. frequency of substance(s) taken over the past month.

24. A characteristic common to most substance abusers is difficulty in effectively
    - o 1. coping with stress and anxiety.
    - o 2. interacting socially.
    - o 3. performing in work-related settings.
    - o 4. setting limits.

25. Signs and symptoms that Mr. Wald is developing impending alcohol withdrawal delirium include diaphoresis, tremors
    - o 1. bradycardia and hypertension.
    - o 2. bradycardia and hypotension.
    - o 3. tachycardia and hypertension.
    - o 4. tachycardia and hypotension.

26. The most widely accepted treatment modality for substance abuse is
    - o 1. individual therapy with a psychodynamically-oriented therapist.
    - o 2. individual therapy with a systems-oriented therapist.
    - o 3. group therapy with others with personality disorders.
    - o 4. group therapy with other substance abusers.

Mr. Norman Koch, age 35, has a history of peptic ulcer disease. He has had numerous bleeding episodes in the past and is admitted to the hospital for evaluation. His physician has prescribed cimetidine (Tagamet).

27. The nurse recognizes that the PRIMARY reason Mr. Koch is taking Tagamet is that it
    - o 1. blocks the secretion of gastric hydrocholric acid.
    - o 2. coats the gastric mucosa with a protective membrane.
    - o 3. increases the sensitivity of H_2 receptors.
    - o 4. releases basal gastric acid.

28. Mr. Koch has been experiencing blood in his feces. The best way for the nurse to assess if the hematochezia is a symptom of gastric bleeding is to
    - o 1. ask him how long he has been bleeding.
    - o 2. check his vital signs.
    - o 3. monitor his laboratory results.
    - o 4. obtain his complete past medical history.

Mr. Koch receives a large volume of blood transfusions.

29. Coagulation disturbances following massive transfusions for GI bleeding are usually associated with
    - o 1. acidification of blood.
    - o 2. infected donors.
    - o 3. poor survival of platelets.
    - o 4. rapid infusion of cold blood.

30. The nurse can decrease the danger of hypothermia in GI bleeding by
    - o 1. administering blood with normal saline.
    - o 2. administering blood products through a central line.
    - o 3. giving only packed cells.
    - o 4. warming blood to body temperature before administering.

Mr. Koch has a Billroth II procedure and does well postoperatively. He is preparing for discharge.

31. Mr. Koch recognizes that symptoms of dizziness, sweating, and weakness in the weeks following the surgery are usually associated with
    - o 1. afferent loop syndrome.
    - o 2. dumping syndrome.
    - o 3. pernicious anemia.
    - o 4. marginal ulcers.

Mrs. Wilma Marshall, age 71, is admitted to the hospital with congestive heart failure. She has shortness of breath and a +3–4 peripheral edema.

32. The care plan to reduce Mrs. Marshall's edema should include nursing strategies for
    - o 1. establishing limits on activity.
    - o 2. fostering a relaxed environment.
    - o 3. identifying goals for self-care.
    - o 4. restricting IV fluids.

33. Mrs. Marshall complains that she is always tired. Which of the following would be an appropriate suggestion by the nurse while the patient is still on bedrest?
    - o 1. Continue to exercise your legs.
    - o 2. Don't think about the fatigue.
    - o 3. Eat larger meals.
    - o 4. Sleep as much as possible.

34. It is determined that Mrs. Marshall has early left-sided failure. Which symptom should the nurse expect to find?
    - o 1. Bradycardia
    - o 2. Jugular vein distension
    - o 3. Liver engorgement
    - o 4. Rales

35. Mrs. Marshall is given digoxin (Lanoxin) 0.25 gm daily. She will need to learn that the signs of digitalis toxicity include
    - o 1. auditory hallucinations and bradycardia.
    - o 2. dry mucous membranes and diarrhea.
    - o 3. heart block and brittle hair and nails.
    - o 4. visual disturbances and premature beats.

36. Which serum potassium level reported for Mrs. Marshall requires NO immediate nursing intervention?
    - o 1. 3.2 mEq/liter
    - o 2. 4.0 mEq/liter
    - o 3. 5.5 mEq/liter
    - o 4. 6.0 mEq/liter

Mrs. Sarah Armstrong, age 45, has a simple goiter. She is being seen by the community health nurse for teaching and follow-up regarding nutritional deficiencies related to her goiter.

37. Mrs. Armstrong's problems are most likely associated with which nutritional deficiency?
    - o 1. Calcium
    - o 2. Iodine
    - o 3. Iron
    - o 4. Sodium

38. To enhance glandular function, Mrs. Armstrong should eliminate which of the following foods?
    - o 1. Corn
    - o 2. Milk
    - o 3. Turnips
    - o 4. Watermelon

39. To meet Mrs. Armstrong's self-esteem needs, the nursing priority is to
    - o 1. encourage her to discuss her disfigurement.
    - o 2. focus her attention on physical problems.
    - o 3. reassure her regarding her general appearance.
    - o 4. suggest she wear make-up daily.

Bryan White, age 12 months, is hospitalized for a severe case of croup and has been placed in an oxygen tent. Today the oxygen order has been reduced from 35% to 25%. His blood gases are normal.

40. Bryan refuses to stay in the oxygen tent. Attempts to placate him only cause him to become more upset. The MOST appropriate action for the nurse is to
    - o 1. restrain him in the tent and notify the physician.
    - o 2. take him out of the tent and notify the physician.
    - o 3. take him out of the tent and let him sit in the playroom.
    - o 4. tell him it will please his mother if he stays in the tent.

41. Bryan is 30 inches tall and weighs 30 lb. The nurse interprets this as
    - o 1. normal height, increased weight.
    - o 2. normal height, decreased weight.
    - o 3. small for age, normal weight.
    - o 4. tall for age, but weight appropriate for height.

12-month-old Barry Kelly had a cleft lip repaired successfully as an infant. His mother brings him to the clinic for a check-up and his MMR immunization. While talking to the nurse, Mrs. Kelly reports that her teenage babysitter has just come down with rubeola.

42. What would be the most appropriate plan of treatment for Barry?
    - o 1. Administer immune serum globulin.
    - o 2. Administer prophylactic penicillin.
    - o 3. Allow him to catch measles from the babysitter in order to develop activity immunity.
    - o 4. Vaccinate him now with MMR.

43. Mrs. Kelly asks the nurse when Barry will be ready for cleft palate repair. The most appropriate response is cleft palate repair is usually done
    - o 1. prior to development of speech.
    - o 2. when the child is completely weaned from the bottle and pacifier.
    - o 3. when the child is toilet trained.
    - o 4. when a large-holed nipple is ineffective for his feedings.

Barry is scheduled for surgical repair of his cleft palate.

44. A priority in the post-op plan of care for Barry would include teaching his mother
    - o 1. to resume toilet training after he is up and around.
    - o 2. to use a cup or wide-bowl spoon for feeding.
    - o 3. that he will be more prone to respiratory infections now that his airway is smaller.
    - o 4. that no further treatment will be needed until his adult teeth come in at age 6.

Ms. Donna Dunn, age 34, is admitted to the psychiatric unit after she was brought to the hospital emergency department by the State Police. She had been wandering on a major four-lane highway with no regard for her safety. On first contact with Ms. Dunn, the nurse observes that her face and hands are very red and excoriated, her hair is matted and dirty, her clothing is dirty and she is quite thin. According to Ms. Dunn, she had been living in a motel with a truck driver, whom she knew by first name only. They had been in the motel for a week, but the truck driver went back to work, and she has been alone for three days. Ms. Dunn cannot specifically relate her activities for those three days. Once the assessment interview was over, Ms. Dunn asked to be excused, went directly to her room, and washed her hands and face. Within a very short while, it became apparent to the nurse that the hand and face washing was quite repetitive and ritualistic and occupied a major portion of Ms. Dunn's time. However, she refused to bathe or wash her clothing.

45. The most thorough way to conduct a nursing assessment of Ms. Dunn's nutritional status would be to
    - o 1. observe her at mealtime.
    - o 2. request a medical consult.
    - o 3. explore her recent dietary intake.
    - o 4. compare current weight with her usual weight.

46. The nursing diagnosis that describes the most prominent difficulty that Ms. Dunn is experiencing is
    o 1. actual impairment of skin integrity.
    o 2. alteration in thought processes.
    o 3. ineffective individual coping.
    o 4. social isolation.

47. Ms. Dunn is constipated and dehydrated. Which intervention would Ms. Dunn most likely comply with?
    o 1. Drinking Ensure between meals
    o 2. Drinking extra fluids with meals
    o 3. Drinking 8 oz water every hour between meals
    o 4. Drinking adequate amounts of fluid during the day.

48. The most effective way for the nurse to intervene with Ms. Dunn's hand and face washing is to
    o 1. allow her a certain amount of time each shift to engage in this behavior.
    o 2. interrupt the activity briefly and frequently.
    o 3. lock the door to her room and restrict access to the bathroom.
    o 4. tell her to stop each time she is observed doing it.

49. The nurse and Ms. Dunn will know that discharge planning is appropriate when Ms. Dunn
    o 1. regains her normal body weight.
    o 2. expresses a desire to leave the hospital.
    o 3. is able to start talking about her guilt and anxiety.
    o 4. limits her hand and face washing to a few times a day.

Mr. Kevin Penn, age 22, is readmitted to the rehabilitation unit after a T4 incomplete spinal cord injury that occurred six months ago. He is about to begin an intensive rehabilitation program.

50. Which of the following statements made by Mr. Penn best indicates that he understands the extent of his injury?
    o 1. I want to use an electric wheelchair.
    o 2. My goal is to be independent in transfers.
    o 3. Soon, I'll be walking.
    o 4. There is little I can do, but I will try.

51. Which activity by Mr. Penn indicates adequate learning regarding urinary tract care?
    o 1. Avoiding the Valsalva maneuver when the bladder is full.
    o 2. Cleaning the urinary meatus every 2 hours.
    o 3. Checking for bladder distension frequently.
    o 4. Limiting fluids to 1000 cc/24 hours.

52. To evaluate the effectiveness of Mr. Penn's bowel program, the nurse should expect him to be able to
    o 1. avoid laxatives and stool softeners.
    o 2. experience no incontinence.
    o 3. move his bowels daily.
    o 4. resume previous bowel habits.

53. The nurse administers diazepam (Valium) 10 mg qid. Which observation is most indicative of the need to reassess this order?
    o 1. Drowsiness
    o 2. Hyperesthesia of the arms
    o 3. Loss of appetite
    o 4. Severe muscle spasms

Mr. Edgar Jefferson, age 57, is being treated in the clinic for hypertension. His blood pressure is 170/92 and he is complaining of fatigue and lassitude.

54. Mr. Jefferson has been taking propranolol (Inderal) 80 mg bid. The best indication that previous teaching about this drug has been successful is that he
    o 1. checks his pulse for bradycardia.
    o 2. makes an appointment as soon as he notices fatigue.
    o 3. stops the drug when he experiences chest pain.
    o 4. takes the drug with breakfast and dinner.

55. To facilitate Mr. Jefferson's ability to lower his blood pressure to a normal range, the nurse should teach him to avoid which of the following foods?
    o 1. Cheese
    o 2. Carrots
    o 3. Catsup
    o 4. Sugar

56. Mr. Jefferson has his blood pressure taken in lying and standing positions. The nurse explains to him that this is a test for
    o 1. central nervous system depression.
    o 2. malignant hypertension.
    o 3. orthostatic hypotension.
    o 4. vascular insufficiency.

Mr. Samuel Rockwood, age 64, has been smoking since he was 11 years old. He has a long history of emphysema. Mr. Rockwood is admitted to the hospital because of a respiratory infection that has not improved with out-patient therapy.

57. Which finding would the nurse expect to observe during Mr. Rockwood's nursing assessment?
    o 1. Electrocardiogram changes
    o 2. Increased anterior-posterior chest diameter
    o 3. Slow, labored respiratory pattern
    o 4. Weight-height relationship indicating obesity

58. When formulating a teaching plan for Mr. Rockwood, the nurse should instruct him to select activities that PRIMARILY
    o 1. avoid movement.
    o 2. build strength.
    o 3. conserve energy.
    o 4. test his limits of tolerance.

59. Supplemental low-flow oxygen therapy is prescribed for Mr. Rockwood. Which is the most appropriate action for the nurse to initiate?
    o 1. Anticipate the need for humidification.
    o 2. Notify the physician that this order is contraindicated.
    o 3. Place Mr. Rockwood in high-Fowler's position.
    o 4. Schedule nursing care to allow frequent observations of Mr. Rockwood.

60. Nursing interventions to facilitate breathing for Mr. Rockwood are considered effective if he
    o 1. deemphasizes expirations.
    o 2. increases his respiratory rate.
    o 3. reduces the use of his diaphragm.
    o 4. utilizes abdominal breathing.

The laboratory notifies the nursing unit that the arterial blood gases on Mrs. Sarah Williams indicate she has metabolic acidosis.

61. Causes of metabolic acidosis include all of the following EXCEPT
    o 1. cardiac arrest.
    o 2. diabetic ketoacidosis.
    o 3. hypokalemia.
    o 4. renal failure.

62. Which set of blood gases should the nurse expect to find in a patient with metabolic acidosis?
    o 1. pH = 7.28; pCO_2 = 55; HCO_3 = 26
    o 2. pH = 7.50; pCO_2 = 40; HCO_3 = 31
    o 3. pH = 7.48; pCO_2 = 30; HCO_3 = 22
    o 4. pH = 7.30; pCO_2 = 36; HCO_3 = 18

Allen Kile, age 24, was admitted on a voluntary basis to psychiatric services. He had agreed to in-patient care as an alternative to a 30-day jail sentence for reckless driving, driving under the influence, and speeding. He has been under psychiatric care for three years; has a long history of petty crimes, and was able, with the help of his therapist, to convince the judge that a higher level of psychiatric care would be in everyone's best interest. Once on the unit, Mr. Kile is difficult to manage because he is arrogant and manipulative. When a scheduled group therapy session is announced, he refuses to go and the nurse has to resort to pleading with him to attend. He uses other patients to his own ends and often pioneers causes that are disruptive to the milieu.

63. The diagnostic title which best describes Mr. Kile's behavior is
    o 1. antisocial personality disorder.
    o 2. borderline personality disorder.
    o 3. passive-aggressive personality disorder.
    o 4. passive-dependent personality disorder.

64. In planning Mr. Kile's care it is important to recognize that all of the following are likely to occur EXCEPT
    o 1. staff and patient agree when setting treatment goals.
    o 2. staff and patient are in a constant struggle for control of the milieu.
    o 3. staff and patient feel threatened by one another.
    o 4. staff and patient use the same defense mechanisms when interacting.

65. Key interventions with a patient like Mr. Kile include all of the following EXCEPT
    o 1. assisting him to identify and clarify his feelings.
    o 2. changing staff assigned to Mr. Kile at his request.
    o 3. making expectations about his behavior clear as well as consequences for same.
    o 4. setting firm limits with clear consequences.

66. At the time of discharge from the hospital, Mr. Kile is most likely to
    o 1. be committed to another facility for a longer length of stay.
    o 2. be committed to a virtuous and socially acceptable life-style.
    o 3. discontinue treatment with the outpatient therapist.
    o 4. revert to prehospitalization behaviors.

Timmy Thomas, age 2 years 6 months, has had one bout of nephrosis (nephrotic syndrome). His mother suspected a recurrence when she observed swelling around his eyes.

67. The nurse helps to confirm this condition by recognizing what additional symptom?
    o 1. Blood pressure of 140/90
    o 2. A history of a positive streptococcal infection
    o 3. Cola-colored urine
    o 4. Marked proteinuria

68. Successful treatment of nephrosis will be characterized by
    o 1. diuresis and weight loss.
    o 2. increase in the sedimentation rate and urine specific gravity.
    o 3. improved appetite and weight gain.
    o 4. return of temperature to normal and signs that Timmy is more comfortable.

While talking with the nurse about Timmy's diet, Mrs. Thomas describes his temper tantrums demanding cookies in the supermarket, and asks how she can best handle these temper tantrums when he is well.

69. The nurse's best response is to
    o 1. buy one box of cookies for each shopping trip.
    o 2. leave him home while you do your shopping.
    o 3. remain calm and ignore his behavior.
    o 4. comment that she seems quite embarrassed by his behavior.

Cynthia Morris, age 25 and in her fifth month of pregnancy, has been taking 20 units of NPH insulin for diabetes mellitus daily for 6 years. Her diabetes has been well controlled with this dosage. She has been coming for routine prenatal visits during which diabetic teaching has been implemented.

70. Which of the following statements indicate that Cynthia understands the teaching regarding her insulin needs during her pregnancy?
    - o 1. Are you sure all this insulin won't hurt my baby?
    - o 2. I'll probably need my daily insulin dose raised next month when I start my third trimester, won't I?
    - o 3. I will continue to take my regular dose of insulin.
    - o 4. These fingersticks make my hands sore. Can I do them less frequently?

Cynthia's prenatal course is problem free and she delivers a full term 9 lb 2 oz girl.

71. At 1 hour after birth, Cynthia's baby exhibits tremors. The nurse performs a heelstick and a Dextrostix test. The result is 40 mg/dl. The nurse concludes that these symptoms are most likely caused by
    - o 1. hypoglycemia.
    - o 2. hypokalemia.
    - o 3. hypothermia.
    - o 4. hypercalcemia.

Julia Dever, age 42, has been in psychiatric hospitals intermittently for 24 years. Her longest period of stability was 18 months; otherwise, the majority of her time has been spent in the hospital. She rarely uses more than three- or four-word sentences to express her needs. She stays by herself in the dayroom and does not necessarily verbally respond when spoken to. She has a fixed delusion that a part of her body is broken and thinks that she is always in danger of being harmed by others. When extremely upset, she will either become aggressive towards others or immobile, remaining in the same position for extended periods of time. When in this state, she will maintain whatever position she is placed in and may not demonstrate spontaneous movement or speech for two or three days at a time.

72. The primary nurse planning interventions to moderate the severity of Miss Dever's symptoms will continually assess her for evidence of
    - o 1. bodily harm inflicted by herself or others.
    - o 2. cheecking or spitting out medications.
    - o 3. insight into her condition.
    - o 4. stressors that trigger periods of extreme behavior.

73. The nursing diagnosis of HIGHEST PRIORITY that most specifically describes Miss Dever WHEN EXTREMELY UPSET is
    - o 1. anxiety.
    - o 2. activity intolerance.
    - o 3. ineffective individual coping.
    - o 4. self-care deficit.

74. To increase Miss Dever's social skills, she and the nurse would probably
    - o 1. maintain a physical distance until Miss Dever shows an interest in talking.
    - o 2. maintain brief and frequent contact focusing on initiating conversations.
    - o 3. meet once a week to discuss Miss Dever's progress.
    - o 4. meet with other patients like Miss Dever twice a week for topically-oriented group therapy.

75. Symptoms of catatonic schizophrenia that Miss Dever demonstrates are
    - o 1. ambivalence, aggression, and delusions of control.
    - o 2. ambivalence, aggression, and somatic delusions.
    - o 3. autism, delusions of control, and waxy flexibility.
    - o 4. autism, somatic delusions, and waxy flexibility.

76. Because medication is a very important component of Miss Dever's treatment, the nurse may recommend
    - o 1. injectable medication.
    - o 2. rapid tranquilization.
    - o 3. oral medication in concentrate form every 6 hours.
    - o 4. oral medication in concentrate form at H.S.

Sally Brady, age 17, is admitted to the hospital with a diagnosis of acute renal failure. She is oliguric and has proteinuria.

77. Sally asks the nurse, "How long will it be until I start to make urine again?" A correct nursing response would be to tell her that this phase of renal failure will last for approximately which of the following time periods?
    - o 1. 1–2 days
    - o 2. 3–7 days
    - o 3. 1–2 weeks
    - o 4. 3–4 weeks

Sally develops pulmonary edema secondary to acute renal failure.

78. Nursing interventions for Sally should include all of the following EXCEPT
    - o 1. administer oxygen.
    - o 2. encourage coughing and deep breathing.
    - o 3. place her in semi-Fowler's position.
    - o 4. replace all lost fluids.

79. The appearance of a U wave on Sally's ECG should alert the nurse to check laboratory values for
    - o 1. hyperkalemia.
    - o 2. hypokalemia.
    - o 3. hypernatremia.
    - o 4. hyponatremia.

Sally develops chronic renal failure as a result of the episode of acute failure. She is placed on hemodialysis three times a week.

80. Which is an attainable short-term goal for Sally when she is placed on hemodialysis?
    ○ 1. Fully understanding the treatment and its implications
    ○ 2. Independence in the care of the AV shunt
    ○ 3. Self-monitoring during dialysis
    ○ 4. Recording dialysate composition and temperature

81. Which finding should Sally expect when assessing the fistula?
    ○ 1. Ecchymotic area
    ○ 2. Enlarged veins
    ○ 3. Pulselessness
    ○ 4. Redness

The remainder of this section consists of individual questions.

82. In evaluating the effectiveness of IV pitocin for a patient with secondary dystocia (uterine inertia), the nurse should expect
    ○ 1. a precipitate delivery.
    ○ 2. cervical effacement without delivery.
    ○ 3. infrequent contractions lasting longer than 90 seconds.
    ○ 4. progressive cervical dilation with contractions lasting less than 90 seconds.

83. George is recovering from chickenpox. At what point will he be allowed to return to school?
    ○ 1. After he has been on antibiotics for 48 hours
    ○ 2. After his temperature is normal and the itching has subsided
    ○ 3. When all lesions are crusted and scabbed
    ○ 4. When his skin is clear of all lesions

84. Florence Hill has had severe preeclampsia. She delivered 2 hours ago. Which nursing action should be included in the plan of care for her postpartum hospital stay?
    ○ 1. Continuing to monitor blood pressure, respirations, and reflexes
    ○ 2. Encouraging frequent family visitors
    ○ 3. Keeping her NPO
    ○ 4. Maintaining an IV access to the circulatory system.

85. Lori Miller had a vaginal delivery with her first child. Her second child was born by cesarean intervention due to a placenta previa. The plan of care to meet her needs postoperatively should include strategies to
    ○ 1. demonstrate gluteal tensing exercises for comfortable sitting.
    ○ 2. encourage her to recover in the same amount of time as with the first delivery.
    ○ 3. encourage her to verbalize any negative feelings she may have about this birth experience.
    ○ 4. keeping the baby in the nursery for longer periods of time to allow her to rest.

86. Jimmy had a tonsillectomy performed earlier in the day. He is now 4 hours post-op. Which of the following is an abnormal finding and a cause for concern?
    ○ 1. An emesis of dried blood
    ○ 2. Increased swallowing
    ○ 3. Pink-tinged mucus
    ○ 4. Jimmy's complaints of a very sore throat

87. The school nurse is assisting a school teacher to understand the classroom capabilities of a child with athetoid cerebral palsy. She explains that the child most probably will demonstrate
    ○ 1. exaggerated hyperactive reflexes.
    ○ 2. normal intelligence levels.
    ○ 3. slow, wormlike, writhing movements.
    ○ 4. unsteady gait and clumsy, uncoordinated upper extremity function.

88. Mrs. O'Toole calls her neighbor (who is a nurse) to say that her 5-year-old has had a stomach virus with vomiting for 24 hours. The doctor recommended the child eat nothing for 4–6 hours. There has been no vomiting during that time and now she wants to know what is best to give him. Her neighbor recommends
    ○ 1. broth and water.
    ○ 2. flat gingerale and tea.
    ○ 3. Jell-O and a soft-boiled egg.
    ○ 4. skim milk and dry toast.

89. Christopher, 2 months old, is suspected of having coarctation of the aorta. The cardinal sign of this defect is
    ○ 1. clubbing of the digits and circumoral cyanosis.
    ○ 2. pedal edema and portal congestion.
    ○ 3. systolic ejection murmur.
    ○ 4. upper extremity hypertension.

90. Susan, age 4, has leukemia. Her mother understands the white count involvement in this disease but doesn't understand why her child has bruises and anemia. The nurse explains that
    ○ 1. all blood cells are made in the bone marrow and therefore all types will be affected.
    ○ 2. the anemia is because her child hasn't been eating well; the bruises are from the multiple needle sticks.
    ○ 3. they are a result of the chemotherapy Susan was receiving.
    ○ 4. this is indicative that the end is near.

ANSWERS AND RATIONALES FOR PRACTICE TEST 1

ANSWER	RATIONALE	NP	CN	CL

#1 4 Bluish discoloration of the umbilicus (Cullen's sign) results from free blood present in the abdomen. It is not a sign of ascites. — A II An

#2 4 A major problem with ascites is fluid retention, and sodium restriction is the main intervention for controlling it. — I II Ap

#3 3 Increased ammonia levels occur in patients with liver damage as a result of the breakdown of blood protein in the intestinal tract. — An II An

#4 4 Rapid blood and fluid administration is necessary to restore vascular volume in the patient with a severe GI bleed. — P II An

#5 1 Airway obstruction will occur if the Sengstaken-Blakemore tube becomes dislodged. The nurse's first action should be to deflate the esophageal balloon in order to oxygenate the patient. — I II An

#6 4 The absence of pancreatic enzymes in cystic fibrosis requires a diet high in protein and calories to meet the child's growth needs. Between-meal snacks, such as skimmed milk shakes, are frequently given to supply additional protein, vitamins, and calories without exceeding the moderate fat restrictions for these patients. — P IV Ap

#7 2 Cystic fibrosis is considered an autosomal recessive genetic disease. If both parents are carriers of the trait, each child has a 25% chance of developing the disease, a 50% chance of being a carrier of the disease, and a 25% chance of being unaffected. — An IV C

#8 1 Leaving an object that the child can identify as his mother's and promising to return in the morning promotes trust between the mother and her child. — I IV Ap

#9 3 Patients with cystic fibrosis are prone to electrolyte imbalances due to increased loss of sodium and potassium in their sweat. Heat prostration will exacerbate these losses. — P I An

#10 4 Probable signs of pregnancy are those that are present on physical examination. A positive urine pregnancy test is an objective, probable sign of pregnancy. — A IV An

#11 3 Nägele's rule for predicting the estimated date of confinement is to add 7 days to the first day of the last menstrual period, subtract 3 months, and add 1 year. — An IV An

#12 1 In pregnancy, constipation results from reduced gastric motility and increased water reabsorption in the colon caused by increased levels of progesterone. Increasing fluid intake to 3 liters a day will minimize drying of feces. — P II Ap

#13 4 Backache in the late months of pregnancy may be prevented by wearing shoes with low heels. — P I C

#14 3 At 8 cm the patient is nearing the end of the first stage of labor. As labor progresses, many women develop hyperesthesia of the skin and the normal response is to reject touch during contractions. — An III An

#15 2 The counterpressure of a back rub during contractions will relieve discomfort. — I I Ap

#16 2 Variable decelerations are characterized by variable onset, occurrence, and waveform, frequently caused by transient pressure on the umbilical cord. — An II C

ANSWER	RATIONALE	NP	CN	CL
#17 2	Changing the position of the mother will relieve transient pressure on the umbilical cord.	I	I	Ap
#18 2	Discomfort while sitting is expected following episiotomy.	An	I	C
#19 1	Lochia rubra, which is moderate red discharge, is present for the first 2–3 days postpartum.	A	II	C
#20 2	The nursing infant can stimulate let-down resulting in milk dripping from the opposite breast.	E	IV	An
#21 4	Nipples should be washed with water only (no soap) to prevent excess drying.	I	I	Ap
#22 3	Breast-fed babies will pass 6–10 small, loose, yellow stools per day.	E	II	C
#23 1	Although a complete substance-use history is valuable eventually, the most important information to determine accurately on admission for detoxification is what the patient last took, when, and how much. In this way, appropriate nursing and medical interventions can be planned and implemented to assure the patient of an optimally safe detoxification.	A	II	Ap
#24 1	While the substance abuser has difficulty in all areas listed, problems handling stress and anxiety underlie all others. Difficulty handling stress and anxiety is often a pre-substance abuse characteristic. The others are more likely to be a result rather than the cause of substance abuse.	An	III	C
#25 3	Delirium tremens is characterized by increased blood pressure, pulse, and respirations, and an increase in psychomotor activity.	A	III	C
#26 4	While some have found treatment on an individual basis with therapists of varying orientations to be beneficial, group therapy with other substance abusers is the most highly prescribed treatment modality. It is the model of Alcoholics Anonymous upon which many other groups have been based.	I	III	C
#27 1	Cimetidine (Tagamet) is an H_2 antagonist that blocks the secretion of gastric hydrochloric acid.	An	II	C
#28 4	Hematochezia may come from a source in either the upper or lower GI tract. The patient's past medical history will give information regarding the presence of disorders that can be localized to either the upper or lower GI tract.	A	II	An
#29 3	Hemorrhagic reactions are a result of banked blood that is low in platelets and coagulation factors.	An	I	C
#30 4	Hypothermia with cardiac arrhythmias may occur when infusing the large quantities of blood that are required in GI bleeding. Blood-warming equipment should be used to prevent this problem.	I	I	Ap
#31 2	Early signs of dumping syndrome include vertigo, sweating, pallor, palpitations, and weakness.	An	IV	An
#32 4	Restricting all fluids is important to reduce the excess vascular volume in CHF. The other nursing interventions are all important but not specific to the problem of edema.	P	II	An

ANSWER		RATIONALE	NP	CN	CL
#33	1	Leg exercises are important for the patient on bedrest, as a measure to prevent thrombophlebitis.	I	I	An
#34	4	Left-sided CHF causes left ventricular dysfunction, resulting in increased pressure in the pulmonary veins, which leads to rales.	A	II	An
#35	4	Visual disturbances and arrhythmias are signs of digitalis toxicity.	I	I	Ap
#36	2	Normal serum potassium levels are 3.5–5.3 mEq/liter. Only 4.0 mEq/liter is within normal limits and does not require immediate nursing intervention.	An	I	An
#37	2	A lack of iodine in the diet is a primary contributor to the development of a simple goiter.	An	IV	An
#38	3	Turnips belong to a classification of foods called exogenous goitrogens. Goitrogens are thyroid-inhibiting substances and therefore should be avoided.	I	IV	Ap
#39	1	Encouraging the patient to discuss her disfigurement allows her to ventilate her feelings and gives the nurse the opportunity to provide appropriate support.	P	III	Ap
#40	2	The energy exerted by the child in resisting the oxygen tent will increase respiratory effort. Removing the child from the oxygen tent will have a calming effect, thus reducing his respiratory effort. The child should be closely observed for his ability to cope outside the oxygen tent. The physician should be notified because the oxygen concentration of room air is 20% and is less than that ordered.	I	II	Ap
#41	1	Normal height for a 12-month-old ranges from 29–32 inches. Normal weight for a 12-month-old ranges from 19–27 lb. Bryan's height is within the normal range, but his weight is above normal for his age.	An	IV	An
#42	1	Administration of immume serum globulin will provide the child with passive immunity to prevent a full-blown case of measles or reduce the severity of symptoms. Active immunization with MMR can be given at a later time.	P	I	Ap
#43	1	Correcting a cleft palate prior to development of speech allows for formation of more normal speech patterns.	E	IV	Ap
#44	2	Care should be taken not to put anything in the mouth that could damage the suture line. Mrs. Kelly may feed Barry with a cup or a wide-bowl spoon that cannot enter the mouth.	I	I	Ap
#45	4	Current weight as it relates to usual weight is a better determinant of nutritional status and weight change when the client is unable to be specific about recent activities.	A	II	Ap
#46	3	The nursing diagnosis that supersedes all others is ineffective individual coping. This area will be the primary focus of the nurse's interventions, and changes in the client's ability to cope will be the criteria for discharge readiness.	An	III	A
#47	3	Building drinking a specific amount of a certain type of fluid into a daily schedule of activities is very consistent with the obsessive/compulsive client's need to control as many aspects of her life as possible.	P	II	Ap
#48	1	Allowing the patient a certain amount of time to engage in the activity alleviates some of the client's anxiety by restructuring how she is to use her time. It is an alternative way for the client to use the same coping mechanism but in a more adaptive way that enables her to engage in other activities.	I	III	Ap

ANSWER		RATIONALE	NP	CN	CL
#49	4	The major issue is control of behavior and thoughts. When Ms. Dunn is able to control her compulsive behaviors (i.e., limit her hand and face washing to a few times a day), she will then be able to resume ADL. Compulsive behavior is often episodic and relates to repression and anxiety.	E	III	An
#50	2	Patients with a T4 injury will have sufficient upper extremity strength to master the techniques of independent transfer.	A	I	An
#51	3	Checking for bladder distention frequently will prevent distension of the ureters and renal pelvis.	I	I	An
#52	2	The major goal of a bowel program is to prevent incontinence by having the patient control defecation.	E	I	An
#53	4	Severe muscle spasms indicate that the Valium is not effective as a muscle relaxant.	E	I	An
#54	1	A common side effect of propranolol is a slowed pulse rate because the drug is a beta blocker.	E	I	An
#55	3	Catsup is a condiment that is very high in sodium and should be avoided.	P	I	Ap
#56	3	Assessments are made of lying and standing blood pressures to detect the presence of orthostatic hypotension, which is characterized by a decrease in systolic blood pressure when the patient moves from a lying to standing position.	I	I	C
#57	2	An increased anterior-posterior chest diameter, commonly referred to as "barrel chest," is seen in patients with emphysema as a result of chronic hyperinflation of the lungs.	A	II	Ap
#58	3	Activities should be planned to conserve energy as the patient must work so hard to breathe. It is important to plan care in a manner that does not worsen breathlessness.	P	II	Ap
#59	4	The respiratory drive in a patient with emphysema is oxygen rather than rising carbon dioxide levels. Frequent nursing observatons are necessary to monitor the patient's breathing pattern.	I	II	Ap
#60	4	Abdominal breathing elevates the diaphragm thereby improving breathing effectiveness in patients with emphysema.	E	II	An
#61	3	Cardiac arrest, diabetic ketoacidosis and renal failure all cause metabolic acidosis. Hypokalemia, if persistent, eventually would lead to metabolic alkalosis.	An	II	An
#62	4	The pH is below the normal range of 7.35–7.45. The pCO_2 is within the normal range of 35–45. the HCO_3 is below the normal limits of 21–28. This indicates metabolic acidosis.	An	II	An
#63	1	A long history of petty crimes, high level of manipulative behavior, using other clients to his own end, and pioneering causes that are disruptive to the milieu all support this diagnosis.	An	III	An
#64	1	The staff and client will most likely disagree when setting treatment goals. All the other responses describe the relationship between the antisocial client and staff that makes it quite challenging to work with such clients therapeutically.	P	III	Ap

ANSWER		RATIONALE	NP	CN	CL
#65	2	Although the client will compare and "split" staff, it is very important that the staff assignment be as consistent as possible. Otherwise, the patient will be in control of the staff, thus repeating early difficulties with authority figures, which would be counter-therapeutic.	I	III	Ap
#66	4	People who have this type of personality disorder typically seek pychiatric care as a lesser of two evils. In this case, in-patient care was preferable to jail. The chance of this patient making any great changes in his life-style as a result of this short-term hospitalization are slim.	E	III	Ap
#67	4	In nephrotic syndrome plasma proteins are excreted in the urine.	A	II	An
#68	1	The primary goal of treatment to control edema. Corticosteroids are used to promote diuresis and subsequent weight loss.	E	II	An
#69	3	Effective techniques for handling temper tantrums include being consistent, remaining calm, and ignoring the behavior.	I	IV	Ap
#70	2	As a result of placental maturation and human placental lactogen production, insulin requirements start elevating in the second trimester and may double or quadruple by the end of the pregnancy. In the insulin-dependent diabetic mother, insulin doses need to be titrated to maternal blood levels.	E	II	C
#71	1	Tremors are one of the many symptoms the hypoglycemic neonoate may exhibit. A Dextrostix below 45 mg/dl in a neonate is an indication for performing a laboratory blood sugar test.	An	II	C
#72	4	The chronically mentally disabled have an exquisite vulnerability to stress. The level of intensity and severity of symptoms is thought to be directly related to the level of stress that the patient is experiencing. The key to treatment is to identify the stressors and to teach the client alternative responses to them or to modify the stressor in some way to make it less threatening to the client's stability.	A	III	An
#73	4	While there may be evidence to support all of the other diagnostic titles, the client's selfcare deficits will be pervasive and extreme, and pose the greatest threat to her well-being.	An	III	An
#74	2	Because the client has marked withdrawal and verbal paucity, meeting with her briefly and frequently with a singular focus on initiating conversations is a specific intervention aimed at increasing her social skills.	P	III	C
#75	4	This client exhibits waxy flexibility (remaining in the position in which one is placed for long periods of time), somatic delusions (part of her body is broken), and autism.	An	III	An
#76	3	Oral medication in concentrated form is very appropriate as the chance of cheeking or spitting out the medication is minimized. HS single dose is preferable over multiple daily doses as it may aid in producing sleep and continue to have therapeutic effects during waking hours.	I	I	Ap
#77	3	The oliguric period ranges from 1–2 weeks.	I	II	C
#78	4	In pulmonary edema, all fluids are not replaced. It is the goal of therapy to reduce the amount of fluid in the body.	E	II	Ap
#79	2	U waves are associated with hypokalemia.	An	II	An

ANSWER		RATIONALE	NP	CN	CL
#80	1	Prior to the start of dialysis, the patient should fully comprehend its meaning and the changes in life-style required.	An	II	An
#81	2	The leaking of arterial blood into an AV fistula causes the veins to enlarge so they are easier to access for hemodialysis.	A	I	Ap
#82	4	IV pitocin for a patient with secondary dystocia should produce progressive cervical dilation with contraction duration not exceeding 90 seconds.	E	I	An
#83	3	Chickenpox lesions are no longer infectious once they are crusted.	E	I	C
#84	1	Postdelivery management of the severely preeclamptic mother includes close observation for blood pressure elevations, CNS irritability, and respiratory function.	P	I	C
#85	3	Encouraging the mother to verbalize any negative feeling about the birth experience allows her to maintain a positive sense of self-worth and self-esteem.	P	III	C
#86	2	Blood flow or hemorrhage from the surgical site will cause increased swallowing.	A	II	C
#87	4	Athetoid cerebral palsy is characterized by involuntary, purposeless, slow, writhing motion.	A	I	C
#88	2	Flat gingerale and tea are well tolerated and nonirritating to the GI tract after acute insult.	P	II	Ap
#89	1	Coarctation of the aorta is characterized by upper extremity hypertension and diminished pulses in the extremities.	A	II	Ap
#90	1	In leukemia, bone marrow is replaced by blast cells resulting in decreased white cells, red cells, and platelets.	An	II	Ap

Practice Test 2

Mr. Harold Porth, age 84, has just returned to the nursing unit after a transurethral resection. A three-way Foley catheter connected to straight drainage is in place.

1. Immediately after surgery, the nurse would expect Mr. Porth's urine to be
   - ○ 1. clear.
   - ○ 2. light yellow.
   - ○ 3. pink with blood clots.
   - ○ 4. bright red.

2. Mr. Porth tells the nurse he has to void. The MOST APPROPRIATE nursing action is to
   - ○ 1. allow him to void around the catheter.
   - ○ 2. irrigate the catheter.
   - ○ 3. notify the physician.
   - ○ 4. remove the catheter.

Mrs. Margaret Toze, age 39, has advanced cancer of the breast. She is admitted to the medical unit for nutritional evaluation. She weighs 101 lb and is 5 ft 8 in tall. She is started on leucovorin (Wellcovorin).

3. Assessment of Mrs. Toze's nutritional health would include all the following EXCEPT
   - ○ 1. a diet history.
   - ○ 2. anthropometric measurements.
   - ○ 3. food preferences.
   - ○ 4. serum protein studies.

4. Mrs. Toze complains of hypogeusia. The nurse should recommend
   - ○ 1. eating dry crackers.
   - ○ 2. monitoring intake and output.
   - ○ 3. using spices to enhance food flavors.
   - ○ 4. weighing Mrs. Toze before and after meals.

Mr. John Dennis, age 26, is admitted to the hospital to undergo a stapedectomy for the treatment of otosclerosis.

5. Which of the following findings elicited during the physical assessment are most indicative of otosclerosis?
   - ○ 1. Bone conduction is greater than air conduction.
   - ○ 2. Bone conduction is equal to air conduction.
   - ○ 3. Air conduction is greater than bone conduction.
   - ○ 4. Sound lateralizes to the unaffected ear.

6. Mr. Dennis is scheduled for the stapedectomy the day after admission. Which of the following nursing actions is the MOST IMPORTANT to include in the post-op care plan?
   - ○ 1. Checking the gag reflex
   - ○ 2. Encouraging independence
   - ○ 3. Instructing Mr. Dennis not to blow his nose
   - ○ 4. Positioning Mr. Dennis on the operative side

7. Post-op communications with Mr. Dennis will be effective if the nursing personnel
   - ○ 1. overarticulate.
   - ○ 2. shout in his affected ear.
   - ○ 3. speak at a moderate rate.
   - ○ 4. use long, easily understood phrases.

Amy Johnson, age 4, is admitted to the hospital for the treatment of an acute asthma attack. Her health history reveals that she has been blind since birth and has had four asthma attacks in the past six months. She received epinephrine (Adrenalin) in the emergency department and was transferred to the pediatric unit with an aminophylline infusion.

8. When evaluating Amy for positive effects of the aminophylline treatment, the MOST SIGNIFICANT finding is
   - ○ 1. a decrease in mucus production.
   - ○ 2. a decrease in wheezing.
   - ○ 3. an increase in blood pressure.
   - ○ 4. a sleeping child.

9. Amy has been attending a nursery program for the visually impaired. To continue independence in her activities of daily living, when her lunch tray arrives the nurse will
   - ○ 1. offer to feed her.
   - ○ 2. explain that foods on her tray are set up like a clock.
   - ○ 3. put food on her fork and hand her the fork.
   - ○ 4. tell her that two foods are in front of her, one at the top of the tray and one at the bottom.

David Freeze, age 26, is admitted involuntarily to the psychiatric unit in a manic state. He has been arrested by the police for indecent exposure, loitering, and disturbing the peace. Prior to his arrest he had visited his mother's grave (she has been deceased for 12 years), where he became hyperactive, stripped off his clothes, and terrorized people living in the area near the cemetery. Upon arrival on the unit, he was unable able to sit, and it was very difficult to follow what he was saying because of the rate and content of speech. He was very provocative and refused to eat or drink. At one point, he took shaving cream from his luggage and put crosses on the door to each room on the unit.

10. The area of disturbance which poses the greatest physical danger to this client is
   ○ 1. activity.
   ○ 2. perceptual.
   ○ 3. sensory.
   ○ 4. social.

11. The nursing diagnosis that would most appropriately describe the behavior which is of greatest concern is
   ○ 1. anxiety.
   ○ 2. potential for violence.
   ○ 3. self-care deficit.
   ○ 4. alteration in nutrition: less than body requirements.

12. During the manic phase found in the initial period of hospitalization, the nurse would most likely
   ○ 1. encourage Mr. Freeze to participate in group and therapeutic activities.
   ○ 2. observe Mr. Freeze closely until he calms down.
   ○ 3. place Mr. Freeze in four-point restraints for protection of self and others.
   ○ 4. place Mr. Freeze in seclusion but maintain frequent one-to-one contact with him.

13. Which of the following is LEAST likely to influence the potential for this client to comply with lithium therapy after discharge?
   ○ 1. The impact of lithium on the client's energy level and life-style.
   ○ 2. The need for consistent blood level monitoring.
   ○ 3. The potential side-effects of lithium.
   ○ 4. What the client's friends think of his need to take medication.

Mrs. Alice Sloane, age 25, has been coming to the prenatal clinic on a regular basis. She is five months pregnant. She suffered from morning sickness early in her pregnancy and is now concerned because the vomiting has continued and she is feeling weak and exhausted. Diagnosed as having hyperemesis gravidarum, she is hospitalized and parenteral fluid therapy is started.

14. Mrs. Sloane has vomited twice within the last hour. The FIRST appropriate nursing intervention would be to
   ○ 1. assist her with mouth care.
   ○ 2. notify the physician.
   ○ 3. change the IV infusion to Ringer's lactate.
   ○ 4. warm her tray and serve it to her again.

Mrs. Sloane responds well to therapy. Now in her seventh month of pregnancy, her only presenting problem is a hemoglobin of 10.5 gm.

15. In evaluating the effectiveness of nutritional teaching with Mrs. Sloane, the nurse would expect her to state that she eats
   ○ 1. an orange for breakfast.
   ○ 2. a green leafy vegetable occasionally.
   ○ 3. liver once a week.
   ○ 4. six small meals a day.

Mrs. Sloane is admitted to the labor room in early active labor.

16. What information should the nurse obtain from Mrs. Sloane to avoid respiratory complications during labor and delivery?
   ○ 1. Family history of lung disease
   ○ 2. Food or drug allergies
   ○ 3. Number of cigarettes smoked per day
   ○ 4. Time and contents of last food ingested

Mrs. Sloane delivers a 6 lb 5 oz (2863 gm) boy. Because his serum bilirubin level is elevated, Baby Boy Sloane is receiving phototherapy.

17. To meet the safety needs of Baby Boy Sloane while he is undergoing phototherapy, the nurse should
   ○ 1. limit fluid intake.
   ○ 2. cover the infant's eyes while he is under the light.
   ○ 3. keep him clothed to prevent skin burns.
   ○ 4. make sure the light is not closer than 24 inches.

18. The nursery nurse carries Baby Boy Sloane into his mother's room. Mrs. Sloane states, "I think my baby's afraid of me. Every time I make a loud noise, he jumps." The nurse should
   ○ 1. encourage Mrs. Sloane not to be so nervous with her baby.
   ○ 2. reassure her that this is a normal reflexive reaction for her baby.
   ○ 3. take the baby back to the nursery for a neurologic evaluation.
   ○ 4. wrap the baby more tightly in warm blankets.

19. Mrs. Sloane asks how much her 3-day-old baby weighs. When the nurse tells her 5 lb 11 oz (2580 gm), she starts to cry because the baby is losing weight. What is the expected weight loss pattern in a newborn?
   ○ 1. None
   ○ 2. 5%
   ○ 3. 5%–10%
   ○ 4. 10%–15%

20. The morning temperature on Baby Boy Sloane is 97.6°F (36.4°C). In order to prevent cold stress, which nursing action should be included in the plan of care? Teach Mrs. Sloane to
   ○ 1. keep the baby's head covered.
   ○ 2. keep the baby unwrapped.
   ○ 3. turn up the thermostat in the nursery.
   ○ 4. use warm water for the bath.

Mrs. Sloane brings her baby in for his one-month check-up. Her only problem is that she has difficulty spreading his right leg when she is diapering him. The nurse suspects a dislocated hip.

21. Further assessment of this child for the possibility of a dislocated hip on the right side would include observing for
    o 1. absence of Ortolani's sign.
    o 2. presence of Trendelenburg's sign.
    o 3. an increase in skin folds on the unaffected side.
    o 4. shortening of the affected femur when supine with knees bent.

Mrs. Elena Smith, age 46, is admitted to an isolation unit in the hospital after tuberculosis was detected during a pre-employment physical. Although frightened about her diagnosis, she is anxious to cooperate with the therapeutic regime.

22. The teaching plan for Mrs. Smith would include information regarding the most common means of transmitting the tubercle bacillus from one individual to another. Which contaminated item is usually responsible?
    o 1. Hands
    o 2. Droplet nuclei
    o 3. Milk products
    o 4. Eating utensils

23. Mrs. Smith is receiving rifampin (Rifadin) and should be alerted to which of the following common side effects?
    o 1. Vertigo
    o 2. Skin rash
    o 3. Tingling in the feet
    o 4. Orange-tinged body fluids

Mrs. Gertrude Borden, age 92, was found at home lying on the floor of her kitchen. She was unable to move without experiencing severe pain in her right hip. She is admitted to the orthopedic unit with a diagnosis of a right intracapsular hip fracture.

24. Mrs. Borden is upset, confused, and repeatedly tells the nurse she is worried about being constipated while in the hospital. To elicit information effectively about Mrs. Borden's bowel status, the nurse should ask
    o 1. Do you realize you are confused?
    o 2. What laxative do you take at home?
    o 3. When was your last bowel movement?
    o 4. Why are you so worried about your bowels?

Buck's extension traction is employed prior to surgery.

25. Mrs. Borden complains of numbness in the right foot. The nurse inspects the foot and notes the traction tapes are lengthwise on opposite sides of the limb. The nurse's response to Mrs. Borden should be
    o 1. How long has your foot been numb?
    o 2. I can adjust it for your comfort.
    o 3. I'll call your doctor about it.
    o 4. There is nothing wrong with the traction.

Three days after her fall, Mrs. Borden goes to the operating room for the insertion of an Austin-Moore prosthesis.

26. Mrs. Borden is told that it is important to keep her hip in good position. Which of the following statements indicates that Mrs. Borden understands her instructions?
    o 1. I shouldn't bend my knees.
    o 2. I will be sure to put my shoes on when I go for a walk.
    o 3. Put a pillow between my legs when you turn me.
    o 4. Put me on the commode chair for my bowel movement.

27. Which of the following nursing measures will best facilitate the resumption of activities for Mrs. Borden?
    o 1. Arranging for a wheelchair
    o 2. Asking her family to visit
    o 3. Assisting her to sit out of bed in a chair qid
    o 4. Encouraging the use of an overhead trapeze

28. Mrs. Borden is preparing for transfer to an extended care facility. She begins to cry and says, "When you're young these things don't happen. Why did I break my hip at this age?" Which response by the nurse indicates the best understanding of risk factors for the elderly?
    o 1. As you age you become less aware of your surroundings and careless about safety.
    o 2. Nothing works as well when we are older.
    o 3. There are no known specific reasons why hip fractures occur more often in your age group.
    o 4. Your age and sex are factors in the loss of minerals from your bones making them more likely to break.

Mr. Brian Kelly. age 68, is admitted to the Emergency Department with a medical diagnosis of closed-angle glaucoma. Mr. Kelly is placed on miotic therapy and receives 75% glycerin (Glyrol).

29. In planning care for Mr. Kelly, which of the following should be a teaching priority during the acute phase of his illness?
    o 1. Eye drop administration
    o 2. Eye patch changes every hour
    o 3. Measuring all intake and output
    o 4. Keeping bright lights on in the room

30. Which of the following nursing actions represents UNSAFE nursing care for Mr. Kelly?
    o 1. Administration of morphine sulfate 8 mg IM PRN for pain.
    o 2. Allowing him to ambulate to the bathroom with assistance.
    o 3. Occluding the puncta during the administration of eye drops.
    o 4. Wearing unsterile gloves when examining the eye.

31. Mr. Kelly recognizes that the primary purpose of medications such as pilocarpine (Pilocar) used in the treatment of his glaucoma is
    o 1. control of increased intraocular pressure.
    o 2. improvement of vision.
    o 3. relief of pain.
    o 4. restoration of peripheral vision.

32. Mr. Kelly tells you he has heard that glaucoma may be a hereditary problem. He is concerned about his children, a son, age 45, and a daughter, age 38. The MOST appropriate response by the nurse is
    - ○ 1. Are your children complaining of eye problems?
    - ○ 2. There is no need for concern because glaucoma is not a hereditary disorder.
    - ○ 3. There may be a genetic factor with glaucoma and your children should be screened.
    - ○ 4. Your son should be evaluated because he is over 40.

Mr. Michael O'Malley, age 34, is involved in many craft projects. While he is burning the paint off some furniture that he is restoring, his shirt catches on fire. In a panic, he runs into his neighbor's yard with his clothes in flames.

33. All the following are appropiate first-aid interventions for Mr. O' Malley EXCEPT
    - ○ 1. dousing the flames with water.
    - ○ 2. removing his burned clothing.
    - ○ 3. removing his jewelry.
    - ○ 4. rolling him on the ground rapidly.

The fire is extinguished and Mr. O'Malley is admitted to the hospital burn unit.

34. During the acute burn phase, the nurse explains to Mr. O'Malley that his nursing care planning is directed toward all of the following EXCEPT
    - ○ 1. strict aseptic techique.
    - ○ 2. proper alignment of all joints.
    - ○ 3. frequent and routine administration of narcotics.
    - ○ 4. maintenance of fluid and electrolyte balance.

35. Nursing care planning is based on the knowledge that Mr. O'Malley's first 24–48 hours post-burn are characterized by
    - ○ 1. an increase in the total volume of intravascular plasma.
    - ○ 2. excessive renal perfusion with diuresis.
    - ○ 3. fluid shift from interstitial spaces to plasma.
    - ○ 4. fluid shift from plasma to interstitial spaces.

36. An acceptable range for hourly urine output during the first couple of days post-burn is
    - ○ 1. 20 cc.
    - ○ 2. 30–50 cc.
    - ○ 3. 50–90 cc.
    - ○ 4. 90–150 cc.

37. The nurse should plan to utilize all of the following interventions to prevent Mr. O'Malley from developing an infection EXCEPT
    - ○ 1. administer hyperimmune tetanus globulin.
    - ○ 2. apply topical antibiotics.
    - ○ 3. cleanse the wounds.
    - ○ 4. place Mr. O'Malley in protective isolation.

Mrs. Susan Findlay, age 38, was admitted to the psychiatric service after a failed suicide attempt by drug overdose. She had been in treatment with a clinical psychologist on a biweekly basis for six weeks. Mrs. Findlay sought help when her husband informed her of his decision to leave her and the

children after 19 years of marriage. Mrs. Findlay's suicide attempt was made after she and her husband had had a fierce argument about property settlement. Upon initial contact with the nurse, the client looked exhausted, affect was sad, movements and responses were slowed, and self-care impairments were evident. She is convinced that a blemish on her face is a melanoma that is invading her brain and eating away at the tissue.

38. Mrs. Findlay's disorder is best classified as
    - ○ 1. bipolar disorder.
    - ○ 2. depression with melancholia.
    - ○ 3. dysthymic disorder.
    - ○ 4. major depression.

39. Which nursing diagnosis is of greatest priority at the time of Mrs. Findlay's admission?
    - ○ 1. Alteration in nutrition: less than body requirements
    - ○ 2. Ineffective individual coping
    - ○ 3. Potential for violence: self-directed
    - ○ 4. Self-care deficit

40. In attempting to stabilize Mrs. Findlay's activities of daily living in a optimally therapeutic way, she and the nurse would most likely plan to
    - ○ 1. allow her to catch up on lost sleep for the first three days of her hospitalization.
    - ○ 2. have her fully involved in all therapeutic activities.
    - ○ 3. have her husband visit for brief periods of time.
    - ○ 4. schedule balanced periods of rest and therapeutic activity.

41. By the end of the third day of hospitalization, Mrs. Findlay's fear of dying from the melanoma had reached psychotic proportions. The most adaptive way she might try to deal with this would be to
    - ○ 1. attempt thought control methods to decrease pervasiveness of thoughts.
    - ○ 2. request PRN medication whenever such thoughts intrude.
    - ○ 3. share her concerns with another patient whenever they arise.
    - ○ 4. withdraw to her room whenever such thoughts arise.

42. The beneficial effects of group therapy for this client would include all of the following EXCEPT
    - ○ 1. a decrease in isolation and an increase in reality-testing.
    - ○ 2. an increase in the sense of belonging and worthiness.
    - ○ 3. focusing strictly on personal situations.
    - ○ 4. the opportunity to ventilate and problem solve.

Ruth Stone, age 28 and 35 weeks pregnant, comes to the Emergency Department with painless vaginal bleeding. This is her third pregnancy and she states that this has never happened to her before.

43. In caring for Mrs. Stone, the nurse should AVOID
    - ○ 1. allowing her husband to stay with her.
    - ○ 2. keeping her at rest.
    - ○ 3. shaving the perineum.
    - ○ 4. performing a vaginal examination.

Mrs. Stone is admitted to the hospital. After three weeks on bedrest her membranes rupture.

44. The nurse notices that the amniotic fluid has a greenish color and that Mrs. Stone has started to bleed again. The nurse should plan to
   o 1. administer oxygen.
   o 2. place her in Trendelenburg's position.
   o 3. call the physician and prepare for a cesarean birth.
   o 4. move her to the delivery room immediately.

Mrs. Stone delivers a 6 lb 4 oz (2835 gm) baby boy.

45. Which of the following statements would indicate to the nurse that the mother has begun to integrate her new baby into the family structure?
   o 1. All this baby does is cry. He's not like my other child.
   o 2. I wish he had curly hair like my husband.
   o 3. My parents wanted a grandaughter.
   o 4. When he yawns, he looks just like his brother.

Mrs. Stone brings her son to the well-baby clinic for his two-month check-up. She reports that he is doing well except that he has a rash on his cheeks, trunk, and extremities that won't heal. A diagnosis of infantile eczema is made and the nurse reviews the care for this problem with Mrs. Stone.

46. When Mrs. Stone returns for her child's three-month check-up, reporting what activity would indicate that she has been properly caring for his skin?
   o 1. She bathes him twice a day to remove crusts.
   o 2. She leaves his skin exposed to air dry whenever possible.
   o 3. She gently pats lubricant into the skin immediately after the bath.
   o 4. She uses only natural fibers against his skin.

Mrs. Janice Backer, age 44, has been complaining of severe back pain that has been treated conservatively for the past year. She is admitted to the hospital for treatment of a herniated disk. A laminectomy with spinal fusion is scheduled.

47. When Mrs. Backer returns to the unit after surgery, she is afraid to turn. Of the following maneuvers she plans to use to avoid pain, which is UNSAFE?
   o 1. Log rolling
   o 2. Asking for pain medication
   o 3. Placing pillows between her legs
   o 4. Sitting up in bed

48. Immediately after surgery, which of the following should the nurse expect Mrs. Backer to manifest?
   o 1. Absence of lower extremity movement
   o 2. Response to pinprick sensation
   o 3. Severe muscle spasms
   o 4. Weak pedal pulses

49. The donor site for the graft begins to hemorrhage and then ooze blood. What is the most appropriate way to determine if nursing interventions to stop bleeding have been effective?
   o 1. Monitoring output
   o 2. Taking hourly vital signs
   o 3. Asking Mrs. Backer if she feels dizzy
   o 4. Outlining drainage on dressing and noting time

50. The teaching plan for Mrs. Backer when she just begins to get out of bed can be considered effective if she
   o 1. bends only from the waist.
   o 2. moves rapidly.
   o 3. thinks through each movement.
   o 4. refuses to use a walker.

Mr. Dan Book, age 45, is admitted to the hospital with Addison's disease. He has a respiratory infection.

51. When Mr. Book's vital signs are assessed, his blood pressure is 90/40. The nurse should notify the physician immediately because
   o 1. blood gases need to be drawn.
   o 2. seizure activity is imminent.
   o 3. shock may be developing.
   o 4. the reading is atypical.

52. Upon further assessment, what manifestation should the nurse expect to find in Mr. Book?
   o 1. Acne.
   o 2. Hyperpigmentation.
   o 3. Moon face.
   o 4. Supraclavicular fat pads.

53. The nurse is teaching Mr. Book about glucocorticoid replacement therapy. What should be included as a reason to increase the dose?
   o 1. Fatigue
   o 2. Abdominal discomfort
   o 3. Emotional stress
   o 4. Loss of appetite

54. In evaluating the effectiveness of teaching regarding drug therapy for Mr. Book, the nurse should expect him to be able to verbalize the need
   o 1. to avoid antibiotics.
   o 2. for lifelong therapy.
   o 3. to taper the steroid dose.
   o 4. to receive alternate day therapy.

Mr. William Wilson, age 24, was seen in the out-patient clinic by the psychiatric nurse clinician for an assessment interview. In establishing the data base, Mr. Wilson related that he hears the voice of his former girlfriend calling to him to help her. In an attempt to find her, he breaks into various buildings and enters homes other than his own uninvited. He rarely sleeps and has lost a job because he is afraid he will miss a visit or telephone call from her. Mr. Wilson lives with his parents who are very upset by his behavior and have threatened to evict him from the house if he does not get help.

55. The component of the mental status examination that tests for the client's ability to abstract as well as reason is the use of
    o 1. proverbs.
    o 2. item identification.
    o 3. presidents' names.
    o 4. serial sevens.

56. All of the following nursing diagnoses apply to this case EXCEPT
    o 1. alteration in thought processes.
    o 2. self-care deficit.
    o 3. sensory-perceptual alteration.
    o 4. sleep pattern disturbance.

57. Using the community mental health model, the nurse would plan to
    o 1. encourage Mr. Wilson to admit himself to a community hospital psychiatric unit.
    o 2. file a petition for involuntary commitment.
    o 3. maintain Mr. Wilson in treatment in a community-based setting.
    o 4. refer Mr Wilson to a psychiatrist for medication as sole treatment.

58. Which of the following will offer the best motivation to engaging Mr. Wilson in treatment?
    o 1. Limited verbal interaction
    o 2. Parent's response to his behavior
    o 3. Potential noncompliance with his appointment schedule
    o 4. Potential noncompliance with his medications

After six weeks of biweekly therapy sessions, Mr. Wilson secured full-time, mimimun wage employment. Within the first week of working, it became apparent that Mr. Wilson was not able to get out of bed in time for work and was jeopardizing his employment.

59. A realistic, initial, client-oriented goal which Mr. Wilson might negotiate with the nurse-therapist is to get to work
    o 1. on time 4 out of 5 days with his parent's assistance.
    o 2. every day with his parent's assistance.
    o 3. on time every day independently.
    o 4. on time 2 out of 5 days independently.

Alice White, age 10, has been hospitalized for two weeks with rheumatic fever.

60. Alice's mother questions whether her other children can catch the rheumatic fever. The nurse's BEST response is
    o 1. The fact that you brought Alice to the hospital early enough will decrease the chance of her siblings getting it.
    o 2. It is caused by a autoimmune reaction and is not contagious.
    o 3. You appear concerned that your daughter's disease is contagious.
    o 4. Your other children should be taking antibiotics to prevent them from catching rheumatic fever.

61. In addition to carditis, the nurse would assess Alice for the presence of
    o 1. arthritis.
    o 2. bronchitis.
    o 3. malabsorption.
    o 4. oliguria.

Mr. John Mooney, age 51, has a 13-year history of heavy alcohol consumption He has been smoking 2 packs of cigarettes a day since he was 15 years old. He complains of a sore throat, weight loss, and increasing hoarseness. After an extensive medical workup, a diagnosis of cancer of the larynx is made and Mr. Mooney is scheduled for a radical neck dissection.

62. When Mr. Mooney returns to the nursing unit after surgery, he is having difficulty breathing. Secretions are visible in the laryngectomy tube. The INITIAL nursing intervention should be to
    o 1. obtain the vital signs.
    o 2. notify the physician.
    o 3. remove the secretions.
    o 4. start oxygen via a tracheostomy collar.

63. The nursing management for Mr. Mooney in the EARLY post-op period is PRIMARILY directed toward
    o 1. alleviation of pain.
    o 2. decreasing Mr. Mooney's concern about appearance.
    o 3. improving the nutritional status of Mr. Mooney.
    o 4. observing Mr. Mooney for hemorrhage.

Mr. James Rubin, age 36, is involved in a multivehicle accident. You are the first professional to arrive at the scene. Mr. Rubin was riding a motorcycle. Upon impact, he fell off the bike and it fell back on his legs.

64. Priority care for Mr. Rubin should be directed toward
    o 1. assessing blood loss.
    o 2. monitoring respiratory status.
    o 3. obtaining vital signs.
    o 4. organizing lay people on the scene.

65. Mr. Rubin has a 4-inch gash on his left leg that is bleeding profusely. Which of the following is the best approach to stop the bleeding?
    o 1. Apply direct pressure to the wound.
    o 2. Move the motorcycle off his legs.
    o 3. Raise the extremity.
    o 4. Wrap a tourniquet above the wound.

Mr. Rubin is admitted to the hospital. X-rays reveal a fractured tibia and a cast is applied.

66. Of the following, which nursing action would be MOST important after the cast is in place?
    o 1. Assessing for capillary refill
    o 2. Arranging for physical therapy
    o 3. Discussing cast care with Mr. Rubin
    o 4. Helping Mr. Rubin to ambulate

67. 1 liter of IV fluid every 6 hours is ordered. Which of the following flow rates indicates the IV calculations are correct for an administration set that delivers 10 gtts/cc?
    o 1. 22 gtts/minute
    o 2. 28 gtts/minute
    o 3. 32 gtts/minute
    o 4. 36 gtts/minute

68. Which observation BEST indicates that Mr. Rubin's IV has infiltrated?
    o 1. Pain at the site
    o 2. A change in flow rate
    o 3. Coldness around the insertion site
    o 4. Redness around the insertion site

Ms. Jennifer Mason, age 19, comes to the gynecology clinic to be fitted for a diaphragm.

69. Which nursing action would best prevent incorrect placement of a diaphragm when Ms. Mason is inserting it for the first time?
    o 1. Allowing her supervised practice time
    o 2. Providing a brochure
    o 3. Teaching her to lie on her back
    o 4. Teaching her sex partner to insert it

70. Ms. Mason tells the nurse that she gets her menstrual period every 18 days. She states that her flow is very heavy and lasts six days. The nurse identifies this pattern as
    o 1. dysmenorrhea.
    o 2. dyspareunia.
    o 3. menorrhagia.
    o 4. metrorrhagia.

71. Ms. Mason returns to the clinic in three months complaining that she has "many little blisters on my privates." After examining her labia and perineum, the nurse finds multiple vesicles, some ruptured and crusted over. There is no unusual vaginal discharge. The nurse should suspect
    o 1. chlamydia.
    o 2. gonorrhea.
    o 3. herpes.
    o 4. syphilis.

Both of Sammy Slater's parents carry the sickle cell anemia trait. Sammy, age 8 months, contracted chickenpox from his brother and now is very weak, febrile, anorexic, and cries with pain when his wrists and elbows are moved. He is admitted to the hospital with a diagnosis of sickle cell crisis.

72. Mrs. Slater asks the nurse why Sammy has not been symptomatic before now. The best response by the nurse would be
    o 1. high fetal hemoglobin protected Sammy against sickling.
    o 2. his red blood cell levels remained normal.
    o 3. maternal antibodies protected Sammy against sickling.
    o 4. sickle cell hemoglobin was not present until about 1 year of life.

As Sammy responds to treatment, Mrs. Slater becomes more receptive to teaching.

73. In planning care for Sammy, his mother should be taught that vaso-occlusive crises may be prevented by
    o 1. prophylactic administration of acetaminophen.
    o 2. eating food with a high iron content.
    o 3. exercising regularly.
    o 4. promoting hydration.

Mr. Richard Olson, age 74, has a 10-year history of Parkinson's disease. He is admitted to the hospital because of deterioration in his condition.

74. The symptom of Parkinson's disease that would be MOST obvious during the admission assessment is
    o 1. confusion.
    o 2. intention tremor.
    o 3. pallor.
    o 4. pill-rolling.

75. Amantadine hydrochloride (Symmetrel) is prescribed for Mr. Olson. He asks how this drug works. In formulating a response, the nurse recalls that the drug
    o 1. allows accumulation of dopamine.
    o 2. corrects mineral deficiencies.
    o 3. elevates the patient's mood.
    o 4. replaces enzymes.

76. A priority in planning care for Mr. Olson is
    o 1. positioning.
    o 2. encouraging independence.
    o 3. increasing activity.
    o 4. preventing aspiration.

77. Nursing care MOST likely to be effective in alleviating Mr. Olson's fatigue includes
    o 1. attention to his bed time.
    o 2. avoiding high-carbohydrate foods.
    o 3. collaborating with him when scheduling activities.
    o 4. morning and afternoon naps while in the hospital.

Mrs. Anna Bowen, age 28, is admitted to the psychiatric unit under an involuntary petition after a perceived suicide attempt. Mrs. Bowen cut the palmar aspect of her arm from the antecubital space to the hand. Immediately before this episode, she had flown across the country to return to her parents' home after her husband of one and a half years left her. Initially, she presented as very tearful and highly anxious. Her affect was more that of intense anger than of sadness. As the staff became more familiar with her, it became apparent that she had had many episodes of self-mutilation and would do so "So I can feel something." While Mrs. Bowen could appear quite intact most of the time, when stressed she would respond very impulsively, report hearing voices of a depreciative nature, and require a high level of observation. As the end of her hospitalization neared, she became increasingly angry, anxious, and hostile stating, "You people (the staff) are useless. You can't help anyone get better. Look at me, I'm no better than when I came in."

78. This case can best be described as fitting which of the following diagnostic categories?
    o 1. Antisocial personality disorder.
    o 2. Borderline personality disorder.
    o 3. Passive-aggressive personality disorder.
    o 4. Passive-dependent personality disorder.

79. All of the following components of a nursing history/data base are extremely important to explore with this client EXCEPT
    o 1. ego strength assessment.
    o 2. social history
    o 3. cognitive aspect of mental status exam.
    o 4. past psychiatric treatment history.

80. Should Mrs. Bowen attempt to self-mutilate while in the hospital, the best plan for the nurse to implement is
    o 1. focus on the how, when, and where of the injury.
    o 2. care for the injury and explore Mrs. Bowen's activities and feelings immediately before the episode.
    o 3. care for the injury and leave Mrs. Bowen alone for a while to let her settle down.
    o 4. care for the injury and seclude, and possibly restrain, Mrs. Bowen to prevent further injury.

81. In evaluating Mrs. Bowen as she nears discharge, the nurse would identify the major issues during this hospitalization to be all of the following EXCEPT
    o 1. cognition.
    o 2. identity.
    o 3. dealing with anger.
    o 4. separation/individuation.

Mrs. Nancy Sampson, age 46, is admitted to the hospital for a panhysterectomy.

82. Which nursing strategy should be included in the nursing care plan for Mrs. Sampson to meet her body-image perceptual changes?
    o 1. Allowing her time to work out her feelings on her own
    o 2. Discouraging fears about weight gain
    o 3. Helping her verbalize her concerns about her femininity
    o 4. Insisting that she look at the scar

Following surgery, Mrs. Sampson is placed on estrogen replacement therapy.

83. The primary purpose of estrogen replacement therapy following surgical menopause is to prevent
    o 1. arthritis.
    o 2. pregnancy.
    o 3. breast cancer.
    o 4. vasomotor instability.

The remainder of this section consists of individual questions.

84. A 1-day-old infant is admitted to the intensive care nursery. She is suspected of having esophageal atresia with a tracheo-esophageal fistula. What symptoms would indicate this?
    o 1. Bile stained vomitus and a weak cry
    o 2. Diarrhea and collicky abdominal pain
    o 3. Excessive drooling and immediate regurgitation of feedings
    o 4. Visible peristaltic waves and projectile vomiting

85. What developmental skill should the parents of a 6-month-old expect to see their child achieving?
    o 1. Language development
    o 2. Sitting alone
    o 3. Social smile
    o 4. Pulling up to a standing position

86. 10-year-old Jamie takes aspirin qid for Still's disease (juvenile rheumatoid arthritis). What symptoms would her mother observe that would be indicative of aspirin toxicity?
    o 1. Hypothermia
    o 2. Hypoventilation
    o 3. Decreased hearing acuity
    o 4. Increased urinary output

87. The Tates have one child with hemophilia. Mrs. Tate wants to have another child and she asks the nurse what her chances are of having another child with hemophilia. The nurse's best response is:
    o 1. All of your daughters will be carriers of the disease.
    o 2. If you have another son, there is almost a 100% chance he will have hemophilia.
    o 3. If you have a son, there is a 50% chance he will have hemophilia but none of your daughters will have it.
    o 4. there is a 25% chance of having another child with hemophilia.

88. A 10-year-old is being prepared for a bone marrow transplant. The nurse can assess how well he understands this treatment when he says
    o 1. I'll be much better after this blood goes to my bones.
    o 2. I won't feel too good until my body makes healthy cells.
    o 3. This will help all of the medicine they give me to work better.
    o 4. You won't have to wear a mask and gown after my transplant.

89. A 4-year-old with tetralogy of Fallot is seen in a squatting position near his bed. The nurse should
    o 1. administer oxygen.
    o 2. take no action if he looks comfortable, but continue to observe him.
    o 3. pick him up and place him in Trendelenburg's position in bed.
    o 4. have him stand up and walk around the room.

90. An autistic child will have a deficit in
    o 1. hearing.
    o 2. speech.
    o 3. vision.
    o 4. intelligence.

ANSWERS AND RATIONALES FOR PRACTICE TEST 2

ANSWER	RATIONALE	NP	CN	CL
#1 3	Up to 36 hours after surgery, the urine is expected to be pink and contain blood clots.	A	II	Ap
#2 2	Blood clots clogging the catheter will produce the sensation of needing to void. Irrigation of the catheter will remove the blood clots allowing the urine to flow freely.	An	II	An
#3 3	Food preferences are considered when planning a program to meet the patient's nutritional requirements after the nutritional assessment has been completed.	A	IV	An
#4 3	It is thought that hypogeusia (altered taste sensation) occurs when cancer cells release substances that resemble amino acids and stimulate the bitter taste buds. Spices and seasonings can mask the taste alterations that are occurring.	I	IV	Ap
#5 1	In the patient with otosclerosis, bone conduction is greater than air conduction because the fixed stapes are unable to conduct air currents to the inner ear.	A	I	An
#6 3	The patient should be taught to avoid blowing his nose because this action could increase the pressure in the eustachian tube and dislodge the surgical graft.	P	I	Ap
#7 3	Speaking at a moderate rate will allow the patient to observe the lips of the speaker and to hear normal tones.	E	I	Ap
#8 2	Aminophylline is a bronchodilator. As it exerts its effects, wheezing will decrease.	E	II	Ap
#9 4	Placing the foods in a recognizable location will foster autonomy as well as reinforce independence with ADL. Four-year-olds have not yet developed a concept of time.	I	I	Ap
#10 1	While the client has sensory overload, altered perception of events, and lacks good judgment, it is the high activity level without proper fluids, nutrition, and rest that can lead to dehydration, electrolyte imbalances, their concomitant effects, and eventual physical collapse.	An	I	An
#11 2	Someone who is in a manic state has many characteristics (increased motor activity, pacing, excitement, irritability, agitation, delusions, hypersensitivity, hyperreactivity, and provocative behaviors) that contribute to the potential for violence. It is not that the person necessarily expresses the intent to be violent towards self or others; rather, by the nature of the manic state, the person is at high risk of being violent. Maintaining the client's safety is of highest priority.	An	III	An
#12 4	Manics cannot calm down without assistance. Decreasing the level of sensory stimulation is of paramount importance and provides the greatest therapeutic effect until lithium levels are established.	I	I	Ap
#13 4	While the client's social network can influence the client in terms of compliance, the influence is typically secondary to that of the other factors presented.	E	III	An
#14 1	Frequent vomiting irritates oral mucosa and leaves the mouth very dry. The first nursing action should be aimed at preventing irritation and drying of oral mucosa by implementing oral hygiene.	I	I	Ap
#15 3	Liver contains more iron than any other food source.	E	IV	C

ANSWER		RATIONALE	NP	CN	CL
#16	4	Gastric motility is decreased in pregnancy. Food eaten several hours prior to the onset of labor may still be in the stomach undigested. This will influence the type of anethesia the patient may receive.	A	II	Ap
#17	2	The infant receiving phototherapy should have patches applied over closed eyes to prevent damage to the retina.	I	I	Ap
#18	2	The startle reflex, normally present in neonates, is characterized by symmetric extension and abduction of the arms with fingers extended. The parent perceives this response as jumping.	An	I	C
#19	3	Within 3–4 days of birth, a weight loss of 5%–10% is normal in this size baby.	A	IV	C
#20	1	Stabilization of the infant's body temperature is accomplished by keeping the baby wrapped in warm blankets and keeping the head well covered.	P	IV	Ap
#21	4	Gravity will cause the head of the femur to drop toward the bed, causing the affected knee to appear to be lower.	A	I	An
#22	2	The most frequent means of transmission of the tubercule bacillus is by droplet nuclei. The bacillus is present in the air as a result of coughing, sneezing, and expectoration by infected persons.	P	I	C
#23	4	Orange-tinged body fluids are a common side effect of rifampin.	I	I	Ap
#24	3	Any initial assessment must have an established baseline. Eliciting when the patient had her last bowel movement provides this baseline information.	A	II	Ap
#25	1	Numbness is symptomatic of circulatory or nerve impairment to the extremity. It is important to know the length of time the patient has been experiencing this sensation.	An	I	An
#26	3	A pillow placed between the patient's legs will keep the affected leg abducted and in good alignment while the patient is being turned.	E	I	Ap
#27	4	Exercise is important to keep joints and muscles functioning and to prevent secondary complications. Use of the overhead trapeze prevents hazards of immobility by permitting movement in bed and strengthening of the upper extremities in preparation for ambulation.	I	I	Ap
#28	4	Elderly females are prone to hip fractures because the cesssation of estrogen production after menopause contributes to demineralization of bone.	An	IV	An
#29	3	Because glycerin, a rapid acting osmotic diuretic, is being used to treat the patient's glaucoma, intake and output need to be monitored as a priority.	P	I	Ap
#30	1	Morphine is contraindicated for the patient with glaucoma because its pupillary action may restrict drainage of aqueous humor.	An	I	Ap
#31	1	Pilocarpine is a cholinergic agent that reduces intraocular pressure by producing miosis, thus increasing the outflow of aqueous fluid.	A	I	Ap
#32	3	There is a strong heredity factor in glaucoma and, if there is a family history of glaucoma, family members shuld have intraocular pressures measured yearly.	I	I	C
#33	2	Removal of burned clothing will cause further trauma to adhering tissue.	I	I	Ap

ANSWER		RATIONALE	NP	CN	CL
#34	3	Narcotics should be given only after careful assessment in this phase due to the danger of respiratory depression and shock.	P	II	An
#35	4	The initial fluid alteration following a burn is a plasma to interstitial fluid shift. The capillary walls become permeable and fluid is lost in significant quantities.	P	I	K
#36	2	A safe range for the hourly urine output post-burn is 30–50 cc. Less than this amount would indicate severely decreased renal arterial perfusion.	E	II	An
#37	1	Tetanus is a potential danger in burn patients and is prevented by administration of hyperimmune tetanus globulin; this treatment will not prevent or control other infections.	P	I	Ap
#38	4	The client shows many signs of classic depression as evidenced by psychomotor retardation, self-care impairment, inability to sleep, and a suicide attempt. There is no indication of mood swings or of melancholia. Typically, dysthymic disorders are chronic and nonpsychotic, whereas this is an acute and psychotic episode.	An	III	C
#39	3	While all the diagnoses listed may be appropriate for this client, the absolute priority at any time in a client's hospitalization is maintenance of the client's safety. This client is at particular risk for self-directed violence because of her recent failed suicide attempt and her obsession with what she perceives to be impending death.	An	I	An
#40	4	The key here is stabilization. While the client might be exhausted, the optimum environment would be provided by scheduling balanced periods of rest and therapeutic activity.	P	I	Ap
#41	1	In terms of adaptation, it is optimal for the client to identify the least restrictive means of achieving symptom control. Thought control methods are applicable in this situation.	I	I	An
#42	3	The strict focus on the individual's personal situation is not appropriate in group therapy. This typically occurs within an individual therapy context.	I	III	An
#43	4	Painless vaginal bleeding is symptomatic of a placenta previa. Vaginal examinations are contraindicated before 37 weeks unless done in the delivery room as a double set-up.	I	I	An
#44	3	Green amniotic fluid is indictive of hypoxia in the fetus and, in the presence of bleeding with placenta previa, may require a cesarean section.	P	I	Ap
#45	4	Family identification of the new infant is an important part of attachment. The first step in identification is defined in terms of "likeness" to family members.	E	III	An
#46	3	Lubricants applied to the skin after bathing seal in moisture and rehydrate, lubricate, and moisturize the skin.	E	I	Ap
#47	4	The patient returning from a spinal fusion should be kept flat in bed; sitting up is an unsafe behavior.	P	I	Ap
#48	2	There should be a normal response to pinprick sensation following a laminectomy.	A	I	An
#49	4	Outlining drainage on the dressing provides a quantitative measure of bleeding.	E	I	An
#50	3	The patient should think through each movement to maintain good body alignment.	E	I	Ap

ANSWER		RATIONALE	NP	CN	CL
#51	3	Any emotional or physical stress, such as a respiratory infection, may precipitate acute adrenal crisis with vascular collapse.	An	I	An
#52	2	98% of patients with Addison's disease will have skin that is bronzed in appearance due to the similarities of ACTH and melanocyte-stimulating hormone.	A	I	An
#53	3	Acute adrenal crisis can be precipitated by physical or emotional stress. Hormone replacement is necessary and the patient titrates the dose.	E	I	Ap
#54	2	Addison's disease cannot be cured but is controlled with lifelong hormonal replacement.	E	I	Ap
#55	1	Use of proverbs tests for the client's ability to abstract as well as reason.	A	III	An
#56	2	There are no data in this case summary to support a diagnosis of self-care deficit.	An	III	An
#57	3	The community mental health model is based upon the philosophy that mental health care can best be delivered within the community context and focuses on prevention. It arose in response to a perceived dehumanizing effect of mental health care institutions such as state hospitals. Thus, it would support caring for this client in a community-based setting such as partial hospitaliation, community support, or out-patient.	P	I	Ap
#58	2	The greatest motivator for this client to stay in treatment is his parents' threat to evict him from their home if he doesn't comply with the prescribed treatment program.	I	I	An
#59	1	The key to this question is "realistic, initial, client-oriented goal." It is highly unlikely that this client will be able to get to work, either on time or late, without assistance. To expect him to get to work on time every day with assistance is probably unrealistic. Because of the ambivalence that pervades much of the schizophrenic's life, this client will be hesitant to consistently accept his parent's help and to consistently accept the responsibiities of the adult role of wage earner.	E	I	An
#60	2	Rheumatic fever is an autoimmune reaction to a streptococcal infection and is limited to the person having the reaction.	An	I	C
#61	1	A major symptom of rheumatic fever is arthritis.	A	I	Ap
#62	3	The secretions visible in the tube may be partially occluding the airway and should be removed immediately.	I	II	Ap
#63	4	Observations for hemorrhage and breathing difficulties are priorities in the immediate post-op period.	An	II	An
#64	2	In the presence of multiple trauma, maintenance of a patent airway must always be the priority in the sequence of care delivery.	P	I	Ap
#65	1	Direct pressure to the wound will aid in the development of a blood clot, which is the initial step in wound healing.	I	I	Ap
#66	1	Good capillary refill indicates that the cast has not caused a circulatory problem in the extremity.	I	I	Ap
#67	2	Using the formula: amount of solution in cc / time in minutes × gtt factor, the correct rate of flow is 28 gtts/min.	E	II	Ap

ANSWER		RATIONALE	NP	CN	CL
#68	3	While pain and a change in flow rate may accompany the infiltration of IV fluids, coldness and swelling around the insertion site are the best indicators that the fluid has extravasated into the subcutaneous tissue.	E	II	An
#69	1	Correct placement of the diaphragm is accomplished best if the patient is allowed time to practice insertion of the device under professional supervision.	I	IV	Ap
#70	3	Menorrhagia is abnormally profuse or excessive menstrual flow.	A	II	K
#71	3	Genital herpes is characterized by multiple little blisters on the cervix, vagina, vulva, and buttocks that rupture and crust over in 2–6 weeks.	A	I	C
#72	1	High levels of fetal hemoglobin inhibit sickling of red cells prior to age 6 months.	An	II	C
#73	4	Promoting good hydration is a major factor in maintaining the blood viscosity needed to maximize the circulation of red blood cells. Good hydration can help to minimize the severity of symptoms should the child develop sickle cell crisis.	P	II	C
#74	4	Rhythmic flexion and contraction of the muscles cause a characteristic tremor called the pill-rolling tremor in the patient with Parkinson's disease.	A	I	Ap
#75	1	Amantadine hydrochloride (Symmetrel) is a synthetic antiviral agent with an unknown mechanism of action that allows dopamine to accumulate in extracellular or synaptic sites.	An	I	Ap
#76	4	Patients with Parkinson's disease may have extreme difficulty swallowing and are in danger of choking. Aspiration pneumonia must be prevented and is therefore the priority nursing problem.	P	I	Ap
#77	3	Scheduling activities in collaboration with the patient will allow him to proceed at his own pace and maximize his strength.	E	I	Ap
#78	2	The clustering of self-mutilation, impulsivity, transient psychosis, intense anger, and feeling empty is most typically found in the borderline personality disorder.	An	III	An
#79	3	The mental status exam is conducted when the nurse suspects the client is disoriented. Borderlines have, for the most part, intact reality testing and, if psychotic, tend to be so quite briefly and transiently. Therefore, in this case, exploring the other areas listed would be of higher priority.	A	IV	C
#80	2	A matter-of-fact approach to the injury with emphasis on the events leading to the episode of mutilation is optimally therapeutic.	P	III	Ap
#81	1	Impairments involving cognition are most commonly found in psychoses. All other responses are found in borderline personality disorders with separation/individuation being most basic.	E	IV	An
#82	3	Loss of the organs of reproduction are often equated with a loss of femininity. The care plan should include helping the patient to explore her feelings and accept body changes.	P	III	Ap
#83	4	Low-dose estrogen therapy is used to relieve the vasomotor symptoms of menopausal women.	I	IV	K

ANSWER		RATIONALE	NP	CN	CL
#84	3	In atresia of the esophagus this structure is normally closed, resulting in the formation of a blind pouch that prevents food and mucus from going to the stomach. When the pouch fills, the food is regurgitated.	A	II	C
#85	2	A 6-month-old is learning to sit alone.	E	IV	K
#86	3	Tinnitus or ringing in the ears is a side effect of aspirin therapy.	A	I	Ap
#87	3	Hemophilia is inherited as an x-linked recessive trait. If this family has another son, there is a 50% chance that he will have the disease. If they have a daughter, she will not have the disease but she will be a carrier.	P	IV	C
#88	2	The goal of a bone marrow transplant is to have the donor cells produce functioning blood cells for the patient.	An	II	An
#89	2	Squatting is a normal response to a cyanotic heart defect. This position increases pulmonary blood flow because it changes the relationship between systemic and pulmonary vascular resistance.	I	II	An
#90	2	Autistic children do not interact with others. They have echolalia (repeating the speech of others) but all other senses are normal.	An	III	C

APPENDICES

Appendix I: Special Diets

by Theresa Marie Giglio, RD, MS

EXCHANGE LISTS FOR MEAL PLANNING

Food Exchange Lists

List	Measure	Carbohydrates gm	Protein gm	Fat gm	Energy kcal
Milk, nonfat (list 1)	1 cup	12	8	trace	80
Milk, whole (list 1)	1 cup	12	8	9	160
Vegetables (list 2)	½ cup	5	2		25
Fruits (list 3)	Varies	10			40
Breads, cereals, and starchy vegetables (list 4)	Varies	15	2		70
Meat, low fat (list 5)	1 oz		7	2.5	50
Meat, medium fat (list 5)	1 oz		7.5	5	75
Meat, high fat (list 5)	1 oz		7	7.5	95
Fat (list 6)	Varies			5	45

Resource: Committees of the American Diabetes Association, Inc., and the American Diatetic Association: Exchange Lists for Meal Planning. Chicago: The American Dietetic Association and the American Diabetes Association, in cooperation with the National Institute of Arthritis, Metabolism and Digestive Diseases and the National Heart, Blood and Lung Institute, Public Health Service, U.S. Department of Health, Education and Welfare, 1976.

List 1: Milk Exchanges

Milk (nonfat, fortified)

Use only this list for diets restricted in saturated fat.

	Amount to Use
Skim or nonfat milk	1 cup
Powdered (nonfat dry)	⅓ cup
Canned, evaporated, skim	½ cup
Buttermilk made from skim milk	1 cup
Yogurt, made from skim milk, plain, unflavored	1 cup

Milk (low fat, fortified)

1% fat, fortified (omit ½ fat exchange)	1 cup
2% fat, fortified (omit 1 fat exchange)	1 cup
Yogurt made from 2% fortified, plain, unflavored (omit 1 fat exchange)	1 cup

Milk (whole)

Whole milk	1 cup
Canned evaporated	½ cup
Buttermilk made from whole milk	1 cup
Yogurt made from whole milk, plain, unflavored	1 cup

List 2: Vegetable Exchanges

One-half cup equals one exchange.

Asparagus*
Bean sprouts
Beets
Broccoli*†
Brussels sprouts*
Cabbage*
Carrots†
Celery
Cauliflower*
Cucumbers
Eggplant
Greens*†
  Beet greens
  Chard
  Collards
  Dandelion greens
  Kale
  Mustard greens
  Spinach
  Turnip greens

Mushrooms
Okra
Onions
Rhubarb
Rutabaga
Sauerkraut
String beans, green or yellow
Summer squash
Tomatoes*
Tomato juice
Turnips
Vegetable juice cocktail
Zucchini

These vegetables can be used as desired: chicory, Chinese cabbage, endive, escarole, lettuce, parsley, radishes, and watercress. *See List 4, Bread Exchanges, for starchy vegetables.*

*Good sources of ascorbic acid.
†Good sources of vitamin A.

List 3: Fruit Exchanges

	Amount to Use
Apple	1 small
Apple juice	⅓ cup
Applesauce (unsweetened)	½ cup
Apricots, fresh†	2 medium
Apricots, dried†	4 halves
Bananas	½ small
Blackberries	½ cup
Blueberries	½ cup
Raspberries	½ cup
Strawberries	¾ cup
Cherries	10 large
Cider	⅓ cup
Dates	2
Figs, fresh	1
Figs, dried	1
Grapefruit*	½
Grapefruit juice	½ cup
Grapes	12
Grape juice	¼ cup
Mango*†	½ small
Cantaloupe*	¼ small
Honeydew*	⅛ medium
Watermelon	1 cup
Nectarine	1 medium
Orange*	1 small
Orange juice*	½ cup
Papaya*†	¾ cup
Peach†	1 medium
Pear	1 small
Persimmon	1 medium
Pineapple	½ cup
Pineapple juice	⅓ cup
Plums	2 medium
Prunes	2 medium
Prune juice	¼ cup
Raisins	2 tbsp
Tangerine*	1 large

Cranberries may be used as desired if no sugar is added.

*Good sources of ascorbic acid
†Good sources of vitamin A

List 4: Bread, Cereal, and Starchy Vegetable Exchanges

	Amount to Use
Bread	
White (including French and Italian)	1 slice
Whole wheat	1 slice
Rye or pumpernickel	1 slice
Raisin	1 slice
Bagel, small	½
English muffin, small	½
Frankfurter roll	½
Hamburger bun	½
Plain roll (bread)	1
Dry bread crumbs	3 tbsp
Tortillas, 6 in	1
Cereal	
Bran flakes	½ cup
Other ready-to-eat unsweetened cereal	¾ cup
Puffed cereal, unfrosted	1 cup
Cereal, cooked	½ cup
Grits, cooked	½ cup
Rice or barley, cooked	½ cup
Pastas, cooked	½ cup
Popcorn, popped	3 cups
Cornmeal, dry	2 tbsp
Flour	2½ tbsp
Wheat germ	½ cup
Crackers	
Arrowroot	3
Graham, 2½ inch	2
Matzoh, 4 × 6 inch	½
Oyster	20
Pretzels, 3⅛ inch × ⅛ inch	15
Rye wafers, 2 × 3½ inch	3
Saltines	6
Soda, 2⅛ inch square	4
Dried Beans, Peas, and Lentils	
Dried beans, peas, and lentils cooked	½ cup
Baked beans, no pork	¼ cup
Starchy Vegetables	
Corn	⅓ cup
Corn on cob	1 small
Lima beans	½ cup
Parsnips	⅔ cup
Peas (green, fresh, canned, or frozen)	½ cup
Potato, white	1 small
Potato, mashed	½ cup
Pumpkin	¾ cup
Winter squash, acorn or butternut	½ cup
Yam or sweet potato	¼ cup
Prepared Foods	
Biscuit, 2 inch diam. (omit 1 fat exchange)	1
Cornbread, 2 × 2 × 1 inch (omit 1 fat exchange)	1
Corn muffin, 2 inch diam. (omit 1 fat exchange)	1
Crackers, round, butter type (omit 1 fat exchange)	5
Muffin, plain, small (omit, 1 fat exchange)	1
Pancake, 5 × ½ inch (omit 1 fat exchange)	1
Potatoes, French fried, 2 inch to 3½ inch (omit 1 fat exchange)	15
Waffle, 5 × ½ inch (omit 1 fat exchange)	1

List 5: Meat and Protein-Rich Exchanges

Lean Meat, Protein-Rich Exchanges

Use only this list for diets low in saturated fat and cholesterol

	Amount to Use
Beef	
Baby beef (very lean), chipped beef, chuck, flank steak, tenderloin, plate ribs, plate skirt steak, round (bottom, top), all cuts rump, spare ribs, tripe	1 oz
Lamb	
Leg, rib, sirloin, loin (roast and chops), shank, shoulder	1 oz
Pork	
Leg (whole rump, center shank), smoked ham (center slices)	1 oz
Veal	
Leg, loin, rib, shank, shoulder, cutlets	1 oz
Poultry without skin	
Chicken, turkey, Cornish hen, Guinea hen, pheasant	1 oz
Fish, any fresh or frozen	1 oz
Canned crab, lobster, mackerel, salmon, tuna	¼ cup
Clams, oysters, scallops, shrimp	5 or 1 oz
Sardines, drained	3
Cheeses containing less than 5% butterfat	1 oz
Cottage cheese: dry or 2% butter fat	¼ cup
Dried peas and beans (omit 1 bread exchange)	½ cup

Medium Fat Meat and Protein-Rich Exchanges

Beef	
Ground, 15% fat; corned beef, canned; rib eye, round, ground (commercial)	1 oz
Pork	
Loin, all cuts tenderloin, shoulder arm (picnic); shoulder blade; Boston butt; Canadian bacon; boiled ham	1 oz
Liver, heart, kidney, and sweetbreads (high in cholesterol)	1 oz
Cottage cheese, creamed	¼ cup
Cheese	
Mozzarella, ricotta, farmer's, Neufchâtel	1 oz
Parmesan	3 tbsp
Eggs (high in cholesterol)	1
Peanut butter (omit 2 fat exchanges)	2 tbsp

High-Fat Meat and Protein-Rich Exchanges

Beef brisket; corned beef brisket; ground beef (over 20% fat); hamburger (commercial); chuck, ground (commercial); rib roast, club and rib steak	1 oz
Lamb, breast	1 oz
Pork; spare ribs; loin (back ribs); pork, ground; country style ham, deviled ham	1 oz
Veal, breast	1 oz
Poultry: capon, duck (domestic), goose	1 oz
Cheese: cheddar type	1 oz
Cold cuts, 4½ × ⅛ inch	1 slice
Frankfurter	small

List 6: Fat Exchanges

For a diet low in saturated fat and higher in polyunsaturated fat, select only from this list.

	Amount to Use
Margarine: soft, tub, or stick (made with corn, cottonseed, safflower, soy, or sunflower oil)	1 tbsp
Avocado, 4 in diam.	⅛
Nuts	
Almonds*	10 whole
Peanuts*	
Spanish	20 whole
Virginia	10 whole
Pecans*	2 large, whole
Walnuts	6 small
Other nuts*	6 small
Oil, corn, cottonseed, safflower, soy, sunflower	1 tsp
Oil, olive or peanut*	1 tsp
Olives*	5 small
Salad dressings, if made with corn, cottonseed, safflower or soy oil	
French dressing	1 tbsp
Italian dressing	1 tbsp
Mayonnaise	1 tsp
Salad dressing, mayonnaise type	2 tsp

* Fat content is primarily monounsaturated

The following fats should not be used on a diet low in saturated fat.

Margarine, regular stick	1 tsp
Butter	1 tsp
Bacon fat	1 tsp
Bacon, crisp	1 strip
Cream, light	2 tbsp
Cream, sour	2 tbsp
Cream, heavy	1 tbsp
Cream cheese	1 tbsp
Lard	1 tsp
Salad dressings (permitted on restricted diets if made with allowed oils)	
French dressing	1 tbsp
Italian dressing	1 tbsp
Mayonnaise	1 tsp
Salad dressing, mayonnaise type	2 tsp
Salt pork	¾ inch cube

HIGH-FIBER DIET

Description

The diet is essentially a normal diet with increased amounts of cellulose, hemicellulose, lignin, and pectin. It increases the volume and weight of the stool; increases gastrointestinal motility; and decreases intraluminal colonic pressure in patients suffering from increased pressure.

General Characteristics

Consume a regular diet with increased fiber content

1. Include raw fruits and vegetables instead of canned or cooked ones.
2. Substitute whole grain bread and cereals for refined grains.
3. Include dried fruits, nuts, and coconut in meals.
4. Prepare soups with high-fiber vegetables.
5. Eat a fresh vegetable or fruit salad daily.
6. Add 1–2 tablespoons of bran to other foods daily.
7. Initiate the high-fiber diet gradually.

Possible Complications

1. Osmotic diarrhea.
2. Decreased serum levels of minerals, such as iron, calcium, magnesium, etc.

1500 KILOCALORIE DIET

Description

A 1500 kcal diet will permit a steady weight loss of body fat without loss of body tissue and other essential body components. The diet meets the Recommended Dietary Allowances for the adult for protein, minerals, and vitamins.

Food Preparation

Foods should be prepared without added sugar and flour, using only that amount of fat allowed in the diet. Meats may be broiled, braised, stewed, or roasted. All visible fat should be trimmed. The measure or weight of food refers to the food in its cooked form.

Diet Guidelines

Food Exchange Lists

Daily Allowance

List 1: Milk: 1 serving = 8 ounces — 2 cups

Skim milk (1% fat)
Buttermilk (1% fat)
Yogurt made from skim milk

List 2: Vegetables: 1 serving = ½ cup — 3 servings

Asparagus	Green peppers
Bean sprouts	Mushrooms
Beets	Okra
Broccoli	Onions
Brussels sprouts	Sauerkraut
Cabbage	Stringbeans
Carrots	Summer squash
Cauliflower	Tomatoes
Celery	Tomato/vegetable juice
Eggplant	Turnips
Greens	
Zucchini	

List 3: Fruits (fresh or unsweetened) — 5 servings

Small apple	12 grapes
⅓ cup apple juice	⅛ honeydew melon
2 apricots	Small orange
½ small banana	½ cup orange juice
½ cup berries	Medium peach
¾ cup strawberries	½ cup pineapple
¼ canteloupe	⅓ cup pineapple juice
10 cherries	2 plums
2 dates	2 prunes
½ grapefruit	¼ cup prune juice
½ cup grapefruit juice	1 cup watermelon
2 tbsp raisins	Medium tangerine

List 4: Bread, Cereal, Starchy Vegetables — 6 servings

1 slice bread	2 graham crackers
½ bagel	6 saltine crackers
½ English muffin	½ matzoh
½ hamburger roll	25 small pretzels (3⅛ inch long, ⅛ inch diam)
¾ cup dry cereal	3 cups popcorn
½ cup cooked cereal	½ cup pastas
½ cup rice, grits	1 small potato
½ cup peas, beans	⅓ cup corn
¼ cup baked beans	
¼ cup sweet potato	

List 5: Meat and Poultry Foods

Lean — 3 oz total or ¾ cup

1 oz beef: leg, round, chipped, rump, loin
1 oz lamb: leg, rib, loin, sirloin
veal: leg, loin, rib, cutlets
1 oz pork: leg, rump, center slice
1 oz poultry: without skin (no duck or goose)
¼ cup tuna, salmon, crab, shrimp, lobster
¼ cup dry cottage cheese

Medium Fat — 3 oz total or ¾ cup

1 oz ground beef (15% fat)
1 oz pork shoulder, boiled ham, Canadian bacon
1 oz liver
1 egg
1 oz mozzarella, ricotta, farmer's cheese
¼ cup cottage cheese

List 6: Fats — 5 servings

1 tsp butter	¾ inch cube salt pork
1 tsp margarine	1 tbsp cream cheese
1 tsp oil	2 tbsp cream
1 tbsp French dressing	1 slice crisp bacon
	1 tsp bacon fat
1 tbsp Italian dressing	5 small olives
	1 tsp mayonnaise
10 peanuts	1 tsp lard

Foods Allowed as Desired

Cucumbers, dill pickles, Chinese cabbage, endive, escarole, lettuce, parsley, radishes, bouillon, unflavored gelatin, coffee, tea, spices

1000 MILLIGRAM SODIUM-RESTRICTED DIET

Description

The aim of this diet is to promote the loss of excess sodium and water from the extracellular fluid compartents of the body. It is used primarily for patients with ascites/edema associated with advanced liver or renal disease, patients in congestive heart failure, as a treatment for essential hypertension, and with patients receiving adrenocorticosteroids.

Food Preparation

All food should be prepared without the addition of salt, regular baking powder, and baking soda. No salt should be used at the table.

General Principles

Select foods that have not been processed or preserved with large amounts of salt. Include all fruits and fruit juices, fresh, canned, frozen, dried. Use only unsalted snack foods.

Diet Guidelines

Type of Food	Allow	Avoid
Milk	Whole or skim milk Limit: 2 cups/day	Milk shakes, malted milk, commercial chocolate, or buttermilk
Eggs	Any form prepared without the addition of salt. Limit: 4/week	
Cheese	Dry cottage cheese and low-sodium American cheese	All types except those allowed
Meat, fish, poultry	Meat or poultry without added salt or sodium products. Fresh or canned fish without added salt. Unsalted peanut butter.	Lunchmeat, sausage, hot dogs, shellfish, organ meats, bacon, ham, corned beef, dried beef, canned meat, anchovies, salted canned fish, dried cod
Soups and sauces	All made with allowed milk and vegetables	Broth, bouillon, gravy, canned soup, consomme and cream sauce
Vegetables Potatoes	Fresh, frozen or canned white and sweet potatoes without added salt	Potato chips

Type of Food	Allow	Avoid
Other vegetables	Unsalted asparagus, green beans, wax beans, corn, fresh or canned lima beans, eggplant, endive, escarole, lettuce, mushrooms, fresh or canned peas, squash, tomatoes. Also, if tolerated: broccoli, Brussels sprouts, cabbage, cauliflower, turnips, onions, parsnips, radishes, rutabagas and cucumbers Following vegetables should be limited to one serving per day: beets, carrots, celery, spinach or turnips	Beet greens, kale, frozen lima beans, olives, frozen peas, pickles, sauerkraut, Swiss chard, mustard greens, dandelion greens
Cereals	Puffed rice, puffed wheat, shredded wheat, and regular cooked whole-grain or enriched cereals	All other ready-to-eat cereals. Quick cream of wheat, quick-cooking farina, hominy
Bread	Regular white, whole wheat or rye. Limit: 3 slices/day If additional bread is desired, use low-sodium bread.	All others
Crackers	Unsalted crackers	All others
Other cereal	Macaroni, spaghetti products, noodles, rice	
Fats	Unsalted butter, margarine, oil	Salted butter or margarine, salad dressings, salt pork, bacon fat

BLAND DIET

Description

This diet excludes foods that may be chemically or mechanically stimulating or irritating to the gastrointestinal tract. Small, frequent meals may be indicated.

Food Preparation

Meats may be baked, broiled, stewed, or roasted. Fruits and vegetables should be cooked or canned. Avoid meat extracts, pepper, and chili powder.

Diet Guidelines

Type of Food	Allow	Avoid
Milk	Milk, buttermilk, cocoa, milk beverages	None
Eggs	Soft cooked, hard cooked, poached, steam scrambled	Fried, deviled
Cheese	Cottage cheese cream, mild cheddar in sauces or in combination dishes	Strongly flavored cheese
Meat, fish, poultry	Tender beef, lamb, pork, liver, poultry, veal, fish, crisp bacon	Smoked, salted or fatty meat or fish
Vegetables Potatoes	Baked (without skin), boiled, creamed, escalloped, or mashed white potatoes	Sweet potatoes, fried potatoes
Other vegetables	Cooked asparagus tips, beets, carrots, peas, chopped spinach, winter squash, green beans, mushrooms, waxed beans, strained corn pudding	All others
Cereals	Cream of rice, cream of wheat, farina, cornmeal, hominy grits, strained oatmeal, cornflakes, puffed rice, Rice Krispies, Special K	Bran, whole-grain cereals
Breads	White, Italian, French, rye bread without seeds, melba toast	Whole grain breads
Crackers	Soda crackers, saltines	Graham crackers, crackers with seeds
Other cereal products	Macaroni, noodles, rice, spaghetti	

Type of Food	Allow	Avoid
Fats	Butter, margarine, cream, salad oil	All others
Fruits	Avocado, ripe bananas, canned peaches, pears, Royal Anne cherries, peeled apricots, applesauce, baked apple (no skin), all strained fruit juices	Raw fruits except avocado and bananas; berries, figs, pineapple
Desserts	Plain sugar cookies, vanilla wafers, lady fingers, angel food cake, sponge cake, plain sherbert, plain ice cream, custard, Jello, Junket, Bavarian cream, simple puddings, fruit whips	Any containing fruits, nuts or spices; pastries, pies, doughnuts
Beverages	Decaffeinated beverages	Caffeine-containing soft drinks, coffee, tea; alcohol

LOW-RESIDUE DIET

Description

The low-residue diet is low in fiber, soft in texture, and easily digested. It decreases the weight and bulk of the stool.

Food Preparation

Fruits and vegetables should be well cooked and pureed. Meats may be baked, broiled, stewed, or roasted. The meats that must be ground may be made from cooked meats that have had the gristle and excess fat removed, or ground meats may be purchased and made into patties or meatloaf. The food may be mildly seasoned.

Diet Guidelines

Type of Food	Allow	Avoid
Milk	1 pint	Any additional
Eggs	Hard cooked, soft cooked, steam scrambled, poached	All others
Cheese	Cottage, cream, mild American	All others
Meat, fish, poultry	Ground lean beef, lamb, veal, liver Sliced white meat of chicken or turkey Fish, crisp bacon Smooth peanut butter	Luncheon meats, sausages; smoked, highly seasoned or highly salted meats and fish
Vegetables Potatoes	White potato, strained sweet potato	Potato chips or fried potatoes
Other vegetables	Cooked and pureed: beets, peas, lima beans, squash, string beans, spinach, asparagus, pumpkin Whole asparagus tips and carrots cooked tender, mushrooms Tomato juice	All others
Cereals	Cream of rice, cream of wheat, farina, cornmeal, strained oatmeal, cornflakes, puffed rice, Rice Krispies, Special K	Whole-grain cereals
Breads	White bread, melba toast, zweiback	All others
Crackers	Soda crackers, saltines	All others
Other cereal products	Macaroni, noodles, refined rice, spaghetti	Whole grain rice

Type of Food	Allow	Avoid
Fats	Butter, margarine, cream, mayonnaise, salad oil, shortening	All others
Fruits	All canned or strained fruit juices. Cooked or canned applesauce, Royal Anne cherries, peeled apricots, peaches, pears, bananas, peeled baked apple	All others
Desserts	Simple puddings, ice cream, sherbert, plain cakes and cookies, flavored gelatin, custards	All others. Allowed desserts with nuts, seeds, or coconut
Beverages	Coffee, tea, Postum, Sanka, carbonated beverages, fruit juices Milk in allowed amount	All others

20 GRAM FAT-RESTRICTED DIET

Description

The 20 gm fat-restricted diet is designed for patients with an acute intolerance for fat. Lean meat is the only source of fat.
For a 40 gm fat-restricted diet, add any combination of 4 teaspoons of the following: butter, margarine, shortening oil, mayonnaise.

Diet Guidelines

Type of Food	Allow	Avoid
Yogurt, milk	Skim milk, skim milk yogurt, skim milk buttermilk	Whole milk, butter-milk, yogurt
Eggs	Egg whites only	Whole eggs and egg yolks
Cheese	Dry cottage cheese, skim milk cheese	Whole milk cheese
Meat, fish, poultry	Two 2 oz servings of 'lean beef, veal, pork, lamb, poultry, liver or fish	Corned beef, sausages, goose, duck, fish canned in oil such as sardines, tuna fish and salmon. Fried meats, fish, and poultry
Vegetables Potatoes	Sweet or white	Those prepared with fat
Other vegetables	All prepared without fat, oil or cream	Frozen vegetables in butter or cream sauces, au gratin; potato chips, casseroles
Cereals	Cooked and ready-to-eat cereals	None
Bread	White, whole wheat and rye bread Hard, water rolls, simple yeast buns	All others
Crackers	Saltine and graham	All others
Other cereal products	Macaroni, noodles, rice and spaghetti	
Fats	None	All
Fruits	Any fruit or juice	Olives, avocados
Desserts	Fruit ices and sherberts, gelatin desserts, puddings prepared with skim milk, fruit whips made with egg whites, and angel food cake	Pies, cakes, pastries, chocolate, rich desserts, ice cream, any containing nuts, whole milk, cream or butter

Type of Food	Allow	Avoid
Beverages	Coffee, tea, carbonated beverages	All beverages made with whole milk
Sauces	Tomato sauce and white sauce made with skim milk. Gravy made with fat-free broth or drippings	Gravies with fat. Cheese sauces, meat sauces, rich dessert sauces
Soups	Fat-free broth soups and creamed soups made with skim milk	Soups made with whole milk, cream or additional fat
Condiments and miscellaneous	In moderation: salt, pepper, spices, herbs, flavoring extracts	Chocolate, nuts
Sweets	Sugar, jelly, honey, jams, syrups, molasses, plain hard candy	Candy with chocolate and nuts

FAT-CONTROLLED DIET

Description

The fat-controlled diet limits foods containing cholesterol and saturated fatty acids and increases foods high in polyunsaturated fatty acids. (Cholesterol intake should be limited to 300 mg daily if diet is followed.)

Food Preparation

Only lean meats, fish, and poultry are used. The allowed vegetable oils may be used in preparing meats, fish, or poultry; used in salad dressings; or in baked products. A portion of the total fat is allowed in the form of margarine each day. Margarine labels should be read carefully to ensure that the one selected contains liquid polyunsaturated oils, preferably corn, soy, or safflower.

Diet Guidelines

Type of Food	Allow	Avoid
Milk	Yogurt made from skim milk, skim milk, skim buttermilk	Whole milk and cream; creamed buttermilk
Eggs	Three whole eggs per week; egg whites as desired	Those prepared with fats other than vegetable oils
Cheese	Dry cottage cheese, skim milk cheese	All others Whole milk cheese
Meat, fish, poultry	Lean beef, veal, lamb, and pork limited to 9 oz/week; fish, poultry without skin	Fat meats such as bacon, duck, goose, sausages, luncheon meats, frankfurters and spareribs. Glandular and organ meats, caviar and shrimp
Vegetables Potatoes	Sweet or white	Those prepared with fats other than a special margarine or vegetable oil
Other vegetables	All	None
Cereals	All	None
Bread	White or whole grain, hot breads made with vegetable oil	Breads made with other shortenings and egg yolk
Crackers	Soda and graham	All others
Other cereal	Macaroni, rice and spaghetti	Noodles made with egg

Type of Food	Allow	Avoid
Fats	Margarine (polyunsaturated), corn oil, safflower oil, soybean oil; salad dressings made with these oils	Butter, mayonnaise, cream, lard, hydrogenated vegetable shortening, olive oil, coconut oil
Fruits	All	None
Desserts	Fruit ices, gelatin, fruits, angel food cake, puddings prepared with skim milk, fruit whips made with egg whites and baked products made with allowed oils	Ice cream; sherbert; baked products made with egg yolk, shortening (other than vegetable oil) or cream Other desserts prepared with same
Beverages	Coffee, tea made with skim milk, carbonated beverages	Beverages made with whole milk or cream
Sauces	Tomato sauce and sauces made with skim milk	Gravies, meat sauces, and rich dessert sauces
Soups	Home-made fat-free soups made with allowed ingredients	Soups made with cream and whole milk
Condiments	All desired	No restrictions
Sweets	All except chocolate	Chocolate

SUMMARY OF DIETS FOR HYPERLIPOPROTEINEMIA

	Type I	Type IIa	Type IIb & Type III	Type IV	Type V
Diet pre-scription	Low fat, 25–35 gm	Low cholesterol Polyunsaturated fat increased	Low cholesterol Approximately 20% kcal protein 40% kcal fat 40% kcal CHO	Controlled CHO Approximately 45% of kcal Moderately restricted cholesterol	Restricted fat, 30% of kcal Controlled CHO, 50% of kcal Moderately restricted cholesterol
Kilocalories	Not restricted	Not restricted	Achieve and maintain "ideal" weight (reduction diet if necessary)	Achieve and maintain "ideal" weight (reduction diet if necessary)	Achieve and maintain "ideal" weight (reduction diet if necessary)
Protein	Total protein intake is not limited	Total protein intake is not limited	High protein	Not limited other than control of patient's weight	High protein
Fat	Restricted to 25–35 gm Type of fat not important	Saturated fat intake limited Polyunsaturated fat intake increased	Controlled to 40% of kcal (unsaturated fats recommended in preference to saturated fats)	Not limited other than control of patient's weight (polyunsaturated fats recommended in preference to saturated fats)	Restricted to 30% of kcal (polyunsaturated fats recommended in preference to saturated fats)
Carbohydrate	Not limited	Not limited	Controlled: concentrated sweets are restricted	Controlled: concentrated sweets are restricted	Controlled: concentrated sweets are restricted
Cholesterol	Not restricted	As low as possible; the only source of cholesterol is the meat in the diet	Less than 300 mg: the only source of cholesterol is the meat in the diet	Moderately restricted to 300–500 mg	Moderately restricted to 300–500 mg
Alcohol	Not recommended	May be used with discretion	Limited to 2 servings (substituted for carbohydrate)	Limited to 2 servings (substituted for carbohydrate)	Not recommended

From Frederickson, D., Levy, R., Jones, E., Bonnell, M., & Ernst, N. (1973). The dietary management of hyperlipoproteinemia: a handbook for physicians and dietitians. Washington, DC: Government Printing Office.

Appendix 2: Drug Administration

by Deborah L. Dalrymple, RN, CRNI, MSN

TECHNIQUES OF DRUG ADMINISTRATION

General Principles for All Medications

A. Check all new orders, expiration dates, and any orders that seem unusual.
B. Prepare medications in a quiet environment.
C. Wash your hands.
D. Collect all necessary equipment including straws, juice or water, stethoscope.
E. Read orders carefully to ensure safety: note medication, dosage, route, and frequency.
F. Be aware of drug compatibilities, drug actions, purposes, side effects, and routes (it is a nursing responsibility to know this).
G. Find medication; calculate dosage accurately.
H. Check expiration date on medication and look for any changes that may indicate decomposition (color, odor).
I. Compare label three times with the medication to decrease risk of error
    1. When removing package from drawer
    2. Before preparing medication
    3. After preparing medication.
J. Always place any removable lids open side up.
K. Be sure medications are identified for each patient.
L. Check for any allergies before administration.
M. Confirm patient's identity by checking at least two of the three possible mechanisms for identification to ensure patient safety
    1. Ask patient his name.
    2. Check patient's identi-band.
    3. Check bed tag.
N. Provide privacy if needed.
O. Inform patient of medication, any procedure technique, purpose; use time for patient teaching as applicable.
P. Stay with patient until medication is gone; do not leave medication at bedside.
Q. Assist patient as needed.
R. Give medication within 30 minutes of prescribed time.
S. Chart administration immediately in ink marking your initials in the appropriate space.
T. Circle initials and document rationale if drug not administered.
U. Report any errors immediately.
V. Observe for any reactions.
W. Observe the five "rights": give the right *dose* of the right *drug* to the right *patient* at the right *time* by the right *route*.
X. To ensure safety do not give a medication that someone else prepared.

Administration of Oral Medications

A. Use mortar and pestle to crush tablets.
B. With the exception of time-release capsules, capsule contents may be mixed with food to enhance swallowing.
C. Unless contraindicated (e.g., cough syrup) give medication with water or juice to aid in swallowing and to increase intake.
D. Prepare solid medications (tablets, capsules, etc.).
    1. All solid medications can be placed in one medicine cup unless an assessment needs to be made before administering a particular medication (e.g., blood pressure, apical pulse).
    2. To reduce chance of contamination place necessary medications into cap of container and transfer to med cup; replace lid and container.
E. Prepare liquid medications
    1. Shake liquid medications if necessary to mix.
    2. Pour away from bottle label.
    3. Read liquid amount at meniscus of med cup at eye level to ensure accuracy.
    4. If needed, a syringe may be used to measure and administer liquid medications.
    5. Wipe lip of bottle with damp towel to prevent stickiness.
    6. Replace lid and container.
F. Sit patient upright to enhance swallowing.
G. Have patient swallow medication except with the following
    1. Sublingual (SL) route: have patient place medication under tongue (high rate of absorption).
    2. Buccal route: have patient place medication between gum and cheek.
    3. Iron or HCl: have patient use straw to prevent staining teeth.
H. Stay with patient until medication is gone.
I. Special concerns
    1. Use an eye dropper to give medications to an infant.
    2. Keep infant at 45° angle.

3. See if medication is available in liquid form if patient is a child or unable to swallow solid medication.

4. If using an NG or stomach tube for medication administration, check for correct placement before administration and follow medication with water.

Administration of Rectal Drugs

A. Remove suppository from refrigerator.

B. Provide privacy.

C. Position patient to expose anus.

D. Put on glove.

E. Moisten suppository with water-soluble lubricant.

F. Insert suppository, tapered end first, approximately 2 inches (to pass internal sphincter).

G. Hold buttocks together.

H. Encourage patient to retain suppository for 10–20 minutes to allow suppository to melt.

I. If drug administered via enema, have patient retain solution 20–30 minutes.

Administration of Nasal Medications

A. Have patient blow nose to clear mucus.

B. Position patient so that head can be tilted back to aid in gravitational flow.

C. Push up on tip of nostril.

D. Place dropper or atomizer angled slightly upward just inside nostril; be careful not to touch nose with applicator.

E. Squeeze atomizer quickly and firmly or instill correct number of drops.

F. Remind patient to keep head tilted for 5 minutes.

G. Inform patient the drops may produce an unpleasant taste.

H. Leave tissues with patient; instruct just to wipe nose, not blow, to allow for absorption.

I. Special concerns
  1. If patient aspirates and begins to cough, sit patient upright, stay until patient's distress is relieved.
  2. If patient is an infant, lie on back.

Administration of Inhalants

A. Have patient inhale and exhale deeply.

B. Have patient place lips around mouthpiece and inhale medication until lungs are fully inflated.

C. Have patient remove mouthpiece, hold breath as long as able, and then exhale completely.

D. If necessary, repeat procedure until medication is gone.

E. Wash mouthpiece with warm water.

F. Special concerns
  1. Monitor vital signs before and after treatment.
  2. Have tissues handy; encourage expectoration of sputum.
  3. Be sure patient is aware that coughing is expected after treatment.

Administration of Ophthalmic Medications

A. Check solution for color and clarity before administering.

B. Warm solution in hands before administration.

C. Have patient lie on back with head turned to affected side to aid in gravitational flow.

D. Cleanse eyelid and eyelashes with sterile gauze pad soaked with physiologic saline.

E. Have patient look up.

F. Assist patient in keeping eye open by pulling down on cheekbone with thumb or forefinger and pulling up on eyelid. Be sure lower conjunctiva is exposed.

G. Place necessary number of drops into lower conjunctiva near outer canthus (less sensitive than cornea).

H. If using ointment, squeeze into lower conjunctiva moving from inner to outer canthus; do not touch eye with applicator.

I. Have patient blink 2–3 times.

J. Wipe away any excess medication starting from inner canthus.

K. Repeat if necessary using clean tissue.

L. Special concerns
  1. Ophthalmic medications are for individual patients; droppers and ointment should not be shared.
  2. Restrain infants and children if necessary.

Administration of Otic Medications

A. Warm medication in hands prior to administration.

B. Have patient turn to unaffected side to aid gravitational flow.

C. Clean outer ear using a wet gauze pad.

D. Straighten ear canal by pulling pinna up and back for adults, or down and back for infants and children.

E. Instill necessary number of drops along side of canal without touching ear with dropper.

F. Maintain position of ear until medication has totally entered canal.

G. Have patient remain on side for 5–10 minutes to allow medication to reach inner ear.

H. Cotton may be used to keep medication in canal, but only if it is premoistened with medication.

I. Repeat procedure for other ear if necessary.

J. Special concern: restrain infants and children if necessary.

Administration of Topical Agents

A. Provide privacy to promote comfort.

B. Cleanse area of old medications using gauze pads with soap and warm water.

C. Use gloves and sterile tongue depressor or sterile gloves.

D. Assess area for any changes.

E. Spread medication over site evenly.

F. If necessary, cover area loosely with a dressing.

G. Special concerns
  1. Patients often receive topical agents for image-altering problems. Applying the medication offers a good opportunity to talk about these problems and to share information about improvements.
  2. When applying nitroglycerin ointment, take patient's blood pressure 5 minutes before and after application.
  3. Wash hands after administration to prevent self-absorption.

Administration of Vaginal Medications

A. Provide privacy.

B. Have patient void.

C. Place patient in dorsal recumbent position on a bedpan.

D. Cleanse perineum with warm, soapy water working from outer to inner position.

E. Moisten applicator tip with water-soluble lubricant.

F. Separate labia to insert applicator approximately 2 inches, angled downward.

G. Instill medication.

H. If giving douche, dry patient's buttocks; otherwise have patient remain in position approximately l5–20 minutes (there is no sphincter to hold suppository in place).

I. Wash applicator with warm, soapy water.

J. Provide patient with pads if needed.

Administration of Parenteral Medications

General Principles

A. Select appropriate needle size and syringe.

B. When medication comes in a vial, cleanse rubber stopper with alcohol pledget.

C. Without contaminating plunger draw up air equal to the amount of medication needed.

D. Inject the air into the vial to prevent negative pressure and aid in aspirating medication.

E. Remove the appropriate amount of medication.

F. Check to ensure no air bubbles are present; if bubbles are a problem, draw up slightly more medication than is needed, return all medication to vial, and withdraw medication again.

G. When using an ampule: tap neck to force medication into ampule, wrap neck with alcohol pledget, snap off top, place needle into ampule to withdraw medication.

H. When mixing a powder, use a filter needle when drawing up medication.

I. Replace protective cover before proceeding.

J. Select appropriate site, avoiding bruised or tender areas; rotate sites as much as possible.

K. Cleanse site with alcohol pledget to decrease contamination.

L. Insert needle quickly with bevel up and release hold (to decrease pain).

    1. With the exception of heparin, aspirate to check for blood.

    2. If blood present, remove needle and start again.

    3. When giving medications IV, a blood return is desired.

M. Inject medication slowly.

N. Place alcohol pledget over site with gentle pressure.

O. Remove needle and massage area; do not massage area if giving heparin.

P. Dispose of syringe in appropriate manner.

Q. Record site when documenting medication administration to assist in site rotation and avoid tissue atrophy.

Subcutaneous (SC) Administration

A. Use size 25 g to 27 g, $\frac{1}{2}$–1 inch needle.

B. Pinch skin to form SC fold.

C. Insert needle at 45° angle (to avoid entering muscle)—for insulin, see pg. 175.

D. Possible sites

    1. Outer aspect of upper arm

    2. Anterior thigh

    3. Abdomen: 1 inch away from umbilicus

Hypodermoclysis

A. A method of giving large volume solutions SC at a slow rate.

B. Reserved for patients unable to receive fluids IV.

Intradermal Administration

A. Use size 25 g, 1 inch needle.

B. Stretch skin taut.

C. Insert needle at 10° angle.

D. Possible sites

    1. Ventral forearm

    2. Scapula

    3. Upper chest

E. When wheal appears, remove needle; do not massage site.

Intramuscular (IM) Administration

A. Use size l8 g to 23 g, 1–2 inch needle.

B. Stretch skin taut.

C. Insert needle at 90° angle.

D. Possible sites

    1. Gluteus minimus: landmarks are anterior superior iliac spine, iliac crest, greater trochanter of femur

    2. Vastus lateralis (anterior thigh): a hand breadth above the knee and below greater trochanter; good site for children

    3. Rectus femoris (medial thigh): a hand breadth above knee and below greater trochanter; good site for infants and self-injection

    4. Gluteus medius: landmarks are posterior superior iliac spine, iliac crest, greater trochanter of femur

    5. Deltoid: landmarks are acromium process, axilla base; for small doses only

E. Z-track injection (IM variation)

    1. Needle size: replace needle used to draw up medication with one 3 inches long.

    2. Pull skin away from site laterally to ensure medication enters muscle.

    3. Wait 10 seconds after injecting medication before withdrawing needle.

    4. Release skin; do not massage (seals needle track).

    5. Encourage physical activity.

    6. Possible sites: gluteus medius best, but may use any IM site except deltoid

Administration of Intravenous (IV) Medications

A. General principles

    1. Check site for complications (redness, swelling, tenderness).

    2. Check for blood return in syringe.

    3. Prepare medication according to manufacturers' specifications.

B. *Intermittent therapy (also known as heparin well, male adaptor, capped jelco, or heparin lock)*

1. Swab injection port with alcohol at each step
2. Use SASH method to give medication
   a. S: flush with 2 cc saline
   b. A: administer medication at prescribed rate using a short needle with a gauge equal to or smaller than catheter (25 g ½ in)
   c. S: flush with 2 cc saline
   d. H: flush with 10–100 units heparin depending on hospital policy

C. *Secondary piggyback/add-a-line* (added to an existing IV line) (Figure A.1)

1. With Flotrol turned off, spike tubing into IV bag with medication.
2. Squeeze drip chamber: fill half way with solution.
3. Run fluid through tubing.
4. If using add-a-line tubing, lower main IV bag on hanger provided.
5. Swab most proximal port with alcohol.
6. Attach 20 g 1 inch needle to tubing, if needed.
7. Insert needle into injection port.
8. Regulate rate with control and watch to count drops.
9. When medication absorbed, main line will start to drip again.
10. Turn off secondary tubing.
11. Return main bag to original position.
12. Special concerns
    a. Be sure to label tubing with date.
    b. Use new tubing every 24 hours (or according to institution policy).

D. Sites

1. Peripheral: jugular, basilic, cephalic, brachial veins
2. Alternatives: Hickman, double- or triple-lumen catheters; subclavian line; subcutaneous ports

MEDICATION CALCULATIONS

Conversions

Conversions need to be made within systems (from one measurement to another) and also among systems (from apothecary to metric or household to metric).

Conversions Within Systems

A. Metric system

1. Based on decimal system, basic unit is 10.
2. Units of measurement are

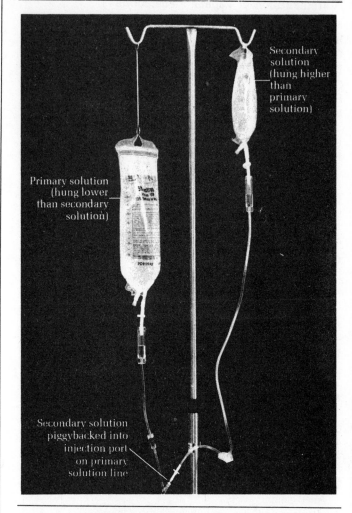

Figure A.1 Piggyback infusion.
(From "Manual for IV Therapy Procedures" 2nd ed., (p. 90) by S. Channell, 1985. Oradell, NJ: Medical Economics. Copyright ©1985 by Medical Economics Company, Inc. Reprinted by permission.)

a. Meter (m) for length
b. Gram (gm) for weight
c. Liter (l or L) for volume.

3. Multiples and fractions of 10 are identified by prefixes (Figure A.2).
   a. 0.001 liter would then be equal to 1 milliliter (ml).
   b. 1000 grams would be equal to a kilogram (kg).

	Multiples			Measure				Factions		Micro
Decimal Metric	1000 Thousands Kilo-	100 Hundreds Hecto-	10 Tens Deka-	L G M	0.1 Tenths Deci-	0.01 Hundredths Cent-	0.001 Thousandths Milli-	.000001 millionth Micro		

Figure A.2 Metric prefixes denoting multiples and fractions of 10.
(Adapted from "How to Calculate Drug Dosages" (p. 18) by A. Pecherer and S. Vertuno, 1978. Oradell, NJ: Medical Economics.)

4. Commonly used terms of weight include kilogram, gram, milligram, and microgram.
5. Commonly used terms of volume include liter and milliliter. *Note:* a cube measuring 1 cm per side holds one milliliter, so a cubic centimeter (cc) equals a milliliter (ml): *1 cc = 1 ml.*
6. To convert within the metric system, set up a ratio with the conversion factor on the right and the desired information on the left, cross multiply, divide to find X, and complete needed math. Remember to keep ratios equal: whatever is done to one side must be done to the other.
7. Example: convert 5000 mg to gm
   a. 1000 mg = 1 gm
   b. $\dfrac{5000 \text{ mg}}{X} = \dfrac{1000 \text{ mg}}{1 \text{ gm}}$
   c. (X) (1000 mg) = (5000 mg) (1 gm)
   d. $\dfrac{(X) (\cancel{1000 \text{ mg}})}{\cancel{1000 \text{ mg}}} = \dfrac{(\cancel{5000}^{\,5} \text{ mg}) (\text{gm})}{\cancel{1000 \text{ mg}}}$
   e. X = (5) (1 gm)
   f. X = 5 gm
   g. 5000 mg = 5 gm

B. Apothecary system
1. Based on arbitrary measure
2. Basic unit of weight is a grain (gr), basic unit of volume is minim (m or min) (Table A.1).
3. Small Roman numerals are often used to identify drug dosages (gr xvi = 16 grains) as are fractions ($\frac{1}{3}$ gr); $\overline{ss}$ is abbreviation for $\frac{1}{2}$ and is used with Roman numerals ($\overline{vss}$ = 5$\frac{1}{2}$).
4. Grain is only common term for weight.
5. Common terms for volume include minim, fluidram (f ʒ), fluid ounce (f ʒ), pints (pt), quarts (qt), and gallons (gal).
6. Conversions within the apothecary system are made the same way as conversions within the metric system
7. Example: convert 360 min to fluidrams
   a. 60 min = 1 f ʒ
   b. $\dfrac{360 \text{ min}}{X} = \dfrac{60 \text{ min}}{1 \text{ f ʒ}}$
   c. (60 min) (X) = (360 min) (1 f ʒ)
   d. $\dfrac{(\cancel{60 \text{ min}}) (X)}{\cancel{60 \text{ min}}} = \dfrac{(\cancel{360}^{\,6} \text{ min}) (1 \text{ f ʒ})}{\cancel{60 \text{ min}}}$
   e. X = 6 f ʒ

Table A.1 Apothecary units of weight and volume

Weight	Volume
60 grains (gr) = 1 dram (ʒ)	60 minims
8ʒ = 1 ounce (℥)	(m or min) = 1 fluidram (fʒ)
12ʒ = 1 pound (lb)	8 fʒ = 1 fluidounce (f℥)
	16 f℥ = 1 pint (pt)
	2 pt = 1 quart (qt)
	4 qt = 1 gallon (gal)

(Adapted from "How to Calculate Drug Dosages" by A. Pecherer and S. Vertuno, 1978, Oradell, NJ: Medical Economics.)

Table A.2 Household units of liquid measure

60 drops (gtts)	= 1 teaspoon (tsp)
3 tsp	= 1 tablespoon (tbsp)
6 tsp	= 1 ounce (oz)
2 tbsp	= 1 oz
6 oz	= 1 teacup
8 oz	= 1 glass
8 oz	= 1 measuring cup

(Adapted from "How to Calculate Drug Dosages" by A. Pecherer and S. Vertuno, 1978, Oradell, NJ: Medical Economics.)

C. Household system
1. Approximate measures that vary according to manufacturer, temperature.
2. Common units include teaspoon (tsp), tablespoon (tbsp), ounce (oz), cup, and drop (Table A.2).
3. Conversions within the system are the same.
4. Example: convert 3 tsp to drops
   a. 60 drops = 1 tsp
   b. $\dfrac{3 \text{ tsp}}{X} = \dfrac{1 \text{ tsp}}{60 \text{ gtts}}$
   c. (1 tsp) (X) = (3 tsp) (60 gtts)
   d. $\dfrac{(\cancel{1 \text{ tsp}}) (X)}{\cancel{1 \text{ tsp}}} = \dfrac{(\cancel{3 \text{ tsp}})^{3} (60 \text{ gtts})}{\cancel{1 \text{ tsp}}}$
   e. X = 180 gtts

Conversions From One System to Another

A. Conversions are done in the same manner. Some of the equivalents must be memorized (Table A.3).
B. Example: convert 90 gtts to cc
   1. 15 gtts = 1 cc
   2. $\dfrac{90 \text{ gtts}}{X} = \dfrac{15 \text{ gtts}}{1 \text{ cc}}$
   3. (15 gtts (X) = (90 gtts) (1 cc)
   4. $\dfrac{(\cancel{15 \text{ gtts}}) (X)}{\cancel{15 \text{ gtts}}} = \dfrac{(\cancel{90 \text{ gtts}})^{6} (1 \text{ cc})}{\cancel{15 \text{ gtts}}}$
   5. X = 6 cc

Table A.3 Approximate equivalents to remember

Household	Apothecary	Metric
1 drop (gt)	= 1 minim (m or min)	= .06 milliliter (ml)
15 drops (gtts)	= 15 min	= 1 ml [1 cc]
1 teaspoon (tsp)	= 1 fluidram (fʒ) [60 min]	= 5 (4) ml
1 tablespoon (tbsp)	= 4 fʒ	= 15 ml
2 tbsp.	= 1 fluidounce (f℥)	= 30 ml
1 ounce (oz)	= 1 f℥	= 30 ml
1 teacup	= 6 f℥	= 180 ml
1 glass	= 8 f℥	= 240 ml
1 measuring cup	= 8 f℥	= 240 ml
2 measuring cups	= 1 pint (pt)	= 500 ml

(Adapted from "How to Calculate Drug Dosages" by A. Pecherer and S. Vertuno, 1978, Oradell, NJ: Medical Economics.)

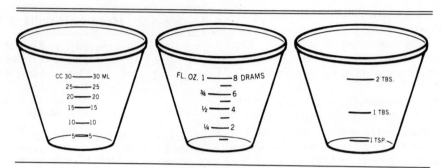

Figure A.3 Disposable medicine containers.
(From "How to Calculate Drug Dosages" (p. 40) by A. Pecherer and S. Vertuno, 1978. Oradell, NJ: Medical Economics.)

Dosage Calculations

A. Calibrated containers are available for oral liquids (Figure A.3) and liquid injectables (Figure A.4).

B. Formula for calculations

$$\frac{\text{desired amount of drug}}{\text{amount of drug on hand}} = \frac{\text{unknown quantity needed (X)}}{\text{known quantity of drug}}$$

C. Be sure all conversions are done first. The technique of using ratios is the same.

Technique

A. Dosage calculation for scored tablet
  1. 30 gr of a drug is ordered; it is available in scored tablets, 4 gm per tablet.
  2. Calculations
    a. 15 gr = 1 gm
    b. $\dfrac{30\,\text{gr}}{X} = \dfrac{15\,\text{gr}}{1\,\text{gm}}$
    c. (15 gr) (X) = (30 gr) (1 gm)
    d. $\dfrac{(15\,\text{gr})}{15\,\text{gr}} = \dfrac{(30\,\text{gr})\,(1\,\text{gm})}{15\,\text{gr}}$
    e. X = 2 gm
    f. Desired amount of drug is 2 gm; amount of drug on hand is 4 gm.
    g. Unknown quantity is X; known quantity is 1 tablet
      1) $\dfrac{2\,\text{gm}}{4\,\text{gm}} = \dfrac{X}{1\,\text{tablet}}$
      2) (4 gm) (X) = (2 gm) (1 tab)
      3) $\dfrac{(4\,\text{gm})\,(X)}{4\,\text{gm}} = \dfrac{(2\,\text{gm})\,(1\,\text{tab})}{4\,\text{gm}_2}$
      4) X = .5 tablet
  3. Give ½ tablet.
B. Dosage calculation for liquid
  1. The order is for potassium chloride (KCl) 20 mEq. The bottle is labeled KCl elixir 10 mEq/cc. How many cc will be given?
    a. Desired amount of drug is 20 mEq; amount of drug on hand is 10 mEq.

b. Unknown quantity is X; known quantity of drug on hand is 1 cc.
  2. Calculations
    a. $\dfrac{20\,\text{mEq}}{10\,\text{mEq}} = \dfrac{X}{1\,\text{cc}}$
    b. (10 mEq) (X) = (20 mEq) (1 cc)
    c. $\dfrac{(10\,\text{mEq})\,(X)}{10\,\text{mEq}} = \dfrac{(20\,\text{mEq})^2\,(1\,\text{cc})}{10\,\text{mEq}}$
    d. X = 2 cc
  3. Give 2 cc potassium chloride.
C. Dosage calculation for a capsule
  1. The order is for Nembutal gr $\overline{\text{iss}}$. The bottle contains Nembutal 100 mg/capsule. How many capsules will be given?
  2. Calculations
    a. First, convert to equal measurements
      1) 1 gr = 60 mg
      2) $\dfrac{1\,\text{gr}}{60\,\text{mg}} = \dfrac{1.5\,\text{gr}}{X}$
      3) (X) (1 gr) = (60 mg) (1.5 gr)
      4) $\dfrac{(X)\,(1\,\text{gr})}{1\,\text{gr}} = \dfrac{(60\,\text{mg})\,(1.5\,\text{gr})^{1.5}}{1\,\text{gr}}$
      5) X = 90 mg
    b. Desired amount of drug is 90 mg; amount of drug on hand is 100 mg
    c. Unknown quantity is X; known quantity on hand is 1 capsule
    d. Now you can calculate dosage
      1) $\dfrac{90\,\text{mg}}{100\,\text{mg}} = \dfrac{X}{1\,\text{capsule}}$
      2) (100 mg) (X) = (90 mg) (1 capsule)
      3) $\dfrac{(100\,\text{mg})\,(X)}{100\,\text{mg}} = \dfrac{(90\,\text{mg})^9\,(1\,\text{capsule})}{100\,\text{mg}}$
      4) X = .9 capsule
  3. Since part of a capsule, drop, or suppository cannot be given, give 1 capsule.
D. Dosage calculation for parenteral medications
  1. The order reads codeine gr $\overline{\text{ss}}$. The vial reads codeine

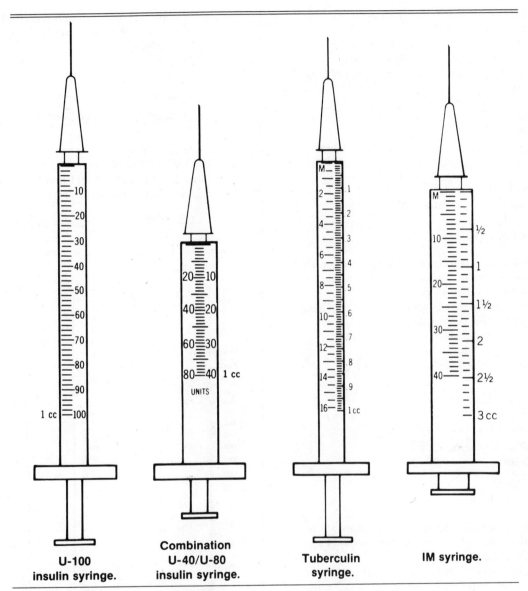

U-100
insulin syringe.

Combination
U-40/U-80
insulin syringe.

Tuberculin
syringe.

IM syringe.

Figure A.4 Different types of syringes.
*(From "How to Calculate Drug Dosages" (p. 45) by A. Pecherer and S. Vertuno, 1978.
Oradell, NJ: Medical Economics.)*

60 mg/cc. How many cc should be given?

2. Calculations

   a. First, convert to like units of measure

      1) 60 mg = 1 gr

      2) $\dfrac{60\,mg}{X} = \dfrac{60\,mg}{1\,gr}$

      3) (60 mg) (X) = (60 mg)(1 gr)

      4) $\dfrac{(60\,mg)\,(X)}{60\,mg} = \dfrac{(60\,mg)\,(1\,gr)}{60\,mg}$

      5) X = 1 gr

   b. Desired amount of drug is .5 gr; amount on hand is 1 gr.

   c. Unknown quantity is X; known quantity on hand is 1 cc.

   d. Then calculate dosage

      1) $\dfrac{.5\,gr}{1\,gr} = \dfrac{X}{1\,cc}$

      2) (X) (1 gr) = (.5 gr) (1 cc)

      3) $\dfrac{(X)\,(1\,gr)}{1\,gr} = \dfrac{.5\;(.5\,gr)\,(1\,cc)}{1\,gr}$

      4) X = .5 cc

3. Give .5 cc codeine.

E. Dosage calculation for units (some medications such as heparin and penicillin are ordered in units)
1. The order is penicillin 750,000 u. The vial reads 300,000 u/2 cc. How many cc will be given?
2. Desired amount of drug is 750,000 u; amount of drug on hand is 300,000 u.
3. Unknown quantity is X; known quantity is 2 cc.
4. Calculations
   a. $\dfrac{750,000\,u}{300,000\,u} = \dfrac{X}{2\,cc}$
   b. $(300,000\,u)\,(X) = (750,000\,u)\,(2\,cc)$
   c. $\dfrac{(300,000\,u)\,(X)}{300,000\,u} = \dfrac{(750,000\,u)\,(2\,cc)}{300,000\,u}$
   d. $X = 5\,cc$
5. Give 5 cc penicillin.

F. Dosage calculation for powders that need to be reconstituted by adding sterile water or normal saline solution (the total amount of solution is used for calculations)
1. Mefoxin 1.0 gm is ordered; mefoxin 2.0 gm is on hand. Add 4.3 cc to equal 5 cc solution.
2. Desired amount of drug is 1.0 gm; amount of drug on hand is 2.0 gm.
3. Unknown quantity is X; known quantity is 5 cc.
4. Calculations
   a. $\dfrac{1.0\,gm}{2.0\,gm} = \dfrac{X}{5\,cc}$
   b. $(2.0\,gm)\,(X) = (5\,cc)\,(1.0\,gm)$
   c. $\dfrac{(2.0\,gm)\,(X)}{2.0\,gm} = \dfrac{(5\,cc)\,(1.0\,gm)}{2.0\,gm}$
   d. $X = 2.5\,cc$
5. Give 2.5 cc mefoxin.

G. Dosage calculation in children (pediatric dosages)
1. Body surface area (BSA): most accurate method for calculating pediatric dosages.
   a. *West nomogram* (Figure A.5) if BSA is not known: draw a line from height on the nomogram; the point of intersection on surface area is the BSA.
   b. Formula for surface area (m²)
      $$\frac{surface\ area\ (m^2)}{1.73\,m^2} \times adult\ dose = X$$
   c. Example of calculating a pediatric dosage using BSA
      1) the adult dose is 100 mg Demerol; the child weighs 20 kg and is 40 inches tall.
      2) BSA is .77 m²
      3) Calculations
         a) $\dfrac{.77\,m^2}{1.73\,m^2} \times 100\,mg = X$
         b) $0.45 \times 100\,mg = X$
         c) $45\,mg = X$
      4) Child's dose is 45 mg.
2. Pediatric dosages may also be calculated by weight (mg/kg)

a. Example: the order is for phenobarbital 20 mg/kg of body weight; the patient weighs 25 kg.
b. Calculations
   1) $\dfrac{2\,mg}{X} = \dfrac{1\,kg}{25\,kg}$
   2) $(1\,kg)\,(X) = (2\,mg)\,(25\,kg)$
   3) $\dfrac{(1\,kg)\,(X)}{1\,kg} = \dfrac{(2\,mg)\,(25\,kg)}{1\,kg}$
   4) $X = 50\,mg$
c. Give 50 mg of phenobarbital.
3. Other, less frequently used, formulas include
   a. Fried's rule (birth to 12 months)
      $$\frac{age\ in\ months}{150} \times adult\ dose = infant's\ dose$$

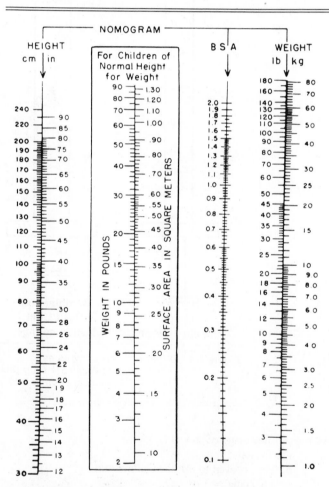

Body surface area (BSA) is determined by drawing a straight line from the patient's height in the far left column to his or her weight in the far right column. Intersection of the line with the surface area (SA) column is the estimated BSA. For infants and children of normal height for weight, BSA may be estimated from weight alone by referring to the enclosed area.

Figure A.5 West's nomogram for estimating body surface area.

b. Young's rule (1–12 years)

$$\frac{\text{age in years}}{\text{age in years} + 12} \times \text{adult dose} = \text{child's dose}$$

c. Clark's rule

$$\frac{\text{weight of child in lb}}{150 \text{ lb}} \times \text{adult dose} = \text{child's dose}$$

H. Dosage calculation for IV medications

1. In order to calculate the flow rate, need to know drop factor: 10, 15, or 20 gtts/cc depending on manufacturer.
2. Microdrop drop factor is always 60 gtts/cc.
3. Formula for calculation

$$\frac{\text{amount of solution in cc}}{\text{time in minutes}} \times \text{drop factor}\left(\frac{\text{gtts}}{\text{cc}}\right) = \text{gtts/minute}$$

4. Example: the order is for 1000 cc NSS over 8 hours; drop factor is 10 gtts/cc.
5. Calculation

   a. $\dfrac{1000 \text{ cc}}{480 \text{ min}} \times \dfrac{10 \text{ gtts}}{\text{cc}} = X$

   b. $\dfrac{1000 \text{ cc}}{480 \text{ min}} \times \dfrac{10 \text{ gtts}}{\text{cc}} = X$ *48*

   c. $\dfrac{1000 \text{ gtts}}{48 \text{ min}} = 20.8$

   d. X = 20.8 gtts/min

6. A partial drop cannot be given so run IV at 21 gtts/min.
7. The same formula can be used for IVs requiring microdrop rates, or the following formula can be used

cc/hour = microdrops/min

This formula works because the drop factor for microdrop tubing is always 60 microgtts/cc and an hour is 60 minutes.

   a. Example: order is for 1000 cc D₅NS over 24 hours. Drop factor is 60 gtts/cc.

   b. Calculation with the first formula

    1) $\dfrac{1000 \text{ cc}}{1440 \text{ min}} \times \dfrac{60 \text{ gtts}}{\text{cc}} = X$

    2) $\dfrac{1000 \text{ cc}}{1440 \text{ min}} \times \dfrac{60 \text{ gtts}}{\text{cc}} = X$

    3) X = 41.66

   c. Cannot give a partial drop, so rate is 42 gtts/min.

   d. Calculation with the second formula

    1) first determine the cc/hour: $\dfrac{\text{total volume}}{\text{total hours}}$

    2) $\dfrac{1000 \text{ cc}}{24 \text{ hours}} = 42 \text{ cc/hour} = 42 \text{ gtts/min}$

8. Readjusting IV rates may be necessary when the rate for an existing IV is changed

   a. Formula for calculation

$$\frac{\text{amount of solution remaining}}{\text{remaining hours in minutes}} \times \text{drop factor}$$

   b. Example: the order is to infuse remaining 700 cc over 3 hours; drop factor is 15 gtts/cc.

   c. Calculation

    1) $\dfrac{700 \text{ cc}}{180 \text{ min}} = \dfrac{15 \text{ gtts}}{\text{cc}} = X$

    2) $\dfrac{700 \text{ cc}}{180 \text{ min}} = \dfrac{15 \text{ gtts}}{\text{cc}} = X$ *12*

    3) $\dfrac{700 \text{ gtts}}{12 \text{ min}} = 58.3 \text{ gtts/min}$

   d. Cannot give partial drop, so run IV at 58 gtts/min.

PRACTICE PROBLEMS

1. The order is dilaudid gr 1/8. The bottle reads dilaudid 15 mg/tablet. Give _____ tablet.
2. The order is chloral hydrate 250 mg. The bottle reads chloral hydrate 0.1 gm/capsule. Give _____ capsules
3. The order is penicillin 50,000 u. The vial reads penicillin 500,000 u. Add 4.3 cc to yield 5 cc. Give _____ cc.
4. The order is ampicillin .4 mg/kg. Patient weighs 38.5 pounds. The bottle reads ampicillin 10 mg/ml. Give _____ cc.
5. The adult dose is Dilantin 150 mg. Give _____ mg to a 6-year-old child.
6. Average adult dose is 200 mg. What is dose for a 4-year-old weighing 40 kg and 100 cm tall?
7. Order is for 2500 cc D₅W over 24 hours. Drop 5 factor is 15 gtts/cc. Run IV at _____ gtts/minute.
8. Order is for 2000 cc D₅W over 24 hours. Drop 5 factor is 60 gtts/cc. Run IV at _____ gtts/minute.
9. Average adult dose is 250 mg. What is dose for 12-month-old infant?
10. Average adult dose is 500 mg. What is dose for 30 lb child?

ANSWERS

1. $\frac{1}{2}$ tablet
2. 3 capsules
3. 0.5 cc
4. 0.7 cc
5. 50 mg
6. 129 mg
7. 26 gtts/min
8. 83 gtts/min
9. 20 mg
10. 100 mg

REFERENCES AND RECOMMENDED READINGS

Gordon, M. (1984). Clinical calculations for nurses. Englewood Cliffs, NJ: Prentice Hall.

McConnell, E. (1986). The subtle art of really good injections. *RN, 45*(2), 25–35.

Pecherer, A., & Vertuno, S. (1978). How to calculate drug dosages. Oradell, NJ: Medical Economics.

Perry, A., & Potter, P. (1986). Clinical nursing skills and techniques. Princeton: Mosby.

Wieck, L.; King, E.; & Dyer, M. (1986). Illustrated manual of nursing techniques (3rd ed.). Philadelphia: Lippincott.

Appendix 3: Standards and Ethics

STANDARDS OF NURSING PRACTICE*

Nursing practice is a direct service, goal directed and adaptable to the needs of the individual, family and community during health and illness. Professional practitioners of nursing bear primary responsibility and accountability for the nursing care clients/patients receive. The purpose of Standards of Nursing Practice is to fulfill the profession's obligation to provide and improve this practice.

The Standards focus on practice. They provide a means for determining the quality of nursing which a client/patient receives regardless of whether such services are provided solely by a professional nurse or by a professional nurse and nonprofessional assistants.

The Standards are stated according to a systematic approach to nursing practice: the assessment of the client's/patient's status, the plan of nursing actions, the implementation of the plan, and the evaluation. These specific divisions are not intended to imply that practice consists of a series of discrete steps, taken in strict sequence, beginning with assessment and ending with evaluation. The processes described are used concurrently and recurrently. Assessment, for example, frequently continues during implementation; similarly, evaluation dictates reassessment and replanning.

These Standards for Nursing Practice apply to nursing practice in any setting. Nursing practice in all settings must possess the characteristics identified by these Standards if clients/patients are to receive a high quality of nursing care. Each Standard is followed by a rationale and assessment factors. Assessment factors are to be used in determining achievement of the standard.

STANDARD I

The collection of data about the health status of the client/patient is systematic and continuous. The data are accessible, communicated, and recorded.

Rationale:

Comprehensive care requires complete and ongoing collection of data about the client/patient. All health status data about the client/patient must be available for all members of the health care team.

Assessment Factors

1. Health status data include:
   - Growth and development
   - Biophysical status
   - Emotional status
   - Cultural, religious, socioeconomic background
   - Performance of activities of daily living
   - Patterns of coping
   - Interaction patterns
   - Client's/patient's perception of and satisfaction with his health status
   - Client/patient health goals
   - Environment (physical, social, emotional, ecological)
   - Available and accessible human and material resources
2. Data are collected from:
   - Patient/client
   - Health care personnel
   - Individuals within the immediate environment and/or the community
3. Data are obtained by:
   - Interview
   - Examination
   - Observation
   - Reading records, reports, etc.
4. There is a format for the collection of data which:
   - Provides for a systematic collection of data
   - Facilitates the completeness of data collection
5. Continuous collection of data is evident by:
   - Frequent updating
   - Recording of changes in health status
6. The data are
   - Accessible on the client/patient records
   - Retrievable from record-keeping systems
   - Confidential when appropriate

STANDARD II

Nursing diagnoses are derived from health status data.

*Reprinted with permission from *Standards of Nursing Practice,* © 1973, Kansas City, American Nurses' Association.

Rationale:

The health status of the client/patient is the basis for determining the nursing care needs. The data are analyzed and compared to norms when possible.

Assessment Factors:

1. The client's/patient's health status is compared to the norm in order to determine if there is a deviation from the norm and the degree and direction of deviation.
2. The client's/patient's capabilities and limitations are identified.
3. The nursing diagnoses are related to and congruent with the diagnoses of all other professionals caring for the client/patient.

STANDARD III

The plan of nursing care includes goals derived from the nursing diagnoses.

Rationale:

The determination of the results to be achieved is an essential part of planning care.

Assessment Factors:

1. Goals are mutually set with the client/patient and pertinent others:
   - They are congruent with other planned therapies.
   - They are stated in realistic and measurable terms.
   - They are assigned a time period for achievement.
2. Goals are established to maximize functional capabilities and are congruent with:
   - Growth and development
   - Biophysical status
   - Behavioral patterns
   - Human and material resources

STANDARD IV

The plan of nursing care includes priorities and the prescribed nursing approaches or measures to achieve the goals derived from the nursing diagnoses.

Rationale:

Nursing actions are planned to promote, maintain and restore the client's/patient's well-being.

Assessment Factors:

1. Physiological measures are planned to manage (prevent or control) specific patient problems and are related to the nursing diagnoses and goals of care, e.g. ADL, use of self-help devices, etc.

2. Psychosocial measures are specific to the client's/patient's nursing care problem and to the nursing care goals, e.g. techniques to control aggression, motivation.
3. Teaching-learning principles are incorporated into the plan of care and objectives for learning stated in behavioral terms, e.g. specification of content for learner's level, reinforcement, readiness, etc.
4. Approaches are planned to provide for a therapeutic environment:
   - Physical environmental factors are used to influence the therapeutic environment, e.g. control of noise, control of temperature, etc.
   - Psychosocial measures are used to structure the environment for therapeutic ends, e.g. paternal participation in all phases of the maternity experience.
   - Group behaviors are used to structure interaction and influence the therapeutic environment, e.g. conformity, ethos, territorial rights, locomotion, etc.
5. Approaches are specified for orientation of the client/patient to:
   - New roles and relationships
   - Relevant health (human and material) resources
   - Modifications in plan of nursing care
   - Relationship of modifications in nursing care plan to the total care plan
6. The plan of nursing care includes the utilization of available and appropriate resources:
   - Human resources—other health personnel
   - Material resources
   - Community
7. The plan includes an ordered sequence of nursing actions.
8. Nursing approaches are planned on the basis of current scientific knowledge.

STANDARD V

Nursing actions provide for client/patient participation in health promotion, maintenance and restoration.

Rationale:

The client/patient and family are continually involved in nursing care.

Assessment Factors:

1. The client/patient and family are kept informed about:
   - Current health status
   - Changes in health status
   - Total health care plan
   - Nursing care plan
   - Roles of health care personnel
   - Health care resources
2. The client/patient and family are provided with the information needed to make decisions and choices about:
   - Promoting, maintaining and restoring health
   - Seeking and utilizing appropriate health care personnel
   - Maintaining and using health care resources

STANDARD VI

Nursing actions assist the client/patient to maximize his health capabilities.

Rationale:

Nursing actions are designed to promote, maintain and restore health.

Assessment Factors:

1. Nursing actions:
   - Are consistent with the plan of care.
   - Are based on scientific principles.
   - Are individualized to the specific situation.
   - Are used to provide a safe and therapeutic environment.
   - Employ teaching-learning opportunities for the client/patient.
   - Include utilization of appropriate resources.
2. Nursing actions are directed by the client's/patient's physical, physiological, psychological and social behavior associated with:
   - Ingestion of food, fluid and nutrients
   - Elimination of body wastes and excesses in fluid
   - Locomotion and exercise
   - Regulatory mechanisms—body heat, metabolism
   - Relating to others
   - Self-actualization

STANDARD VII

The client's/patient's progress or lack of progress toward goal achievement is determined by the client/patient and the nurse.

Rationale:

The quality of nursing care depends upon comprehensive and intelligent determination of nursing's impact upon the health status of the client/patient. The client/patient is an essential part of this determination.

Assessment Factors:

1. Current data about the client/patient are used to measure his progress toward goal achievement.
2. Nursing actions are analyzed for their effectiveness in the goal achievement of the client/patient.
3. The client/patient evaluates nursing actions and goal achievement.
4. Provision is made for nursing follow-up of a particular client/patient to determine the long-term effects of nursing care.

STANDARD VIII

The client's/patient's progress or lack of progress toward goal achievement directs reassessment, reordering of priorities, new goal setting and revision of the plan of nursing care.

Rationale:

The nursing process remains the same, but the input of new information may dictate new or revised approaches.

Assessment Factors:

1. Reassessment is directed by goal achievement or lack of goal achievement.
2. New priorities and goals are determined and additional nursing approaches are prescribed appropriately.
3. New nursing actions are accurately and appropriately initiated.

CODE FOR NURSES (ANA, 1985)*

1. The nurse provides services with respect for human dignity and the uniqueness of the client, unrestricted by considerations of social or economic status, personal attributes, or the nature of health problems.
2. The nurse safeguards the client's right to privacy by judiciously protecting information of a confidential nature.
3. The nurse acts to safeguard the client and the public when health care and safety are affected by the incompetent, unethical, or illegal practice of any person.
4. The nurse assumes responsibility and accountability for individual nursing judgments and actions.
5. The nurse maintains competence in nursing.
6. The nurse exercises informed judgment and uses individual competence and qualifications as criteria in seeking consultation, accepting responsibilities, and delegating nursing activities to others.
7. The nurse participates in activities that contribute to the ongoing development of the profession's body of knowledge.
8. The nurse participates in the profession's efforts to implement and improve standards of nursing.
9. The nurse participates in the profession's efforts to establish and maintain conditions of employment conducive to high quality nursing care.
10. The nurse participates in the profession's effort to protect the public from misinformation and misrepresentation and to maintain the integrity of nursing.
11. The nurse collaborates with members of the health professions and other citizens in promoting community and national efforts to meet the health needs of the public.

*Reprinted with permission from *American Nurses' Association, Code for Nurses with Interpretive Statements*, Kansas City, American Nurses' Association, 1985.

Appendix 4: Answers and Rationales for Sample Questions

UNIT 2: ADULT NURSING

1. The correct answer is 2. The protruding bowel is expected to be contaminated; therefore, obtaining a culture is unnecessary and will delay appropriate nursing actions. Loops of bowel should be covered with a wet, sterile towel to protect them. If the patient is in pain, the administration of analgesics will assist the patient to lie still and avoid increasing intra-abdominal pressure. An IV line should be inserted for infusion of fluids and blood.

2. The correct answer is 1. There are numerous mechanisms of action for chemotherapeutic drugs, but they all affect rapidly dividing cells. Cancer cells are characterized by rapid division. Some, but not all, chemotherapeutic drugs affect molecular structure. Chemotherapy slows, not stimulates, cell division. All cells are sensitive to drug toxins, but not all chemotherapeutic drugs are toxins; there are several different mechanisms of action.

3. The correct answer is 3. Severe vomiting results in a loss of hydrochloric acid and acids from extracellular fluids, leading to metabolic alkalosis. It is rare that a loss of base intestinal fluids results in metabolic acidosis.

4. The correct answer is 3. It has been demonstrated that positioning the patient with the head elevated to 30° decreases ICP. Gravity aids in venous drainage from the head. Pronounced angulation of the neck can obstruct venous return. Pain, airway problems, and a Valsalva maneuver will all increase ICP and will not directly benefit from proper head alignment.

5. The correct answer is 3. Cheyne-Stokes respirations are a pattern of breathing in which phases of hyperpnea regularly alternate with apnea. The pattern waxes (crescendo) and wanes (decrescendo). Ataxic breathing is a completely irregular breathing pattern. Apneustic breathing is a pattern with prolonged inspiration with pauses. Central neurogenic hyperventilation is a sustained, regular, rapid respiratory pattern of increased depth.

6. The correct answer is 1. Anginal pain is of short duration. It is usually relieved by rest. The usual treatment for anginal pain is nitroglycerin. Anginal pain and the pain of an acute MI can both radiate to other locations.

7. The correct answer is 3. The nurse should assess both Mr. and Mrs. Heath's understanding of the disease and rehabilitation processes. They both exhibit the need for information in order to be able to make rational decisions.

8. The correct answer is 3. Louder breath sounds on the right side of the chest indicate that the endotracheal tube may be misplaced and is aerating only one lung. Dullness to percussion is normal in the third to fifth intercostal spaces as the heart is located there. Decreased paradoxical motion is a desired effect when the patient has a flail chest. A pH of 7 is within normal limits.

9. The correct answer is 2. Fluctuation in the water-seal chamber demonstrates that the tubing system is patent. Bubbling in the water seal is normal only if is is gentle and occasional. Vigorous bubbling indicates that air is being pulled into the system and is not normal. The fact that suction tubing is attached to a wall unit provides no information about function. Vesicular breath sounds should not be heard in the upper chest.

10. The correct answer is 4. The nurse should explore the patient's motivation for posing the question and establish what his current knowledge is. "Ask your physician" is a response that ignores the role of the nurse in dealing with patient concerns. The response "It is rarely fatal" is not accurate. "It depends on the form of the disease" is a true statement, but does not give the patient an opportunity to express his concerns.

11. The correct answer is 2. The patient is placed in Trendelenburg's position to aid in the filling of the subclavian veins. Supine, reverse Trendelenburg's, and high-Fowler's positions do not allow for subclavian filling.

12. The correct answer is 3. Cleansing the peristomal skin is critical to maintenance of skin integrity. The appliance should be changed in the morning when urinary drainage can be expected to be scant. A $\frac{1}{2}$ inch gap between the stoma and the wafer is too large and encourages skin excoriation. Aspirin is not appropriate for odor control and may irritate the stoma.

13. The correct answer is 2. Attaching a larger bag at night helps to prevent reflux of urine into the stoma during a period when the bag is emptied less frequently. Allowing the bag to fill completely will cause the seal to be broken but will not prevent urinary tract infection. Fluids should be encouraged, not restricted, in a patient with a urinary stoma. Changing an appliance every 8 hours is too frequent and may cause skin irritation.

14. The correct answer is 2. Chrysotherapy often requires a 3- to 6-month period before effects are seen. Cushing's syndrome is associated with steroid therapy, which is also utilized in rheumatoid arthritis. Side effects such as blood dyscrasias and renal damage are not rare, and the patient must be carefully monitored. Daily doses of this drug are usually not required.

15. The correct answer is 4. Small joint involvement is common in rheumatoid arthritis. All of the other symptoms listed (asymmetric joint involvement, Heberden's nodes, and obesity) are symptoms that are seen in osteoarthritis.

16. The correct answer is 1. Type I diabetes, also known as insulin-dependent diabetes, occurs in individuals whose pancreatic beta cells do not function at all. Metabolic processes are interfered with in diabetes, therefore fat metabolism is incomplete. Although type I diabetes can occur in an obese individual, obesity is more characteristic of type II diabetes. Diet and insulin therapy can be effective in controlling blood sugar.

17. The correct answer is 4. As NPH insulin is an intermediate-acting insulin, the result of mixing regular and NPH insulin is a total duration of action of 24 hours. Onset of the regular insulin does not occur immediately, regardless of what it is mixed with. NPH insulin peaks in 8–12 hours.

18. The correct answer is 2. A yellow discoloration of the nails is frequently seen in psoriasis. The pain of psoriasis produces discomfort, but it is usually not described as intense. The lesions of psoriasis are usually distributed on the extremities; these lesions are raised macular-papular areas with erythema rather than hyperpigmentation.

19. The correct answer is 1. Sunlight should be avoided after a coal tar treatment. Special diets and other activity restrictions are not required. The coal tar is applied topically, not ingested.

UNIT 3: PEDIATRIC NURSING

1. The correct answer is 3. This child may have a physiologic or psychologic problem; all others answers indicate age-appropriate situations.

2. The correct answer is 1. All Down's syndrome children are retarded and care must be geared to their mental age. The other measurements of age do not reflect the special needs of these children.

3. The correct answer is 2. In Down's syndrome there is an extra chromosome on the 21st pair, which is why the disease is also called trisomy 21. The mutation is spontaneous, and not inherited.

4. The correct answer is 4. Pressure must be kept off the spinal sac. As there is paralysis of the lower extremities, the legs should be abducted. Trendelenburg's position is contraindicated in hydrocephalus.

5. The correct answer is 3. With improved draining of CSF, the head circumference should become smaller. All the other signs indicate increased ICP.

6. The correct answer is 2. Dilantin is an anti-epileptic drug that controls seizures. All the other signs and symptoms are side effects of the medication.

7. The correct answer is 4. The apical pulse is taken for 1 full minute and the medication is withheld if the pulse is less than 100 beats/minute.

8. The correct answer is 3. Crying expends already decreased energy. All the other measures help to compensate for the decreased cardiac output.

9. The correct answer is 3. Iron is given with a straw to prevent staining the teeth. It is best absorbed on an empty stomach in an acidic environment. Do not ask toddlers if they want to take their medication. They are likely to say no.

10. The correct answer is 2. Aspirin interferes with the clotting mechanism. All the other measures listed will help decrease bleeding or alleviate the associated pain.

11. The correct answer is 2. Chest percussion is done prior to meals to prevent vomiting. It follows aerosol therapy and positioning. Suctioning may be needed afterwards to remove thick secretions after they have been loosened by percussion.

12. The correct answer is 4. The affected lobe must be uppermost to be drained by gravity.

13. The correct answer is 1. There is increased excretion of chloride in the sweat of children with cystic fibrosis. A chloride level of over 60 mEq/liter is diagnostic for the disease.

14. The correct answer is 1. Enemas, cathartics, and heat to the abdomen should all be avoided in appendicitis because they may cause perforation of the appendix. All the other measures are appropriate pre-op interventions.

15. The correct answer is 2. The prescribed diet for children with celiac disease is gluten free; crackers contain gluten, but the other foods do not.

16. The correct answer is 4. Palpation of the abdomen may cause the tumor cells to spread.

17. The correct answer is 2. If the testes remain in the abdomen beyond the age of 5, damage resulting from exposure to internal body temperature can result in sterility.

18. The correct answer is 2. In Bryant's traction both legs are in traction at a 90° angle and the buttocks are raised off the mattress. The child's weight provides the counter-traction; he should not be pulled down towards the bottom of the bed.

19. The correct answer is 3. The patient in a hip spica cast should be turned as a unit. The stabilizing bar should not be handled.

20. The correct answer is 4. Weight loss is associated with juvenile diabetes, whereas weight gain develops in maturity-onset diabetes. The other three signs appear in both forms of the disease.

21. The correct answer is 3. Jenny is having a hypoglycemic reaction from the NPH insulin and needs an afternoon snack.

22. The correct answer is 3. Juvenile diabetics need lifetime insulin. Jenny will never be able to switch to oral hypoglycemics.

23. The correct answer is 2. Adolescents may want to give away their belongings. The other interventions are all inappropriate and may increase Louise's fears and anxiety.

24. The correct answer is 4. Selecting hats to cover his head will help Jack deal with the change in his body image. The other suggestions are all inappropriate.

UNIT 4: MATERNITY AND GYNECOLOGIC NURSING

1. The correct answer is 3. The dates of the last menstrual period, especially the first day of that period, will be utilized in applying Nägele's rule to determine the estimated date of delivery. The other information may be gathered as part of a general health history.

2. The correct answer is 4. A frequent cause of backache in the third trimester of pregnancy is the combined effect of relaxation of the sacroiliac joints and the change in the center of gravity of the pregnant woman due to the enlarging uterus. Wearing low-heeled shoes, especially when on her feet for extended periods of time, will help to minimize this discomfort.

3. The correct answer is 1. Convulsions are associated with an eclamptic condition. The other findings are usual for severe preeclampsia.

4. The correct answer is 3. A quiet room, in which stimuli are minimized and controlled, is essential to the nursing care of the severely preeclamptic patient. Because she will need continuous monitoring, the room farthest from the nursing station is inappropriate. Additionally, this patient may not need to be in the labor suite; the first goal of care is to prevent the condition from worsening.

5. The correct answer is 2. With the baby in a vertex, LOA presentation, and no other indicators of distress, amniotic fluid should have a clear to straw-colored appearance. Too much or too little amniotic fluid may be indications of congenital anomalies in the fetus.

6. The correct answer is 3. Immediately after the rupture of membranes, fetal heart tones are checked, then checked again after the next contraction or after 5–10 minutes. With the fetus in a LOA presentation, there is less chance for a prolapsed cord. However, if the FHR drops significantly at any of the above times, a sterile vaginal exam is indicated.

7. The correct answer is 4. Oxytocic medications such as Pitocin, Methergine, and Ergotrate are administered to stimulate uterine contractility and reverse fundal relaxation in the postdelivery patient.

8. The correct answer is 2. An episiotomy is an incision made in the perineum to enlarge the vaginal opening, allowing additional room for the birth of the baby.

9. The correct answer is 1. A well-fitting, supportive bra with wide straps can be recommended for both the nursing and the non-nursing mother, for the support of the breasts and for comfort. The nursing mother's bra should have front flaps over each breast for easy access during nursing periods.

10. The correct answer is 2. Afterbirth cramps are most common in nursing mothers and multiparas. Gerry falls into both of these categories. The release of oxytocin from the posterior pituitary for the "let-down" reflex of lactation causes the afterbirth cramping of the uterus. The other choices represent potentially pathologic symptoms on the second day postpartum, and require further investigation.

11. The correct answer is 4. During the first few days after delivery, the mother is in a dependent phase, initiating little activity herself, and is usually content to be directed in her activities by a health care provider. The other choices represent behaviors that are seen after this dependent phase.

12. The correct answer is 3. Both parents will need education about the new baby: how to care for the baby, information about the baby, and how to be a parent. This education will have an information component, a skills component, and a psychologic component.

13. The correct answer is 3. Acrocyanosis, where hands and feet are still slightly blue for the first 24 hours, is a normal variant in the newborn, but it rates a "1" on the Apgar scale. All the other descriptors are rated "2" on the Apgar scale, giving this newborn a total of "9".

14. The correct answer is 1. Meconium is usually passed during the first 24 hours of life. The respiratory rate at rest is usually between 30 and 60; early jaundice indicates RBC breakdown before birth, and umbilical bleeding should not be occurring.

15. The correct answer is 2. Caput succedaneum (scalp edema) will regress in a few days without interventions such as rubbing or applications of cold. Parents need to have this explained to them as well as what caused it, how it will regress without residual damage, etc. They also need time to express their feelings about this occurrence.

16. The correct answer is 4. Time is one of the most important criteria in differentiating physiologic from pathologic jaundice. Physiologic jaundice appears after 24 hours. When jaundice appears earlier, it may be pathologic. No matter what the cause, the newborn must be observed closely for rising bilirubin levels so that appropriate interventions may be implemented.

17. The correct answer is 1. Because of the complex interaction between the hypothalamus, the ovary, and the amount of body fat, women who are underweight, or who engage in strenuous physical activity over prolonged periods of time may experience changes in their menstrual cycle and their fertility.

18. The correct answer is 3. The patient must be instructed to clean the diaphragm with mild, plain soap and warm water, dust it lightly with cornstarch, and store it in a cool, dry place. She should also be instructed to check it regularly for perforations or defects.

19. The correct answer is 4. The ingestion of sufficient amounts of water by a woman taking calcium supplements is crucial to the prevention of renal calculi.

20. The correct answer is 2. Postmenopausal women who are experiencing vasomotor instability may have "night sweats" and interrupted sleep. Some physicians prescribe estrogen replacement therapy (ERT) for women with severe postmenopausal vasomotor instability.

UNIT 5: PSYCHIATRIC-MENTAL HEALTH NURSING

1. The correct answer is 3. Upon hearing her son's diagnosis, Eddie's mother is experiencing emotional turmoil and projecting blame. Acknowledging her feelings would build further trust and encourage her to discuss her thoughts and feelings.
2. The correct answer is 2. Patients diagnosed with eating disorders have difficulty establishing trust. Confronting the patient's manipulation assists the patient to deal with this maladaptive behavior.
3. The correct answer is 4. Responding factually provides the patient with reality orientation. The alternative responses belittle the patient.
4. The correct answer is 3. The nurse should be someone a confused patient can turn to for direction and guidance. The alternative strategies are appropriate when Nellie is oriented.
5. The correct answer is 4. Millie's short-term memory loss may increase her frustration and anxiety during the other activities. Providing her with structured exercises permits her to release tension.
6. The correct answer is 4. Including the family in the plan of care ensures a more effective plan.
7. The correct answer is 2. A delusion is a fixed false belief.
8. The correct answer is 2. The nurse needs to present reality to the patient and not encourage the delusion.

9. The correct answer is 2. Assessing increasing signs of anxiety and agitation gives clues to the patient's ability to maintain control and suggests further nursing interventions to protect the patient and others.
10. The correct answer is 3. Paranoid patients develop this delusional system to defend against anxiety. Arguing with the patient would increase his anxiety.
11. The correct answer is 4. Daily walks provide time for the nurse to develop trust. The alternative activities are too competitive and would increase the patient's paranoia.
12. The correct answer is 1. Obsessive-compulsive behavior represents displacement of anxiety. A concrete, measurable goal is to decrease the number of handwashings.
13. The correct answer is 4. Providing ample time for Lillian to complete her handwashing rituals will lessen her anxiety.
14. The correct answer is 2. Planning a structured schedule of activities provides the patient with other ways to decrease anxiety.
15. The correct answer is 2. Legal statutes require health professionals to report suspected cases of child abuse.
16. The correct answer is 4. Because Tammy's mother is only 17 years old, she needs information and role modeling on how to provide an emotionally and physically safe environment for her child.
17. The correct answer is 1. A sexual assault is a crisis situation that requires immediate intervention.
18. The correct answer is 2. The goal of adjustment is to have Marilyn return to her precrisis level of functioning.
19. The correct answer is 4. AIDS is an illness that generates intense emotional reactions and fears. Acknowledging these feelings allows the family to discuss them with the nurse in a nonthreatening environment.
20. The correct answer is 1. Because Larry's illness has no cure and the progression is dependent on the body system affected, the primary goal is to ensure his personal dignity and make plans to fulfill personal goals.
21. The correct answer is 2. Research has found that many patients with AIDS are most fearful of the debilitating effects of the disease.

Index

Index

NOTES

NOTES

NOTES